'77

Women's Bodies, Women's Wisdom

ALSO BY CHRISTIANE NORTHRUP, M.D.

The Wisdom of Menopause
Creating Physical and Emotional Health and
Healing During the Change

Mother-Daughter Wisdom
Understanding the Crucial Link Between
Mothers, Daughters, and Health

Women's Bodies, Women's Wisdom

Creating Physical and Emotional
Health and Healing

REVISED AND UPDATED

Christiane Northrup, M.D.

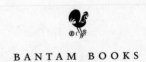

BANTAM BOOKS

WOMEN'S BODIES, WOMEN'S WISDOM
A Bantam Book

PUBLISHING HISTORY
Bantam hardcover edition published July 1994
Bantam revised edition published March 1998
Bantam third edition / November 2006

Published by
Bantam Dell
A Division of Random House, Inc.
New York, New York

Author photo by Barbara Peacock
Jacket and cover design by Beverly Leung

Book design by Glen Edelstein

Grateful acknowledgment is made for permission to quote the following:
Excerpt from *Circle of Stones: Woman's Journey to Herself,* by Judith Duerk. Copyright © 1989
by LuraMedia. Reprinted by permission of LuraMedia, Inc., San Diego, CA; excerpt from
Guided Meditations, Explorations and Healing, by Stephen Levine. Copyright © 1991 by
Stephen Levine. Used by permission of Doubleday, a division of Random House, Inc.; excerpt
from *Mothering Myself,* by Nancy M. Sheehan, M.Ed.; excerpt from *When Society Becomes an
Addict,* by Anne Wilson Schaef. Copyright © 1987, HarperSanFrancisco.

Bantam Books is a registered trademark of Random House, Inc., and the colophon is
a trademark of Random House, Inc.

Library of Congress Cataloging-in-Publication Data
Northrup, Christiane.
Women's bodies, women's wisdom : creating physical and emotional health and healing /
Christiane Northrup.
Revised and updated edition
p. cm.
Includes bibliographical references (p. 813).
ISBN-13: 978-0-553-80483-6 (hc); 978-0-553-38410-9 (tp)
ISBN-10: 0-553-80483-9 (hc); 978-0-553-38410-4 (tp)
1. Gynecology—Popular works. 2. Holistic medicine. 3. Generative organs, Female—
Diseases—Popular works. 4. Women—Health and hygiene. I. Title.
RG121 .N59 3005
618.'1 22   2006048271

Printed in the United States of America
Published simultaneously in Canada

www.bantamdell.com

10 9 8 7 6 5
BVG

This book is for all who believe that it is possible to live our lives fully regardless of our present or past circumstances.

It is for all who acknowledge the daily presence in our lives of mystery, uncertainty, and hope.

It is for those who yearn to be well and know that there is something more to healing than simply external substances or techniques.

This book is for every physician, nurse, health care practitioner, healer, or patient who has ever honestly acknowledged how much we don't know.

It is for those who know that our healing will not be complete until we bring the sacred back into our daily lives.

This book is dedicated with gratitude to the scientists and healers of the past, present, and future who have dared and continue to dare to go forward in faith, hope, and joy despite the deadening effects of conventional thinking.

Contents

Part One
From External Control to Inner Guidance

Part Two

The Anatomy of Women's Wisdom

Part Three
Women's Wisdom Program for Vibrant Health and Healing

List of Figures

List of Tables

Acknowledgments

A book as big as this one has required a dedicated staff of midwives to help with this current incarnation.

I'd like to acknowledge all of those who contributed to the first two editions of this book back in 1994 and 1998 and helped lay the original foundation upon which this book is built. Leslie Meredith, Mona Lisa Schulz, M.D., Ph.D., and Joel Hargrove, M.D. My original partners at Women to Women, Marcelle Pick, R.N.C., Annie Rafter, R.N.C., and Ellen Fenn, M.D. Thanks also to Bethany Hays, M.D., Susan Doughty, R.N.C., and Hector Tarrazza, M.D. And to Helen Rees, the agent who first championed this book.

For this third edition, special thanks and appreciation go to Toni Burbank, my editor extraordinaire at Bantam Books whose editing skills continue to amaze and delight me.

Irwyn Applebaum, president of Bantam, who has believed in my message from the start.

To Barb Burg and Theresa Zorro of the Bantam Publicity Department for your consummate media skills.

To my agent Ned Leavitt, with whom I share such a rich history and spiritual kinship.

To Sue Abel for helping keep the home fires burning, the wood stacked, and the cats happy during this writing process.

To Regena Thomashauer for having the courage to live a new story for women and show all of us a better way of relating to men.

To Chip Gray, the Gray family, and the staff of the wonderful Harraseeket Inn. Your beautifully prepared and delicious organic meals served in such a warm and cozy atmosphere have sustained me through the writing of two books and two revisions. I am deeply grateful.

To the staff of the Royal River Grillhouse for making my business lunches so delicious and fun. And for serving the best bread, cappuccino, and mussels I've ever enjoyed anywhere.

To Katy Koontz, scribe extraordinaire, whose writing, organizational, and research skills—not to mention sense of humor—made this project go along more smoothly and with more fun than I dreamed possible!

To Dixie Mills, M.D., breast surgeon and friend, whose careful review of the appropriate sections in this book was a real blessing.

To Fern Tsao and her daughter Maureen Manetti for providing me and my family with phenomenal knowledge and skill with Traditional Chinese Medicine through all these years.

Julie Hofheimer for your healing bodywork skills.

To Deena Spear, vibrational healer and good friend. Our conversations about the Hogwash School of Healing and other extraordinary happenings, plus my personal "tunings" with you, have been not only a blessing but, most important, a lot of laughs!

To Ina May Gaskin for your vision of childbirth as a ecstatic life-changing event—plus the research that backs that up!

To Donna Abate and Judie Harvey—my newsletter and e-letter editors. You two are a fabulous team with whom I adore working.

Mike Brewer for your property maintenance skills and good heart.

Abby Shattuck for your winning ways with flowers and gardening.

To Louise Hay, Reid Tracy, Ron Tillinghast, Margarete Nielson, Nancy Levin, and all of the Hay House staff. You have shown me that work, pleasure, and prosperity go together beautifully. I give thanks every day for our association.

Paulina Carr, my girl Friday, for doing whatever needs to be done—including bringing in her truck when necessary.

To Janet Lambert for your incredible bookkeeping and business skills.

To Diane Grover, whose organizational skills, intuitive gifts, loyalty, friendship, and personal cheerleading on behalf of my business, personal health, happiness, and prosperity are Divine gifts in my life. I don't know what I ever did to attract someone as extraordinary as you as my first office nurse twenty-five years ago. Thank you for stepping up to the plate and daring to grow and change along with me, becoming the CEO of Everything. Not to mention surrogate mother to my children. Thanks also for lending me your husband, Charlie, to take tango lessons with!

I thank my parents for the enormous support they have always provided: my indomitable mother, Edna, and my late father, Wilbur, whose work I have carried forth in my own way. My heart is full of gratitude and appreciation to my sister Penny, her husband, Phil, my brother John, his wife, Annie, and also my brother Bill and his wife, Lori. You all create an incredibly strong first chakra that makes my immunity and sense of belonging really solid and secure. I appreciate you more now than ever before.

And finally, I acknowledge and thank my two daughters, Annie and Katie, who are living the legacy of this work in their own lives and passing it on in their own unique ways. I am filled with gratitude for your beauty, your vibrant good health, your enthusiasm for life, and your loud and boisterous laughter (which is not unlike my own!).

Christiane Northrup, M.D.

Introduction to the Third Edition

The Medicine of Empowerment

Two decades have passed since my experiences as an OB/GYN physician, woman, and new mother led me to see the need for a revolutionary new approach to women's health and wellness that acknowledges the seamless unity of our bodies, minds, and spirits. Though this wasn't obvious back in the '80s and '90s when I was first field-testing the approaches outlined in this book, it is no longer a secret that the state of a woman's health is highly influenced by the culture in which she lives, her position within it, her experiences, and her day-to-day thoughts, beliefs, and behaviors.

It has taken me nearly thirty years to know in my bone marrow the truth about what keeps us healthy and what makes us sick. And here's what I want you to know: regardless of our individual circumstances, our pasts, or our age, each of us has inner guidance available which we can tune into to create vibrant health daily—right now. We are born with this inner guidance, which comes in the form of the desire for a better life, a good education, more love, more joy, and more fulfillment every day. It comes through the pursuit of freedom, pleasure, and joy. Though we've too often been talked out of our desires as children, I've learned that we can trust those things that bring us sustainable pleasure and make us want to get up in the morning. Our desires are the way that the healing life-force comes through us and replenishes our bodies. They are what make life worth living. They make up our hopes and dreams. And they invariably hold the key necessary to help us heal not only our bodies, but our entire lives. As a physician, I've seen time and time again how our inner guidance also comes in the form of bodily symptoms and illnesses—especially when we are living lives devoid of pleasure, joy, and hope. Our illnesses are designed to stop us in our tracks, make us rest, and bring our attention back to the things that are really important and that give our lives meaning and joy—aspects of life that we have often put on the back-burner until "someday."

The insights catalyzed by more than twenty years of medical practice as well as my own health problems challenged everything I had learned in medical school and residency training about women's health. I began to see that PMS, pelvic pain, fibroid tumors, chronic vaginitis, and menstrual cramps were related to the contexts of an individual woman's life and her beliefs about herself and what she thought was possible in her life. Learning about their diets, work situations, and relationships often provided me with clues to the source of women's distress. I learned to appreciate the life patterns behind medical conditions in ways that I had never noticed before. Once I did notice, however, I knew that these insights held the key to true health and healing.

Over the years, as I developed more sensitivity to these patterns of health and illness in myself and in my patients, I came to realize that without a commitment to looking at all aspects of our lives and accessing our power to change them, improving habits and diet alone is not enough to effect a permanent cure for conditions that have been present for a long time. For nearly three decades, I've worked with many women whose illnesses cannot be ascribed simply to what they eat and cannot be cured solely through medication or surgery. Following a special diet or running three miles a day won't make a woman feel well if her health is being unconsciously and adversely influenced by a subconscious belief that she isn't good enough, or that she is the wrong gender, or that it's a woman's lot in life to suffer! If she has experienced incest and hasn't allowed herself to feel the emotions that are often associated with that history, or if she was unwanted or abused as a child, then there are no prescription drugs that will heal that wound and the physical aftereffects that often result. Trying dietary changes and alternatives to drugs and surgery, however, are often very powerful and health-enhancing first steps that open us up to new ways of looking at our bodies. With a new outlook that we are not simply victims of our bodies and the reassurance that we all have within us the ability to heal from anything and go on to live joy-filled lives, we are empowered to heal mentally, emotionally, and spiritually as well as physically. Eventually we come to see that pleasure, not pain, is our birthright! Stories of such healings and awakenings are found throughout this book. When we finally make the connection between our thoughts, our beliefs, and our subsequent physical health and life circumstances, we find that we are in the driver's seat of our lives. Nothing is more exhilarating or empowering.

One of my readers recently wrote to tell me that, "*Women's Bodies, Women's Wisdom* is a love letter to women and their bodies." She is right! As you read this new edition, please know that it is designed to help you fall in love with your own flesh and blood and to help you wake up to the preciousness of your female body and its Divine processes. Let it help you become the physical embodiment of your soul so that you discover the woman you were always meant to be. Let it help you find the best possible health care for your individual situation. But above all, let it fill you with the courage necessary to make radical and life-giving changes in your mind and life that will get and keep you vibrantly healthy and happy for your entire life. The most fundamental of these changes is learning how to love and accept your precious self—warts and all!

Speaking Our Truth

During the month after this book was initially published, I had a series of nightmares that someone was in my bedroom about to kill me. For five consecutive nights I woke up screaming in terror, scaring my children as well as myself. My dreams were my not-so-subtle inner guidance system letting me know how terrified a part of me was to actually put what I knew out into the world. I was shocked by the power of this fear. Though I'd known intellectually that many women have a wall of fear within them that arises when they dare to speak their truth, I hadn't realized how much of that fear I also shared. I dreaded going to the hospital for the regular OB/GYN meeting in June 1994, after the book went on sale, because I was sure that my colleagues would reject me and my work. Until then I had lived a professional double life: One part of me told patients what I really believed, in the privacy of my personal office, and the other part, the "official" me, held back a bit (or a lot) in the hospital or around many colleagues. My socialization as a doctor had taught me well what was acceptable to my colleagues and the hospital staff. I'd been treading a fine line for years. In fact, back in 1980, right after the birth of my first child and before I took my oral exams for board certification in OB/GYN, I was featured in a cover story on holistic women's health for *East West Journal* (now *Natural Health*). In order to ensure that nobody at the hospital where I worked saw the article, I went to the co-op where *East West* was sold locally and personally purchased all the copies there. No one at my hospital ever saw it—or if anyone did, they never said anything about it. But in 1994, it was not going to be possible to purchase every copy of a mass-marketed book! I had to face the music and bring the two parts of myself together publicly—and in front of conventional medical groups—for the first time.

My first step was to go to my weekly hospital meeting. When I walked in, I was relieved when almost no one said anything about the book and I wasn't treated any differently. It was as though nothing had happened. I had to laugh, for at that moment I learned a lesson about self-centeredness—believing that everyone around me is interested in what I'm doing or saying, when in fact they have their own lives to live. My biggest lesson was that my fear was just that . . . all mine, and it was time to let it go. This has been a gradual process: On the book's first anniversary, I had a series of dreams in which someone was videotaping me naked. I was still feeling vulnerable, but at least I wasn't about to be killed! Since then, the dreams have gradually disappeared.

Since 1994, I've been invited to speak to hospital staffs and doctors all over the country and abroad, and I have received an overwhelmingly positive and heartwarming response from women and men in the United States and around the world. Clearly, the world is ready for women's wisdom. The comment I hear most often, from women, men, and even many doctors, goes something like this: "Somewhere deep within me, I've always known the truth of what you were saying . . . but I didn't have words for it. And I certainly had never heard a doctor say it."

I have come to see that medical science, when combined with the wisdom of our hearts and our minds, is powerful medicine indeed. And that's why, almost as soon as this book was published, I found myself itching to revise it. Though there is no replacement for developing and honing our intuitive women's wisdom—that inner guidance that helps us choose which roads to take and which ones to avoid—I've found that this inner guidance works best when it's balanced with good, solid, up-to-date information.

And though the principles of true wisdom don't change much over time, useful and practical information does. We need both—just as we need both our left and right brain hemispheres. And with the burgeoning acceptance of alternative medicine into mainstream culture (a phenomenon that still surprises and delights me), more and more scientifically documented natural solutions to women's health problems become available every day. Simultaneously, good technological solutions, such as new devices to help stress urinary incontinence, as well as better surgical techniques to remove fibroids, are also helping many women. And each time I have updated my thinking and my recommendations, I have wanted to get that new information out to my readers so that they too can use it to improve their lives and their health.

Writing the first edition of *Women's Bodies, Women's Wisdom* opened up to me a larger world of women's wisdom that is growing all over the planet. Because of this, I have more support from more people and places than I ever dreamed possible. This has allowed me to become more of who I really am. I know from all the letters I receive that the same thing is happening to others across the globe. The original book is being used as a text in nursing schools and hospitals around the country—and this helps women's wisdom gather steam and momentum.

I've learned the power of telling my personal truth. It has been a very significant part of my healing process. And I have emerged feeling stronger and freer than ever before. I hope this book will inspire other women to speak their personal truths, too. I know that as each of us does this, the world—and our health—changes for the better.

Physician, Heal Thyself

In 1981, while I was trying to breast-feed my first child full time and simultaneously work sixty or more hours a week, I developed a severe mastitis that eventually led to the loss of function of my right breast. Instead of taking a day or two off from work at the first sign of infection, which is what I would have told any patient to do, I neglected myself and continued to work. I did this because I was torn in two directions. I believed then, and I still believe today, that breast milk is the best food for babies, and I was determined to feed my children optimally. I treated myself with antibiotics because I was sure I'd be told to stop nursing if I went to another doctor. At the same time, I knew that women doctors had been accused by our male colleagues of being weak or incapable of pulling our weight, and I didn't want that label. At the time, I was working in a well-respected group OB/GYN practice. At the age of thirty-one I had made it in a male-dominated field of medicine, and I worked among colleagues I respected. I did not want to jeopardize my career path. So I neglected myself and continued working—and I got sicker and sicker.

Though I took medication, my infection was severe enough to be resistant to common antibiotics. My condition progressed over several days until one night I began running a high fever and had shaking chills and delirium. During this time, I found out later, the infection was walling off in my body as an abscess deep in my breast. Even then, I went to work and continued to perform my duties. Being both a mother and a doctor, I felt I had no choice. All my years of training had taught me to put my own needs last.

After several weeks of trying to treat myself, I finally called a surgeon, who agreed to meet me in his office after I finished seeing patients (while popping Tylenol with codeine throughout the day to fight off the pain). That same evening I ended up in surgery—the very thing that I had been determined to avoid.

The surgeon told my husband, who is also a doctor, that the abscess cavity under my breast was so large, it was penetrating into my chest wall—the worst he'd seen in thirty years of practice. He didn't know how I had managed to continue working in spite of it. I had ignored the age-old teaching "Physician, heal thyself." I was embarrassed that I had not successfully treated myself as a doctor, that I had myself become an ill person, a patient. I also felt my self-esteem as a mother was threatened if I could not breast-feed. (By this time my milk supply had dwindled significantly anyway from stress.) Yet I remember thinking that night in the hospital that I had to get back to work as soon as possible.

When my second child was born two years later, I assumed that the old damage had healed. Although I'd had to supplement the breast milk for my first child with formula, I figured I wouldn't have to do that again. But no milk could get out of my right breast for my new baby daughter, even though the milk came in on schedule. The prior infection had destroyed the duct structure of that breast. I was again afraid that I would be unable to nurse my baby. I had paid a price with my body for trying to prove myself two years earlier. Though I took full responsibility for this situation, I could see how I had learned to neglect myself. Ignoring my own physical needs and my own body was built right into the fabric of my life.

On the third postpartum day, in the depths of despair about my situation, I called La Leche League International in Chicago to ask for advice. The woman who answered the phone had had the same problem and informed me that I could nurse from only one side, as long as I nursed more frequently and didn't mind being lopsided! Following her advice, I was able to nurse enough to maintain my milk supply. Though I had to supplement with formula when I was away from my daughter at work, my milk was adequate for her needs whenever I was with her for long periods of time. I will be forever grateful to this grassroots organization of women, which was started in Chicago by a group of homemakers who wanted to nurse their babies in an era when the medical profession was less than supportive. (To this day, most OB/GYN residents are not given a formal course on breast-feeding and are therefore not as knowledgeable as they could be about this important function.)

Although I knew that the breasts are often the physical metaphor for giving, receiving, and nurturing, in my rush to nurture everyone else

I had left myself out. My body, however, would not let me get away with my neglectful treatment of it and had communicated an important lesson to me: Our body symptoms have meaning beyond the immediate health problem they are warning us about. Carl Jung said that the gods visit us through illness, and I've come to believe that we can benefit emotionally, physically, and spiritually by paying attention to our body's messages.

While I had always believed this intellectually, to become effective as a healer I had to experience it personally. Only by living through a serious health problem did I become understanding of what other women with health and life problems are living through. As long as I was an overachieving, never-sick white female fully living inside the male-dominant worldview, I was not able to see the patterns that are so commonly associated with women's health problems. As long as I saw myself as separate from other women, I could never understand that these patterns were part of many women's struggles to be whole.

THE PERSONAL IS POLITICAL

Having babies and struggling to balance my work and my family changed me in ways that nothing else could. Instead of learning from books and professors, I was now learning from direct experience what feminists mean by "the personal is political." I learned that there is no such thing as a part-time mother. Once a woman has a baby, that child is a part of her twenty-four hours a day in ways that no one can explain until it happens to her. I was not prepared for the ache in my heart that occurred when I left my baby to go to work every day. I also began to question my longtime assumption that child care and motherhood were not real work.

I noticed right away that being at work was in many ways infinitely easier than being at home with two young children. I could get so much done! As a good daughter of patriarchy, I worshiped at the altar of efficiency and productivity. I began to rethink why it felt okay to care for other people's bodies but not for my own or my children's. Why did I feel so guilty whenever I rested? Even though I had a lot to do, why did I have trouble getting down on the rug and playing with my children for a half hour? Why did I feel that this was wasting time? I also wondered why this whole child care thing was considered a women's issue—why were my children primarily *my* worry? My husband and I had equal educations and equal incomes. Why hadn't his life changed much when the children were born?

As I noticed how my own and other women's well-being is affected by their family life, I had to step back and reassess everything I had ever believed about success, medicine, and myself. Up until my second child's birth, I had never considered myself a feminist. I had always been able to accomplish whatever I'd set my mind to. I didn't know what "those" women were talking about when they spoke of the injustices of society toward women. I didn't know that women and men were treated any differently, because I hadn't experienced (or more accurately, I hadn't noticed) those differences personally.

But my life became unglued when I was a doctor and a mother living in a society that suggests that a woman has to choose between those two roles if she wants to do at least one of them well. Nothing had prepared me for this. Superwoman was dying.

The insights catalyzed by my breast abscess affected not only my beliefs about my own health but my work as a doctor. I began to reassess my beliefs about and understanding of disease. I began to see that the PMS, pelvic pain, fibroid tumors, chronic vaginitis, and other problems that my patients had were often related to the contexts of their lives. Learning about their diets, work situations, and relationships often provided me with clues to the source of their bodies' distress. I appreciated the life patterns behind these conditions in ways that I had never even noticed before.

Over the years, as I developed more sensitivity to these patterns of health and illness in myself and my patients, I came to realize that without a commitment to looking at all aspects of one's life, improving habits and diet alone is not enough to effect a permanent cure for conditions that have been present for a long time. For almost two decades, I've worked with many women whose illnesses cannot be ascribed simply to what they eat and cannot be cured solely through medication or surgery. Following a special diet or running three miles a day won't make a woman feel well if she's still living with an active alcoholic or workaholic, or if she has experienced incest and hasn't allowed herself to feel the emotions that are often associated with that history. Trying dietary changes and alternatives to drugs and surgery, however, can be first steps that open women to new ways of looking at their health. With a new outlook on their bodies and themselves, they often begin to heal mentally, emotionally, and spiritually as well as physically. Stories of such healings and spiritual awakenings are found throughout this book.

We can look at the illnesses in these women's stories, like my own breast abscess, as wake-up calls. Though these experiences were painful for the women involved, they brought us back to our bodies and grounded us again in a consciousness of what is important in life. My own illness showed me that my health is a process of balance and that, having ignored my body and inner self for so many years, I would have to look inward for the answers to the questions raised by my own and other women's health problems and challenges. Since Everywoman's problem occurs in part because of the nature of being female in this culture, which programs us to put the needs of others ahead of our own, we need to make radical changes in our minds and lives to get and stay healthy.

WOMEN TO WOMEN

Because of these revelations, I left my group practice in 1985, determined to create a practice in which I could incorporate into treating my women patients not only medical care but what I knew about nutrition, lifestyle, and the experience of being female in this culture. Three other women and I decided to open a health care center for women that would value what it means to be female. We knew there had to be alternatives to the conventional ways of creating health and treating women's health problems. We wanted to do more than just treat symptoms—we wanted to help women change the basic condition of their lives that had led to their health problems. For us, it would not be enough to "privatize" and isolate each woman's situation. We wanted to teach women that their wounding—physical, psychological, and spiritual—is part of a larger cultural wound that potentially affects all of us.

So the four of us—two nurse-practitioners and two female OB/GYNs—founded Women to Women in December 1985 in a small town in Maine. There were no models for what we set out to do. We wanted to practice within the context of conventional medical care, which has a great deal to offer. I had watched far too many women make an entire career out of trying to heal a condition by avoiding conventional surgery, which could have been extremely helpful to them in making it easier for the physical body to regain and maintain health. (When a woman focuses too much on healing a condition, she often does so to avoid facing the issues that led to the condition in the first place. Thus, the healing process itself becomes addictive.) But we also wanted to reeducate our patients about health-enhancing behaviors. We all had experienced firsthand the power of thoughts and body symptoms to lead us to healing and to a deeper understanding of our bodies and ourselves. We wanted to lead our patients to this, too. In essence, that is also what I try to do in this book.

Women to Women was a leap of faith from the beginning. Over the years of my practice there, I have learned that it is no small task to change one's focus from what can go wrong to what can go right and to empower women to shift from destructive behaviors to those that are generally associated with health. Over the years we all had to acknowledge how entrenched our own habitual fears and health-destroying patterns had become. Our frustration with our patients' self-destructive habits gradually lessened as we came to appreciate that we all shared these same patterns to some degree. All the people (including me) who have come to practice at Women to Women since its inception have found it necessary to work on themselves and on their own behaviors and ways of communicating in order to become better health care practitioners and healers and to keep themselves open to the practice of medicine and nursing as constant learning processes. We worked for years to break down the hierarchical barriers between ourselves and our patients so that the patients participated in their own healing in conscious ways, such as figuring out the best diet or combination of holistic treatments. We would not play doctor god or nurse god with them. Starting in 1986, we enlisted the help of a skilled therapist to help us be honest with each other—instead of hiding our true feelings behind the veil of "niceness" that most of us have been taught—when we discuss and decide on our business duties, shifts, on-call time, vacation, time off, and other necessary issues of practice and communication.

CREATING HEALTH

During the first five years of Women to Women, we learned that our original instincts had been correct. The state of a woman's health is indeed completely tied up with the culture in which she lives and her position within it, as well as in the way she lives her life as an individual. Our formal medical training had not acknowledged what now seems obvious to us.

But acknowledging that the cultural context of a woman's life affects her health is only the first step in creating a new model for women's wellness. The next step we took was to commit ourselves to improving women's health by actively changing the circumstances of our and their lives.

In 1991 we formulated a credo for Women to Women: "We are committed to living, creating, and enjoying health, balance, and freedom on all levels, personally and professionally, while providing educational and medical services." I'm uplifted just reading it. This vision doesn't require perfection. It requires each of us to do our best, remembering that no one can fix our lives *for* us. Only we can do this for ourselves, and we need to set out consciously to do it. I'm not suggesting it is easy. Each of us needs support and guidance. Women to Women has been a source of support and guidance for thousands of women— a place where we tell our stories, creatively dream up our futures, heal our wounds, and then go forth to create health and joy in our own lives.

It is my goal that *Women's Bodies, Women's Wisdom* will also be a source of support and guidance, as it presents healing stories of women who have been patients, colleagues, family, and friends. These women have found their voices and begun to heal and create health daily in their lives. Together they are part of the greater women's consciousness— giving voice to our real identity and needs, reclaiming femininity, and being female in our own way.

These stories are told in women's own words and images and depict women's often individually created but collectively valuable rituals. Most of the women are composite portraits. Though based on real people, their names and other identifying details of their stories have been changed. I hope that by reading these stories, you will be inspired to remember your own life history—not just your medical history—and will reflect on it in a new way. I hope that you will also be moved to write down your life and medical history—to see what patterns emerge, what links there are between the two. By examining, naming, and then reclaiming your life, you, too, can heal.

You will also learn from these stories how to listen to your own body and trust its wisdom so that you can grow into wellness physically and spiritually. Medically speaking, this book addresses women's health issues, the care of our female systems and organs. I explore the diseases, discomforts, and dysfunctions of all the female systems and give suggestions on how to heal them. But beyond this explicit medical focus and advice, the most important guidance I hope to present—with the help of my advisers, my colleagues, and most of all my patients' examples—includes information that speaks to women's "insides." I want to awaken that still, small, wise, intuitive voice in all of us, that voice of our own body that we have been forced to ignore through our culture's illness, misinformation, and dysfunction. And I want to give you the courage to listen to that voice and act on it.

I've come to see that we're all in this together, and that women everywhere are birthing a new vision of women's health and wellness—and of identity. Central to this vision is that we trust what we know in our bones: that our bodies are our allies, and that they will always point us in the direction we need to go next.

May this book be a source of guidance, information, and support in your own healing journey.

Part One

From External Control to Inner Guidance

1

The Patriarchal Myth: The Origin of the Mind/Body/Emotion Split

The world we have created is a product of our thinking. It cannot be changed without changing our thinking.

—Albert Einstein

Belief becomes biology.

—Norman Cousins

Consciousness creates the body, pure and simple. Consciousness isn't just in the head. It is far more vast than our brains and bodies and exists beyond time and space. On a practical day-to-day level, however, our consciousness is the part of us that chooses and directs our thoughts. Thoughts that are uplifting, nurturing, and loving create healthy biochemistry and healthy cells while thoughts that are destructive to self or others do just the opposite. We are born with innate love and acceptance of our bodies. Over time, our bodies and states of health are molded by the habitual thoughts and beliefs that guide our behavior. To improve our lives and our health, we must acknowledge the seamless unity between our beliefs, behaviors, and physical bodies. Then we must critically examine and change any health-eroding beliefs and assumptions that we have unconsciously inherited and internalized from our parents and our culture.

OUR CULTURAL INHERITANCE

Western civilization is characterized by the belief that the intellect is superior to emotions, the mind and spirit are superior to and entirely separate from the body, and that masculinity is superior to femininity. Western civilization has also rested for the last five thousand years on the mythology of patriarchy, the authority of men and fathers. Cultural historian Riane Eisler calls this the dominator mode. If, as Jamake Highwater says, "all human beliefs and activities spring from an underlying mythology," then it is easy to make the connection that if our culture is "ruled by the father," our views of our female bodies and even our medical system also follow male-oriented rules.[1] Yet patriarchy is only one of many systems of social organization.

Even so, we will not be able to create another kind of social organization until we heal ourselves in our own culture. I have been in the delivery room countless times, for example, when a female baby is born and the woman who has just given birth looks up at her husband and says, "Honey, I'm sorry"—apologizing because the baby is not a son! The self-rejection of the mother herself, apologizing for the product of her own nine-month gestation period, labor, and delivery, is staggering to experience. Yet when my own second daughter was born, I was shocked to hear those very words of apology to my husband come right up into my brain from the collective unconscious of the human race. I never said them out loud, and yet they were there in my head—completely unbidden. I realized then how old and ingrained is this rejection of the female by men and women alike! I also know that this is changing.

Still, our culture too often gives girls the message that their bodies, their lives, and their femaleness demand an apology. Have you noticed how often women apologize? I was walking down the street recently when a man ran into a woman who was walking by, causing her to drop a package. *She* apologized profusely. Somewhere deep inside many of us is an apology for our very existence. As Anne Wilson Schaef writes, "The original sin of being born female is not redeemable by works."[2] No matter how many degrees you get in college, no matter how many awards you earn, somehow you can never measure up. If we must apologize for our very existence from the day we are born, we can assume that our society's medical system will deny us the wisdom of our "second-class" bodies. In essence, patriarchy blares out the message that women's bodies are inferior and must be controlled.

Our culture habitually denies the insidiousness and pervasiveness of sex-related issues. I first learned in my medical practice that abuse against women (and the feminine aspects of men) is epidemic, whether subtle or overt. And I saw how abuse sets the stage for illness in our female bodies. Consider the following: more than 40 percent of women in the U.S. have likely been the victim of violence, including childhood sexual abuse (almost 18 percent), physical assault (more than 19 percent), rape (more than 20 percent), and intimate partner violence (almost 35 percent).[3] Some 6 percent of all pregnant women experienced violence during their pregnancies, as well.[4] Despite how widespread such violence against women remains, less than 10 percent of primary care physicians normally screen for domestic violence during routine office visits.[5] Yet if the violence is not addressed, it is likely to escalate, putting victims at increased risk for committing suicide, being murdered, and suffering a host of serious injuries (such as brain damage) and chronic health conditions (including contracting sexually transmitted diseases and HIV/AIDS and abusing drugs and alcohol).[6]

Abuse against girls has been connected not only with early death and disability later in their lives, but also with such diseases as cancer, diabetes, and heart disease, according to research by the Southern California Kaiser Permanente Medical Group and the Centers for Disease Control and Prevention (CDC).[7] The relationship, the researchers report, is cumulative.

A 2003 report from the United Nations Educational, Scientific and Cultural Organization (UNESCO) documents that more than two-thirds of the world's 860 million illiterates are women, and that when societies are faced with limited resources, females are more likely than males to be deprived of basic necessities, including food and medicine, increasing the risk of physical or mental impairment.[8]

Some of the abuse against women in other parts of the globe is even more shocking. Consider these findings:

～ The World Health Organization estimates that between 100 and 140 million females have undergone female genital mutilation worldwide and that each year, an additional 2 million girls are at risk for becoming victims of this practice (most commonly performed in twenty-eight African countries).[9]

～ In India, the practice of sex-selective abortions in favor of male babies has become so widespread that the male-female balance is beginning to be thrown off. One Indian fetal medicine specialist estimates that a million female fetuses are aborted every year in India. The danger is greatest in urban areas with greater access to amniocentesis and ultrasound, yet illegal traveling, laptop ultrasound units are now appearing in areas so remote that they don't yet have electricity or running water.[10]

~ In some Middle Eastern countries, the practice of honor killings (the murder at the hand of family members of women suspected of adultery) is alive and well. Incest perpetrators have used such "honor killings" to cover up their crimes when their victims become pregnant, and others have even used it to solve disputes over inheritance. Some victims have even been forced to commit suicide.[11]

~ A 2003 report by a division of the Cyprus government recently reported that more than two thousand women a year, particularly those arriving from Eastern Europe and the former Soviet republics hoping for a better life, end up forced into prostitution and trafficked to other European and Arab countries.[12]

~ Due to widespread exploitation, sexual abuse, and discriminatory practices, teenage girls in southern Africa and the Caribbean are infected with AIDS four to seven times more often than are boys.[13]

In a 2005 presentation in New York City, UNESCO decreed that violence against women and girls (including rape and torture as "a new strategy of warfare") has become not only a major human rights problem affecting one in three females worldwide but also "a major public health emergency" of global proportions.[14]

Cultural historian and evolutionary theorist Riane Eisler, author of *The Chalice and the Blade* (Harper & Row, 1987), wrote in a recent e-mail to supporters, "The world at large is finally waking up to the fact that we can no longer ignore the victims of intimate violence and the link between intimate violence and international violence, including terrorism." After much research, Eisler cofounded the nonprofit Center for Partnership Studies (with social psychologist and futurist David Loye) to introduce a new model of human rights that she calls partnership, and "to show the link between 'women's and children's issues' and social violence, poverty, and other global problems, [as well as] to put an end to gender inequality and intimate violence." (For more information on how she is helping to effect global change, see the Spiritual Alliance to Stop Intimate Violence program on the website of the Center for Partnership Studies at www.partnershipway.org.)

PATRIARCHY RESULTS IN ADDICTION

The Judeo-Christian cosmology that informs Western civilization sees the female body and female sexuality in the person of Eve as responsible for the downfall of *mankind*. In her book *Healing Eve: The Woman's Journey from Religious Fundamentalism to Spiritual Freedom* (Ampersand, Inc., 2005), Jimmy Laura Smull, Ph.D., shares a typical quote from Adrian, a woman brought up in a fundamentalist family: "The first thing I knew about myself was that I made a big mistake being female, and I shouldn't have done that. From the very beginning I knew it. You know—Eve, the bad bad apple, Eve." For thousands of years, women have been beaten, abused, burned at the stake, and blamed for all manner of evil simply because of their sex. We forget, in this era of rapid change, that American women did not even win the right to vote until 1920!

In 1953, in her book *The Second Sex*, Simone de Beauvoir wrote, "Man enjoys the great advantage of having a God endorse the code he writes. And since man exercises a sovereign authority over women it is especially fortunate that this authority has been vested in him by the Supreme Being. For the Jews, Muslims, and Christians among others, man is master by Divine right; the fear of God will therefore repress any impulse towards revolt in the downtrodden female."[15] The belief that men are meant to be rulers of women runs deep in many Western traditions.

The patriarchal organization of our society demands that women, its second-class citizens, ignore or turn away from their hopes and dreams in deference to men and the demands of their families. Instead of learning how to pay attention to the genius of our intuition and inner guidance, we instead internalize the belief that we are not worthy enough, smart enough, or good-looking enough to live lives of freedom, joy, and fulfillment. Little boys learn early on how to shut down their feelings to avoid being called a "sissy" or otherwise being compared to an inferior girl. The systematic stuffing or denying of the universal human need for emotional expression, love, support, partnership, self-actualization, and self-expression causes enormous emotional pain and also uses up a great deal of energy. Lacking a way to name and change their situations, many women (and men) instead turn to addictions such as overwork, overcare, smoking, and overeating that result in an endless cycle of abuse that we ourselves help perpetuate. Being abused or abusing ourselves, we become ill. Then we turn to a medical system that is set up to deliver mostly quick-fix pharmaceutical solutions to problems that can't be healed until we change our core beliefs and thoughts!

Anne Wilson Schaef writes that "anything can be used addictively, whether it be a substance (like alcohol) or a process (like work). This is because the purpose or function of an addiction is to put a buffer between ourselves and our awareness of our feelings. An addiction serves to numb us so that we are out of touch with what we know and what we feel."[16] Schaef renamed patriarchy the "addictive system" and described the characteristics of societies that squelch people's inner knowing and emotions—thus favoring the use of addictive substances or processes to keep them going. (See table 1, page 19.)

Whether you call it patriarchy, the addictive system, the dominator society, or the mind/body split, it is abundantly clear that the way in which our society functions is harmful to both men and women (men die on average seven years sooner than women) and that both genders participate fully in keeping it going. Yet the good news is that when we acknowledge and release our emotional pain we are put immediately in touch with our feelings and our inner guidance system. Our intellects and thoughts can now assume their rightful role: being of service to our hearts and our deepest knowing, not the other way around. Now healing can happen. This shift results in a new kind of medical attitude and wisdom that helps put us in touch with the message behind our pain as a first step toward healing.

FUNDAMENTAL BELIEFS OF THE
DOMINATOR SYSTEM

I encourage you to get a handle on how you participate in the beliefs and behaviors characteristic of a dominator society. As you become more conscious of your own role in this feedback loop and then change your thoughts and behavior patterns, both your health as an individual and our health as a society will improve. See if the following descriptions of our cultural attitudes toward women and health ring true for you. They may help you become more conscious of your own body and health issues.

Belief One: Disease Is the Enemy

Dominator societies have been properly described as societies that are either preparing for war or recovering from war. Such societies elevate the values of destruction and violence over values of nurturing and peace. We have only to look at what our society spends on defense to see where its values lie, since the amount of money this society spends on something is a measure of its worth in that society. The amount spent on weapons every minute could feed two thousand malnourished children for a year, while the price of one military tank could provide classrooms for thirty thousand students.[17]

It's no mistake that the medical establishment describes our bodies not as natural systems homeostatically designed to tend toward health but rather as war zones. Military metaphors run rampant through the language of Western medical care. The disease or tumor is "the enemy," to be eliminated at all costs. It is rarely, if ever, seen as a messenger trying to get our attention. Even the immune system, which works to keep us in balance, is described in militaristic terms with its "killer" T cells. Recently, at a conference on a tumor held in our center, one of the radiologists said, "The previous bullets we've fired at that area [the pelvis, in this case] have failed to sterilize it from disease."

The modern medical preference for drugs and surgery as treatments stems seamlessly from the ideology of our culture. That which is natural and nontoxic is seen as inferior and ineffective compared to "real medicine"—the "big guns" of drugs, chemotherapy, and radiation. Drug-free, natural methods of treatment with well-studied, well-documented benefits, such as massage, therapeutic touch, and prayer are ignored at worst[18] or tolerated as "probably not harmful" at best. A classic example of this in the field of OB/GYN is the impeccable research of Marshall Klaus, M.D., and John Kennell, M.D., on the effect of continuous labor support by doulas (women whose job is to sit with laboring mothers and provide emotional support). In a series of six different studies, Dr. Kennell found that the mere presence of a doula shortened laboring time in first-time mothers by an average of two hours, and reduced the need for cesarean delivery by 50 percent. It also decreased the need for pain medication and increased the chances of successful breastfeeding. Back in the early 1990s, Dr. Kennell estimated that having a doula to support birthing mothers would save the health care system over two billion dollars per year in unnecessary medical costs from epidurals, surgery, fevers, etc. Dr. Kennell quipped, "If the doula effect were a drug, it would be considered unethical not to use it." But the effect of one caring human on another falls outside of the paradigm of standard medicine where the current rate of cesarean birth has now risen to an all-time high of 30 percent in many hospitals![19]

The medical literature is loaded with similar examples, including many that show a striking benefit from prayer and also the power of the placebo to heal. Given these benefits and the total absence of side effects, a true scientist would be fascinated and want to study the effects further. Bernie Siegel, M.D., the famous Yale pediatric surgeon and author of *Love, Medicine & Miracles*, once told me that when he posted a study in the doctors' lounge about the beneficial effect of prayer on heart attack sufferers, within a few hours one of his colleagues had written *BULLSHIT* across the front page.

Our culture considers the body to be inferior to the mind and its dictates of reason. It often teaches us to ignore fatigue, hunger, discomfort, and our need for caring and nurturing. It conditions us to see the body as an adversary, particularly when the body is giving us messages we don't want to hear. I saw a T-shirt the other day that said it all: "Pain is weakness leaving the body—U.S. Marine Corps." We're encouraged to try to kill the body—as messenger—along with the message. Though it's important to stretch and challenge the body to keep fit and healthy, it's important to know the difference between stretching yourself and overextending. A dead giveaway that you are overextending, rather than stretching yourself, is the inability to nurture yourself or rest without a drink, a smoke, or overeating.

Belief Two: Medical Science Is Omnipotent

We have been taught that our disease-care system is supposed to keep us healthy. We have been socialized to turn to doctors whenever we have concerns about our bodies and our health. We have been taught the myth of the medical gods—that doctors know more than we do about our bodies, that the expert holds the cure. It's no wonder that when I ask women to tell me what's going on in their bodies, they sometimes reply, "You tell me—you're the doctor!" Doctors are authority figures for some women, right up there with their husbands and religious leaders. Yet each woman is more knowledgeable about herself than anyone else.

Women's ambivalence toward our bodies and our own judgment takes a toll on us psychologically. As one woman said to me recently, "I don't trust doctors. I don't like medicine. Yet I'm obsessed with them and am always drawn to looking at what's wrong with me. I go to a lot of doctors looking for answers, then I'm angry when they offer only drugs or surgery." Other women, when they are offered alternatives, reject them, firmly believing that only drugs or surgery will help. Either way, most women are trained to look outside themselves for answers because we live in a society in which so-called experts challenge and subordinate our own judgment and in which our ability to heal or stay healthy without constant outside help is not honored, encouraged, or even recognized.

As a physician, I was trained to be paternalistic, the all-knowing outside expert. The public, in turn, is conditioned to believe that doctors are the paragons of healthy behavior who will judge them for their shortcomings. It always astounded me that my patients expected me to yell at them for missing an annual Pap smear or mammogram appointment—something I (and most of my colleagues) have done!

Medicine itself has a very pathological focus. Scientists rarely study healthy people, and when people with chronic or terminal conditions manage to recover completely, defying the statistical medical prognosis, health professionals too often think that their initial diagnosis must have been wrong, instead of investigating why these people have done so well.[20] In medical school, I practiced on sick or dead people. I was trained in what could go wrong. I was taught to anticipate everything that could possibly go wrong and to plan for it. As an OB/GYN, I was taught that the normal process of labor and delivery was a "retrospective diagnosis" and that it could randomly become a disaster at any moment without warning. When this kind of training goes unquestioned by doctors, the fear and tension that the doctor carries into the room of a laboring woman can increase her anxiety, resulting in hormonal changes in her body that, if not interrupted, favor a cascade of physiological events that ultimately lead to a high rate of dysfunctional labors and cesarean deliveries.

Our culture and its conventional medical system believe that technology and testing will save us, that it is possible to control and quantify every variable, and that if we just had more data from more studies, we'd be able to improve our health, cure diseases, and live happily ever after. Americans and their doctors equate doing more with improving care. We also believe that we can "buy" an answer by throwing money at it. Again, we ignore or don't trust our inner guidance system and our own healing ability.

Physicians order lots of tests because they are uneasy about being uncertain. They are taught to behave as if it were intolerable to be uncertain. The more information physicians get, the more confidence they feel in the validity of their diagnoses, even when their confidence in the information is not justified. Health care consumers, for their part, are just as uncomfortable with uncertainty as their doctors are. They want to know things in absolute ways. When people ask me about genital herpes, for instance, they want to know, "How did I get it?" "How do I know I won't give it to anyone else?" These questions are essentially unanswerable with absolute certainty.

When it comes to ourselves, doctors know all this. And it leads to a "do as I say, not as I do" attitude. A very telling report from the University of California found that 50 percent of female physicians don't do monthly breast self-exams even though they tell their patients to do them (more on this in chapter 10, "Breasts"). My personal experience with both myself and my colleagues bears this out. I believe that the discrepancy between what doctors tell patients to do and what they do themselves has to do with "insider" knowledge. We know too much. We're far more clear on the limitations of medical science than are our patients. But we don't dare let on lest we destroy the placebo effect of our patients' faith in us! The answer to this dilemma is for both doctors and patients to acknowledge the unknown and also heed the message behind the symptom. This awakens inner guidance and is compatible with any and all treatment choices!

Belief Three: The Female Body Is Abnormal

Because being male has always been considered the norm in our culture, most women internalize the idea that something is basically "wrong" with their bodies. They are led to believe that they must control many aspects of their bodies and that their natural odors, shapes, and processes such as menstruation are simply unacceptable. Women are socialized to think that their bodies are essentially dirty—requiring constant surveillance for "freshness" so that we don't "offend." Females naturally have more body fat than men, and because of better nutrition than in past decades, women today are also bigger than were their mothers and grandmothers. Yet the average fashion model, our cultural ideal, weighs 17 percent less than the average American woman. No wonder anorexia nervosa and bulimia are ten times more common in females than in males and are on the rise.[21]

This denigration of the female body has made many women either afraid of their bodies and their natural processes or else disgusted by them. Many never touch or get to know what their breasts feel like, for instance, because they're afraid of what they might find. They may feel guilty for touching them, equating this with masturbation, since breasts are erotic for men—another sign of how thoroughly we have turned our bodies over to men.

Health practitioners and women alike have been acculturated to view even normal bodily functions such as menstruation, menopause, and childbirth as medical conditions requiring treatment. The attitude that our bodies are accidents waiting to happen seems to get internalized at a young age and sets the stage for women's future relationships with their bodies. Given what we are taught, it is no wonder that so many women feel ill prepared to deal with and trust ourselves. Our bodies have been "medicalized" since before we were born!

Our culture fears all natural processes: birthing, dying, healing, living. Daily, we are taught to be afraid. When my older daughter was seven, she was out with her father chopping down some brush in our backyard. Suddenly she started to cry and came running into the house with a bleeding finger. She had cut herself on a blade of grass. As I calmly held her finger under some cold water and saw that it was only a tiny cut, she looked up at me and uttered what I consider a major healing principle: "It didn't hurt until I got scared."

Because our culture worships science and believes that it is "objective," we think that everything labeled "scientific" must be true. We believe that science will save us. But science as it is currently practiced is a cultural construct rife with all the biases of the culture in general. There is actually no such thing as completely objective data. Cultural bias determines which studies we believe and which we ignore. No one is immune to this behavior. We all have our sacred cows. A presenter at a medical conference once said, "The human mind is an organ uniquely designed to create antibodies against new ideas."

Many procedures that have been routinely performed on women's bodies in particular are not based on scientific data at all but are rooted in prejudice against the body's innate wisdom and healing power. Some procedures have their origins in emotional views of women handed down from previous generations. Routine episiotomies at delivery (cutting of the tissue between the vagina and rectum to allegedly make more room for the baby's head) are an example. Despite the fact that studies have shown for the past ten years that episiotomy increases blood loss, pain, and risk of long-term pelvic floor damage and tears (something that midwives have been saying for years), episiotomy is still too common. It wasn't until 2005 that a study published in the *Journal of the American Medical Association* on the outcomes of routine episiotomy was widely publicized, thus causing both women and their doctors to question the procedure more thoroughly.[22]

The reason this practice has persisted so long despite scientific data to the contrary is that obstetricians have truly believed that the birthing female body required the procedure to protect the pelvic floor and also to ensure a suitably "tight" vagina postpartum. One of the first things I was taught in my OB/GYN residency was how to place what was called the "husband's stitch" in the episiotomy incision.

RECLAIMING OUR OWN AUTHORITY

While true science is based on observation, experimentation, and continuous readjustment of thought processes and beliefs, depending upon its empirical findings, the same is true for trusting our inner guidance. Ultimately, I've found it enormously empowering to realize that no scientific study can explain exactly how and why my own particular body acts the way it does. Only our connection with our own inner guidance and our emotions is reliable in the end. That is because we each comprise a multitude of processes that have never existed before and never will again. Science must acknowledge truthfully how much it doesn't know and leave room for mystery, miracles, and the wisdom of nature.

My father used to say, "Feelings are facts. Pay attention to them." Yet in my scientific training I quickly learned that feelings, intuition, spirituality, and all experiences of life that cannot be explained by the logical, rational parts of our minds or measured by our five senses are suspect or discounted as "magical thinking." Because our culture places such emphasis on our intellects, we learn to fear our emotional responses and highly value the control of the emotions we're out of touch with. It took me years and years to break out of this pattern within myself! In his groundbreaking book *The Biology of Belief* (Mountain of Love/Elite Books, 2005), cellular biologist Bruce Lipton, Ph.D., who has done pioneering research on the effect of consciousness on cells, writes, "Bio-scientists are conventional Newtonians—if it isn't matter . . . it doesn't count. The 'mind' is a non-localized energy and therefore is not relevant to materialistic biology. Unfortunately, that perception is a 'belief' that has been proven to be patently incorrect in a quantum mechanical universe." Female bodies, long associated with cycles and subject to the ebb and flow of natural rhythms, are seen as especially emotional and in need of management. Our entire society functions in ways that keep us out of touch with what we know and feel.

In a dominator system, in which the intellect is seen as superior to the body and to emotions, people in general and women especially are

put on the defensive and often act negatively. When I examined a pregnant woman and her blood sugar test came back with an elevated reading, for example, she would almost invariably become very defensive
about her eating habits. She would usually deny that she had consumed
any nonnutritious or sweet foods at all, because she felt ashamed that
she'd been "caught" sneaking sweets, a common enough impulse that
pregnant women have. She'd then get defensive and feel that her body
had betrayed her through her blood sugar. To teach her, or anyone else
about nutrition and how to substitute healthy foods for junk, you usually have to get through the individual's defensiveness, which often
takes up time and energy that can be better spent on addressing her
overall health. In psychiatry they have a name for people who aren't
ready to do what it takes to get better. They're labeled "pretreatment."
And we've all been there.

Remaining unconscious about our acculturated habits takes an
enormous emotional and physical toll on our bodies and spirits. These
habits keep us from being connected with our inner guidance and our
emotions. This disconnection, in turn, keeps us in a state of pain that
increases the longer we deny it. It takes a lot of energy to stay out of
touch with this pain, and we often turn to acculturated habits, such as
addictive substances, to keep us from confronting that unhappiness and
pain.

Almost everyone understands that physical destruction results from
abusing alcohol and drugs. Fifty percent of the accident victims in most
emergency rooms are there because of alcohol abuse. As one of our staff
anesthesiologists once said, "If it weren't for cigarettes and alcohol, I'd be
out of a job!" What many people don't appreciate, however, is the enormous and equally deadly toll taken by compulsive behaviors such as overwork and overeating, used to avoid or deny one's feelings.

Sexual and relationship addictions have gynecological implications
and result in the epidemics of sexually transmitted diseases, such as
venereal warts, herpes, and cervical cancer. A former patient of mine
was married to a recovering alcoholic and was suffering from chronic
vaginitis, for which I could find no cause. She finally came to the realization that her husband had been "medicating himself through sex
with me every day for years. I saw that my body was his bottle—he was
using it and sex the same way he had used alcohol, and I thought it was
my duty as a wife to comply."

My experiences in my own practice have led me to believe that
health promotion and education won't do a thing to decrease health
care expenses unless we as a society acknowledge the enormity of our

own addictive behaviors and the personal pain hidden behind them. Only then can we begin to participate in our own recovery and create health. Every overweight woman I know is clear about what she "should" eat. She doesn't need more nutrition information. She needs first to *feel* the pain that the excess food is chronically pushing down. This can only happen when she takes control of her own health and allows her own inner guidance to prevail—when she learns, in essence, to trust her own body's wisdom.

The Power of Naming

A first step toward making a positive change in your life or your health is to name your current experience and allow yourself to feel it fully—emotionally, spiritually, and physically. Back in the 1980s, it was crucial for me to see how often I used the caretaker and rescuer role to stay out of touch with my own feelings. It was crucial for me to name this behavior "relationship addiction." Before I did this, I looked to others to affirm me and tell me that I was okay. I took their cues for how to act, feel, and look: I was always seeing myself in terms of other people. I believed that if I said no to someone who needed me, I wouldn't be valued and loved. Looking back over my life, I see not only how persistent this pattern has been but also how much it has improved through insight and behavior change. My own life and health have improved enormously as a result of naming and changing this behavior. Simple. Not easy.

I came to see that my tendency to rescue people in need, my acquiescence to others, and my saying yes to everyone came out of my attempt to exercise a form of control: I believed that if I said yes, I would earn their love. This wasn't good either for me or for them, since by putting myself in the position of being someone's rescuer, a substitute for their own higher power or inner guidance, I allowed them to remain out of touch with their own strengths. My behavior actually helped to create victims who needed me. Now I can see and name this behavior as a relationship addiction. Now when someone says they need me, a red flag immediately goes up within me. I wait, check out the situation, and see what my inner guidance tells me before I decide how to respond.

One of the most common characteristics of people in our addictive society is dependence. "Dependency is a state in which you assume that someone or something outside you will take care of you because you cannot take care of yourself," writes Schaef. "Dependent persons rely on others to meet their emotional, psychological, intellectual, and spiritual needs.[23] For centuries women have relied on men to meet their economic needs (not that they were given much choice, since they were owned like property for centuries), while men have relied on women to meet their emotional needs. As one patient of mine said about her former marriage, "Our agreement was, he would make the money and I would do the emotions." Clarissa Pinkola Estes points out that one of the reasons women have not been more in touch with their creative instincts is that they have spent so much time succoring others who have been at war—either on the battlefield or in corporate America.[24]

The problem with this way of relating to others is that it prevents true intimacy. Intimacy can take place only in a partnership relationship, not one based on intersecting dependencies. My parents once cautioned me, "If a man ever says, 'I need you,' run the other way." It's good advice.

Naming the addictive characteristics in our daily life offers us a way out of the culturally induced trance that affects all women—the culture's definition of what it means to be a "good" woman as one who meets everyone's needs but her own. This is a setup for resentment, anger, and eventually illness. Though it earns love and acceptance in the short run, it always backfires because our bodies were designed to be healthy to the extent that we follow our hearts' desires! When you name an experience intellectually, be aware of how that experience actually feels in your body. Allow yourself to feel it physically. Otherwise, your own behavior—and your health—will not change. *Once an experience is consciously named and internalized, physically and emotionally, it can no longer influence us unconsciously.* When we change our perception, every cell in our bodies changes! We then begin to see how we have been influencing and perpetuating our own problems. Naming something that has affected us adversely is part of freeing ourselves from its continued influence. Many times healing cannot begin until we allow ourselves to feel how bad things are (or were in the past). Doing this frees emotional and physical energy that has been stuffed, stuck, denied, or ignored for many years. When we can allow ourselves to feel exactly how we feel without judgment, we begin to free our energy. Only then can we move toward what we want. Table 1 can help you name your addictive characteristics.

One of my former patients had a chronic and painful vaginal and vulva herpes condition that didn't respond to conventional drug therapy or even to alternatives such as dietary changes. After three years of un-successfully searching for a way to stop her recurrent outbreaks, she came to the following conclusion: "Maybe I just need to walk around for a while saying that my vagina hurts. I was never able to say that to my mother when I was little." From the moment she spoke this truth out loud, she began to heal. She told me that her father had sexually abused her for years and her mother hadn't believed her. Layer by layer, she be-gan to uncover her wounds, name them, and heal. With great compas-sion for herself, she acknowledged the pain of her past and moved beyond judgment of herself and her parents. As she did this, her pain gradually decreased while her creative life as a writer began to blossom. Today, she no longer has herpes outbreaks.

Whether you call our society "the addictive system" or not, you'll find it very empowering to check out your behaviors in table 1 with as much honesty as possible. The degree to which we notice these character-istics in ourselves, name them, and then choose to change our habitual thoughts and behaviors is the degree to which we are healthy. As individ-uals do this work, society as a whole becomes healthier.

Over time I came to see that what society calls being a "good woman" or a "good doctor" or a "good mother" came dangerously close to an invitation for me to lose myself in serving others at my own expense! I've learned that I can't get tired enough to help those who are tired, sick enough to help those whose are sick, or poor enough to help those who are poor. I am able to provide optimal service and friendship to others only to the degree that I'm also tuning in to what I need to do for me! Over time I've created a life in which my family, colleagues, and loved ones have all committed themselves to living in balance as well. As a result of learning how to care for myself and listen to my own inner guidance, I have become far more effective at helping others than I ever dreamed possible!

Part of creating health is allowing others to go through their own learning processes. No one can create health for another person. I have re-alized that I don't have the answers for everyone—and neither does any-one else. Only the individual herself can gain access to her inner guidance when she is ready. After years of feeling that I was responsible for having all the answers for others at the expense of myself, I no longer try to con-vince anyone of anything (most of the time).

Many women are not in jobs and families that fully support their health. But if enough of us learn to value ourselves deeply, name our addictive behaviors, and commit to living our lives fully and joyfully, our jobs and circumstances will begin to change. Changing our thoughts and consciousness is always the first step toward healing.

TABLE 1

CHARACTERISTICS OF AN ADDICTIVE SYSTEM

Characteristic	Definition	Examples
BLAME	Believing that someone or something outside of yourself is the cause of whatever is happening to you	"I can't help the way I am. My mother was an alcoholic." "I married a man who is completely incapable of having an intimate relationship."
DENIAL	Being out of touch with your feelings, needs, or other information	"My parents weren't alcoholics, they were heavy social drinkers." "There's a fine line between drinking too much and being an alcoholic." "I don't know why I've gained twenty pounds. I never eat a thing that isn't healthy."
CONFUSION	Lacking clarity about a situation or your emotions	"Nobody ever tells me anything." "I never know what's going on around here."
FORGETFULNESS	Putting out of your mind, ceasing to notice	Forgetting appointments, car keys, personal belongings, bodily needs
THE SCARCITY MODEL (ZERO-SUM MODEL)	Believing that there's a limited amount of everything that's desirable: love, money, men, happiness	"If I am successful, someone else has to suffer." "It is not okay to spend time or money on oneself or to admit it."
PERFECTIONISM	Having an extreme need for external order to cover internal chaos	Relentless pursuit of a perfect body, home, mate, job
THE ILLUSION OF CONTROL OR OBJECTIVITY	Fearing your needs and feelings, and creating an illusion that you can somehow control yourself; separating yourself from your emotions, and believing that it is possible to be completely objective and unemotional	"If I could find the right drug, I could get rid of these panic attacks." "Premenstrually I become a different person. I'm like Dr. Jekyll and Mr. Hyde. I'm not myself." "The ozone level is high today. Please stay inside."

Characteristic	Definition	Examples
NEGATIVISM	Seeing life from a lackful viewpoint	"I always catch whatever is going around." "Now that I'm forty, everything is starting to fall apart." "You can't have that, it costs too much."
DEPENDENCY	Believing that someone or something outside of you will take care of you because you can't do it for yourself	"I can't leave my husband. Who would support me?" "I can't live without him."
CRISIS ORIENTATION	Using or creating an external crisis as a socially acceptable way to distract yourself from your feelings	"There's no question that we really look forward to the next multiple trauma. It gets the juices flowing." —Emergency room nurse
DEFENSIVENESS	Being unable to accept feedback and make positive adjustments	"Who are you to tell me that PMS is related to my family? My childhood was perfect."
DISHONESTY	Not telling the truth	"Do I need a break? No, I'm fine." "It wasn't that bad. I can handle it."
DUALISTIC THINKING	Believing that there are only two choices: one is right or good, the other is wrong or bad	"Vitamins and herbs are good. Drugs and surgery are bad."

Sources: Anne Wilson Schaef, *When Society Becomes an Addict* (New York: Harper & Row, 1987), p.72; Anne Wilson Schaef and Diane Fassel, *The Addictive Organization* (New York: Harper & Row, 1988).

Naming and Healing Emotional Pain and Its Physical Consequences

Our emotions and thoughts have such profound effects on us because they are physically linked to our bodies via our immune, endocrine, and central nervous systems. All emotions, even those that are suppressed and unexpressed, have physical effects. Unexpressed emotions tend to "stay" in the body like small ticking time bombs—they are illnesses in incubation.

A culture that is unsupportive of women sets the stage early on for health problems because the context of a woman's life contributes greatly to the state of her health. Millions of women suffer from chronic pelvic pain, vaginitis, ovarian cysts, genital warts, endometriosis, and cervical dysplasia (abnormal cells on the cervix that are picked up by a Pap smear)—all diseases of organs that are unique to females. These conditions are the language through which our bodies speak to us. Through these our bodies are telling us that we need to heal from a deeper, often unconscious wounding—that we are never enough and that we are somehow tainted.

A forty-one-year-old executive came to see me because she was having uncomfortable hot flashes. She was on four times the normal dose of estrogen and was still getting no relief. In addition to being related to decreased estrogen levels, hot flashes are a neuroendocrine problem and increase with stress. When a woman feels that she is under stress, the frequency and severity of her hot flashes increase both objectively and subjectively. My patient had already had a hysterectomy and removal of her ovaries for uncontrollable pelvic pain as a result of severe endometriosis two years before. Now she seemed beyond relief. It took this patient two years to tell me that when she was six, she had been sexually molested in the basement of a candy store by the man who ran the store. While this was happening to her, she had felt frozen, unable to speak. She said, "I just went numb. He told me never to tell anyone, because if I did they'd never like me. I felt completely ashamed." On the day she did tell me, she still felt that she had done something wrong and that she was bad. She later said that she drove away from the office certain that once I knew the truth about her, I'd never like her again.

My patient, trying to redeem "the original sin of being female" and the emotional pain that stemmed from it, had continually worked two jobs since high school and earned an M.B.A., and she is very successful in her work. She had used work, constant striving, and earning more degrees as a way to "prove herself" and to stay out of touch with that early emotional pain and feeling that she was unworthy and bad. Her beliefs stemmed directly from the addictive system and were reinforced by it. She still hasn't been able to shed a tear about her experience, an emotional release that I feel will help her once she's ready.

I agree with my patient that the seeds for her physical problems were planted by her emotional traumas. I am not saying that her childhood sexual abuse "caused" the endometriosis or chronic pelvic pain. What I'm suggesting is that her early abuse, common to so many of my patients, inserted a set of destructive beliefs about her worth and her lovability that have persisted to the present, creating discomfort in her bodymind. The truth is that every one of us was imprinted in the womb by our parents with beliefs and behaviors, as were their parents before them. This is inevitable. The only way for any one of us to begin the healing process is to affirm our own preciousness and lovability while simultaneously allowing ourselves to feel the old unhealed emotional pain. The human heart has an almost endless capacity to transform emotional pain through the process of grieving, forgiving, and letting go. This isn't an intellectual process. It happens in the body. When she was going through a very difficult divorce, one of my friends started a meditation practice. One day, while in meditation, she had the realization that to doubt the beauty within herself was to doubt God. This was a turning point in her health and her healing.

Only by tuning in to how we feel in our bodies can we appreciate our inner guidance. Yet we look to our schools to tell us what is worth learning, our governments to take care of our communities, and our doctors to immunize us against the latest germ. We learn that we will be okay if we follow the rules. One of our patients who recently developed vulvar cancer said, "I can't understand how this happened. I've come in for an exam every year, had normal Pap smears, and yet I still got cancer." Like this patient, we often believe that the tests themselves will prevent us from getting ill.

In first grade my younger daughter was told on the first day of school what were the acceptable times for students to go to the bathroom. I went in and told her teacher that in my practice I regularly see adult women with constipation and urinary problems who cannot move their bowels in public restrooms because early "rules" from home and school like these had damaged their ability to know when their bodies needed to perform a normal function. I didn't want this to happen to my daughter. I made sure she heard my conversation with her teacher so that she felt supported in going to the bathroom when she needed to go.

Healing Means Leaving Wounding Behind

We can't make a new world for ourselves as long as we hold on to old self-destructive beliefs about ourselves and our worth—or about the worth of others. If we fail to notice the ways in which we daily co-operate with the system that's destroying us, we're in danger of operating out of the perpetual-victim mode, always blaming someone "out there" for our problems. Much like the battered woman who finally gets out because one day she realizes that if she stays she will die, each of us must recognize when and where we're cooperating with our own oppression.

One of my friends who was brought up Catholic in the 1950s describes the effect of confession on her body. "I remember having to go to confession," she says, "beginning at age seven, searching my conscience for crimes and misdemeanors, feeling caught in the horrible dilemma of being unable to speak the unspeakable—about sexual wonderings, masturbation—who had the language for that? And were girls even capable of it? Was I the only one in this dilemma? It was suggested on a plastic card that guided the confessional process that these failings fall into the category of 'impure thoughts and deeds.' Even given this sanitized version, I could not confess to some man, semivisible behind the confessional grill, whose breath smelled of cigarettes and alcohol, the sensual dimensions of myself. Without a complete confession, however, you were not allowed to take Holy Communion, or if you did, you would be condemned to hell, with a mortal sin on your soul. (They sort of had you coming and going.) This was my first encounter with an ethical dilemma.

"And so I unconsciously and ingeniously devised a way out. When I was at the entry of adolescence, around age eleven, I began systematically to faint during mass, right before communion. I had to be carried out of church, and there on the entryway steps I remember being able to breathe, to hear the birds and feel the sun. This went on for over a year. I had no control over these fainting sessions. I was embarrassed by them and bewildered by what my body was doing—cold sweats, ringing in my ears, and the inevitable blackness closing in on me. (I have ever since felt oppressed in the confines of a church.) The intolerable and contradictory demands simply knocked me unconscious.[25]

Many women have been knocked unconscious by the conflicting demands of our culture. And many of us are waking up to it. Healing from conditions such as pelvic pain, PMS, and chronic fatigue syndrome is almost always enhanced when we realize that we are not alone in our suffering and that our problems occur in a cultural context that is often unsupportive to us. Recovering our health and then learning to create health on a daily basis involves naming our experiences for what they are—no matter how painful—and then learning that the motor for our lives is within us, regardless of our past.

Though it is extremely helpful to have a physician or health care provider who acknowledges the mind/body connection, it is even more important that we ourselves appreciate that our bodies and their symptoms are part of our inner guidance. We can free ourselves from our

TABLE 2

THE BODY AS A PROCESS VS. MEDICAL WORLD VIEW

The Body as a Process	Medical World View
~ The female body reflects nature and earth.	~ The female body and its processes are uncontrollable and unreliable. They require external control.
~ Thoughts and emotions are mediated via the immune, endocrine, and nervous systems. They are biochemical events.	~ Thoughts and emotions are entirely separate from the physical body.
~ The physical, emotional, spiritual, and psychological aspects of an individual are intimately intertwined and cannot be separated.	~ It is possible to separate an individual into entirely separate, unrelated compartments.
~ Illness is part of the inner guidance system.	~ Illness is a random event that just happens. There is very little a woman can do to prevent illness.
~ The body creates health daily. It is inherently self-healing.	~ The body is always vulnerable to germs, disease, and decay.
~ Illness is best prevented by living fully according to one's inner guidance while creating health daily.	~ Illness prevention is not possible in this system. So-called prevention is really disease screening.
~ Concerned with living fully. Focuses on what is going well without denying death.	~ Concerned with avoiding death at all costs. Focuses only on what can go wrong.
~ Our true selves don't die.	~ Death is seen as failure and final.

overdependence on the medical system by seeing the ways in which our own beliefs and behaviors perpetuate the parts of this system that do not help us create health. If we ourselves persist in thinking that our diseases and symptoms, such as endometriosis, fibroids, and PMS, are "just medical" and not related to the other parts of our lives, we are participating in and thus perpetuating the addictive system in medical care.

On the other hand, when we learn how to tune in to the language of our bodies, we're more able to make informed decisions about medical testing and technology, which can lead to more satisfactory relationships with our health care providers. We must begin to trust ourselves and our experience as much as we trust laboratory data. One of my patients who had infrequent periods came to see that she always got a period whenever she was "in love." She came to trust that she didn't need a lot of hormonal testing every time her period ceased for several months. Instead, she became interested in the meaning behind those periods and what emotions were associated with them. Working in partnership with such women is a true joy for me and for their other physicians as well. Both doctor and patient acknowledge our areas of expertise, our areas of ignorance, and the unknown that lies beyond.

As you read this book, remember that we all have choices—and we all have inner guidance and spiritual help available that can help us move toward optimal health and fulfillment. Recovery from the mind/body split means learning to live fully from the inside out in a culture that often negates this way of being in the world. Our bodies and their symptoms are our biggest allies in this endeavor, because nothing gets our attention as quickly. Our bodies never lie. They are impeccable barometers of how well we're living in the present and taking care of ourselves.

Germaine Greer said in an interview about her book *The Change*, "Nobody knows what a well woman would look like. How can you treat women if you don't know what femaleness is?" I see increasing numbers of well women all over the world, and I'm becoming one myself, more and more every day. I know what wellness looks like, and it starts by embracing our bodies and knowing that they are manifestations of thoughts and beliefs that can always be changed and updated. Imagine yourself whole, healed, and deeply in touch with the wisdom of your female body. Know that to be healthy and whole, you must have enough courage to follow your desires and your heart. What do you know in your bones? Nothing is more exciting than knowing that our bodies and our feelings are a clear, open pathway toward our destinies.

2

Feminine Intelligence and
a New Mode of Healing

In the end I find I can't separate brain from body. Consciousness isn't just in the head. Nor is it a question of mind over body. If one takes into account the DNA directing the dance of the peptides [the] body is the outward manifestation of the mind.

—Dr. Candace Pert, former chief brain biochemist,
National Institute of Mental Health

The mind and the body are intimately linked via the immune, endocrine, and central nervous systems. Today, mind/body research is confirming what ancient healing traditions have always known: that the body and the mind are a unity. There is no disease that isn't mental and emotional as well as physical.

ENERGY FIELDS AND ENERGY SYSTEMS

Humans are made out of energy and sustained by energy. Our bodies are ever-changing, dynamic fields of energy and vibration, not static physical structures. Cellular biologist Bruce Lipton, Ph.D., author of *The Biology of Belief* (Mountain of Love/Elite Books, 2005), writes that when we truly understand the effect of thoughts, emotions, and energy on the body, "we will no longer fractiously debate the role of nurture and nature, because we will realize that the fully conscious mind trumps both nature and nurture. And I believe we will also experience as profound a paradigmatic change to humanity as when a round world reality was introduced to a flat-world civilization." I couldn't agree more!

The truth is that our bodies are holograms in which every part contains information about the whole. We know from quantum physics that at the subatomic level, matter and energy—which can also be called spirit—are interchangeable. The best expression of this that I have heard is that matter is the densest form of spirit and that spirit is the lightest form of matter. We can view our bodies as manifestations of spiritual energy. Our mind and daily thoughts are part of this energy, and they have a well-documented effect on matter and our bodies. The quality of our daily thoughts and emotions actually sets up an electromagnetic field around us (and every cell in our bodies) that attracts to us our vibratory equivalent. This tendency is known as the law of attraction and is the most fundamental law that governs the universe. Like is attracted to like. As we vibrate, so we attract. Or to state it more simply, birds of a feather flock together!

Psychological and emotional factors influence our physical health greatly because our emotions and thoughts are always accompanied by biochemical reactions in our bodies, which are mediated by cell membranes, which are the actual "brains" of each cell. The mind/body continuum can be adequately understood only when we appreciate ourselves as an ever-changing energy system that is affected by, and also affects, the energy surrounding it. We don't end at our skins. This fact has been beautifully illustrated by the work of Dr. Masaru Emoto, a Japanese researcher who has done groundbreaking work on the effect of emotions on the crystalline structure of water. In his book *The Hidden Messages in Water* (Beyond Words Publishing, 2004), and also in the movie *What the Bleep Do We Know!?* Dr. Emoto documents the effects of different emotions on the structure of frozen water crystals, showing beyond a shadow of a doubt that the energy of loving appreciation creates the most profoundly beautiful crystalline patterns. Given that our bodies are over 70 percent water, Emoto's research has profound implications for health. How we think about, talk to, and feel about ourselves creates an imprint on our cells that affects not only us, but also everyone around us!

Though we cannot see this vibrational energy that makes up the body/mind and sustains us, it is nevertheless a vital part of us. It is the life-force that keeps our hearts beating and our lungs breathing even when we are asleep. Anyone who has had the experience of being with a dying person will tell you that after the moment of death, something changes. Though the physical body is still present, the person they knew is no longer there. Their life-force has gone elsewhere.

Vibrational fields interact within an individual person. They also interact between one person and another, and between one person and the world in general. These interactions, whose existence is well documented, are important for lifelong human growth and healthy development. A study at the University of Miami on premature babies, for example, found that babies who were stroked regularly gained weight 49 percent faster than did those of the same weight who weren't stroked. (Both groups of babies were fed exactly the same amount of food.) The stroked babies were longer and had larger heads and had fewer neurological problems at eight months of age than did the controls.[1] Babies who are not touched and cuddled, even though they are fed and cared for physically, are at great risk of death from the elusive diagnosis "failure to thrive."[2]

Even accidents, which we think of as "random" events, have been shown in a number of studies to be related to the emotional and psychological states (or vibrational fields) of the "victims." Several studies have indicated that accident-prone individuals have certain personality features that include impulsiveness, resentment, aggressiveness, unmet dependency needs, depression, sadness, loneliness, and unresolved grief. They tend to punish themselves when they feel anger toward others. In his book *Traffic Safety* (Science Serving Society, 2004), for example, Leonard Evans, president of Science Serving Society, presents exhaustive research on factors contributing to auto accidents including safety standards, road conditions, etc. One part of his analysis shows that drivers who are at higher risk for automobile accidents are, among other traits, less mature, intellectual, and concerned with aesthetics while they are more emotionally unstable, unhappy, antisocial, impulsive, openly hostile, and aggressive. They also have lower self-esteem and lower aspirations and are more likely to have had unhappy childhoods. So in the language of vibrational systems, it appears that the vibrational field of certain individuals interacts with the environmental vibrational field in a way that increases their incidence of accidents.

Clearly, human interactions have profound effects on health. These effects can be either positive or negative, depending upon the state of mind of the people involved in those interactions. When we begin to appreciate ourselves as vibrational fields of energy with the ability to affect the quality of our own experience, we will be getting in touch with our innate ability to heal ourselves and create health every day of our lives.

Our bodies are influenced and actually structured by our thoughts and beliefs. Every thought is accompanied by an emotion or feeling, and every emotion creates a specific biochemical reality in our bodies. Thoughts that are reinforced over and over become beliefs. Beliefs drive our behavior. We inherit many of these beliefs from our parents and the circumstances of our upbringing. Scientific studies conducted by Dr. Leonard Sagan, a medical epidemiologist, underscore this and show that social class, education, life-skills, and cohesiveness of family and community are key factors in determining life expectancy. Of all these factors, however, education has been shown to be the most important. A review of *all* the major epidemiological data on health makes clear that the major determinants of health are not immunization, diet, water supply, or antibiotics. In fact, the dramatic decline in death rates from infectious disease earlier in this century began long before the routine use of penicillin and antibiotics. *Hope, self-esteem, and education are the most important factors in creating health daily,* no matter what our background or the state of our health in the past.[3] All illnesses are affected by our emotional state. Dr. Jeanne Achterberg has shown that the course of cancer can be better predicted by psychological variables such as hope than by medical measurements.[4]

The huge 1998 ACE (Adverse Childhood Experiences) study, which has documented the dramatic adult health consequences of childhood abuse and family dysfunction, has shown beyond a shadow of a doubt the health effects of one's often inherited beliefs about their worthiness and lovability.[5] This study was initially triggered by observations made in the mid-1980s in the obesity program at the Kaiser Permanente Department of Preventive Medicine in San Diego. This program had a very high drop-out rate—and, surprisingly, the people dropping out were successfully losing weight. Detailed life interviews of almost two hundred such individuals unexpectedly revealed that childhood abuse was remarkably common and antedated the onset of their obesity. Many patients spoke openly about this. Obesity was not their problem: it was their protective solution to problems that they had previously never discussed with anyone. For example, a woman who gained 105 pounds in the year after being raped said, "Overweight is overlooked. And that is exactly what I need to be."

The ACE study found that adverse childhood experiences are vastly more common than is recognized or acknowledged. Slightly more than half of the 17,000 middle-class, middle-aged study participants in the ACE study had grown up in dysfunctional alcoholic homes, homes with a depressed or mentally ill person, or homes in which they had experienced sexual, physical, or emotional abuse. And these events were highly correlated with pharmacy costs, doctor visits, emergency room visits, hospitalization, and premature death.

In reflecting on the enormity of all this, ACE researcher Vincent Felitti, M.D., wrote: "If the treatment implications of what we found in the ACE study are far-reaching, the prevention aspects are positively daunting. The very nature of the material is such as to make one uncomfortable. Why would one want to leave the relative comfort of traditional organic disease and enter this area of threatening uncertainty that none of us has been trained to deal with?"

I know what Dr. Felitti is talking about. It's ever so much easier for both doctor and patient to ignore what's really going on, but it's ever so much more satisfying to get to the heart of the matter. After all, our bodies never lie and they're always trying to get us to see the truth. So I suggest a middle ground. It's prudent to use symptomatic medical treatments as a bridge across the river to true health. But we need to understand that in order to truly heal on the deepest level and give our cells the "live" message that creates health, we need to change and update our beliefs and behaviors. This includes releasing emotions that we have stuffed. Our past is not our destiny. Our power to change is now. This power within is engaged by affirming our worthiness and lovability, updating our beliefs, feeling our true feelings, and choosing thoughts that are more uplifting and healing.

One of my patients told me, "I had a flash of insight on the way to your office today. When I was little, the only way I could get my mother's attention was to be sick. So I've had a lot of broken bones, then cancer, and now an abnormal Pap smear. I just realized today that I don't have to get sick to get her attention anymore!" She added that at the moment she had that insight in the car, the sun broke through the clouds, reinforcing her insight with its brilliance.

UNDERSTANDING THE BODYMIND

The medical community is beginning to view patients as physical beings who constantly renew themselves. The body is like a river of information and energy, and all its parts have a dynamic communication with all the other parts. Radioisotope studies have shown, for example, that red blood cells replenish themselves every twenty-eight days, while we regenerate all our liver cells over a six-month period. In this continual restructuring of our physical bodies, we have daily opportunities to create health.

Though each of us is bombarded by millions of stimuli daily, our central nervous system and sense organs function in such a way as to choose and process *only those stimuli that reinforce what we already believe about ourselves*. A Nobel Prize–winning experiment underscores the importance of this concept: Scientists raised kittens to adulthood in an environment that contained only horizontal lines on the walls of their cages and in the rooms where they were kept. Once they grew into mature cats, they were placed in a normal environment and proceeded to run into anything with vertical lines. The cats literally didn't "see" anything vertical. The opposite proved true with kittens raised within an environment of only vertical lines. Once they grew up, they bumped into everything horizontal. We can apply this insight to people, too. For instance, women who are abused as children are much more likely to be abused repeatedly as adults. They have been conditioned to being abused and have difficulty recognizing loving people and environments. As adults, our nervous systems function to reinforce what we were exposed to in our early years, unless we consciously change the effects of our early programming. The seeds of many later illnesses are sown in our childhoods, then fertilized regularly by our beliefs and thoughts that expect these experiences to be repeated.

The science of the mind/body connection, or psychoneuroimmunology (PNI), helps explain how the circumstances of our lives can affect our bodies. PNI and related research show that the hormonal and neurological events within the body and the subtle electromagnetic fields around and within the body form a crucial link between the cultural wounding, which we think of as "psychological" and "emotional," and the gynecological or other problems women have, which we think of as "physical."

Many women who've survived sexual abuse, for example, divorce themselves from their bodies. Some experience themselves in their bodies only from the neck up. As one of my patients with continual menstrual spotting said, "I don't want to think about anything below my waist. I hate that part of my body. I wish that part of me would just go away." This was an important understanding for her; it indicated where she needed to take a step toward healing. Her menstrual spotting continually drew her attention back to a disowned part of her body that needed healing. An associate of mine sometimes has patients draw pictures of themselves. She told me of a patient with chronic pelvic pain who drew a self-portrait only from the waist up. My associate pointed out to this woman that maybe her pelvis, through pain, was trying to get her attention. She was leaving it out!

If the science of the mind/body connection helps explain how our

emotional and psychological wounding becomes physical, it also supports our ability to heal from those conditions. All distress, all healing
of distress, and all creation of health are simultaneously physical, psychological, emotional, and spiritual.

Up until fairly recently, scientists believed that information was
passed linearly in the nervous system from nerve to nerve, just like electrical hard wiring. But now we know that our body organs communicate directly with the brain and vice versa, through chemical
messengers known as neuropeptides. These neuropeptides pass messages between nerve cells; neuropeptide receptor molecules then receive
messages that are triggered to be released by emotions and thoughts. It
used to be believed that receptor sites for neuropeptides were located
only in the body's endocrine and immune system cells, as well as in
nerve cells. Now we know that body organs such as the kidney and
bowel also have receptor sites for these so-called brain chemicals. And
so do blood cells! These chemicals are part of the way in which
thoughts and emotions affect our physical bodies directly.

Not only do our physical organs contain receptor sites for the neurochemicals of thought and emotion, our organs and immune systems
can themselves manufacture these same chemicals. What this means is
that our entire body feels and expresses emotion—all parts of us
"think" and "feel." It is well documented, for example, that the gut
makes more neurotransmitters than the brain.[6] Moreover, white blood
cells produce morphinelike pain-relieving substances, and they in turn
contain receptor sites for the same substances. This gives a person the
capacity to modulate her own pain without medication. Studies are beginning to document the fact that the uterus, ovaries, and breast tissue
make the same neurochemicals of thought and emotion as the brain
and the other organs. Hormones, for example, are messenger molecules
for emotions and thoughts. The immune cells, too, have receptors for
neuropeptides, the messenger molecules. Ovaries and probably the
uterus make estrogen and progesterone—hormones that are also neurotransmitters that affect emotions and thoughts. And these organs,
too, have receptor sites that receive messages from the brain and the
immune system. It's easy, then, to understand that when we are sad, our
female organs "feel" sad and their functions are affected.

Our thoughts, emotions, and brains communicate directly with our
immune, nervous, and endocrine systems and with the organs of our
bodies. Moreover, although these bodily systems are conventionally
studied and viewed as separate, they are, in fact, aspects of the *same*
system! If the uterus, the ovaries, the white blood cells, and the heart
all make the same chemicals as the brain makes when it thinks, then

where in the body is the mind? The answer is, *the mind is located throughout the body* and even beyond.[7] In fact, an extensive body of research on prayer has documented that our minds are nonlocal and have profound effects at a distance from our bodies![8]

Our entire concept of "the mind" needs to be expanded considerably. *The mind can no longer be thought of as being confined to the brain or to the intellect; it exists in every cell of our bodies.* Every thought we think has a biochemical equivalent. Every emotion we feel has a biochemical equivalent. One of my colleagues says, "The mind is the space between the cells." So when the part of your mind that is your uterus talks to you, through pain or excessive bleeding, are you prepared to listen to it?

When I asked a married thirty-five-year-old lawyer who had a sudden onset of bleeding between her periods what was going on in her life, she bristled. "I think this problem is medical," she said. By that, she meant that the problem was purely physical and was not related in any meaningful way to the rest of her life. I gently explained to her that I would have asked her the same question had she broken her leg, and I pointed out that all symptoms are "physical." My patient then calmed down and told me the truth: Recently she had had an extramarital affair and was feeling guilty, and she was terrified that she had acquired a sexually transmitted disease. Her irregular bleeding had started soon after her affair began. This additional history enabled me to give her better and more appropriate medical care, while she learned that she didn't have to separate herself into unrelated parts.

One of my patients went to see a biofeedback therapist about shoulder pain caused by chronic muscle tension. While she was learning to relax the muscles of her shoulder, she noticed that her muscle tension increased whenever she was thinking certain thoughts. One of these thoughts was of being spanked as a child. Another was of her husband's ill health and its possible implications for her. On the other hand, when she thought of the positive aspects of her life, her muscle tension lessened. She came to see that her fears and beliefs were encoded in her body. Through biofeedback, she learned that her muscle tissue had feelings, thoughts, and memories that were part of her body's wisdom.

The mind and the soul, which permeate our entire body, are much vaster than the intellect can possibly grasp. Our inner guidance comes to us through our feelings and body wisdom first—not through intellectual understanding. When we search for inner guidance with the intellect only—as though it exists outside of ourselves and our own deepest knowing—we get stuck in the search, and our inner guidance is effectively silenced. The intellect works best *in service* to our intuition, our heart, our inner guidance, soul, God, or higher power—whichever term we choose for the spiritual energy that animates life. Once we have acknowledged that we are *more* than our intellect and that guidance is available to us from the universal mind, we have accessed our inner healing ability. As William James once said, "The power to move the world is in the subconscious mind."

FEMININE INTELLIGENCE:
HOW THOUGHTS BECOME EMBODIED

Women have the capacity to know with their bodies and with their brains at the same time, in part because their brains are set up in such a way that the information in both hemispheres and in the body is highly available to them when they communicate.

In school I was taught to distrust my own thinking process because it never fit with the dualistic way in which education is set up. On a multiple-choice test, for example, I could always find a reason why almost every choice given might be correct. I could always see "the big picture," and I could see how everything was related to everything else. In going over my wrong answers, my teachers often told me, "You're reading too much into it. The correct answer is obvious." It was not always obvious to me. Now that I have learned to appreciate how intimately my thoughts, emotions, and physical body are connected, I have begun to reclaim my full intelligence. It is staggering to realize how many highly intelligent women think that they are stupid because so much of their intelligence has been undervalued. Dr. Linda Metcalf says, "Women think that their intellects are a male construct sitting inside their heads."

I have learned that like many women, I speak and think in a multimodal, spiral way using both hemispheres of my brain and the intelligence of my body all at the same time. Anthropologist and visionary writer Jean Houston describes the evolution of multimodal thinking like this: "For centuries, women stood in their caves, stirring the soup with one hand, bouncing the baby on one hip, and kicking the woolly mammoth out the door with the other foot." We evolved having to focus on more than one task at a time—understanding innately the consequences of our actions, not just on ourselves but on our entire family unit or tribe. It makes sense that this brain structure would evolve in the gender whose bodies carry and grow babies who are separate individuals who think and feel even before birth! By having to focus on more than one thing or person at a time, women have, over the centuries, developed a brain structure and style of thinking that are characteristically different from most men's.[9]

In most women, the corpus callosum, the part of the brain that connects the right and left hemispheres, is thicker than it is in most men. That is, male and female brains are "wired" differently. Men characteristically use mostly their left hemispheres to think and to communicate their thoughts; their reasoning is usually linear and solution-oriented. It gets to "the point." Women, in contrast, recruit more areas of the brain when they communicate than do most men. They use both the right and the left sides of their brain simultaneously. Because the right hemisphere has richer connections with the body than the left hemisphere, women have more access to their body wisdom when speaking and thinking than do most men.

This doesn't mean that male brains inherently lack this capacity. It's just that for centuries they haven't been encouraged to develop it. For the last five thousand years, Western society has believed that a linear, left-brain approach is the superior mode of communication and that a woman's more embodied way of speaking and thinking is inferior and "less evolved." Anne Moir and Daniel Jessel, the authors of the book *Brain Sex*, point out, "Men, it seems, are the sex who say the first thing that comes into their heads, while women communicate by calling on a much wider repertoire. Taken all together the evidence paints a comprehensive picture of a busier and wider interchange of information in the female brain."[10] Unfortunately, instead of developing embodied thinking deliberately as an inherent strength, we learn to reject and denigrate this capacity.

In a dialogue with sociolinguist Deborah Tannen, Robert Bly said, "Words are in one lobe of the brain and feelings in the other." "So that means," Bly continued, "that women have an ability to mingle those much quicker than men can. Women have a superhighway going on there. And, as Michael Mead remarked, men have this little corked country road, and you're lucky if a word gets over."[11]

My ex-husband used to say to me, "Can't you say that in fewer words? Can't you get to the point?" This expresses a stereotypically male communication style. When I think or speak, I use language to express the richness of what goes on in my mind and body while I'm communicating my thoughts. I like to hang out with language and wander around in it. I often come to understand how I'm feeling by talking about it for a while, letting my thoughts arise from my whole body and whole brain before speaking them. Processing ideas verbally or writing down my thoughts helps me to know more of myself.

In contrast, my ex-husband used as few words as possible. He and men like him want to get to the point, the product or solution, and everything has to have one, otherwise it is not worth talking about. Most men view and experience the *process* of getting to the point as tedious and worthless. Dr. George Keller, a colleague in holistic medicine, says, "When men talk, they leave out the verbs. When women talk, they leave out the nouns." Alluding to quantum physics, which teaches that particles and waves are simply different aspects of matter, Dr. Keller observes, "Men speak particle language. Women speak wave language."

Multimodal, embodied thinking makes it possible for most women to go to the grocery store without a list and still remember everything they came to buy, plus other stuff that they suddenly remember they need. When my children were little and I was doing a lot of surgery, I was able to do the surgery and simultaneously know what my kids were doing, and that I needed to pick up paper towels and bread on the way home. My husband, on the other hand, was able to hold only one or two thoughts and tasks in his mind simultaneously—and often forgot what he was going to the store for in the first place.

The differences between male and female communication styles come up repeatedly in daily life. When I am explaining a woman's condition to her male partner, I often tell him, "Listen, when I talk to you about what your wife [or partner] has, I may seem to be talking in circles. I'll be going out here, out here, and over there." I move my finger in a circle. "It may feel like a digression to you, and you may not see the relevance of all that I'm saying. But it is all related. Stay with me— I'm coming back to the main point and will tie it all together for you."

It's very healing and empowering for women to understand the fullness of their intelligence, appreciating the crucial role that inner guidance, intuition, and emotions all play in feminine intelligence. Once we embrace these aspects of ourselves, our perception changes. We can then celebrate the differences between male and female intelligence without making men, or ourselves, wrong or inferior.

BELIEFS ARE PHYSICAL

Thoughts are an important part of our body's wisdom because we have the ability to change our minds (and our thoughts) as we learn and grow. A thought held long enough and repeated enough becomes a belief. The belief then becomes biology. Beliefs are vibrational forces that create the physical basis for our individual lives and our health.

If we don't work through self-destructive thoughts and subsequent feelings (I am worthless. I'll never be good enough), our destructive thoughts and suppressed emotions set ourselves up for physical distress because of the biochemical effect that emotions have on our immune and endocrine systems. Diseases such as rheumatoid arthritis, multiple sclerosis, certain thyroid diseases, and lupus erythematosus, for example, are all called autoimmune diseases, meaning that the immune system attacks the body. Why would the immune system attack the cells of the person in whom it is functioning, unless it is getting some kind of destructive message from somewhere very deep within the body? Mental depression has been associated not only with self-destructive behaviors but with depression of immune system functioning.[12] Depression is also an independent risk factor for heart disease and osteoporosis. Many women with autoimmune diseases also suffer from depression. Studies have shown, for example, that stress and loneliness can help cause latent (inactive) herpes virus to become active.[13] The same is true for those with Epstein-Barr virus, the virus linked with chronic fatigue syndrome. This is one reason why, even though over 90 percent of the population have been exposed to and have antibodies to Epstein-Barr virus, only a small percentage actually suffer from the disease. The same is true for those suffering from gastric ulcers associated with *H. pylori* bacteria and from yeast-related diseases. This information is especially relevant to women, since at least 80 percent of all autoimmune disease occurs in us.[14] Even endometriosis, epilepsy, premature menopause, infertility, and chronic vaginitis have autoimmune components.

What an individual believes is heavily influenced by the culture in which she lives. Beliefs held in common perpetuate the type of society in which we live. Given our society, it is not surprising that women have so much perceived stress. In several scientific studies, inescapable stress has been associated with a distinct form of immunosuppression (suppression of immune system response). Emotional shock is associated with the release of endogenous opiates (morphinelike substances) and corticosteroids (hormones from the adrenal glands), which prevent white blood cells from protecting the body from cancer and infection. People who have a sense of hopelessness or despair and who perceive their situation as being uncontrollably stressful have higher levels of corticosteroids and immune suppression than do those who have more resilient coping styles.[15] People who are exposed to what they perceive as inescapable stress actually release opioidlike substances (enkephalins) that literally numb the cells of their bodies (in stress-induced analgesia),[16] rendering them incapable of destroying cancer cells and bacteria if this goes on chronically.[17] *The most crucial thing to understand is this: It is not stress itself that creates immune system problems.* It is, rather, the *perception* that the stress is inescapable—that there is nothing a person can do to prevent or change it—that is associated with immune system suppression. *Perception can always be changed. And that is the key to getting and staying well!*

It is important to understand that our beliefs go much deeper than our thoughts, and we cannot simply will them away. Many beliefs are completely unconscious and are not readily available to the intellect. Most of us aren't aware of the destructive beliefs that undermine our health. They don't come from the intellect alone, the part that thinks it's in control. They come from the other part that in the past became lodged and buried in the cell tissue.

Jean, a lovely dark-haired graphics designer, came for a consultation with me. She was forty-five years old and was concerned that her periods had changed over the years from a pattern of every twenty-eight days to every twenty-five to thirty-four days. She had no spotting in between and no other symptoms. This history sounded completely normal to me, but another doctor had told her that her cycle change might represent cancer. He had recommended a uterine biopsy. Because her cervical opening was too small to allow a biopsy instrument to enter, a D&C under general anesthesia was suggested. Jean decided to seek a second opinion. Her exam was normal, but she did in fact have a very small cervical opening and therefore could not have an office biopsy. Her ultrasound showed a normal uterine lining.

I told Jean that I thought she was a very unlikely candidate for uterine cancer and that I wouldn't recommend a D&C. If she was really worried and wanted one, I said, it could certainly be done to be sure she didn't have cancer. To help her make her decision, I asked her what her childhood experience of illness had been, since a woman's childhood experience tends to profoundly influence her beliefs around health and disease. Jean said, "I was an only child, and my mother was always sick. She constantly had bowel problems. I had to take care of her. As a result, I personally react to everything that happens in my body as though it's a catastrophe—just as my mother did."

Then I said, "If you decided to have a D&C and it turned out to be normal, would you be able to relax and stop obsessing over cancer?" She said that it wouldn't make any difference. She'd still worry. We agreed then that she had to change her belief system about her body and its vulnerability, which had been so firmly influenced by her early years.

To do this, Jean now needs to understand that her fear is not entirely accessible to her intellect. Much of it is in her body and her subconscious mind. Telling Jean, or women with similar problems, to "just relax, you're fine, it's nothing" and that "it's all in your head" is not scientifically accurate. Jean's belief is in her mind, but her mind is located throughout her body and in every organ in it.

For Jean to stop obsessing about cancer (or anything else), she will have to go through a process that every one of us must also go through to heal. To explain this process to patients, I used the first three steps of the twelve-step program, which originated with Alcoholics Anonymous. Since these twelve steps are based on spiritual truths, I've found them applicable to nearly every aspect of life about which I or my patients are seeking guidance. Step one is: "We admitted we were powerless over alcohol and that our lives had become unmanageable." Instead of the word *alcohol,* you can substitute anything that you currently are obsessing about or feel powerless over. In Jean's case, she must admit that she is powerless to change her belief and obsession about cancer with her intellect alone. She must also admit that this belief is not healthy and that it is making parts of her life unmanageable. Her belief won't go away if she beats herself up about it or tries to force herself to change it with her intellect alone. She must also understand that the obsessive thought is trying to keep her from feeling something she may not want to feel. (The intellect likes to think it's in control at all times.) But you have to feel in order to heal.

The second step is: "We came to see that a power greater than ourselves could restore us to sanity." This power "greater than ourselves" is a part of our inner guidance and bodily wisdom. You can even think of it as your soul—the part of you that lives beyond time and space. The word *sanity* means the same thing as inner peace or serenity. Acknowledging that we have access to guidance from a power greater than our own intellect is a very positive step toward actually accessing that guidance. The third step is: "We made a decision to turn our will and our lives over to the care of God *as we understood Him.*" (You can change the word *Him* to *inner guidance* or *divine wisdom, higher self, or Divine Mother.*) This step bypasses the intellect entirely. It is a leap of faith that acknowledges the fact that all of us have inner guidance available within us and that that guidance has the power to remove our harmful beliefs. The words *made a decision* are very important. To create health, a woman needs to make a decision to do it. Then she must be willing to stay with the process. Participating in twelve-step meetings and working the steps around a fear, a belief, or even an illness that you've found your intellect to be powerless over can be very helpful and practical. I also love the affirming work of Louise Hay, who wrote *You Can Heal Your Life*.

For Jean and thousands of women like her, the knowledge that she is not alone in her fears and obsessions is itself very helpful. I've never met anyone who didn't inherit at least some health-destroying beliefs either from their families or from the culture in general. By choosing to move forward into health and joy, we can uncover the deep programming of our bodies and change it to support health. The reason this works is that the very process of deciding to be happier or healthier will automatically bring up the thought patterns that have prevented greater happiness and health in the first place! Many of my patients have been able to change their states of health and their lives once they understand that although their diseases are very real and physical, these diseases are often accompanied and reinforced by unconscious beliefs. Uncovering these and healing from them is a continuous, exciting, and empowering process. It is part of the process of creating health. It requires patience and compassion. And it works.

Beliefs and memories are actually biological constructs in the body. Think of your mind as an iceberg. The conscious part—the part that thinks it's in control—is what peaks above the surface. But it amounts to only about 25 percent of the total iceberg. The so-called subconscious part of your mind is the much larger part—75 percent of it lies below the surface. Our personal histories are stored throughout our bodies, in muscles, in organs, and in other tissues. This information, like the submerged portion of the iceberg, is not generally recognized by the part of the iceberg on the surface, our conscious intellect. Our cells contain our memory banks—even when the conscious mind is not aware of them and actually battles to deny them.

Once when I called a bellman to my hotel room to help me with my bags, he noticed a bottle of Chinese cough syrup near the sink. He made a face, held his stomach, and said, "I thought that was castor oil, and I remember that my mother gave it to me often as a child. I used to have stomach pains after taking it. Just looking at the bottle now gives me a stomachache!" This man had no conscious control over his body's memory of his childhood pain. His body automatically reacted to the sight of a familiar bottle that wasn't even related.

Once I was hiking with a woman who told me that two weeks before, she had gotten some sunscreen in her eye and her eye had watered all day from the irritation. Several days later, she merely smelled the same sunscreen when someone else was using it, and her eye started to water again. Her biological memory was already encoded in her eye. Her intellect had been bypassed entirely!

How Beliefs Become Physical

At any given time, our state of health reflects the sum total of our beliefs since birth. Our entire society functions under many shared and sometimes harmful beliefs. (One that I hear regularly is, "Well, now that I'm thirty [or forty, or fifty], I suppose it's normal to have aches and pains.") All living things respond physically to the way they *think* reality is. Dr. Deepak Chopra, an authority on consciousness and medicine, uses the example of flies placed in a jar with a lid on top. But once the lid is removed, they will not leave the jar except for a few brave pioneers. The rest of the flies have made a "commitment in their body-minds" that they are trapped. It has been shown that in aquariums if two schools of fish are separated with a glass partition for a certain amount of time, the fish will not swim into each other's space after the partition is removed.

So it is that we can be sure the events of our childhood set the stage for our beliefs about ourselves and therefore our experience, including our health. For a woman to change or improve her reality and her state of health, she first has to change her beliefs about what is possible. This is a simple enough process. But it requires discipline and persistence.

That we have the wherewithal to overcome our destructive and unconscious patterns is a truth that I see proved daily. This power has also been documented experimentally in a study of the effects of beliefs on the aging process. Dr. Ellen Langer studied a group of male volunteers over the age of seventy at a retreat center for five days. They all had to agree that they would live in the present as though it were 1959. Dr. Langer told them, "We are not asking you to 'act as if it were 1959' but to let yourself *be* just who you were in 1959." They had to dress as they had then, watch TV shows from 1959, read newspapers and magazines from that time, and talk as if 1959 were right now. They also brought pictures of themselves from that year and put them around the center. Dr. Langer then measured many of the parameters that often deteriorate with aging (but don't need to), such as physical strength, perception, cognition, taste, and hearing. The parameters reflected biological markers that experts in geriatric medicine often cite. Over the course of the five days, many of the chosen parameters actually improved. Serial photographs showed that the men looked about five years younger as well. Their hearing and memory improved. As they changed their mindsets about aging, their physical bodies changed as well! Yale researcher Becca Levy, Ph.D., has also documented the profound effect that belief has on how we age. She found that older people with more positive self-perceptions of aging, measured up to 23 years earlier, lived 7.5 years longer than those with less positive self-perceptions of aging.

The most compelling part of this study is the fact that the 7.5 year higher longevity for those with the more positive attitudes toward aging remained even after other factors were taken into account, including age, gender, socioeconomic status, loneliness, and overall health. The researchers used information from the 660 participants aged fifty and older from a small town in Ohio who were part of the Ohio Longitudinal Study of Aging and Retirement (OLSAR). Dr. Levy and her coauthors compared mortality rates to responses made twenty-three years earlier by the participants (338 men and 322 women). The responses included agreeing or disagreeing with such statements as "As you get older, you are less useful." These beliefs often operate subconsciously without our awareness, often beginning in childhood. Commenting on their research, the study's authors said, "The effect of more positive self-perceptions of aging on survival is greater than the physiological measures of low systolic blood pressure and cholesterol, each of which is associated with a longer lifespan of four years or less. It is also greater than the independent contributions of lower body mass index, no history of smoking, and a tendency to exercise; each of these factors has been found to contribute between one and three years of added life."[18]

There isn't a drug, exercise regimen, or vitamin that comes anywhere near the potential of our beliefs to add 7.5 years to our lives! And that's why examining our beliefs critically is crucial to getting and staying healthy. Dr. Langer writes, "The regular and 'irreversible' cycles of aging that we witness in the later stages of human life may be a product of certain assumptions about how one is supposed to grow old. *If we didn't feel compelled to carry out these limiting mindsets, we might have a greater chance of replacing years of decline with years of growth and purpose*" [emphasis mine].[19]

If we have the power to reverse the effects of aging, what might be possible with health? The hopefulness that these data raise cannot be overestimated. It suggests that if we can leap out of our collective cultural jars, life holds possibilities that we've not imagined before. But before we get there, we must first acknowledge the horizontal or vertical stripes that many of us keep running into. Once we *see* what has been there all along, we can create alternative routes.

HEALING VERSUS CURING

Freedom and fate embrace each other to form meaning; and given meaning, fate—with its eyes, hitherto severe, suddenly full of light—looks like grace itself.

—Martin Buber

There is a difference between healing and curing. Healing is a natural process and *within* the power of everyone. Curing, which is what doctors are called upon to do, usually consists of an *external* treatment; medication or surgery is used to mask or eliminate symptoms. *This external treatment doesn't necessarily address the factors that contributed to the symptoms in the first place.* Healing goes deeper than curing and must always come from within. It addresses the imbalance that underlies the symptoms. Healing brings together the often hidden aspects of a person's life as they relate to her illness. Healing is different from curing, though curing and the restoration of physical function may accompany healing. One can be healed completely and go on to die of her illness. This is a key understanding that is often missing from treatises on holistic medicine: healing and death are not mutually exclusive. As a physician, I've been trained to improve and preserve life. But sometimes we need to let go of that training and accept death as a natural part of a process that is much bigger and more mysterious than we realize. Patricia Reis, who worked with many of my patients' dreams and body symptoms, put it this way: "The bigger meaning of healing is a 'wholeing,' a filling out of the missing pieces of a person's life. Sometimes this may even mean facing death in a more fully realized way. Certainly it is an opportunity to come more deeply and fully into life."

Although our entire bodies are affected by our thoughts and emotions and their various parts talk to one another, each individual's body language is unique. *No matter what has happened in her life, a woman has the power to change what that experience means to her and thus change her experience, both emotionally and physically. Therein lies her healing.* There are no simple formulae for deciphering the message behind a symptom, and only the patient herself can ultimately know what the message is about. Sometimes a woman's body, through chronic vaginitis, asks her to leave a relationship. Sometimes headaches that occur premenstrually are a sign that she needs to give up caffeine. In other women, these symptoms may be related to something entirely different. It is up to each woman to "sit with" her symptoms in a completely receptive, nonjudgmental way so that she can begin to appreciate the unique language of her body.

We don't yet understand completely why it is that one woman who has been abandoned by her husband, for example, will seem to deteriorate emotionally, mentally, and physically, blaming this particular trauma for a lifetime of woes, while another woman with a similar background will recover fully and live a productive life. Some people can name an initially painful and traumatic circumstance as the stimulus from which major personal growth later arose. Childhood abuse, incest, loss of a parent, and other traumas are not absolutely linked in a cause-and-effect way with subsequent distress in adulthood. The effect of trauma on our physical, mental, and emotional bodies is determined largely by *how we interpret the event and give it meaning.*

Emotional factors are usually involved in common gynecological problems, along with diet, behavior, and heredity. I have found that most women with persistent genital warts, herpes, or ovarian cysts have experienced or are continuing to experience emotional and psychological stress or unrest. In these cases, a history of sexual abuse, abortions that haven't been resolved emotionally, or some conflict involving relationships or creativity is almost always present. These conflicts live in the body's vibrational field until they're resolved—they are healing opportunities simply waiting for our attention.

One of my OB/GYN colleagues, Dr. Maude Guerin, illustrates this beautifully by using the example of a woman named Joan who had severe endometriosis and pelvic pain. Dr. Guerin "cured" Joan with a total abdominal hysterectomy and removal of both ovaries and tubes—a standard treatment for her problem. Following surgery, however, Joan developed back pain, depression, and incapacitating hot flashes, requiring many times the regular dose of hormones. Although her pelvic pain had been "cured," in many ways she was no better off than she had been before. Instead of being healed, she had simply traded one group of symptoms for another. The surgical removal of her uterus and ovaries had not resolved the emotional conflicts in her body's vibrational field that were the root cause of her problem.

Dr. Guerin discovered that Joan had been sexually abused at the age of six, had lived through the death of her sister at the age of sixteen, and had turned to workaholism to avoid her feelings. Despite these major traumas in her life, she had never been able to cry. Dr.

Guerin writes, "This patient has been a wonderful teacher for me. Although I never discounted the concept that thoughts and feelings influence physical health, I had always perceived that influence to be relative. This patient taught me that consideration of the mind/body link is obligatory in the case of every patient, no matter how cut-and-dried their course seems to be.

"I certainly felt that I had cured this woman, and was proud of myself at her six-week checkup. It took the two of us years to learn that although she had been 'cured' by surgery, she was not healed by it.

"Looking back on her first visit with me, which I remember vividly, and her subsequent course, there were many, many clues to a much larger picture that I was unable to see at the time. On her initial office visit, she was sitting on the examination table while still wearing her panty hose. Not only did she have trouble getting undressed for the exam, she also had a great deal of difficulty even getting her body in the examination position. Once she was there, I found that placing the speculum in her vagina was nearly impossible because of her extreme anxiety and muscle tension. Since then my patients have continued to help me see the big picture, for each of them. I know that you can 'cure' many patients without acknowledging the mind/body link, but I also know that you will 'heal' very few."[20]

One of my own patients had an abnormal Pap smear. She already knew that simply removing the abnormal cells from her cervix ("curing") would not address the underlying energy imbalance in her body that was at the root of the abnormality. She began working in her journal every morning with the intention of affirming her inherent ability to be whole and healthy. At the same time, she became receptive to what was necessary for her healing. She meditated on what this symptom was trying to teach her so that she could release any patterns that no longer served her. After she had been engaged in this inner healing work for several weeks, she uncovered a key belief that she felt was important to her. This belief was that the abnormal cervical cells were a punishment for her sexuality. Having discovered and named this belief, she proceeded to schedule standard medical therapy so that her "healing" and her "curing" would be in partnership. On her way to the appointment to have laser treatment for this condition, she experienced a wave of forgiveness toward herself and her sexuality that moved her to tears. She even felt a shift take place in her body. When she was examined at the office, all traces of the abnormality had gone, and she didn't require the surgery. She is very grateful for the physical cure, as well as the psychological and emotional healing that took place.

In this society, when a physician acknowledges a woman's innate healing ability, she or he often seems to be saying that she *caused* her illness to begin with. But our illnesses aren't based on simple cause and effect. It is simplistic and potentially harmful to believe that we consciously and intentionally create illness or any other painful life circumstance. Our illnesses often exist to get our attention and get us back on track. Feeling that we are to blame keeps us stuck and unable to move forward in our healing. The part of us that "creates an illness" is not the part of us that feels the pain of the illness. It is not a conscious part of us, but it can be affected by our consciousness once we put our healing process to work. When it comes to taking responsibility, there is a balance. We must learn to take responsibility for the things we caused or are perpetuating. On the other hand, it is equally important to let go of responsibility for those things which have nothing to do with us. Far too many women get sick because they have taken on the mistaken notion that it is their job to take care of everyone in their families or jobs—even those who are old enough to take care of themselves!

Many physicians, however, equate taking responsibility for illness with being to blame for it. Our culture in general assumes that taking responsibility means you are to blame. At the opposite extreme, other physicians feel that since their patients didn't cause their disease, they should not be overly involved in their own treatment. It is important that you have a doctor or health practitioner whose beliefs can reinforce your healing. Recent studies have shown that the expectations that physicians have about their patients' healing potential are picked up consciously and unconsciously by their patients and do affect their ability to get well. Of course all relationships, including those with our doctors, are two-way streets. As Dr. Phil McGraw says, "We teach people how to treat us." When women become more empowered and able to ask for what they need, they find that they can evoke the healer that lives within the hearts of most doctors, whether conventional or alternative. And they get better care.

All relationships begin with how we treat ourselves. We can begin to heal our lives at the deepest levels when we begin to value our bodies and honor their messages instead of feeling victimized by them. Trusting the wisdom of the body is a leap of faith in a culture that fails to acknowledge how intimately the mind and body are connected. By *the wisdom of the body* I mean that we must learn to trust that the symptoms in the body are often the only way that the soul can get our attention. Covering up our symptoms with external "cures" prevents us from healing the parts of our lives that need attention and change.

I used to run into what I call "blame walls" when I asked my patients to participate in their own health care. Once, for example, when

I explained to a woman that her fibroid (benign uterine tumor) might be related to how she was using her creativity within her relationships, she became angry and thought I was blaming her. "Do you mean I caused this?" she said. I told her that she must move beyond blame, beyond cause-and-effect thinking. To heal from the problem she needed to relate to her fibroid in a new way, seeing it not as the enemy to be "cured" but as an aspect of her own inner guidance that was trying to direct her attention toward health-enhancing changes in her life. Responding to and learning from an illness is a very empowering way to achieve permanent healing and a transformed life.

For healing to occur, we must come to see that we are not so much responsible for *our illnesses as responsible* to *them.* The healthiest people I know don't take their diseases or even their lives too personally. They spend very little time beating themselves up about their illnesses, their life circumstances, or anything else. They take their life one day at a time, as it unfolds in its own way and its own time. A young woman stated this attitude beautifully when she wrote, "I take full responsibility not for getting cancer in the first place, nor for ultimately surviving it, but rather for the quality of the way I am responding to this bit of chaos thrown into my life."

The story of Martha, a close family friend, provides a most striking example of the mystery of illness and body symptoms. Though unusual in many ways, her story illustrates the range of experiences available to us when we are open to healing in whatever way it presents itself.

When Martha was in her late fifties, a series of painful childhood memories began to surface spontaneously. She allowed herself to feel fully how painful her childhood had been. She expressed and released these feelings through sobbing for hours over several days within the space of about a week. During this process she fully remembered the details of being taken to run-down bars by her bootlegger father. While she was at these places she had often watched him kissing women who were strangers. She recalled being left with an aunt for a few days while her mother broke her father out of jail. The aunt, who had only one eye, kept her and her younger sister in a cockroach-laden room with only crackers to eat and a single lightbulb hanging from the ceiling. As Martha let herself remember those and many other things that she had "deep-sixed" fifty-five years before, she was able to cry and wail for as long as she needed to as a trusted friend sat with her. This cleansing went on for several days, off and on. Afterward, she said, "I realized that there was nothing of beauty in my life when I was a child. It was worse than I ever let myself remember."

Once she was able to see this part of her life for what it really was and express her emotions around it, the chronic neck and shoulder pain that she'd had for years and that had been ascribed to "degenerative changes in her spine" went away completely. It has never come back.

One spring, Martha called me to say that she was experiencing terror of death to a degree she'd never known possible. Based on her past experience of trusting her symptoms, she decided to stay with her feelings and symptoms to see what they could teach her rather than running away from them or trying to suppress or "cure" them with drugs.

Martha is no stranger to death, having lived through the deaths of two of her children and her husband—two of these in the space of one year. Her fear of her own death, which she told me followed her to bed at night and confronted her in the morning, was accompanied by vague left-sided upper abdominal pains, which she at first misinterpreted as being related to taking penicillin for a dental infection. Her terror was so awful that she couldn't really talk about it for quite some time.

As her terror and the stomach pain became worse, her intuition suggested that she should drive across the country from New England to Taos, New Mexico, where one of her daughters lived. She wanted to be alone, and she felt that driving a long distance would be the right thing. I had never heard her so upset, but I was not worried. I trusted that she had something to work through and that I would hear from her afterward, when she was ready to talk to me. Several days later she called, still quite shaky. "It all started out on the prairie," she said. "For a couple hundred miles I drove, and then I felt this enormous emotional and physical pain. I was driving past the stockyards. There were all these cattle up to their bellies in the excrement. It hit me how we all live in all this crap and then gloss it over with scented toilet paper. I felt such sadness for the state of the world, for all the environmental problems. I thought of all the fear we always have. I found myself trudging across the prairie as a pioneer woman. I 'saw' thousands and thousands of women, of all races, all ages, trudging across the prairie, holding up the world through their labors. I felt the fear and the pain of all those women, the endless work. [As these images were washing over her, her stomach pain was getting worse and worse so that she had to stop the car and pull her legs up to her chest. She tasted blood in her mouth, and when she spat into a tissue, nothing was there.]

"Then the flash came. I was a Viking, a male Viking. I had a huge sword. I killed a woman about to have a child. I killed them both with this sword. It was so awful to think of that. I just kept driving with tears and agony. To think that I was capable of doing such a thing! I felt such compassion for men because they were trained to do this. This pain in my stomach, the tears, the agony—this went on for about four hours. When I went over the mountain pass in the Rockies, the sun came out and I thought the pain would go away. But the horror still came. It was like some horrible dream that was real, but it wasn't.

"I needed to do this alone in an environment that wasn't 'home.' All night Friday on the day I left, the pain was on the left and seemed to be leaving. But on Saturday as I continued my trip, I'd get these waves of dread in the left side of my abdomen. That's exactly where I [the Viking] put the sword.

"When I got to Taos, I had a session with Mary, a gifted intuitive. She did a reading and felt it was not necessary for me to go any farther. This vision of the pioneer women and me as a Viking killing a pregnant woman has helped me to release my fear of death.

"I know I need to put a closure on this, I need to acknowledge it and close it. Perhaps it was necessary for the female to be killed. It was the worst thing I have ever done, the thing that I have tried to hide from God and from myself. The other thing I realized is that all of mankind has done this. We have all killed and murdered. I feel as though I have just died from another lifetime. Now I'm giving birth to myself. I can never go back to what I was before, because too much has happened to me. I can't be what I was before.

"I haven't felt my full physical energy for some time. I've always been at a physical high pitch. This experience helped me in a realization of my own death. The environment, the earth, and what we've done to it is very deep in me. I think that now I have also successfully dropped my ties to my children in the sense of holding on too tightly out of fear. I can move on now."

Martha realized that a full intellectual understanding of what had just happened to her was not necessary for her healing. She did not have to interpret the vision or experience of "being a Viking" as a past-life experience or anything else in order to heal. What was necessary was that she *feel* all of what was coming up from deep within her. After she acknowledged the act of murder, she felt freed of its burden and thus renewed. She also realized that she had to change the way she had been living. She needed to stop spending time with friends who contributed nothing to her life, in friendships that were based on habit, not mutual enrichment.

When Martha returned to her home a week later, she still felt some residual fear and dread from the experience and wanted to be free of it. She wrote down the whole thing, then went out into the backyard under a night sky full of stars, dug a hole, and burned her writing. She buried the ashes and stood up, and finally, after weeks of dread, she felt completely released.

About three weeks later, she was visiting her aunt and uncle in Ohio. Her uncle Roy took her aside and said that he didn't feel that he had much longer to live and that he had something he wanted to give her. He took her into a back room, reached up on a shelf, and handed down a bronze statue. It was a Viking with a sword.

We share our amazement at this bit of synchronicity. ("Synchronicity is God's way of remaining anonymous," says Dr. Bernie Siegel.) Martha said, "I can have this statue in my house now. It is a symbol for me of healing. I know that if I had not allowed myself to experience this memory or dream or whatever it was, I would have developed a fatal stomach condition. I am certain of this."

This story illustrates profoundly that the notion that we are to blame for our illnesses in any conventional sense is irrelevant and narrow. In some mysterious way, our conscious intellect is *not* in control. Another part of us—our highest power, soul, or inner wisdom—is. The concept of the self needs to be expanded. Studies have documented the power of prayer to heal at a distance, instantaneously. Time and space are not absolute. We are acted upon by forces outside of our conscious control. We can be open to learning from all of life, from our inner selves, and from all that with which we are connected.

We have the body we have because it is precisely the vehicle in which we can best do what we came to do. Stevie Wonder has said that his blindness helped him feel the love that is all around him more than he would if he were sighted. Perhaps he couldn't do the creative work he's doing if he were in a "normal" body. The late Elisabeth Kübler-Ross pointed out that when our bodies are sick or nonfunctioning, our spiritual and mental capacities often expand way beyond what they would normally. She used the example of children with leukemia who seem wise beyond their years.[21] I accept the truth of this on faith. We can't really hope to figure it out with our logical, intellectual selves. There are indeed more things in heaven and earth than are dreamt of in our philosophies.

Be open to the messages and mysteries of your body and its symptoms. Be eager to listen and slow to judge. What you learn can save your life.

3
Inner Guidance

R ight after Mary Lu was diagnosed with breast cancer, she called me to discuss her treatment options. I told her that part of her healing would be to learn how to trust herself to make her own decisions about her treatment after gathering information from a number of experts. She later wrote me, "I remember that I felt scared when I heard you affirm that in recovery, I would know what to do to deal with the cancer. I remember thinking that these were life-and-death choices and not on par with deciding how to spend some weekend. Then what flashed for me was that my soul has always been at stake all these years. Anne [Schaef] reminded me that I had come to my first group session with her back in 1981 concerned about my health. It was right after a diagnosis of ulcerative colitis and I was afraid I was killing myself. I do believe in the mind-body-soul connection. With decisions to make concerning my cancer treatment, *I had this sense that I would have a real chance to trust my inner guidance.* Trusting myself at such a deep level was frightening to me, but I gratefully say now several months later that this 'stuff' really does work, that I have trusted my process a lot through this. And each time that I have guided myself to my own healing, it gives me renewed courage to continue to trust."

Our inner guidance can direct us toward that which is most life-enhancing and life-fulfilling for us. Mary Lu learned that she could find the surgeon she needed to work with and the treatment that worked best for her, even in the face of breast cancer. Not only that, she learned that she could even enjoy her life at the same time. She did this by *allowing herself to be led by how she was feeling in each moment of the day*. Each step of the way, she moved toward the decision that *felt best* to her. When you move toward that which is most fulfilling and life-enhancing, healing follows regardless of what your health is like in the moment.

Our inner guidance system is mediated via our thoughts, emotions, dreams, and bodily feelings. Our bodies are designed to act as receiving and transmitting stations for energy and information. Living in touch with our inner guidance involves feeling our way through life using *all* of ourselves: mind, body, emotions, and spirit. When I refer to this process in this book, I mean the various ways we listen and use our inner guidance to make conscious changes in our lives, behavior, relationships with others, and health.

TABLE 3

SOURCES OF GUIDANCE

External Guidance: Dominant Cultural View	Inner Guidance
Physical world is inferior to spirit.	Spirit informs everything.
Nature is inferior to God and must be controlled.	Nature is a reflection of Divine spirit.
Human beings are superior to the natural world.	Human beings are co-creators with spirit and nature.
Behavior is based on fear and judgment.	Behavior is based on respect for self. Respect for self results in respect for others.
Difference is suspect and must be controlled.	Difference is celebrated as a reflection of the creativity of spirit.
There's only one right way to live and to be.	There are many paths to fulfillment and joy. None are superior.
Delayed gratification; enjoyment and fulfillment must be earned.	Live in the moment and enjoy the process of creating.
The inherent worth of an individual is arranged in a hierarchy of superior to inferior.	Life is an interdependent cooperative adventure with all beings connected holographically.

External Guidance: Dominant Cultural View	Inner Guidance
⁓ Guidance for behavior dictated by laws and institutions from external sources.	⁓ Guidance for behavior comes from connection with inner guidance.
⁓ There is such a thing as purely objective reality separate from consciousness.	⁓ The whole universe is a projection of consciousness.
⁓ Action and pushing against what we *don't* want is the only way to accomplish anything.	⁓ Consciousness creates all that is. Thoughts and feelings create reality. We can use them deliberately to improve our lives.
⁓ Support and nourishment must be earned from people and institutions outside oneself.	⁓ The individual is self-nourishing through her connection with her inner being and guidance system.
⁓ Approval from others is the basis for happiness.	⁓ Self-approval and self-acceptance are the keys to happiness.
⁓ Humans are inherently flawed. Worth must be earned.	⁓ We are inherently worthy and precious by virtue of our existence. We have nothing to prove.
⁓ Spiritual guidance comes only from priests, ministers, or churches.	⁓ Our internal guidance and spirit are inherently loving and beneficent. They speak to us directly.
⁓ God and spirit are the ultimate judges of worth.	⁓ The universe is continually unfolding.
⁓ It is possible to control everything and everyone.	⁓ Humans are not capable of understanding everything from a strictly physical viewpoint. Mystery is part of the wonder of life.

LISTENING TO YOUR BODY AND ITS NEEDS

We can generally trust our "gut feeling" about someone or something to be accurate information. This is because the solar plexus, the place in the body where we generally feel the gut reaction, is in fact a primitive brain. It is also a major intuitive center, the part of our body that lets us know whether we are safe and whether we are being lied to. Columbia researcher Michael Gershon, M.D., is a pioneer in the field of neurogastroenterology. In his book *The Second Brain*, he details the discovery and gradual scientific acceptance of the enteric nervous system, which actually operates independently from the brain in the head. Dr. Gershon also points out that 95 percent of the body's serotonin is made in the gut!

Each of us must develop ways to tune in to our body's needs. We can start with simple things. When you're tired, rest. When you have to go to the bathroom, go. If you feel like crying when you read a certain passage in this book, let yourself cry. If you simply can't read certain parts of the text, notice them—they may refer to subjects that are painful to you. Just make a note of your reactions. Notice your breathing as you read: does it speed up or slow down depending upon the material you're covering? What is your heart doing? Is it racing or is it slow? Does reading about the uterus or the menstrual cycle unearth any old memories of body feelings?

I often ask women to pay attention to what their bodies feel like in the moment. In order to heal our bodies, we have to reenter them and experience them. (Right after I wrote that, I noticed that my legs were numb. I'd been sitting too long and had ignored my need for movement. After a ten-minute barefoot walk on the lawn and some deep breathing, my body felt much more alert and happy.)

We have to give our bodies credit for their innate wisdom. We also don't need to know exactly why something is happening in our bodies in order to respond to it. You don't need to know *why* your heart is racing or *why* you feel like crying. Understanding comes *after* you have allowed yourself to experience what you're feeling. Healing is an organic process that happens *in the body* as well as in the intellect. So if you are feeling "out of sorts" or "off balance," just be with that feeling; allow it to come up. After you have allowed yourself to experience it, take a moment and go back over the events of the last few hours or days. If you are feeling ill or having symptoms, reflecting on recent events may give you a clue about what preceded the symptoms.

Here's an example from my own experience. While writing this book, I woke up with the visual signs and numbness of hand and face that are the symptoms of an impending migraine headache. I had developed classic migraines at the age of twelve, had one or sometimes two headaches approximately every month until my sophomore year in college, and then didn't get another one for twenty years. While growing up, I was a definite migraine personality, pushing myself mercilessly in school and in all my activities. Stress "shorted out" my body's electromagnetic system on a regular basis.

So when I began to get that old, familiar, sickening feeling, I immediately used it as an opportunity to learn. I put an ice pack under my neck, lay down, kept the room quiet, and concentrated on making my hands warm. (I had learned from a biofeedback therapist that migraines can often be aborted by relaxing totally and warming the hands.) By doing this I managed to avoid getting a full-blown headache that would have left me in pain, nauseated for most of the day, and very weak. After about one hour, I was able to resume my activities but felt very subdued. I thought back on the previous three days.

I had been tearing around the house, trying to pick up and organize years of clutter in two days. Toward the end of the weekend, my temper had been short, I had scarcely taken time to eat or go to the bathroom, and I hadn't taken a break from the bending and cleaning for hours. I had gone to bed with a dull headache. The next morning, I woke up with the migraine symptoms. It was clear to me that my ability to put my bodily needs for rest, recreation, and nurturing aside for long periods of time was intact. Only now my body wouldn't let me get away with it nearly as much as it used to. Hence the migraine. I took it as a warning.

The healing principle that summarizes this learning is this: *if you don't heed the message the first time, you get hit with a bigger hammer the next time.*

The purpose of emotions, regardless of what they are, is to help us feel and participate fully in our own lives. To become aware of our inner guidance system, we must learn to trust our emotions. This isn't always so easy, because many of us have been taught to live our lives as though we were in a constant emergency situation. We think, "Oh, I'll deal with that painful emotion later. Right now I don't have time. I have to get that report out," or cook dinner, or whatever it is. This delay or denial requires our bodies to speak louder and louder to get our attention. The next time you feel moved to tears or moved to laughter, stop and experience it. It doesn't take that long. And it improves the quality of life enormously!

Many women have been taught to "think"—not feel—that we should be upbeat and happy all the time. Sadness or pain are natural parts of life. They are also great teachers. No one gets through life without experiencing sadness or pain. Yet our culture teaches us that there is something wrong with pain, that it must be drugged, denied, or otherwise avoided at all costs—and the costs are very high.

We are not taught that we have an innate ability to deal with pain, that our bodies know how to do this. Crying is one of the ways in which we rid our bodies of toxins. Crying allows us to move energy around our body and sometimes to rechannel it or understand it in a different way. When we don't allow ourselves to feel our emotions and instead use addictive processes such as running or tranquilizers to "get a high," we actually create hormones (enkephalins) that repress tears (and our full emotional expressions).[1] Tears contain toxins that the body needs to get rid of.[2] Tears of joy and tears of sorrow have different chemical compositions and are influenced by hormones. They also serve different purposes. When we allow ourselves a full emotional release, our body, mind, and spirit feel cleansed and free. Insight about what to do in a given situation often comes *only after* we feel our emotions about it and shed tears if necessary. Interestingly, tears of joy and tears of sorrow are physiologically and chemically distinct from each other, even though sadness and joy are very much related. We cannot feel the height of our joy unless we have allowed ourselves to feel the depths of our sadness. Though joy and sadness express different emotions, both are natural parts of how our body processes and "digests" feelings. Making sounds (like moaning, crying, or singing), moving, and deep full breathing are also part of the body's way to move through painful emotions more quickly and efficiently.

Many illnesses are quite simply the end result of emotions that have been stuffed, unacknowledged, and unexperienced for years. One of my former patients with a long history of migraine headaches told me, "I finally hit bottom with my headaches when my neurologist wanted to put me on lithium. I knew I didn't want to deal with the effects of that drug on my body. I started biofeedback so that I could learn to relax. I had a childhood that was so painful, I had nowhere else to go but into the pain. Now I realize that I don't have to have the pain anymore. I notice that I start to get a headache the minute I stop taking care of myself. If I don't rest or get enough sleep, or if I don't stand up for myself with my family, the headaches start. I see that all along the headaches have been trying to show me something."

EMOTIONAL CLEANSING: HEALING FROM THE PAST

Healing can occur in the present only when we allow ourselves to feel, express, and release emotions from the past that we have suppressed or tried to forget. I call this *emotional incision and drainage*. I've often likened this deep process to treatment of an abscess. Any surgeon knows that the treatment for an abscess is to cut it open, allowing the pus to drain. When this is done, the pain goes away almost immediately, and new healthy tissue can re-form where the abscess once was. It is the same with emotions: they, too, become walled off, causing pain and absorbing energy, if we do not experience and release them.

Children release emotion naturally and immediately, and each of us is born with the innate ability to do this. Yet because our culture worships emotional control and extols the virtues of suffering in silence, we learn early on how to suppress our natural emotional releases, and also to distance the messages behind them. When a woman is having panic attacks or crying spells, I know that some emotional material is coming to the surface to be processed. To observers who haven't experienced deep process (or emotional release), she may appear to be "losing it," "going off the deep end," or "getting out of control." She is not "out of control," however; she is simply allowing a healing process to arise within the body. Only the intellect has lost control—it has taken a backseat to the innate wisdom of the body.

Too often, health care providers prescribe drugs in cases like this. As a result, a woman's natural healing process can get stagnated for months or years. And even if drugs are not prescribed, most people in our culture are uncomfortable with the emotions that arise when they are watching another person feel their emotions. They therefore rush to comfort the person who is beginning to cry or "lose it." This stops the person's emotional process and at the same time protects the comforter from feeling his or her own feelings. The healing process stops for both of them.

On the other hand, if a woman is encouraged to stay with what she's feeling, to go into it, to make the sounds she needs to make, and to cry or yell as long as necessary, staying completely with her innermost self, she'll often discover that her body has the innate ability to heal even very painful memories and events from her past. When we are willing to be with "what is" instead of running away from it, we will often be able to work through painful experiences that have lain dormant and taken up our energy for years. Stephen Levine, a meditation teacher and author of *Healing Into Life and Death* (Anchor Press, 1987), calls this experience "the pain that ends the pain."

When we have allowed ourselves a full emotional release, the body, mind, and spirit feel cleansed and free. Insights come up and long-buried self-understanding returns. I've watched people forgive themselves and others after deep process work because they are finally at peace with painful events in their past. This can happen even after years of intellectualizing that never really healed them. They naturally "lighten up" and are eventually able to laugh at themselves and their past.

One striking example of this was the deep process of an infertility surgeon I'll call Carol. Carol had found it very painful when she was not able to help a woman become pregnant, in spite of using all of the current technology at her disposal. Though infertility is not an exact science, she took her couples' failures to conceive very personally. This made her emotional attitude toward her professional life fraught with sadness.

During a workshop I was leading, the discussion turned to the subject of mothers, and many of the participants began to cry. Carol got down on a mat and allowed herself to cry and wail. During this process she kept repeating, "I don't need to create any more mommies. I don't need to create more mommies." When she was finished, she realized that she herself had never really had a mother in an emotional sense. She had been beaten repeatedly by her mother when she was a child. She had made her career choice as an infertility physician in part because of her unresolved early-childhood pain: on an unconscious level, she was trying to "create mommies" in an attempt to create the mother she emotionally needed but never had. Following this deep insight, she was able to go back to her work refreshed and free, finally released from assuming complete responsibility for her patients' conceptions.

DREAMS: A DOORWAY TO THE UNCONSCIOUS

Dreams are another part of our inner guidance system. Scientific evidence shows that the amount of activity in our brain when we dream is identical to the amount when we are awake. During dreaming, our inner guidance works with our brain to lay down a map of the activities or goals that we desire or need for a healthy balanced future. Dreams also show us the beneficial and nonbeneficial directions toward which we are focusing our energy and how and where we need to make adjustments.

One of my former patients who was healing from chronic pelvic pain related to me that, as she healed, she became more and more competent and powerful in her dreams. She said it was fun to go to sleep at night to see what she'd be capable of next.

Another patient, recovering from incest, said, "I recently dreamed that a little four-year-old girl was trying to tell me about someone who hurt her. I know that I am that girl—and that I need to listen to her in my dreams."

Another woman, suffering from chronic vaginitis, asked her dreams for guidance about what to do, since none of our physical treatments was helping. She came back a week later and said, "I had the dream. Everything was black, and I heard a voice say, 'When you get rid of Larry, the problem will go away.'" She eventually was able to tend to her relationship problems, and her condition began to clear.

Learn to pay attention to your dreams by writing them down first thing in the morning. Plan to remember them before you go to bed at night. Keep a notebook and pen beside your bed.

INTUITION AND INTUITIVE GUIDANCE

Intuition is the direct perception of truth or fact *independent of any reasoning process*. It is the ability to make the right decision with insufficient information. A very good example of intuition is when you walk into a dark room and somehow know that someone is in there, even when you can't see them and haven't been told they are there. We are all born with this ability, and all of us were highly intuitive as children. Most of us, however, were trained out of this way of knowing by the age of seven when the frontal lobe reasoning centers come on board and tend to drown out the intuitive voice. The more education we get in this culture, in general, the less we trust our natural intuition. Because our society glorifies mostly logical, rational, left-brain thinking, we are taught to discount other forms of knowing as primitive or ignorant.

Thus, our intuitive capacity has become suspect and underutilized. Yet it is a skill that can be relearned at any time because it is a completely natural way of knowing. Although addictions keep us out of touch with *what we know and what we feel* and most of us are out of touch with our intuition much of the time, as we become more inner-directed and more in touch with our inner guidance system, we automatically gain access to our intuition. Our society admits that even the geniuses among us use only about 25 percent of their brain capacity. To use intuition is simply to use more of our intelligence than we are accustomed to using.

Intuitive guidance is the ability to read our own (or another's) energy field. Intuitive guidance is centuries old and has been part of many ancient healing systems. Every traditional shaman has worked in this way, as have healers in the Wicca tradition.[3] Intuitive guidance can help us detect energy blockages *before* they become physical. We can act on this information and keep ourselves healthy.

HOW INNER GUIDANCE WORKS

One of my medical student friends who has a bad back has noticed that her back pain always emerges when she has to do something that she doesn't want to do. (This is true in spite of the fact that she has a so-called physical problem that should, by itself, explain her symptoms.) Currently, she is contemplating writing a research paper. Whenever she even thinks about writing this piece and about the colleagues with whom she will be involved, she gets neck pain and feels sick to her stomach. All her training has taught her that publishing this research paper is what she *should* do for her career. Yet her inner guidance, which speaks to her through her body's feelings, is telling her something quite different. She knows that she must take the radical step of choosing between her inner guidance and what society is telling her is best if she is to remain healthy. Update: this friend eventually created a very satisfying career quite different from what she always thought she'd be doing—working in a hospital for a lab! Her body led her to it.

Our bodies are designed to function best when we're doing work that feels exactly right to us. If we want to know God's will for us, all we have to do is look to our gifts and talents—that's where we will find it. Health is enhanced in women who engage in work that satisfies them. If a woman wants to know what her gifts and talents are, she can think back to when she was age nine to eleven, before the culture really put her into a trance. What did she love to do? What did she want to be? Who did she think she was?

Another way to get in touch with our gifts and talents is to ask ourselves what we would do or be if we knew we had only six months to live. Would we stay at our current job? With our current partner?

We are meant to move toward whatever gives us fulfillment, personal growth, and freedom. We are born knowing what activities, things, thoughts, and feelings are associated with these qualities. We must learn to trust ourselves and know that we can naturally move toward that which is healing and fulfilling.

Many people have been taught that they can't have what they want and that a life full of struggle is somehow more honorable than one full of joy. We have also been taught to distrust something if it is considered "too" fulfilling or if it is associated with too much pleasure or with having "too" much fun. How many times have you been laughing in a restaurant or at home and had someone say, "You're having too much fun over there!" This belief is reflected in our bodies. An eminent hypnosis researcher once noted that negative effects, like blisters, were twice as easy to induce as positive outcomes.[4] Yet when we can clearly state what we want and why, we are instantly in alignment with our inner guidance. This is because it feels good in our bodies to think about and dwell upon what we want and why. We get excited and are inspired automatically by these thoughts and feelings, which in turn keep us in touch with our inner knowing and spiritual energy. The result is enthusiasm and joy—the feeling of heaven on Earth.

Our culture has too often taught us that it is selfish to have our own wants and dreams and to enjoy ourselves. Many girls, when they are in touch with their inner power, have been told, "Who do you think you are, the Queen of Sheba?" Too many of us have heard "Don't break your arm patting yourself on the back" when we have done a job we're proud of or have given ourselves credit for something that we loved to do, just for us. All of our lives, this kind of statement has stopped us dead in our tracks. We are accused of being selfish when we've given our own lives and interests priority. We have been brought up to avoid being seen as selfish at all costs. We learn to earn love and acceptance through self-sacrifice because we don't feel worthy of the best that life has to offer.

In general, women in our culture have a difficult time going after what they personally want and need in an atmosphere in which it is assumed that they will perform and be responsible for all of the tasks of daily living such as child-rearing and housekeeping. On the other hand, if these activities are precisely what a woman wants to do the most, she may find that these activities are undervalued and underpaid. However, nothing will change in a woman's outer circumstances until she learns to value her own life and her own gifts as much as she has been taught to value and nurture the lives of others. As a friend of mine says, "If you want to be one of the chosen, all you have to do is choose yourself!"

Nearly every woman I know has been socialized to believe that putting everyone else before herself is the right thing to do. Just the opposite is true—we can't really be there for others unless we're there for ourselves first. Dana Johnson, a researcher friend of mine and a registered nurse, even recovered from Lou Gehrig's disease (amyotrophic lateral sclerosis, or ALS) by learning to respect all aspects of her body. After she had had the disease for some years, she began to lose control over her breathing muscles as well as the rest of her body. Her breathing difficulties made her think she was going to die. But she decided at that point that she wanted to experience unconditional love for herself at least once before dying. Describing herself as a "bowl of Jell-O in a wheelchair," she sat every day for fifteen minutes in front of a mirror and chose different parts of herself to love. She started with her hands because at that time they were the only parts of herself that she could appreciate unconditionally. Each day she went on to other body parts. Day by day, her physical body began to get better as she learned to appreciate it. She also wrote in a journal about insights she had during this process, and she came to see that since childhood she had believed that in order to be of service, acceptable to others, and worthy herself, she had to sacrifice her own needs. It took a life-threatening disease for her to learn that service through self-sacrifice is a dead end. In fact, the effect of psychological factors has been strongly correlated with the length of survival from ALS. Given that ALS has no known cause and no known cure, the importance of these factors can't be underestimated![5] Although feeling good about being of service simply for its own sake is health-enhancing, far too many women bake cookies, make coffee, and clean up because it's expected of them and they would feel guilty (and unworthy) if they didn't do it. Service to others done under obligation creates exhaustion and resentment.

Knowing What We Don't Want

In addition to knowing what we *do* want, we have the capacity to know what we *don't* want. Knowing what we don't want is inborn. Every baby knows what feels good and what doesn't feel good, and up until about the age of six, a child will automatically go toward what feels good and away from what feels bad. This capacity is seen in its purest form in a two-year-old child who has just learned how to say no.

The ability to say no to what doesn't support us is an essential part of our inner guidance system. It is never too late to start saying no to those things that drain you and yes to those that replenish you.

~ When a friend calls and asks for help, stop for a moment and ask yourself, "Do I really want to help right now, or would I prefer to do something else?" Say to your friend, "Let me get back to you on that." If the answer is no, and your friend gets resentful, it's time to question the validity of that friendship.

~ Check your body when someone asks you to do something. Are there areas of tension? Do you get a "gut reaction" of any kind? Does your body say, "Yes, this would be fun," or does it say, "No, doing this would be draining"?

~ If you find yourself tired or irritable at the end of a day, ask yourself what thoughts, activities, or people drained your energy during the day.

~ On the days when you are feeling wonderful, ask yourself what thoughts, activities, or people enhance your energy flow.

~ Keep a journal, and begin to notice and write down everything that contributes to a positive energy flow that replenishes you. Paying attention to these things will draw more of them into your experience.

~ Practice appreciation and gratitude, writing down all the blessings in your life. Remember that what we pay attention to expands!

~ Tap into the power of attention. Consciously directing our attention to thoughts, emotions, and circumstances that feel good and uplifting is powerful medicine. Paying attention to and appreciating what is working well in your life changes your vibration rate—the frequency at which you resonate. And you will attract more good things.

One of my former patients, a social worker, originally came to see me complaining of PMS and mild anxiety attacks. In going over her history, I noticed that she never had any time to herself and that her life was overrun with taking care of others' needs while neglecting her own. I told her that she must practice noticing what activities replenished her energy and which ones drained her. Then I told her that in order to reverse her symptoms, she had to spend at least one hour each day recharging her own energetic batteries by resting or doing something she liked. She did so, and a month later all her symptoms were gone. She told me that she was learning how she drained her energy in her daily life. She said, "When I lie down or sit down to write in my journal, I can literally *feel* the energy coming back into my body. Knowing how crucial this is to my physical and emotional well-being is a revelation."

All of us receive messages from our bodies regularly about what serves our health and well-being and what doesn't. Our bodies know immediately when we are doing something or even thinking about something that doesn't support us fully. One of my friends gets diarrhea and stomach cramps when she just thinks about going to visit her parents. She was abused both physically and emotionally throughout her entire childhood, and this abuse has continued into adulthood. Her body knows that visiting her parents will not be good for her, and it gives her symptoms as messages to stay away. When she gives herself permission to stay away, her stomach problems go away immediately.

(She has also had to learn how to soothe the anxiety that arises from the ingrained belief that not visiting or doing what her mother expects makes her a "bad" daughter.) In time, she may well be able to visit without it having to "cost" her anything. But that's Ph.D.-level healing work!

In order to create health daily, long before illness ensues we need to pay attention to the subtle signals from our bodies about what feels good and what doesn't. Foggy thinking, dizziness, heart palpitations, acne, headaches, and back, stomach, and pelvic pain are a few of the common but subtle symptoms that often signal that it is time for us to let go of what we don't want in life and start using our own power to improve things. Here's an example from my own life.

Back in the 1980s, when I had two young children, I was working too many hours, and I often felt that aspects of my work weren't respected by my colleagues. My face often broke out in large blemishes, which I had never had as an adolescent or at any other time in my life until then. I tried taking vitamins, changing my diet, and using a variety of skin creams. Nothing helped—until I left my place of work. Within six months the problem cleared and has never returned.

Clearly, my face was a barometer of my well-being during those years. Through my skin condition, my body had been telling me that my work setting was not supporting me optimally. My complexion had been registering my "thin-skinned" sensitivity and my anger at not being completely accepted by my colleagues. (I hadn't completely accepted myself, either, at this point, and my work environment was a reflection of that.) All of these emotions lay just below the surface, though I couldn't appreciate this at the time. Once I faced my innermost needs and left the situation that simply was not supporting me, my complexion improved automatically. As my life cleared up, so did my face.

Negative emotions exist to let us know that we are not facing the clearest path to what we want. When we realize that our bodies and their symptoms—feelings—are our allies, pointing out what serves our highest good and what doesn't, we become free. Whenever you feel angry or upset, have a headache or a bodily symptom, take a moment to reflect upon what the symptom is trying to say to you. When I am caught up in a downward spiral of negative feelings, I instantly know that I am out of touch with my inner guidance and that I'm giving too much attention to what I don't want. I have learned to notice when I'm feeling bad and stop for a moment. If I can catch myself at the beginning of the bad mood, I can often get my energy flowing positively again by doing the following process:

1. I acknowledge what I am feeling *without making any judgment about it.* I avoid wallowing around in the negative emotions and prolonging them, but I definitely *feel* them fully. I "stay with the feeling."

2. I acknowledge that there is a reason why I am feeling the way I am.

3. I spend twenty seconds or so identifying what is causing my energy to flow negatively. For example, yesterday I was angry because a staff member didn't get an important message to me in time for me to return a phone call promptly.

4. Having identified the source of my negative emotion, I then ask myself what I *do* want. (I have a friend do this with me if I need help clarifying my wants in a positive, nonreactive way.) What I want is usually the opposite of what I am experiencing the moment I'm feeling bad. Asking myself what I want shifts my focus back to positive thoughts and thus moves my energy toward my wants.

5. I then name what I want. Stating our wants is powerful because it defines them clearly, allowing our creative energy to flow toward them. Thus, in the example in step 3, I would say, "I want to receive my telephone messages on time so that I can respond to them promptly and efficiently." This statement reflects positive energy flowing toward what I want. Because it is a statement of pure positive energy with no negativity in it, it helps draw what I want into my experience. When I am thinking about or talking about what I want, the negative emotion often goes away by itself.

6. Finally, I affirm that I have the power within me, via my inner guidance and my power of intent, to get what I want.

7. Remember the law of attraction. The people and circumstances we attract to us are always a reflection of our own thoughts and beliefs. In my early days of practice and work, I quite often felt unsupported both at work and at home. I operated under the belief "If you want it done right, you have to do it yourself." Over the years, I slowly changed my beliefs about support and realized that I deserve it. I can ask for it, and I will get it. As a result of this inner change, I now enjoy an amazing staff and support system both at home and at work. I call it "assisted living."

Going through this process is *not* a way to deny my emotions or stuff them. Rather, it helps me acknowledge them, feel them fully, and use them as guidance toward what I *do* want. I regularly sit down with a notebook and make a list of exactly what I want in a given situation.

(I also write down goals regularly that act as beacons for manifesting heaven on Earth!) This aligns my thoughts with my inner guidance, and it feels good. Inspiration about what to do generally follows. Please note that I don't try to figure out what to *do* about a certain situation until I've gone through the entire process of looking in the direction of what I want. The reason for this is that directed thought creates vibration, which then results in inspiration. I remind myself that whenever I am creating *against* something I don't want, I just create *more* of what isn't working, and my actions are based on fixing what I don't want instead of creating what I do want. In the past, for example, my former husband would often spend many hours at the hospital and wouldn't come home for dinner on time. I used to look out the window and wait for him, trying to keep the dinner warm, feeling angry at him and sorry for myself. The more I demanded that he show up on time, the more of a problem it became in our relationship. One day, I simply decided to go ahead and eat dinner myself and then get on with the evening's activities and enjoy myself. I did this whenever he wasn't home when he said he would be. Eventually, he began coming home on time spontaneously. I realized that my attention to his continued absence was actually holding the painful pattern in place. When you acknowledge that you are attracting your experiences vibrationally, you have put yourself in the driver's seat of your life. You also have to be willing to let go of any expectations and stop making the behavior of others your reason for unhappiness.

Unfortunately, instead of using our feelings as inner guidance, we're brought up to fear or deny our negative emotions and feelings or judge them as "bad." Most of us were taught that being able to control ourselves and our emotions is commendable and a mark of achievement. When John F. Kennedy was assassinated, my mother thought that Jackie Kennedy was an inspiration and a role model to the nation because she walked behind the casket with such dignity, never shedding a tear or showing any emotion. Though remaining emotionally calm and collected under pressure can be admirable, all too often this control becomes such an ingrained habit that women are out of touch with their emotions even when it would be healing and safe to acknowledge and express them. Men are even more at risk for being out of touch with their feelings than women, since they learn early on that "big boys don't cry." A friend of mine was taught that if she had to cry, she should bury her face in a pillow so that the rest of the family wouldn't have to hear it. Yet crying and making sounds are all a part of our emotional "digestive" system and a way to keep energy flowing evenly throughout our bodies.

Our culture has a kind of "nonliving" orientation. This orientation encourages us to "keep a lid on it," as in "Don't make waves." By learning very early on that emotions are bad or shameful, we learn not to trust our inner guidance or our bodies. When we are encouraged to be out of touch with what we know and what we feel in general, we are systematically trained out of moving toward fulfillment of our innermost desires and saying no to what we don't want. Even our religions teach us to squelch our innate joy and creativity and that feeling good is a sin. As Matthew Fox points out, "Our civilization has not done a good job with the energy called delight and joy."[6] We need to know that the very essence of a life based on inner guidance is abundant delight and joy!

Every smiling, laughing three-month-old baby I've ever met reflects the true, joyous nature with which we were all born. The famous anthropologist and social biologist Dr. Ashley Montagu once said that most adults are nothing more than "disintegrated children." Fortunately, our inner guidance is always available to remind us of our direction toward fulfillment. When we realign with our inner guidance and stop judging our bodies and our feelings as bad when they are offering us information, we are on the pathway to a life filled with growth and delight.

4
The Female Energy System

Understanding that thoughts and emotions affect how energy works in our female bodies can help us decipher our individual body's unique language. The location of disease within the body—where it occurs—has psychological and emotional meaning and significance. Specific mental and emotional patterns are associated with specific body locations. Our thoughts, emotions, and behaviors are reflected or patterned simultaneously in the brain, the spinal cord, the various organs, the blood, and the lymphoid (immune) tissue, and in the electromagnetic field that surrounds and penetrates all those areas. Understanding the different dynamic patterns of energy that our bodies give rise to and operate within can help you appreciate how positive or negative energies can manifest themselves in your individual body.

THE MATTER/ENERGY CONTINUUM

Our body's vibrational system is always changing, and the *potential* for healing or disease is present at all times. Precancerous cells, for example, arise regularly in our bodies. They form invasive cancers only when our own internal controls break down.[1] Mental and emotional energy goes in and out of physical form regularly, bouncing on the continuum between energy and matter, particle and wave.

Vibrational healer Deena Spear says, "Cancer moves in and out of physical reality constantly. But once you get a diagnosis, it really takes root and becomes established." Quite simply, emotional and mental energy can become physical in our bodies.

When we have unresolved chronic emotional stress in a particular area of our lives, this stress registers in our vibrations as a disturbance that can manifest in physical illness. Here is how it happens: When we obsess about someone or something, or keep participating in self-destructive thoughts or behaviors, our life-energy leaks away from our body. When we obsess, we tie up energy—*chi, ki, prana,* or *qi*—in a negative process that diverts it from our cells. Vital cellular processes thereby become depleted. We leak energy in any situation in which our anger, fear, depression, or sadness is controlling our ability to move forward in our lives. While most doctors do not view the onset of disease in terms of these energy leaks, it is interesting to note that more and more medical research supports this observation. In one study, for instance, cancerous cells were shown to "steal" energy (in the form of the ATP-like molecule DPN) from adjacent normal tissue.[2]

Appreciating our bodies in terms of energy fields and energy leaks can help us understand and begin the healing process. When we persist in being angry with someone who has hurt us, for example, a part of our spirit is occupied with that person and is not available to us for healing. When a person has been severely abused, shamans believe that part of the person's spirit may flee in order to escape the abuse. One of the healing traditions of shamanism is called "soul retrieval," in which the missing spirit is called back. Many women who have been sexually abused as children relate that they "left" their bodies during the abuse. Some remember that a part of themselves actually left and went up to the ceiling and "watched." This split-off part of their spirit may not be available to them in the present for healing.

Many times we are not conscious of these energy leaks. But if these leaks continue without being healed, bodily distress is often the result. Bodily symptoms can serve to bring our attention to that area so that healing can begin. One of my former menopausal patients who came to see me with insomnia and depression told me of her sexual abuse as a child—something she had not been consciously aware of until a week before her visit with me. She had gone through a painful divorce in her forties and had had a recent breakup with her lover of seven years. She said, "I realize now that I've spent my entire life trying *not* to remember that I was sexually abused. Now that I know it happened, I realize why I've never had a satisfactory relationship. I've always pushed people away. I didn't know how to be fully present in a relationship. But I didn't know any better. I'm grieving from my early life and the fact that it has taken me this long to remember and release the past. But finally the chronic knot in my stomach is gone. I feel free. I am so relieved." Her sleep problem and depression cleared up spontaneously as her memories of abuse arose and were released from her energy field.

How to Heal Energy Leaks

To stay or become healthy, it is useful for each of us to notice where we are "leaking" our energy. A good time to do this is when you go to bed each night. To begin the process of healing your energy leaks, simply notice who or what you are thinking about, worrying about, or obsessing about. What thoughts, emotions, events, or people keep coming into your mind? Are there any emotions or thoughts over which you are obsessing? See who you're holding resentments against. When you find these areas, you must call your spirit back. One way to do this is by using your will and your power of intent to call back the parts of you that are caught in past or present situations that don't serve your highest good. It is helpful to do this out loud. Simply state, "Spirit, come back here—I need you with me." As you're calling your spirit back, it also helps to affirm your spiritual connection verbally. Repeat the following affirmation (or something similar), really feeling the truth of it: "I am always being Divinely guided toward my Highest Good on all levels. Divine love now dissolves everything that is not on my Divinely designed path." The split-off parts of yourself are not used to this calling, but eventually they will respond to your efforts and your energy will return.

Most of the blockages in our vibrational systems are emotional in nature. It's helpful to think of your vibrational system as being like a stream of water flowing along. As long as this energy flow is healthy and you are feeling good about yourself, there's much less risk of disease. Environmental toxins, dietary fat, and excess sugar or alcohol (to name a few) usually don't manifest in disease unless other factors have already set up the pattern of blockage in the body's energy system in the first place.[3] Environmental or dietary risk factors can be likened to debris carried along in the body's energy flow. This debris stays afloat unless there is a felled tree or other blockage to the water flowing in the stream. When there is, the debris collects in the branches of the felled tree and accumulates. Over time, similar accumulations in the body's energy flow can result in physical illness. In fact, scientific research has associated a failure of the flow of information between cells with the induction of cancer in those cells. A physical barrier of any kind that blocks communication between cells is a carcinogenic influence.[4] The fat and connective tissue that form a fibroid, for example, do so only when the energy flow around and through the uterus is already blocked in some way.

Our emotions are often stuck at the childhood level, when we were not allowed to experience them fully. In this culture, which teaches us to split our adult intellectual knowledge from our emotional reality and needs, one can have a Ph.D. from Harvard but an emotional body that is only two years old. The emotions, unexpressed and unacknowledged, become energetically stuck. Emotions that are expressed, felt, and named, on the other hand, simply flow through our energy system, leaving no residual "unfinished" business.

We do not have to wait to develop cancer or other diseases in order to get the message that we need to change our vibrational point of attraction and begin creating health. None of us is completely free from the fear, anger, and stress that come and go as part of normal life. When these emotions become intense enough to affect our psychological and emotional well-being on a regular basis, we are heading for physical illness unless we resolve them in a healthy way. When our daily unresolved pain, anger, and frustration rob our bodies of vital health-producing energy, it is essential to bring healing and understanding into our daily thoughts, emotions, and actions.

Here is a crucial point: it is completely possible for a woman to go through her entire life free from physical illness, even though she was abused, beaten, or neglected as a child. Early-childhood problems do not *necessarily* cause energy disturbances and physical illness. These problems often occur only after a woman begins to develop as an individual and form her own identity and opinions *separate* from those of her family and her background. At this point she may realize that what happened to her as a child was not acceptable. However, she is realizing this from the perspective of a mature individual, not of the child she was then.

Hurts and wounds from a woman's past do *not* become potentially devastating to her, physically or emotionally, *until* she gets the idea that what happened to her in the past was *wrong,* that it shouldn't have happened, and that she was abused purposely and consciously by her family members. She has now introduced into her emotional and psychological pattern a conflicting model of how her life *should have been.* This sets the stage for the toxic effects of blame. Though a woman may have been terrified or abused as a child, this early abuse will not adversely affect her or her body *unless* she starts to believe that she was *entitled* to a different life. At this point she begins to relive and reevaluate her early life experiences from the perspective of an individual reviewing a crime scene. Energy disturbance and subsequent illness may well result at this point if she is unable to work through her emotional and psychological pain with forgiveness and understanding for herself and others.

The chemistry of conflict, or righteous indignation, requires two major energies: The first is when a woman begins to remember that she was indeed violated in some way. The second is when she interprets those events from the point of view that her family deliberately and of conscious mind chose to do that to her. This mindset, not the abuse, is what creates disease.

I've learned how to recognize the poisoning effects of righteous indignation in my own body. Getting stuck in this energy for a long time becomes self-destructive. Feeling rage and anger from past violations is a necessary first step toward healing. Anger mobilizes and energizes us to make long overdue, life-enhancing changes. It's far preferable to the stasis of depression. The key is to feel it and then move on. Anger and blame are a necessary stop on the road of life but they make a lousy destination. The longer we stay in this mode, searching for a perpetrator to blame for what happened to us—be it men, our mothers, the government, or doctors—the more our bodies are energetically depleted.

Female circumcision, for example, is routinely carried out by elder women in cultures in which it is practiced. The tribal wisdom is that the young girl will be considered "tainted goods" if she hasn't been circumcised. The entire tribe shares in this belief system, so those who have had it done don't necessarily feel abused. From our Western cultural standpoint, this is barbaric. Because consciousness of the physical, psychological, and spiritual effects of female circumcision is now growing, the entire subject is being brought out into the open, discussed, and reevaluated. Incest and other human rights abuses have been the norm for the last five thousand years. "These did not become the crimes they are today," says theologian and medical intuitive Caroline Myss, Ph.D., "until we began to reevaluate our personal boundaries within our tribal settings." In my view, this collective reevaluation constitutes recovery from the addictive system in which we have been caught up.

Our early family life clearly has a profound influence on our character and health. A famous prospective study by Dr. Caroline Thomas, for example, indicates that a man's lack of closeness to his parents, or having a father who was physically and emotionally less involved, could predict early disability and death from suicide, hypertension, coronary artery disease, and tumors.[5] This certainly corroborates the ACE study findings discussed in chapter 2.

EARTH'S ENERGY

Traditional Eastern philosophies describe the profound interaction between the Earth's energy and that of the physical human body, and the strong connection between female energy and the Earth's own natural pull. Understanding women's nature, with its natural ebbs and flows, as positive and powerful gives us a chance to heal and live in a balanced, healthy way.

According to some Eastern beliefs, women's bodies are different from men's in that the Earth's energy moves up through our bodies and inward. This female energy is "drawing-in" energy, or centripetal force. This centripetal female energy is irresistible. It is so powerful that if one lives in a family setting, most of the household will want to be around the person with the most centripetal energy—usually the mother—and will be acutely aware when she is gone. Children will save up their complaints for their mother at the end of the day if she hasn't been around. My children always needed to know where I was in the house. If I walked out of a room, they called, "Mom, where are you?" after about one minute. When they were younger, they always had to be in the same room with me. I couldn't take a bath alone until the older one was about nine. In contrast, when the children were small, my former husband could have been away for much longer before they'd notice. A woman's inward-pulling energy is at work when she puts the baby to the breast, accepts the penis into the vagina (if she is heterosexual), and sends chemical signals to encourage sperm to swim toward the egg. This powerful energy is present not only in our biology but also in our hearts and minds in the form of our unique dreams and desires. When a woman finds the courage to articulate these desires to herself and also share them with others, she will soon find that her irresistible drawing-in energy will help her to fulfill them.

Michio Kushi, the macrobiotic teacher who first discussed and illustrated this energy pattern for Western readers, points out that the
Earth's centripetal force coming up through the feet is present in men
as well as women, just as heaven's force, coming downward from the
sky through the head and the body (centrifugal force), is present in
women as well as men. What differs is the degree to which each energy is present. In women, in general, more "Earth's energy moving
up," or centripetal force, is present. I've been told that Navaho
women wear skirts because doing so increases the body's access to this
Earth energy through the circle that the skirt creates on the Earth in
relationship to the body (see figure 1). The Lakota tradition holds that
the energy of women during menstruation (called "moon time") spi-
rals counterclockwise and downward, into the Earth. (Because of this,
menstruating women don't participate in sweat lodges because their
energy conflicts with the upward spiraling energy of the sweat lodge
ceremony.)[6]

Centripetal energy is a grounding force that affects everyone
around us because women tend to be the centers of their households,
taking on psychological responsibility for the well-being of other
family members. Therefore, when a woman changes her life for the
better, her entire family (whether or not she has children) generally
benefits. She sets the tone. The well-being of the family and of society itself depends upon women becoming and remaining healthy.
Part of creating health is understanding the power of female energy
and its implications. The health of a woman's loved ones is directly
linked to her own personal health. So we owe it to ourselves first to
take the time we need to heal and to become healthy, happy, and
whole. You can't quench another's thirst if your own cup is empty.

THE CHAKRAS

Centripetal "drawing-in" force is only one way to characterize female energy. We also have seven specific vibrational centers in our
bodies known as *chakras*. Emotional-psychological patterns commonly affect women's bodies and their energy centers, the chakras.
Every human being, male or female, has the same chakras, and each
of them is affected by specific emotional and psychological issues.
These energy centers connect our nerves, hormones, and emotions.
Their locations run parallel to the body's neuroendocrine-immune
system and form a link between our vibrational anatomy and our
physical anatomy. The vibrational system of the human body is a

FIGURE 1: EARTH'S ENERGY GOING UPWARD

Female energy = centripetal or "drawing-in" force. Earth's energy coming upward through the feet, then spiraling around the uterus, breasts, and tonsils.

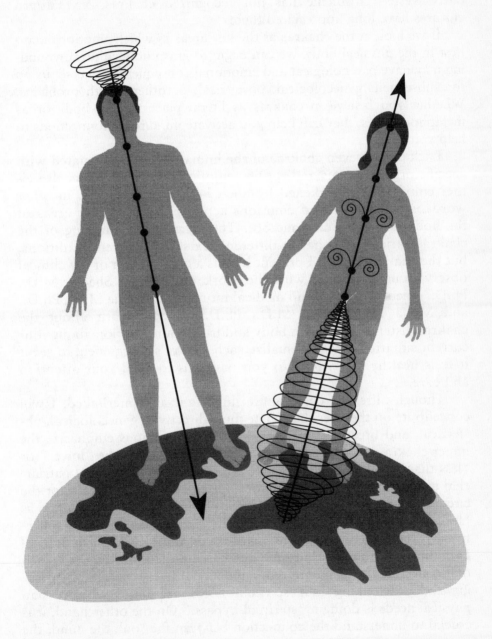

Source: Adapted from Michio Kushi

holographic field that carries information for the growth, development, and reproduction of the physical body. This holographic field guides the unfolding of the genetic process that transforms the molecules of our bodies into functioning organs and tissues. Though standard Western medicine has not recognized chakras yet, Eastern cultures have long appreciated them.

If we look at the chakras as the key areas in which emotions manifest in the physical body, we can begin to grasp how cultural wounding may have psychological and emotional consequences that set us up for subsequent gynecological, obstetrical, or other health problems. Whether you believe in chakras as literal places in the body or as metaphoric ones, they can help you activate mind/body connections to help you heal.

Each of the seven chakras of the human body is associated with specific organ systems and specific emotional states. Each is also either enlivened or weakened by one's beliefs and feelings. In other words, specific fears and emotions actually target specific areas of the body (see figure 2, page 80). The location and naming of the chakras varies somewhat in different texts and different traditions, but the chakras system I present here is a compilation of my clinical observations combined with the work of Norman Shealy, M.D., Ph.D., a neurosurgeon; and medical intuitives Caroline Myss, Ph.D., and Mona Lisa Schulz, M.D., Ph.D.[7] As you learn about the chakras, listen to your own body and trust your intuition about your current situation. Try to visualize each chakra's energy field to see if it feels healthy and whole to you or seems to need your attention and care.

Though all seven chakras are important and interlinked, I will concentrate on the ones that relate most directly to gynecological, obstetrical, and breast health. Some spiritual traditions emphasize the upper chakras as "more important" or "holier" than the "lower" or "less-than" chakras, but I want to stress that this is a typical patriarchal misunderstanding. We cannot hope to improve our health or the circumstances of our lives if we think of our body's lower centers as "less worthy" or "beneath our dignity." If humankind had collectively taken care of its lower-chakra needs and viewed them as vital parts of the whole, instead of subordinating them to "higher" spiritual concerns, our planet and our individual lives would be flourishing today. Thinking that spiritual needs are more worthy than physical needs is doing a "spiritual bypass." On the other hand, it is crucial to understand the connection between the soul, the mind, the emotions, and the physical body. As you work through the chakras, notice which ones you would like to spend less time on and examine why. You may want to review them until you become comfortable with them.

In each chakra area, there are two basic polarities, or extremes, that are associated with ill health. To stay healthy or to regain our health in a certain area, we must learn how to strike a healthy balance between the two extremes of emotional expression represented in each area. Our inner body wisdom, through each of these emotional centers, is always leading us toward health and balance by requiring that we develop a full repertory of skills encompassing the entire range of emotional expression.

One more thing: though the energies associated with blame, guilt, rage, and loss have been associated only with certain areas of the body by other authors, a thorough search of the psychosomatic medical literature indicates that this view is incomplete. These energies affect each area of the body simultaneously, though they may be expressed as health problems in the area of your body that is most vulnerable. The same is true for the health-enhancing energies associated with love, hope, and forgiveness.

THE LOWER FEMALE CENTERS: CHAKRAS ONE TO THREE

The bottom three chakras are related to our physical life: the people, events, memories, experiences, and physical objects within our environment, past and present. All three of the lower female centers are inextricably linked and interacting. Therefore, although I address each one separately, understand that they all affect one another. (Ultimately, all seven chakras affect one another and are interactive.)

The *first-chakra* area is affected by how secure and safe we feel in the world and how well we can balance trust versus mistrust, independence versus dependence, and standing alone versus belonging to groups. This area is also affected by the balance we strike between feeling fearless and allowing ourselves to feel our fear fully. The first-chakra area is, quite literally, affected by how connected we feel to the Earth and the processes of the Earth. The body areas that correlate with this chakra are the spine, the rectum, the hip joints, the blood, and the immune system. The foundation for our sense of safety usually is formed in childhood when we get a sense about whether or not this planet is a safe place to be. Therefore, unresolved family and physical survival issues—such as problems concerning one's house, family, sexual identity, and race—are represented in the first chakra. A person with a first-chakra issue would be likely to say or think regularly: "No one is here for me"; "I'm all alone"; "Nobody cares"; "I'll starve."

The health of the *second-chakra* area has to do with two separate issues. The first involves our outer drives in the world and includes both how we go about getting what we want and the actual things we go after. When we go after what we want, do we do so actively or passively? Are we considered a "go-getter," or do things "come to us"? Finally, when we go after what we want, do we do so "shamelessly," or are we filled with shame, believing that we're not worthy to have what we'd like?

The other second-chakra issue has to do with relationships and understanding that they are a basic human need. Are we dependent or independent? Do we take more in relationships, or do we give more? What is our balance between needing others to fulfill our needs and relying solely on ourselves? Do we give to others to earn love? Do we know how to receive and accept support? Do we have well-defined boundaries, or are they poorly defined? Are we assertive or submissive? Do we protect others, or do others protect us? Do we tend to oppose others, or do we acquiesce to their opinions or actions?

The pelvic and reproductive organs (vulva, vagina, uterus, cervix, and ovaries) are associated with the second chakra, and so are the bladder and the appendix. The health of this area is affected by the degree to which our relationships are based on issues of trust or, alternatively, control, blame, and guilt. If we use sex, money, blame, or guilt to control the dynamics of our relationships (including our relationship with ourselves), then the organs of the second chakra may be adversely affected. A person with a second-chakra issue might often say or think: "I don't feel heard by you"; "You never come to visit"; "He doesn't write, he doesn't call"; "No one will ever love me"; "You're never there for me."

The *third chakra* is associated with a person's self-esteem, self-confidence, self-respect, and sense of responsibility. In other words, how do we balance our feelings of adequacy or worthiness with inferiority in what we do in the outer world of work or achievement? Are we hyperresponsible or irresponsible? Are we aggressive, or do we tend to be defensive? Are we prone to threatening and intimidating others? Are we territorial? Or do we feel trapped and want to escape? In our work, are we overly dependent upon boundaries, or do we have issues around limitations? Finally, do we know how to balance our competitiveness? Do we know how to both win and lose with grace? How do we handle gains and losses? All of these issues affect the health of this area. The foundation for a woman's sense of herself is formed by the emotions, memories, and wisdom stored in the energy fields of the first and second chakras. In order to have good self-esteem, a woman must feel secure in the world (first chakra) and have relationships based on mutual respect and support (second chakra). The gall bladder, liver, pancreas, stomach, and small bowel are the organs associated with the third chakra. Familiar health-damaging statements here would be: "If I don't do it, it won't get done"; "I'll never be good enough"; "It's okay, I'll do it myself."

All of the unresolved stresses of our early physical life related to people, events, memories, and experiences pull energy *primarily* from the three lower power centers, the first three chakras.

STRESS IN WOMEN IN THE FIRST THREE CHAKRAS

- Any unresolved anger
- Resentments and feelings of rejection
- The need for revenge
- Wanting to leave a relationship but fearing the financial consequences
- Shame about one's body
- Shame about one's family background or one's husband's social status
- Being either a child abuser or an abused child
- A history of incest or rape
- Guilt over an abortion
- Inability to conceive
- Inability to launch one's creations

FIGURE 2: CHAKRA DIAGRAM WITH FEMALE FIGURE

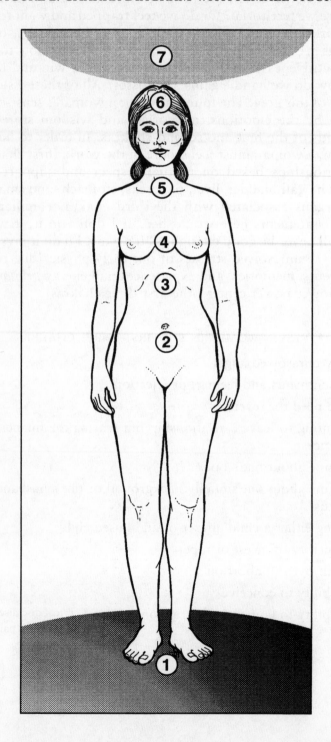

TABLE 4

ENERGY ANATOMY: MENTAL AND EMOTIONAL PATTERNS,
THE CHAKRAS, AND THE PHYSICAL BODY

Chakra	Organs	Mental, Emotional Issues	Physical Dysfunctions
7	Can involve any organ system	Clear sense of life's purpose vs. trusting that life has a purpose that may not be clear Connection to God or universal source of energy Understanding the paradox that an individual can influence her life's events and also trust that things happen as they should and that some things are out of one's control	Developmental disorders (cerebral palsy) Genetic disorders Multiple sclerosis Amyotrophic lateral sclerosis (ALS) Multiple-system abnormalities Any life-threatening illness or accident that serves as a wake-up call
6	Brain Eyes Ears Nose Pineal gland	Perception: clarity vs. ambiguity Thought: left brain vs. right brain—rational vs. nonrational, linear vs. homographic, rigid vs. flexible Morality: conservative vs. liberal, following the rules vs. understanding that rules have exceptions Repression vs. lack of inhibition	Brain tumors/ hemorrhages/stroke Neurological disturbances Blindness/deafness Ménière's disease Dizziness Tinnitus (ringing in ears) Parkinson's disease Learning disabilities Seizures
5	Thyroid Trachea Neck vertebrae Throat Mouth Teeth and gums	Communication: expression vs. comprehension (speaking vs. listening) Timing: pushing forward vs. waiting Will: willful vs. compliant	Bronchitis/hoarseness Chronic sore throats Mouth ulcers Gum difficulties Temporomandibular joint problems (TMJ) Cervical disc disease Chronic neck pain Laryngitis Swollen glands in neck Thyroid problems

Chakra	Organs	Mental, Emotional Issues	Physical Dysfunctions

4	Heart/lungs
	Blood vessels
	Shoulders
	Ribs/breasts
	Diaphragm
	Upper
	  esophagus
		Emotional expression,
		  including capacity to
		  feel fully, express, and
		  resolve anger, hostility,
		  joy, love, grief, forgiveness
		Capacity to form mutual,
		  reciprocal partnerships
		  with balance of giving,
		  receiving, nurturing of
		  self vs. nurturing of
		  others, intimacy with
		  others vs. capacity to
		  be alone (intimacy
		  with self)
			Coronary artery disease
			Myocardial infarction
			  (heart attack)
			Hypertension
			Cardiac arrhythmias
			Chest pain
			Mitral valve prolapse
			Cardiomegaly
			Congestive heart failure
			Asthma/allergy
			Lung cancer
			Pneumonia
			Upper back, shoulder
			  problems
			Breast problems,
			  including cancer

3	Abdomen
	Upper intestines
	Liver, gall
	  bladder
	Lower
	  esophagus
	Stomach
	Kidney,
	  pancreas
	Adrenal gland
	Spleen
	Middle spine
		Self-esteem, self-confidence,
		  or self-respect
		Adequacy vs. inferiority
		  relating to competence
		  and skills in the
		  outer world
		Responsibility vs.
		  irresponsibility
		Substance abuse
		Aggression vs.
		  defensiveness
		Competitiveness vs.
		  noncompetitiveness;
		  winning vs. losing
		Territoriality/too many
		  boundaries
		Fear of assuming
		  responsibility or making
		  decisions for self
		Feeling overly responsible
			Gastric or duodenal ulcers
			Colon/intestinal problems
			Ulcerative colitis, irritable
			  bowel syndrome
			Heartburn/gastritis
			Pancreatitis/diabetes
			Constipation and diarrhea
			Indigestion, chronic
			  or acute
			Anorexia and bulimia
			Liver dysfunction
			Hepatitis
			Adrenal dysfunction

Chakra	Organs	Mental, Emotional Issues	Physical Dysfunctions
2	Uterus, ovaries	Balanced drives in the outer	OB/GYN problems
	Vulva, vagina,	world toward sex,	Pelvic/lower back pain
	cervix	money, and relationships	Creativity
	Large intestine	Capacity to co-create	Sexual potency
	Lower vertebrae	with others	Urinary problems
	Pelvis	Fertility and generativity	Appendicitis
	Appendix	Relationship dynamics	
	Bladder	including: dependency	
		vs. independence,	
		giving and taking,	
		defined boundaries	
		vs. poor boundaries,	
		assertiveness vs.	
		passivity	
1	Physical body	Safety/security in the world;	Chronic spinal problems
	support	knowing when to trust or	Back pain
	Hip joints	mistrust	Sciatica
	Spine	Knowing when to feel fear	Scoliosis
	Blood	and when not to	Rectal tumors/cancer
	Immune system	Balance between	Chronic fatigue
		independence and	Fibromyaglia
		dependence	Autoimmune diseases
			Arthritis
			Skin problems

Sources: C. N. Shealy and C. M. Myss, *The Creation of Health: Merging Traditional Medicine with Intuitive Diagnosis* (Walpole, NH: Stillpoint Publications, 1988). Scientific documentation of the human energy system and updated information from Mona Lisa Schulz, M.D., Ph.D., *Awakening Intuition Using Your Mind-Body Network for Insight and Healing* (New York: Harmony Books, 1998).

These issues all have the potential to affect the organs "below the belt" because of the way in which the first three chakras work together. Now I'll discuss the issues of each chakra in more detail.

The First Chakra: How Family Wounds Are Stored in the Body

Our first-chakra health is related to our upbringing and early life. This includes our immediate and extended family, race, social status, educational level, family legacy, and family expectations as these were handed down through the generations. To describe the breadth of the issues involved in the first chakra, Caroline Myss uses the word *tribe*. For example, we all learn very early what it means to be a member of a defined group: a Smith or a Jones, a Catholic or a Jew. Another first-chakra "inheritance" is the tribal programming of many first- and second-generation immigrant families in the United States, who often pass on the belief that to accomplish anything worthwhile, one must suffer and sacrifice personal happiness and pleasure. Family scars and the social and familial information that form a person's idea of reality are connected to the first-chakra area.

The tribal mind is not an individual's mind. The tribal mind is primarily a collective brain that seeks to hold on to its own and fight for its own survival in the world. The tribal mind is concerned with *loyalty,* not love, kindness, or tenderness. What the tribe refers to as "love" is really obligation to the tribe. An example of this is a family member who says to another, "If you really loved me, you'd come to visit your family and me more often." Tribal consciousness, then, is not a high-level, highly evolved consciousness. Yet we all share it to some degree, and many women admit that as they get older, they can hear that tribal mind within themselves. "I sometimes hear my mother's words coming right out of my mouth, and I can't believe it," patients often tell me. Above all, the tribal mind seeks stability by keeping everything the same, e.g., family holidays and birthdays become "obligations," not joyful times of sharing.

I sometimes refer to the tribal mind as "crabs in the bucket." If you have a bunch of crabs in a bucket and one crab tries to escape over the edge, the other crabs will always pull the escapee back down with the rest of them. The same sort of thing often happens to women and their families as the women decide to break free from limiting patterns. Almost invariably, family members try to sabotage her efforts—at least initially.

Countless women have had the experience of confronting their parents about abuse or incest soon after remembering these events, only to find that their parents deny these allegations outright. The unconscious motive to preserve the tribe is the reason so many parents deny having ever violated a tribe member. At some level, their tribal memory bank has absorbed the memory very differently from the way the individual member records the same event. The person who is waking up from the tribal trance is almost invariably seen as a "traitor" to the family.

FIRST-CHAKRA ISSUES THAT CAN SET THE STAGE FOR ILLNESS

- ~ Unfinished business with parents
- ~ Incest (This is a second-chakra issue as well.)
- ~ Abuse or neglect in childhood
- ~ Psychological programming from one's early years that is limiting, such as:
  - ~ "You're stupid." "You're useless." "You're a bad girl."
  - ~ "Only Catholics go to heaven."
  - ~ "Your body is something to hide out of shame."
  - ~ "Girls are meant to serve men."
  - ~ "Men always come first." (For example, in many families the men get the best cuts of meat, and the women get what is left over.)
  - ~ "Girls should not be ambitious or bright."
  - ~ "Women can't make money. They must marry it."

Most tribes or families *do not deliberately* try to poison their members—they are merely handing down what they recognize as tribal wisdom, even in the form of limiting and painful ideas. It is useful to think of yesterday's tribe as today's dysfunctional family.

My friend Carla recently realized, after resolving her many physical illnesses, that the seeds for these illnesses had been planted in her childhood. Her mother had repeatedly beaten her, not out of malice or lack of love but simply following her own tribal programming of how to love and prepare a daughter for life. She had told Carla that the beatings were how she showed her love. Whenever Carla's mother saw another woman beating a child in the supermarket or elsewhere, she used to remark to Carla that obviously that woman really loved her child. Carla's mother deeply believed that life is very difficult and filled with pain and that to accomplish anything, Carla would have to suffer. Later, each time Carla reached a cherished goal, she developed a serious illness. She is now realizing that she can reach her goals joyfully by using her innate gifts and talents and her inner guidance, and that repeated illness and suffering need not be part of her experience.

The Second Chakra: Symbolic Creative Space

The second chakra is concerned with the day-to-day physical aspects of living, with the people to whom we relate, and with the quality of our relationships. The second chakra also relates to everything we own: money, relationships, and passions. Since most of our early programming is to serve the tribe, most men and women automatically move into the roles of their second chakras in an unconscious way. They choose the partners that fulfill the needs of their second chakra. Women thus tend to marry for physical security, money, children, and social status, and out of fear of abandonment. We then carry out our roles within these needs accordingly. We are programmed to tend to the needs of our personal tribe and often become completely controlled by the fears of the second chakra.

SECOND-CHAKRA ISSUES: HOW RELATIONSHIP
WOUNDS MANIFEST IN THE BODY

- ~ Fear of abandonment
- ~ Financial security
- ~ Social status
- ~ Children
- ~ Creativity

The uterus and ovaries are the major organs in the second chakra. This area is both literally and figuratively creative space, out of which women can produce babies, relationships, careers, novels, insights, and other creative or artistic works. When our energy is not flowing smoothly in this area of the body, gynecological problems, such as fibroid tumors, can result.

When I think of the uterus as "potential space," I also think of what we as women are usually expected to "store" in there. A slang term for the uterus is "the bag," and as humans who have or have had a uterus, we are also the ones who carry all the stuff that others don't want to carry. Women who are married and have children often notice that their children give them, not their husband, the half-eaten food, gum wrappers, and other garbage that they no longer want to carry. We have all heard older women referred to as "old bags." When I was pregnant, nursing, and caring for small children, I felt like the "multiple-bag lady."

Not only do women carry physical excess, we are also expected to carry emotional excess for others—usually for men, but not always. One sixty-year-old former patient of mine with three grown children was living alone with her husband, who had recently retired. She told me she was now chomping at the bit to do other things in her life that she had long wanted to do, such as traveling and writing. But her husband was not enthusiastic about her endeavors. He wasn't sure what to do with his newly acquired freedom from work. My patient said, "But my husband still wants me to carry his anima—his moods, his enthusiasm, his fun. And when I let down and allow any of my own feelings to show, other than enthusiasm, *he* gets depressed." *Anima,* a term coined by the famous psychologist Carl Jung, is a man's inner feminine aspect that often gets projected onto the real-life women in his life when he is unwilling to feel his own emotions and work through them. What unconscious material do we store in our body centers that neither we nor anyone else really wants to carry around? When unresolved second-chakra-related issues surrounding relationships, creativity, and/or a sense of security exist, the pelvic area of the body as well as the lower back can become vulnerable to disease.

A number of second-chakra experiences can set the stage for illness. The studies of Dr. Gloria Bachmann indicate that childhood sexual abuse is associated with eating disorders, obesity, and somatic complaints in the genitourinary system, as well as substance abuse and other self-destructive behaviors.[8] Studies by Dr. Robert Reiter and others have found that previous sexual abuse is a significant predisposing risk factor for chronic pelvic pain.[9]

Whenever I see a woman with a uterine problem such as fibroid tumors—which are present in 40 percent of American women—I ask her to meditate upon her relationships, creativity, and sense of security. Is her creative energy being routed into any dead-end jobs or relationships? What is her fibroid telling her about these areas? Fibroids, endometriosis, diseases of the ovaries, and other pelvic disorders are manifestations of blocked energy in the pelvis. In a misogynist culture in which at least 20 percent of women are sexual abuse survivors and approximately one in four gets physically raped, it's not hard to figure out how this happens.

During her annual exam, I found a small fibroid in Gina, a former patient who was thirty-eight years old at the time. I asked her to meditate on blocked energy in her pelvis, and she later told me, "When I got home and took some time with this question, I realized that when my brother died in an accident, I was furious with him for leaving. I was twenty-five and really couldn't allow myself to feel that rage. So I just stuffed it in my pelvis. I hadn't thought about that for years." On a follow-up exam three months later, I found that her fibroid was gone. I believe that by expressing and experiencing the full impact of her anger for the first time, she changed the energy pattern in her pelvis and actually dematerialized the fibroid, transforming it from matter into energy. She told me, "I had a feeling that when I came in today, you'd say it was gone. I literally felt it let go." I've seen other women decrease or eliminate their fibroids when they remembered and released old experiences.

Third Chakra: Self-Esteem and Personal Power

The foundation for a woman's sense of herself, her self-esteem (third chakra), is formed by her sense of security and safety in the world (first chakra) combined with the quality of her relationships (second chakra). If we feel safe and secure and have supportive relationships, we will be in a good position to achieve our goals in the outer world and to complete tasks that help us develop a sense of self-esteem and self-worth. Third-chakra strength or weakness is related to feelings of adequacy and competence in the world versus inferiority, and to our ability to assume responsibility for our lives and our choices versus the degree to which we relinquish this power to others. The ability to learn from both winning *and* losing creates health in this area. On the other hand, excessive competitiveness and needing to win all the time can weaken the third chakra. It is also affected by the balance one strikes between being aggressive and being defensive.

As a result of the collective and individual histories of most women, many of us have low self-esteem. For centuries women haven't been validated or valued except in their capacity as servers and pleasers of others. Our natural desire to create and achieve in the outer world has often been thwarted at an early age. Thus, as women have become individuals in their own right, their families often do not support them in becoming all of who they can be.

This is because families usually hold an unconscious tribal fear that their female members will abandon them to serve their own needs and live out their personal dreams without the family. We've all inherited the belief that a woman cannot develop herself fully without simultaneously sacrificing her ability to serve her family. And because we've been socialized to see the family as a woman's primary job, we have difficulty expecting and getting the support we need.

Besides undertaking the classic struggle to balance our personal interests and our responsibilities, women often pace our self-esteem to our mate's cycle. If a woman's partner becomes highly successful, she may become depressed because she can't keep pace with him, or she may not back her partner's new adventure into different thoughts or creative new territories for fear that he (or she) will leave her. On the other hand, when a mate is unsuccessful in the outside world and becomes depressed or abusive, this also affects the woman in her third (and also first and second) chakra. Conflicts such as these cause energy-system dysfunction in the third chakra and can result in eating disorders (anorexia nervosa and bulimia) or physical illness in the stomach (ulcers), gall bladder, small intestine (irritable bowel), liver, and pancreas (diabetes).

Archetypes and the First Three Chakras

When a woman feels that she is being forced to participate in an activity she doesn't like, her body, mind, and spirit are at risk for harm.[10] When she unwittingly participates in a pattern of self-abuse and abuse from others, she is acting under the influence of what in vibrational medicine is called the rape archetype.

Archetypes are psychological and emotional patterns that influence us unconsciously until we become aware of their power. Archetypes are universal ideas, images, and patterns of thought that we all share in our subconscious. Though the concept of archetypes may at first seem elusive, these unconscious patterns of thought and behavior have a very real effect on our bodies and emotions.

To help you understand the concept of archetype more clearly, I'll use an example—the mother archetype. A woman who is unconsciously operating under the influence of the mother archetype (as it currently exists in this culture) thinks obsessively about the needs of her children while forgoing her own. Even when her children are old enough to care for most of their physical needs themselves, the woman under the influence of the mother archetype focuses her thoughts on whether they've had enough to eat, whether they are happy, and whether they are warm enough or cool enough, ignoring or suppressing her own needs to do something for them. I know this one well. Up until very recently, I've felt bad about myself if my daughter asked for a tissue and I didn't have one! This culturally encouraged behavior of worrying can become a damaging stereotype. Another example of an archetype is the hero. When we see the word *hero,* we instantly think of a person who is strong, bold, and brave. A hero is one who may fearlessly rescue others and neglect his or her own safety and needs because of a compulsion to "save" someone else. If unconscious, this kind of behavior, too, can be detrimental to health.

When we are unconsciously participating in archetypal patterns of behavior, we lose touch with our deepest selves and our inner needs. When a woman is not following her own heart's desires and instead acts only to fulfill others' needs, she may be under the influence of either the rape archetype, the prostitute archetype, or the mother archetype, depending upon the circumstances.

The rape and prostitute archetypes are very closely related. When a woman engages in sexual activity that she doesn't really want but feels unable to do anything to prevent, she is under the influence of the rape archetype. The same archetype is present if she denies herself sexual pleasure because she feels that this is what her partner wants—and again feels unable to alter her situation. The rape archetype may occur when a woman participates in her own violation, when she participates in such things as an abortion that her mate wants but that she doesn't. A woman who resents her partner but stays in the relationship anyway for financial or other reasons is not acting from her individual strength but is under the spell of the prostitute archetype. Women often handle this archetype by blaming ourselves or by absorbing our own anger and rage, lest telling of these feelings result in being abandoned.

A woman's second-chakra organs are also put at risk when she herself becomes an aggressor or victimizer. Women participate in the rape archetype, for example, when they violate their children's physical and psychological boundaries. Daily enemas and rough washing of the genitalia are other common examples of women as violators. Women use emotional weaponry, while men add to that their fists. Women who victimize pay for it not only through energy of their female organs in the second chakra but with organs in the first and third chakras as well. According to Caroline Myss, aggressive behavior can be associated with cancer in the organs of the first three chakras.

It is important for us to understand and accept that women do have the potential for aggression. When we refuse to acknowledge a problem, we simply perpetuate it. Recovering from patriarchal influences isn't about blaming men, because in our culture we're all potential victims and potential perpetrators. When I first had a reading with Caroline Myss, for example, she told me that my body registered a rape between the ages of twenty-one and twenty-nine—the years that I was in medical school and doing my residency. Though I had not been physically raped, my body's energy system had been emotionally and psychologically "raped" by my medical training—something I had not been consciously aware of at the time. Myss states that almost everyone in this culture has suffered from a psychological or emotional rape of their innermost self at least once. That is one reason why so many women who have not suffered from overt sexual abuse nonetheless have chronic pelvic pain and other second-chakra problems. Many women feel stuck in jobs in which the rape or prostitute archetype is a daily reality.

When we continually see women only as victims, we do not acknowledge the damage women do to themselves and to others. If you've ever borne the brunt of female abuse or been an abuser yourself, you'll understand the significance of this point of view.

Shame and the First Three Chakras

Another issue for many women is shame. Shame hits the first three female centers and the associated interior organs, including the uterus and ovaries. Shame can be a result of social programming that tells a woman she's inferior, and it can be a result of family relationships, such as unhealthy relationships with her children or shame at her partner's social status. Shame over a rape, whether it was physical, emotional, or psychological rape, affects the vaginal area. Shame about one's sexuality can be a setup for vaginitis, pelvic pain, etc.

Research supports these energy dysfunctions. Henry Dreher, author of *Mind-Body Unity: A New Vision for Mind-Body Science and Medicine* (Johns Hopkins University Press, 2003), points to a very large body of research showing that women who have experienced sexual abuse are significantly more likely to develop gastrointestinal disorders, including irritable bowel syndrome (IBS).[11]

Other research points to differences in personality between women who develop interior cancers and those who develop exterior cancers.[12] An individual's perception of whether her body is permeable and easily penetrated by external influences, either physical or emotional, is related to whether she is susceptible to cancer. Those women who perceive their bodies as permeable are subject to cancers that are located more deeply in their bodies—for example, in the ovaries or uterus. Those women who believe that their bodies are strong and protected against external influences are more prone to cancers in the external genital areas.

Research by Lydia Temoshok, Ph.D., author with Dreher of *The Type C Connection: The Mind-Body Link to Cancer and Your Health* (Plume, 1992), found that women with more aggressive and life-threatening cancers (including both breast and cervical cancer) tend to be more self-sacrificing and less aware of their needs and feelings, including physical sensations, than other women.

The Fourth Chakra

The bodily areas associated with the fourth chakra are the heart, breast, lungs, ribs, upper back, and shoulders. The fourth chakra is related to our capacity to express ourselves emotionally and participate in true partnerships in which both members are equally powerful and equally vulnerable. When we express ourselves emotionally, we need a balance between anger and love, joy and serenity. Can we be stoic at times and at other times "lose it" emotionally? Can we allow ourselves to feel grief and loss fully? In partnership, can we allow ourselves times of intimacy balanced with time alone? Can we both nurture others and allow others to nurture us? The emotional and psychological issues associated with ill health in the fourth-chakra area are an inability to give or receive love from self or others (nurturance), lack of forgiveness, unresolved grief, and/or hostility.

The second and fourth chakras have a unique interrelationship. The uterus is sometimes called the "low heart," while the heart in the chest is the "high heart." It's been said that if the low heart has been closed, through rape, incest, abuse, or shame, a woman cannot truly open her high heart. In this culture, women also tend to shut down their low hearts, or their sexuality and erotic needs, because we're taught that "nice" girls aren't sexual. We're also taught, however, that it's fine for us to be in touch with our emotions and feelings, and so we're set up for second- and fourth-chakra conflicts. In addition, women are taught that if we are powerful and successful financially, we'll be isolated from others and won't be able to experience intimacy fully. In addition, we women are often socialized to believe that if we become powerful and successful with money and career (second chakra), no one will love us and we will lose out on intimacy (fourth chakra). Men, on the other hand, have been socialized to believe that their masculinity depends upon being able to bring home the bacon and make the major financial decisions in a relationship. We're now at a historic crossroads as men and women learn how to renegotiate these inherited (and often obsolete) partnership and intimacy beliefs and behaviors.

Energy dysfunctions often arise when a woman is confused about how to use both her loving (fourth chakra) and her creative (second chakra) energies optimally. The major conflict within women is that most of us still believe that in order to be loved, to receive love, and to guarantee that someone will need us, we must care for our loved ones' external physical needs. But such love relationships, dependent upon ties of family obligations and tribal tradition, are recognized as relationship addictions once a woman begins to individuate and become conscious of her patterns. Energy dysfunctions that arise in the second- and fourth-chakra areas at the same time are very common in our culture. They often result when women unconsciously participate simultaneously in both the rape archetype and the mother archetype.

Sally, a twenty-six-year-old waitress, had very-early-stage cervical cancer (second chakra) and multiple breast cysts (fourth chakra). When she was a girl, her father had been both emotionally and physically distant. In her early teenage years, to fill up this emptiness, she had multiple sexual partners, boys whom she neither loved nor respected. This addictive pattern of behavior (the rape and prostitute archetypes) disrupted the energetic patterns of her second-chakra area, and she suffered from very painful and frequent herpes outbreaks in her vagina. She also had genital warts.

Like Sally's distant father, Sally's mother took care of neither her own nor her daughter's physical or emotional needs. Sally never learned how to care for her own emotional needs, in that no one ever demonstrated this behavior to her. Both Sally and her mother had energy disruptions in their fourth-chakra areas related to lack of self-respect and self-nurturance. Both mother and daughter had breast problems. Sally's mother had already had breast cancer, and Sally had had two breast biopsies for benign lumps.

Neither Sally nor her mother is unique in our culture. I've seen many women like them. When a woman neglects her own inner needs, when she addictively cooks, cleans, and cares for the physical needs of her family to "earn" love, when she works obsessively at her job to "prove" her self-worth, and when she provides sex on demand because of feelings of obligation or guilt, she becomes susceptible to disease in both her second and fourth chakras. Quelling her insecurities about abandonment or about being good enough, about self-esteem, uses up her emotional energy. Her life-force gets drained by her fear of abandonment and her belief that she's not good enough.

Supporting these theories of energy-system dysfunctions, research has shown that the personality patterns of women who have disease only in the second chakra differ from those of women with disease only in the fourth chakra. (An extensive literature search reveals no studies on the personality patterns of women who have malignancy in *both* the second- and fourth-chakra areas.)

Patients with malignant tumors in the breast (the high heart) have different personality patterns from those with cancer of the cervix (the lower heart). In one study, 50 percent of patients with cervical cancer (a second-chakra disease) had physically lost their fathers due to death or desertion during their early years (a second chakra–related emotion). In contrast, in the homes of those with breast cancer (a fourth-chakra disease), the father was emotionally distant (a fourth chakra–related pattern).[13] Other studies have shown that significantly more cervical cancer patients have behaviors that suggest a second-chakra energy imbalance: They had married multiple times, had a high incidence of sexual activity with partners whom they neither loved nor respected, and were very concerned with body shape and size. They also had a feeling that they had been neglected as children. In contrast, studies of breast cancer patients suggest behavior patterns associated with fourth-chakra dysfunction: they had a greater tendency to stay in a loveless marriage, had a relatively high likelihood of carrying a heavy load of responsibility for younger siblings during childhood, and had a greater chance of denying themselves medical care and physical nurturance.[14]

Caroline Myss's and Mona Lisa Schulz's observations further substantiate the research above. In general, they find that emotions that are of the raging variety hit below the belt. Sadness that cannot be expressed, on the other hand, is associated with disease above the belt. I will be covering this in more detail in chapters 5 through 10.

How to Heal Lower-Chakra Wounding

Lower-chakra wounds *don't heal until they're witnessed*. Someone has to say, "Yes, this happened to you." One of the functions of this book is this witnessing process. As a physician, I represent an authority figure. When I or another person validates a woman's woundings, she can use that as a very powerful catalyst for healing. But it is even more important that the *woman herself* acknowledge her wounding and need for healing. As long as a woman is stuck in denial ("It wasn't really all that bad, he never hit me," or "My family loved me very much—my father would never have done that"), she won't be able to tell the truth to herself. Her secrets will remain locked in her cells, unavailable for witnessing and healing.

After the witnessing of her wounds, a woman must then investigate how these wounds have affected her life. This is the naming stage—the stage when she realizes that her life has indeed been adversely affected by someone or something. Denial has now left. Many women in our society are currently at this stage. The final stage required for healing and the optimal functioning of the woman's energy system involves *releasing* the power of the wound to control her life. Forgiveness and acceptance is now required, for both herself and others. At the same time, she is now ready to assume personal dominion over her life and choices for the future as she understands her past.

OTHER CHAKRA ISSUES

The *fifth chakra* is related to communication, timing, and will. When you communicate your ideas in the outer world, do you talk as much as you listen? Do you express yourself as well as you comprehend others? As far as timing goes, do you push forward or do you wait? Finally, do you tend toward willfulness, or are you overly compliant? Associated with this chakra are the throat, mouth, teeth, gums, thyroid, trachea, and neck vertebrae. Dysfunctions in this chakra include chronic sore throats, throat and mouth ulcers, gum disease, neck pain, temporomandibular joint disease (TMJ), thyroid disease, cervical disc problems, swollen neck glands, and laryngitis. Women with fifth-chakra problems such as hypothyroidism often have difficulty speaking up for themselves and holding their own point of view, and may have overly soft voices, making it difficult for them to be heard. On the other hand, an overdeveloped will can result in disease such as hyperthyroidism and the exertion of one's intellectual will without acknowledging "higher will" or "higher power"—for example, "I don't care what my body is telling me, I'm going to do it anyway."

The *sixth chakra*, sometimes known as the third eye, is related to perception, thought, and morality. When we perceive the outer world, do we have the capacity to see clearly while also tolerating ambiguity? Can we allow ourselves to have razor-sharp focus sometimes and at other times become relaxed and unfocused? Do we know when to be unreceptive to the ideas of others and when to be receptive? Can we accumulate knowledge but also allow ourselves to be open to what we still need to learn? Can we acknowledge our areas of ignorance? Can we appreciate rational and logical thought from the brain's left hemisphere but also acknowledge the gift of the right hemisphere: the nonrational and the nonlinear? Are our thought processes rigid, obsessive, and ruminating, or do we have flexibility in our thinking? Finally, how do we apply our moral beliefs to ourselves and others? Do we tend to be repressed and overly conscientious model citizens who judge ourselves and others according to rigid standards, or do we allow ourselves, in some cases, to be more liberal, risk-taking, and uninhibited?

This chakra is located between the eyes, near the ears, nose, brain, and pineal gland. Dysfunctions associated with this chakra are vision problems, brain tumors, blood clots (blood clot formation is related to stopping the flow of intuitive information), neurological disorders, blindness, deafness, seizures, and learning disabilities. Health-detracting statements associated with losing energy in this area are: "I don't care how you feel. Tell me what you think"; "I don't have enough information to make a decision"; "Can't you see that I know what I'm talking about? Why are you arguing with me?"; "I'm surprised that you believe in that mind/body nonsense, given that you are an intellectual, educated person."

The *seventh chakra* is related to seeing the larger purpose in our lives. It's also related to our attitudes, faith, values, conscience, courage, and humanitarianism. Do we have a clear sense of purpose? Do we acknowledge that we as individuals have the power to create our lives, while simultaneously acknowledging the larger forces at work in the universe? Do we understand the paradox of knowing that we can influence some events, while also knowing that things happen that we can't control, that we may not like, but which may ultimately serve a purpose we don't understand at the time? This chakra is located near the crown of the head. The seventh chakra is the metaphysical framework around which you build your morals, your values, and your conscience.

Any life-threatening event in your life or any serious illness holds the potential to awaken wisdom in this area by connecting you with a larger view of the universe and your purpose in it. Those individuals who've undergone a near-death experience often relate how this changed their lives on every level and left them with a deep certainty about how best to spend the rest of their lives. Although all life-threatening illness can have seventh-chakra meaning, those that are specifically related to awakening wisdom in this chakra include paralysis and multisystem disease affecting the muscular and nervous systems, such as multiple sclerosis and Lou Gehrig's disease (ALS). An individual may be born with a seventh-chakra challenge such as genetic disease. Life-threatening accidents are also related to this chakra and can be major wake-up calls.

Understanding vibrational anatomy and the law of attraction holds the key to true healing, rather than just masking our symptoms, because it offers a comprehensive and holistic view of how each of us co-creates health or disease.

Regardless of our past, our power to heal and stay healthy is in the present moment, right now. When we're truly present, we can heal almost anything. But most people tie up the bulk of their energy in woundings from their past, while the rest of it is consumed by worrying about the future. You cannot heal anything unless a significant amount of your energy and spirit is available in the present moment. Dr. Lewis Thomas of the Memorial Sloan-Kettering Cancer Center in New York City once said that he had come to believe that cancer was the physical metaphor for the extreme need to grow. Healthy growth involves getting as many parts of yourself as possible available in the present moment—*the now*—the only place that healing can happen. Rarely is a person always present right now, today. Living in the now is a skill that is developed through introspection, meditation, and taking leaps of faith into freedom and joy—one small leap at a time, one day at a time.

Part Two

The Anatomy of Women's Wisdom

5

The Menstrual Cycle

How might it have been different for you if on your first menstrual day, your mother had given you a bouquet of flowers and taken you to lunch, and then the two of you had gone to meet your father at the jeweler, where your ears were pierced, and your father bought you your first pair of earrings, and then you went with a few of your friends and your mother's friends to get your first lip coloring; then you went,
    for the very first time,
      to the Women's lodge,
        to learn
          the wisdom of women?
How might your life be different?

—Judith Duerk, *Circle of Stones*

We can reclaim the wisdom of the menstrual cycle by tuning in to our cyclic nature and celebrating it as a source of our female power. The ebb and flow of dreams, creativity, and hormones associated with different parts of the cycle offer us a profound opportunity to deepen our connection with our inner knowing. This is a gradual process for most women, one that involves unearthing our personal history and then, day by day, thinking differently about our cycles and living with them in a new way.

TABLE 5

The Anatomy of Women's Wisdom

Body Organ or Process	Encoded Wisdom	Energy Dysfunction	Physical Manifestation
MENSTRUAL CYCLE	Cyclic intuitive wisdom and emotional recycling and processing	Refusal to embrace both difficult and pleasant emotions: the dark and the light Not allowing shadow side to be seen and worked through Belief that menstrual cycle is bad or shameful	Lack of periods Heavy periods Irregular periods Painful periods PMS
UTERUS	Creative center in relationship to self	Bondage of the emotions of others Unable to birth most creative self	Fibroids
OVARIES	Creative drives in outer world Assertiveness in outer world Excessive, insufficient, or imbalanced drive toward financial, creative, or relationship goals	Addiction to external authority or approval Disbelief in creative ability	Ovulation abnormalities Ovarian cysts Ovarian cancer Endometriosis
BREASTS	Emotional expression and partnership	Inability to fully feel, express, and resolve emotions Inability to participate in balanced partnerships Imbalance between intimacy with self (time alone) and with others	Breast cysts, pain Breast cancer Lung problems Shoulder problems

Body Organ or Process	Encoded Wisdom	Energy Dysfunction	Physical Manifestation
PREGNANCY	Capacity to conceive an idea or a life with another, hold it, nurture it, and allow it to be born	Insufficient energy to create and maintain new life Inability to trust the process of giving birth Ambivalence about effect of pregnancy and child care on work life, body image, and personal needs Hanging on to grief and loss	Infertility Miscarriage Dysfunctional labor
CERVIX/VAGINA, VULVA	Discretion about intimacy Ability to create healthy boundaries	Poorly defined boundaries in relationships Sexual or other relationships (e.g., work) that detract from well-being Guilt or shame about sexual pleasure or sexuality	Herpes Warts Chronic vulvar pain (vulvodynia) Vaginal infections Abnormal Pap smears Cervical cancer
URINARY TRACT, BLADDER	Capacity to feel emotions fully and discharge completely	Being chronically "pissed off" at life in general Stagnated flow of emotions in relationships Dependency in relationships Inability to release outmoded thoughts Inability to "go with the flow"	Chronic urinary tract infection Interstitial cystitis

Body Organ or Process	Encoded Wisdom	Energy Dysfunction	Physical Manifestation
MENOPAUSE	Passage into the wisdom years	Unfinished business from past that is unaddressed	Incapacitating hot flashes
	Capacity to be open to constant intuitive knowing	Fear of aging process	Melancholia Depression Palpitations
	Reseeding the community		Anxiety Forgetfulness

OUR CYCLICAL NATURE

The menstrual cycle is the most basic, earthy cycle we have. Our blood is our connection to the archetypal feminine. The macrocosmic cycles of nature, the waxing and waning, the ebb and flow of the tides and the changes of the seasons, are reflected on a smaller scale in the menstrual cycle of the individual female body. The monthly ripening of an egg and subsequent pregnancy or release of menstrual blood mirror the process of creation as it occurs not only in nature, unconsciously, but in human endeavor. In many cultures, the menstrual cycle has been viewed as sacred.

Even in modern society, where we are cut off from the rhythms of nature, the cycle of ovulation is influenced by the moon. Studies have shown that peak rates of conception and probably ovulation appear to occur at the full moon or the day before. During the new moon, ovulation and conception rates are decreased overall, and an increased number of women start their menstrual bleeding. Scientific research has documented that the moon rules the flow of fluids (ocean tides as well as individual body fluids) and affects the unconscious mind and dreams.[1] The timing of the menstrual cycle, the fertility cycle, and labor also follows the moon-dominated tides of the ocean. Environmental cues such as light, the moon, and the tides play a documented role in regulating women's menstrual cycles and fertility. In one study of nearly two thousand women with irregular menstrual cycles, more than half of the subjects achieved regular menstrual cycles of twenty-nine days' length by sleeping with a light on near their beds during the three days around ovulation.[2]

The menstrual cycle governs the flow not only of fluids but of information and creativity. We receive and process information differently at different times in our cycles. I like to describe menstrual cycle wisdom this way: from the onset of menstruation until ovulation, we're ripening an egg and—symbolically, at least—preparing to give birth to someone (or something) else, a role that society honors. Many women find that they are at their peak of expression in the outer world from the onset of their menstrual cycle until ovulation. Their energy is outgoing and upbeat. They are filled with enthusiasm and new ideas as well as being quite willing to fold the towels and fulfill their perceived role of helping others. At midcycle, we are naturally more receptive to others and to new ideas—more "fertile." Sexual desire also peaks for many women at midcycle, and our bodies secrete into the air pheromones that increase our sexual attractiveness to others.[3] (Our male-dominated society values this very highly, and we internalize it as a "good" stage of our cycle.) One woman, a waitress who works in a diner where many truckers stop to eat, has reported to me that her tips are highest at midcycle, around ovulation. Another man described his wife as "very vital and electric" during this time of her cycle.

The Follicular and Luteal Phases

The menstrual cycle itself mirrors how consciousness becomes matter and how thought creates reality. On the strictly physical level, during the time between menses and ovulation (known as the follicular phase) an egg grows and develops, while deep within the wall of the uterus circular collections of immune system cells, known as lymphoid aggregates, also begin to develop.[4] On the expanded level of ideas and creativity, this first half of the cycle is a very good time to initiate new projects. A researcher friend of mine tells me that she has the most energy to act on ideas for new experiments during this part of her cycle. Ovulation, which occurs at midcycle, is accompanied by an abrupt rise in the neuropeptides FSH (follicle stimulating hormone) and LH (luteinizing hormone). The rise in estrogen levels that accompanies this has been associated with a rise in left-hemisphere activity (verbal fluency) and a decline in right-hemisphere activity (visual-spatial ability, such as the ability to draw a cube or read a map).[5] But this may be offset by the simultaneous peak in testosterone production, which enhances visual-spatial ability while also increasing libido. Ovulation represents mental and emotional creativity at its peak; FSH-LH surge and subsequent rise in hormone production that accompanies ovulation may be the biological basis for this. The weeks following ovulation lead up to the menses; this is evaluative and reflective time, looking back upon what is created and on the negative or difficult aspects of our lives that need to be changed or adjusted. My researcher friend notes that during this part of her cycle, she prefers to do routine tasks that do not require much input from others or expansive thought on her part.

Our creative biological and psychological cycle parallels the phases of the moon; recent research has found that the immune system of the reproductive tract is cyclic as well, reaching its peak at ovulation, and then beginning to wane. From ancient times, some cultures have referred to women having their menstrual periods as being "on their moon." When women live together in natural settings, their ovulations tend to occur at the time of the full moon, with menses and self-reflection at the dark of the moon. Scientific evidence suggests that biological cycles as well as dreams and emotional rhythms are keyed into the moon and tides as well as the planets. Specifically, the moon and tides interact with the electromagnetic fields of our bodies, subsequently affecting our internal physiological processes. The moon itself has a period when it is covered with darkness, and then slowly, beginning at the time of the new moon, it becomes visible to us again, gradually waxing to fullness. Women, too, go through a period of darkness each month, when the life-force may seem to disappear for a while (premenstrual and menstrual phases).[6] We need not be afraid or think we are sick if our energies and moods naturally ebb for a few days each month. In many parts of India, it's perfectly acceptable for women to

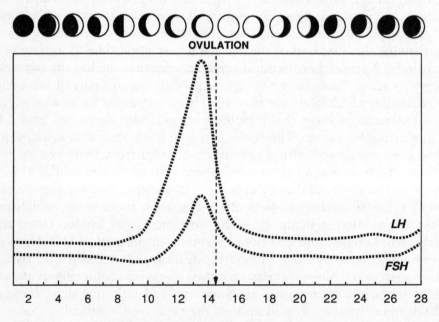

FIGURE 3: MENSTRUAL CYCLE (DAYS)

slow down during their periods and rest more. I have come to see that all kinds of stress-related disease, ranging from PMS to osteoporosis, could be lessened a great deal if we simply followed our body's wisdom once per month. Demetra George writes that it is here, at the dark of the moon, that "life cleanses, revitalizes, and transforms itself in its evolutionary development, spiraling toward attunement with its essential nature."[7] Studies have shown that most women begin their menstrual periods during the dark of the moon (new moon) and begin bleeding between four and six A.M.—the darkest part of the day.[8] Many women, including me, have noticed that on the first day or two of our periods, we feel an urge to organize our homes or work spaces, cleaning out our closets—and our lives. Our natural biological cleansing is accompanied by a psychological cleansing as well.

If we do not become biologically pregnant at ovulation, we move into the second half of the cycle, the luteal phase—ovulation through the onset of menstruation. During this phase, we quite naturally retreat from outward activity to a more reflective mode. During the luteal phase we turn more inward, preparing *to develop or give birth to something that comes from deep within ourselves*. Society is not nearly as keen on this as it is on the follicular phase. Thus we judge our premenstrual energy, emotions, and inward mood as "bad" and "unproductive." (See figure 4, page 108.)

Since our culture generally appreciates only what we can understand rationally, many women tend to block at every opportunity the flow of unconscious "lunar" information that comes to them premenstrually or during their menstrual cycle. Lunar information is reflective and intuitive. It comes to us in our dreams, our emotions, and our hungers. It comes under cover of darkness. When we routinely block the information that is coming to us in the second half of our menstrual cycles, it has no choice but to come back as PMS or menopausal madness, in the same way that our other feelings and bodily symptoms, if ignored, often result in illness.[9]

The luteal phase, from ovulation until the onset of menstruation, is when women are *most in tune with their inner knowing and with what isn't working in their lives*. Studies have shown that women's dreams are more frequent and often more vivid during the premenstrual and menstrual phases of their cycles.[10] Premenstrually, the "veil" between the worlds of the seen and unseen, the conscious and the unconscious, is much thinner. We have access to parts of our often unconscious selves that are less available to us at all other times of the month. In fact, it has been shown experimentally that the right hemisphere of the brain— the part associated with intuitive knowing—becomes more active

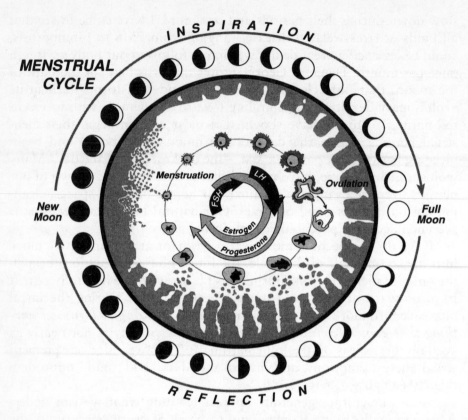

FIGURE 4: LUNAR CHART FOR MENSTRUAL CYCLE

premenstrually, while the left hemisphere becomes less active. Interestingly enough, communication between the two hemispheres may be increased as well.[11] The premenstrual phase is therefore a time when we have greater access to our magic—our ability to recognize and transform the more difficult and painful areas of our lives. Premenstrually, we are quite naturally more in tune with what is most meaningful in our lives. We're more apt to cry—but our tears are always related to something that holds meaning for us. The many studies of Dr. Katerina Dalton have documented that women are more emotional premenstrually, more apt to act out their anger, and more prone to headaches and fatigue, and they may even experience exacerbations of ongoing illnesses such as arthritis. To the extent that we are out of touch with the hidden parts of ourselves, we will suffer premenstrually. Years of personal and clinical experience have taught me that the painful or uncomfortable issues that arise premenstrually are always real and must be addressed.

Women need to believe in the importance of the issues that come up premenstrually. Even though our bodies and minds may not express these issues and concerns as they would in the first part of our cycle—on our so-called good days—our inner wisdom is clearly asking for our attention. One woman told me, for example, that whenever she becomes premenstrual, she worries that the house, car, and investments are in her husband's name only. When she mentions this to her husband, he replies, "What's wrong? Don't you trust me?" I'd call that a premenstrual reality check that needs attention! One husband reported that in the follicular phase of his wife's cycle, she was great, was always cheery, kept the house in order, and did the cooking. But after ovulation she "let herself go" and talked about wanting to go back to college and get out of the house more. I told him that these issues that arise premenstrually should be treated seriously, and I asked him to consider that his wife's needs were for her full personal development. I pointed out that her difficult behavior premenstrually was her way of expressing those needs. She, of course, also needs to learn how to articulate her needs directly!

There is an intimate relationship between a woman's psyche and her ovarian function throughout the menstrual cycle. Before we ovulate we are outgoing and upbeat, while ovulating we are very receptive to others, and after ovulation (premenstrually) we are more inward and reflective. An astounding study done in the 1930s supports my observations. The psychoanalyst Dr. Therese Benedek studied the psychotherapy records of a group of patients, while her colleague Dr. Boris Rubenstein studied the ovarian hormonal cycles of the same women. By looking at a woman's emotional content, Dr. Benedek was able to predict where she was in her menstrual cycle with incredible accuracy. The authors wrote, "We were pleased and surprised to find an exact correspondence of the ovulative dates as independently determined by the two methods"—that is, psychoanalytic material compared with physiological findings. They found that before ovulation, when estrogen levels were at their highest, women's emotions and behavior were directed toward the outer world. During ovulation, however, women were more relaxed and content and quite receptive to being cared for and loved by others. During the postovulatory and premenstrual phase, when progesterone is at its highest, women were more likely to be focused on themselves and more involved in inward-directed activity. Interestingly, in women who had periods but did not ovulate, the authors saw similar cycles of emotions and behavior, except that around the time when ovulation should have occurred, these women missed not only ovulation but the accompanying emotions;

that is, they were not relaxed, content, or receptive to being cared for by others.[12]

Given our cultural heritage and beliefs about illness in general and the menstrual cycle in particular, it is not difficult to understand how women have come to see their premenstrual phase not as a time for reflection and renewal but as a disease or a curse. In fact, the language that our culture uses regarding the uterus and ovaries has been experimentally shown to affect women's menstrual cycles. Under hypnosis, a woman who is given positive suggestions about her menstrual cycle will be much less apt to suffer from menstruation-related symptoms.[13] On the other hand, one study found that women who were led to believe that they were premenstrual when they weren't reported more adverse physical symptoms, such as water retention, cramps, and irritability, than another group who were led to believe they were not premenstrual.[14] These studies are excellent examples of how our thoughts and beliefs have the power to affect our hormones, our biochemistry, and our subsequent experience.

Healing Through Our Cycles

Once we begin to appreciate our menstrual cycle as part of our inner guidance system, we begin to heal both hormonally and emotionally. There is no doubt that premenstrually, many women feel more inward-directed and more connected to their personal pain and the pain of the world. Many such women are also more in touch with their own creativity and get their best ideas premenstrually, though they may not act on them until later. During the premenstrual phase, we need time to be alone, time to rest, and time away from our daily duties, but taking this time is a new idea and practice for many women. Premenstrual syndrome results when we don't honor our need to ebb and flow like the tides. This society likes action, so we often don't appreciate our need for rest and replenishment. We would do well to remember that all the functions of our bodies have both an active (yang) and receptive (yin) phase. The heart actively contracts during systole, sending the blood out into the vessels. (This is the top number we measure when taking blood pressure.) The space between heart contractions, known as diastole (the lower number of blood pressure), is equally important. Without adequate relaxation in this phase, the entire cardiovascular system suffers under too much strain—the same is true in our lives and during our menstrual cycles. The menstrual cycle is set up to teach us about the need for both the in-breath and the out-

breath of life's processes. When we are premenstrual and feeling frag-
ile, we need to rest and take care of ourselves for a day or two. In the
Native American moon lodge, bleeding women came together for renewal and visioning and emerged afterward inspired and also inspiring
to others. I think that the majority of PMS cases would disappear if
every modern woman retreated from her duties for three or four days
each month and had her meals brought to her by someone else.

I personally found that simply and *unapologetically* stating my
needs for a monthly slowdown to my former husband was all that was
needed. When I showed respect for myself and the processes of my
body, he showed respect as well, and my body responded with comfort
and gratitude. Indeed, my experience of my own menstrual cycle began to change after I noticed that my most meaningful insights about
myself, my life, and my writing came on the day or two just before my
period. In my mid-thirties, I began to look forward to my periods, understanding them to be sacred time that our culture didn't honor.
When I was premenstrual, the things that made me feel teary were the
things that were most important to me, things that I knew tuned me in
to my power and my deepest truths. My increased sensitivity felt like
a gift of insight. I didn't become angry, though if I did, I knew to pay
attention and not chalk it up to "my stupid hormones." I liked to keep
track of the phases of the moon in my daily calendar to see if I was
ovulating at the full moon, the dark of the moon, or in between. When
I ovulated at the full moon and menstruated at the dark of the moon,
my inner reflective time was synchronized with the moon's darkness.
Getting my period at the time of the full moon resulted in a more intense period: I was more emotionally charged than usual, and my
bleeding was often heavier than normal. I found that sometimes simply intending to bleed at the dark of the moon tended to move my cycles in this direction, though not always. (I didn't "try" to control
this.) Noting my individual cycle in relationship to the moon's cycle
consciously connected me with the earth and helped me to feel connected with women past and present. Truly welcoming and appreciating my cycles in this way also made the transition into menopause
much easier.

OUR CULTURAL INHERITANCE

The menstrual cycle and the female body were seen as sacred until
five thousand years ago, when the peaceful matrilineal cultures of Old
Europe were overturned.[15] The original meaning of the word *taboo* was

"sacred," and women having their periods were considered sacred; now in some societies they are considered unclean. Often their dreams and visions were used to guide the tribe. Native cultures the world over have honored young women with coming-of-age ceremonies. First menstruation has meant being initiated into the "offices of woman-hood" by mothers, aunts, and other initiated women.[16] Archaeological evidence from more than six thousand years ago points to the fact that the original calendars were bones with small marks on them that women used to keep track of their cycles.[17] Yet throughout much of written Western history, and even in religious codes, the menstrual cycle has been associated with shame and degradation, with women's dark, uncontrollable nature. Menstruating women were thought of as unclean. In A.D. 65, in his encyclopedia, *Natural History*, Pliny the Elder wrote:

> But nothing could easily be found that is more remarkable [note the ambivalent word choice!] than the monthly flux of women. Contact with it turns new wine sour, crops touched by it become barren, seeds in gardens dry up, the fruit of trees fall off. The bright surface of mirrors in which it is merely reflected is dimmed, the edge of steel and the gleam of ivory are dulled. Hives of bees will die. Even bronze and iron are at once seized by rust and a horrible smell fills the air. To taste it drives dogs mad and affects their bite with an incurable poison.[18]

The taboo associated with the menstrual cycle has continued to this day. Generations of women have been taught that we are more physically vulnerable during our periods—that we can't swim, bathe, or wash our hair during those days. These beliefs were originally based on the Victorian theory that bathing, shampooing hair, or swimming might "back up" menstrual flow, resulting in stroke, insanity, or rapid onset of tuberculosis.[19] More recently, it has been felt that contact with water during this time would result in catching a cold. There is no scientific basis for any of these taboos, yet they have served to keep women afraid of a natural bodily process for generations.

If we are to reclaim our menstrual wisdom and honor our cyclic natures, we must at the same time acknowledge the negative attitudes that most of us have internalized concerning our menstrual cycles. We must acknowledge the pain and discomfort that many women experience monthly. Our cyclic nature has borne the brunt of all kinds of jokes about being "on the rag" or having "the curse." Puberty and the first menstruation for many women have been saturated with shame and humiliation. Nothing in our society—with the exception of violence and fear—has been more effective in keeping women "in their place" than the degradation of the menstrual cycle. It's gratifying to see that this attitude is now changing as our culture realizes that the first menses is an important rite of passage.

Replacing the harmful inherited myths about our menstrual cycles with accurate information is part of women's healing. After menarche (the first menstruation), which generally occurs around the age of twelve in this society, a young woman reaches sexual maturity. A certain body composition is required for the onset of menarche. Usually the body mass must be about 17 percent fat for a young woman to start having periods. Studies have indicated that a body fat level averaging about 22 percent is necessary for sustained ovulatory cycles in most females.[20] This is one reason why anorexic young women and female dancers and athletes who are very thin don't have regular periods, though emotional factors that affect the hypothalamus of the brain also play a key role in these situations. Though a young woman's first cycles are usually not ovulatory, she gradually becomes fertile over the next several years, producing an egg each month from her ovaries. If the monthly egg is not fertilized at midcycle, this results in a menstrual period about fourteen days after ovulation. In the flow, the lining of the uterus (the endometrium) is shed. Each month, the lining, or endometrium, builds up and is shed cyclically, stimulated by a complex and amazing interaction between hormones produced by the ovaries, the pituitary gland, and the hypothalamus. (See figure 5, page 116.) Because of the complexity of this hormonal interaction, many areas of a woman's life affect the menstrual cycle. The cycle in turn affects many areas of a woman's life.

Most girls learn about the menstrual cycle in a sterile, clinical way, without respect for their female bodies and their own sexuality. How their bodies and sexuality are linked to the menstrual cycle is rarely discussed. In the past, very few girls were introduced to menstruation as a positive rite of passage. My mother told me the "facts of life" and explained eggs and sperm. I recall being very upset by this information. I was in the fourth grade. My sister, eleven months younger than I, had said earlier that day, "Mom, I know where babies come from, but how do they get there?" My mother took us into her bedroom and read us a book that said that girls get a menstrual period around the age of twelve, and that after they get their period they could have a baby if they had sex.

I was not happy with this information. I continued to hope that women could get pregnant by kissing rather than by the disgusting act my mother described. Why I found the whole thing so disgusting might have had something to do with my own mother's initiation into puberty. She was not concerned with the meaning of the menstrual cycle and the sacredness of the female body, though she was and is a woman who is truly wise and ahead of her time. My mother had learned that once she got her period, somehow she could no longer enjoy herself in the same way. Her favorite girlhood activities had been playing baseball and climbing trees with the boys. But once she "became a woman," she was no longer allowed to play with the boys. Years later, she told me that she begged her mother to take her to the hospital to "get her fixed" so that she wouldn't have periods anymore and could go back to baseball. Because my mother didn't completely resolve her adolescent feelings about her menstrual cycle until she was in her sixties, I absorbed some of her unconscious feelings around menstruation, even though she presented it to me as a normal part of life.

Instead of celebrating our cyclic nature as a positive aspect of our female being, our culture teaches us that we shouldn't acknowledge our periods at all, lest we neglect the needs of our spouses and children. Consider this excerpt from a 1963 insert inside a tampon box:

WHEN YOU'RE A WIFE

Don't take advantage of your husband. That's an old rule of good marriage behavior that's just as sensible now as it ever was. Of course, you'll not try to take advantage, but sometimes ways of taking advantage aren't obvious.

You wouldn't connect it with menstruation, for instance. Yet, if you neglect the simple rules that make menstruation a normal time of month, and retire for a few days each month, as though you were ill, you're taking advantage of your husband's good nature. He married a full-time wife, not a part-time one. So you should be active, peppy, and cheerful every day.[21]

Always cheery—just like those old Doris Day movies. No wonder so many women have PMS! When I think of the indoctrination represented by that 1963 insert, in the year I got my first period, I wonder how we women have come as far as we have.

The Menstrual Cycle, Birth Control Pills, and Women's Intuition

Our intuition works differently during the various phases of our menstrual cycle. It changes again after menopause. One of my colleagues, an osteopathic physician, noticed this connection between intuition and the menstrual cycle when he referred a patient to me for a change in birth control method. She had been on the pill for a number of years, but he felt that continued use of the pill was interfering with her ability to know what her next steps in life should be. The referral note to me read: "Birth control pills are interfering with intuitive function. Suggest alternatives." I applaud this doctor for his insight.

In an age in which millions of women's bodies, due to the use of birth control pills, are more in tune with pharmaceutical companies than with the moon, it is no small task to rethink a medication that has offered so many women such highly touted advantages. After all, the pill provides women with periods that need never ruin their weekends, it often decreases menstrual cramps, and it is associated with a decreased risk of ovarian and endometrial cancer. Women are now being sold on the benefits of Seasonale, a birth control pill that results in only four periods per year. One for each season! But then, no one is sure whether the pill increases the risk of breast cancer, although studies have shown that it can increase the risk of cervical cancer.

Laurie, one of my colleagues in OB/GYN, was on the pill for over nine years before she changed her mind about its advantages. She had routinely pushed the pill as a panacea for all her patients, using her own experience as coercion. When she lectured them on why they should all be on the pill, she always ended her talk with the statement "They'll never get my pills away from me." Only after Laurie began to see her own illnesses as physical manifestations of the diseases in her spirit was she able to reevaluate her position on the pill. The breakthrough for her happened in part because her relationship with her husband had begun to deteriorate. They were having frequent arguments around the subject of sex. "It drove me crazy," she said, "that he seemed to separate it completely from everything else that was going on in our relationship. At the same time, my own confusion about my body, my feelings of discomfort with its size and shape, my inhibitions about noise and awkwardness during sex, and mixed messages from my childhood about sex and seduction made sex something fraught with negative connotation and sometimes insurmountable obstacles."

Laurie was learning about how different parts of our bodies talk to

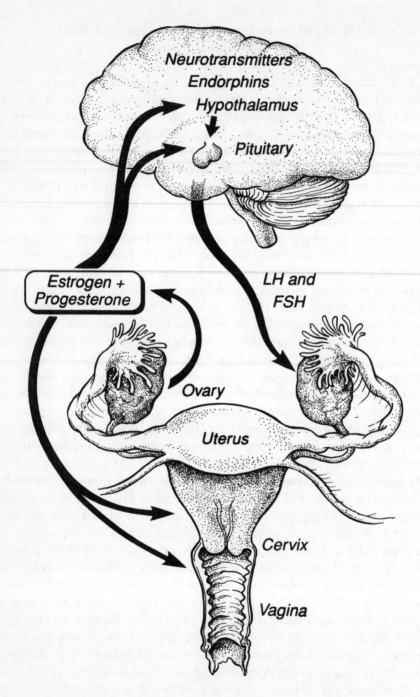

FIGURE 5: THE FEMALE MIND/BODY CONTINUUM:
INTERACTIONS BETWEEN THE BRAIN AND THE PELVIS

us through symptoms as part of our inner guidance system. As she did, she realized that remaining on birth control pills might prevent her female organs from optimally communicating with her, especially in a personal crisis around her own sexuality. She began to awaken to how she had inadvertently become separated from her body by following the dictates of the culture instead of her inner guidance. This awakening was accompanied by an interest in feminism for the first time in her life. Up until then, she had considered herself highly successful and functional, which is how she seems on the surface. Yet she had had a benign ovarian cyst, operated on several years before, and during her OB/GYN residency she had been operated on for thyroid cancer. Her emerging inner wisdom showed her that these conditions had been her body's way of trying to get her attention and let her know that something was off balance in her life. Now she was willing and eager to pay attention to what her body was saying, especially since she was healthy.

"I felt sadness," Laurie says, "that I had taken for granted, drugged away, or labeled a 'curse' all the wondrous workings of my brain, my hormones, my uterus, and my ovaries. No one ever celebrated my first period. No one had helped me connect the power of giving birth to my sexuality. I longed to recapture some of that lost magic and mystery. But it took me almost two years of pulling down the curtains of my life and dusting away the cobwebs before I felt that I could tentatively trust my body."

After these two years of personal struggle, Laurie decided to take a year off from her busy obstetrical practice in a large city. She was exhausted from the demands of three children, her practice, and now a marriage that was ending. She knew that she needed to reflect on her life and explore some new directions. She said that when she finally got around to doing it, going off the pill was "something of an act of celebration and rebellion." It was clear to her that a divorce was imminent. "Since I did not need contraception anymore," she observed, "it occurred to me that now might be the time to allow myself the luxury of my hormones. So I threw away the last dial-pack and waited. I was pretty sure that after nine years of instruction from Ortho Pharmaceutical, my ovaries would be totally confused, so I was willing to be patient. I was prepared for swelling, irritability, wild emotions, and confusion. I was not prepared for what happened."

Two weeks after stopping the pill, Laurie was sitting with a group of women and relating the events of the past two years. She noted, "Suddenly, I was in tears and I could hardly speak. I remember thinking, 'Now isn't this strange?'" It took her a while to realize that even though she did indeed feel sadness about the changes under way in her life, she had in fact told others about these changes and feelings before, while she was on the pill, without any emotional or physiological reaction whatsoever. She discovered that for her, ovulation was associated with an increased ability to feel and express her deepest emotions. She wrote, "I didn't realize for two more days that the excessive cervical mucus [a very common sign of ovulation] and the sudden opening of the emotional floodgate were signs of ovulation. Even when I did put it together, I refused to trust my body. 'Well,' I thought, 'I'll just wait two weeks and see.' Two weeks later, there I was in my red dress—my first spontaneous period in over nine years, never a more welcome sight. I felt as though I had been given a wondrous gift from a long-lost friend. This body, which I had abused for so long and in so many ways, was suddenly talking to me again, giving me encouragement and reassurance. All was not lost."

In addition to finding that her emotions were now more available to her, Laurie found that she was more in touch with anger that she would have previously denied. She related that shortly after her own periods resumed, "I found my anger. My righteous, fiery, white-hot anger. Of course, my husband was the unwitting recipient of what felt like twenty years of suppressed emotions. I don't know if he deserved all of it—certainly not all at once. But as it came pouring out, I remember thinking, 'This is amazing! This is really me. My hormones. My magic!' I think now that if I had been feeling that anger as it came up all those years, I might still be married—or I would have divorced much sooner. Either way would have been better than what had happened. It was not okay that I had missed so much of myself."

Laurie knew to honor and pay attention to what was happening to her, even though some of it was painful. She later reflected, "Since then I have learned to expect to hear regularly from my hormones. They teach me where I still need to put my attention. When I am suddenly in tears, I know to pause and consider what emotional work I still have to do in that area. When anger comes, I remind myself that being able to push it down inside myself is not a gift. Anger unexpressed produces disease. It belongs outside my body."

The other thing that Laurie noticed was the connection between her menstrual cycle and her inherent sexuality. I have heard similar stories from many women. She told me, "There is this wild desire racing around in my brain for several days every month around ovulation. My friends told me about it, but this is amazing. And I thought all those years that the pill was helping my sex life by getting rid of all those messy barrier contraceptives!" (The pill suppresses the midcycle testosterone surge, thus decreasing sex drive in many women.)[22] She had used the diaphragm only while breast-feeding, and she realized she had blamed her lack of sexual desire on the messiness of diaphragm use. But now she understood that her lack of desire was most likely related to breast-feeding hormones and energy drain, not the diaphragm. Many nursing mothers simply are not interested in sexual intercourse, for complex reasons related to lack of support and sleep as well as conventional birth practices that lower oxytocin and endorphin levels. This needn't be the case. Sexual desire resumes gradually as the baby gets older, but this is not inevitable.[23]

Laurie noted another change that is very common. After going off the pill, her body tended to make up for lost time, with ovulations coming more frequently for a while, then adjusting to approximately once per month. "When I first reclaimed my cycles," she wrote, "they were very short, about every three weeks. Although the thought flashed through my head briefly that it would be a pain to be bleeding one week out of every three, I realized that the thought was a conditioned one. How many forty-year-old women had complained to me about the increasing frequency of their periods and begged me to 'do something' about it? Now I realized that I had been given a gift of short cycles to 'catch up.' I loved getting to cycle more often. I got to ovulate every three weeks. I got more lessons about my body. It was like a crash course in female physiology—my own. I began to celebrate getting my periods every three weeks and hoped that menopause would not come until I was sixty-five. Having given myself permission to enjoy all these new lessons, I once again learned that I was not in control—my cycles began to spread out to three and a half, then four weeks. I think it was just a test, having three-week cycles. It was to see if I really wanted this part of my body back. I do."

Laurie's story illustrates what reclaiming our menstrual wisdom and power feels like. Though the pill has been a boon to many women, it has also taken them out of touch with some essential parts of their female wisdom. When people are in close contact with one another, for example, one way they communicate is via pheromones. Oral contraceptives, however, have been shown to eliminate part of our pheromonal communication pathway, including our sexual communication with men. It has now been well established that women secrete pheromones around ovulation that are definitely associated with greater romantic interest from men. The birth control pill blocks these.[24] Women who live together often cycle together, in a process one of my friends calls "becoming ovarian sisters." This doesn't happen to women on the pill. Studies have shown that women who have close relationships with other people have shorter and more regular cycles, whereas women who isolate themselves are more likely to have irregular cycles.[25]

MENSTRUAL CRAMPS (DYSMENORRHEA)

As many as 60 percent of all women suffer from menstrual cramps. A smaller percentage are unable to function for one or more days each month because of the severity of their pain. The fact that the majority of women in our culture suffer from menstrual cramps is a very clear indication that we have something wrong with our relationship to our bodies. It testifies that we have lost much of our connection to our menstrual wisdom. The psychological gynecological literature of the 1950s was filled with studies that suggested that menstrual cramps were mainly psychological, related to being unhappy about being a woman. Caroline Myss says that cramps and PMS are classic indications that a woman is in some kind of conflict with being a woman, with her role in the tribe, and with the tribal expectations of her. Given our current society's traditional expectations for women, it's amazing that 100 percent of us don't have cramps and PMS.

Cramps are not the same as PMS, although women often suffer from both. Dysmenorrhea is divided into two types. Primary dysmenorrhea is cramps that are not secondary to another organic disease in the pelvis. Secondary dysmenorrhea is cramps that are caused by endometriosis or other pelvic disease. Treatments that help primary dysmenorrhea usually help secondary dysmenorrhea as well.

I had primary dysmenorrhea in my teens and up until after the birth of my first child. I sometimes had to call my mother from school and leave class because of the pain. Once during my residency I even had to leave a major surgical case because of menstrual cramps. One of my fellow residents said to me, "Gee, Chris, *you* have cramps? Must be it's not all in women's heads!" (Remember, I was "one of the guys" back then and was doing everything in my power to maintain that position. You can imagine what a blow it was to have to leave the operating room because of that dreaded female weakness, *cramps*!)

Beginning in the late 1970s, studies showed that women with cramps have high levels of the hormone prostaglandin F2 alpha (PGF2 alpha) in their menstrual blood. When this hormone is released into the bloodstream as the endometrial lining breaks down, the uterus goes into spasm, resulting in cramping pain.[26] (Menstrual cramps are not in the head after all—they're in the uterus! Actually it's not either/or. What goes on in the head does affect what goes on in the uterus.)

When I first got my period, I developed astigmatism and myopia and had to get glasses. I resented this—no one else in the family had glasses. I now know there was something I didn't want to see. I was unmistakably a girl in a family where male pursuits reigned supreme! My vision problem was exacerbated by reading without adequate breaks to rest my eyes. I was conflicted about growing up in general and growing up as a girl in particular, just as my mother had been. The increased stress of puberty produced high levels of the stress hormones cortisol, norepinephrine, and subsequently insulin, the hormone that helps the body process glucose. High stress hormone levels, in combination with my diet of too much dairy food and too many refined carbohydrates, resulted in an overproduction of insulin, and the overproduction of the inflammatory chemical PGF2 alpha in the lining of my uterus. Bad cramps were the result! The cramps disappeared for a while after the birth of my first child, but they came back, though much milder and not with every period, when my second daughter was about five. This time of no cramps taught me that when my life was in balance, I didn't have cramps. When I became too busy or stressed out, producing too much cortisol, norepinephrine, and insulin, my body produced too many inflammatory chemicals and I'd have a few hours of cramps on the first day of my period. They slowed me right down and were a good reminder that I needed to make some adjustments and to tune in to the wisdom of my body.

Treatment

Diet. A nutrient-poor diet that contains too many refined foods that raise blood sugar levels too quickly (known as high glycemic index foods) favors the production of inflammatory chemicals throughout the body that result in pain and tissue damage. These inflammatory chemicals (also known as eicosanoids) go by a wide variety of names including cytokines, bradykinins, interleukins, and prostaglandins (including PGF2 alpha) and prostacyclins. Many of the most common drugs on the market, including aspirin, block the effects of these substances! When high glycemic index foods are consumed in an individual who also has high circulating levels of stress hormones, the production of inflammatory chemicals is made even worse. Menstrual cramps are just one manifestation of this vicious cycle. Others include fluid retention, headaches, insomnia, and muscle aches and pains. In fact, all of the symptoms of PMS (see page 128) are caused, in part, by cellular inflammation from the overproduction of inflammatory chemicals.

Therefore, a dietary approach that decreases the production of these inflammatory chemicals is the backbone for treatment of cramps and many other health problems. (For a full discussion, see chapter 17.) The basic approach is the following: Eliminate or greatly reduce all "white foods" such as those made with white sugar and white flour. Decrease grain products to no more than two or three servings per day. Diet should consist mostly of fresh vegetables and fruits along with lean protein such as chicken, fish, tofu, eggs, beans, and soy products. Essential fatty acids are also crucial for producing hormonal balance and eliminating cellular inflammation. And so are an adequate amount of vitamins C and E, magnesium, and many other nutrients. (See chapter 17 for vitamin recommendations.)

NUTRITIONAL TREATMENTS

~ Stop dairy foods, especially ice cream, cottage cheese, and yogurt.

It has been my clinical experience that many women get relief of symptoms such as menstrual cramps, heavy bleeding, breast pain, and endometriosis pain when they stop consuming dairy foods. This is not true for everyone, but it works often enough to be worth a try. Though it's not clear why dairy foods seem to be associated with women's pelvic symptoms, I have a few theories. One possible explanation is that most milk today is produced by cows treated with BGH (bovine growth hormone), which overstimulates the cow's udder. These cows are more likely to have infected udders and thus require antibiotics. Both hormone and antibiotic residues in the milk may stimulate the female hormonal system in some way we are not yet able to pinpoint. We do know that antibiotics fed to livestock make their way into the human food chain. Antibiotics change the way hormones are metabolized in the bowel and thus can change hormonal levels. Other research suggests that the milk sugar lactose may have a toxic effect on the ovaries. The research of Daniel Cramer, M.D., Sc.D., at Brigham and Women's Hospital in Boston has linked milk sugar lactose consumption with increased risk of ovarian cancer. He found that women who consume one or more servings of skim or low-fat milk daily had a 32 percent higher risk of epithelial ovarian cancer compared with those who consumed three or less servings monthly.[27]

Dairy foods produced organically, without BGH, antibiotics, or pesticides in the cow's feed, don't seem to have the same adverse effect on uterine and breast tissue. Many women have noted that when they change to organically produced dairy foods, their symptoms go away. Experiment and discover what works for you. But be willing to stop dairy foods for a while to see if you notice any benefits. Make sure you get your calcium from other sources.

~ Cut way down on or eliminate refined carbohydrates. More than any other food, excess carbohydrates—especially refined ones such as those in cookies, cake, chips, crackers, and so on—can trigger high blood sugar and insulin levels, which result in an increase in prostaglandins, setting the stage for cramps.

~ Limit red meat and egg yolks to no more than two servings per week, or eliminate them. If you do eat red meat, use low-fat cuts from organically raised animals. Red meat and egg yolks are very rich in arachidonic acid (AA), which can result in increased cellular inflammation and uterine cramps in susceptible individuals. Not all individuals are sensitive to AA, so this recommendation will not apply to everyone; to find out if you are sensitive to AA, avoid all red meat and egg yolks for three weeks, then eat several servings in one day and see if your symptoms return. Red meat can be very high in saturated fats, which also can increase cellular inflammation—that's why you need to stick with the low-fat cuts.

~ Take essential fatty acids. Omega-3 fatty acids in the form of fish oil, which contains DHA (docosahexaenoic acid), and EPA (eicosapentaenoic acid) have been shown to work well for menstrual cramps even in those who didn't change other aspects of their diets. A recent study suggested a dosage of 1,000 mg EPA, 720 mg DHA, together with 1.5 mg vitamin E; you can use any amount that approximates this. Because fish oil degenerates with exposure to oxygen, take capsules that have added vitamin E (to prevent oxidation). A much cheaper and often healthier alternative is to eat sardines packed in their own oil or in olive oil two to three times per week. Other coldwater fish such as mackerel, salmon, and swordfish are also good sources of fish oil.[28] DHA made from marine algae is also available (the brand name is Neuromins, and the usual dose is 400 mg one to two times per day). Flaxseed oil—500 mg two to four times per day—can also be used if fish oil is not available or if it is unacceptable. You can also buy fresh flaxseed and grind it in a coffee grinder just before adding it to soups, salads, or cereals. Usually one to two tablespoons per day of the fresh ground seeds will be enough.

~ Take a multivitamin-mineral supplement. The antioxidant effect of vitamins and minerals helps prevent cellular inflammation.

~ Take 100 mg vitamin B_6 per day, in combination with B complex. B_6 has been shown to decrease the intensity and duration of menstrual cramps.[29]

~ Take magnesium, as much as 100 mg every two hours during the menstrual cycle itself, and three or four times per day during the rest of the cycle. Magnesium relaxes smooth muscle tissue. Use a chelated form.[30] (See chapter 17.)

~ Take 50 mg vitamin E three times a day during the entire cycle. Vitamin E has also been shown to improve dysmenorrhea.[31] Vitamin E must be in the form of d-alpha tocopherol for it to have any biological effect.

~ Eliminate sources of trans-fatty acids whenever possible. These increase production of inflammatory chemicals associated with cramps. Trans-fatty acids are found in all foods containing partially hydrogenated oils. Margarine and solid vegetable shortening are examples. Check labels on all prepared foods.

Medication. Nonsteroidal anti-inflammatory drugs, such as Advil, Nuprin, Anaprox, and Motrin, block the synthesis of prostaglandin F2 alpha when taken just at the onset of periods, *before* the pain starts, or as soon after as possible. Once the endometrial lining begins to shed and prostaglandin F2 alpha (and other inflammatory chemicals) gets released into the bloodstream, it's much harder to interrupt the resulting uterine spasms that cause the pain.

Birth control pills, which eliminate ovulation and therefore the hormonal changes associated with cramps, work well for many women who are not interested in making lifestyle or dietary changes. Some women, however, get cramps even on oral contraceptives. The newer pills can be safely used by most women over thirty-five, as long as they do not smoke.

Energy Medicine.

⁓ Reduce stress.

⁓ Learn to appreciate the rhythms of your menstrual cycle.

⁓ Castor oil packs to the lower abdomen at least three times per week for several months improve immune system functioning and decrease stress and adrenaline levels. (See page 148.) Packs should not be used when you are bleeding heavily.

⁓ Acupuncture has been shown to eliminate or greatly decrease menstrual cramps, and I refer women for this regularly. The usual course of acupuncture is ten treatments, but many women feel relief after as few as three treatments.[32]

⁓ Moderate exercise helps lower stress hormone levels, which decreases cellular inflammation. Yoga is also good and often relieves cramps.

Herbs. In Chinese medicine, menstrual cramps are often associated with what is called "liver stagnation." Bupleurum (Xiao Yao Wan, also known as Hsiao Yao Wan) may help.[33] This Chinese herbal formula is available from any practitioner of Chinese medicine, and many of my patients have done very well with it. Take four or five of the tiny tablets four times per day two weeks before the period is due and continue through the first day of bleeding. It may take two or three months to experience optimal results. (See Resources for sources.)

Menastil, a roll-on product, is also very effective. (See Resources.)

⁓ Black cohosh, or "cramp bark," can also be used as a preventive. This herb is available in tablet or tincture form in natural food stores. Follow directions on the bottle.

Many women are helped by other measures such as massage, yoga, or homeopathy. Homeopathic remedies are best prescribed by a competent practitioner who is familiar with the field. The Wurn Technique, a noninvasive, nonsurgical type of deep tissue massage performed by specially trained physical therapists, can also be helpful in treating dysmenorrhea. (For more information, contact Clear Passage Therapies at 866-222-9437 or visit www.clearpassage.com.)

Maya Traditional Massage. Indigenous Mayan healers in Central America have long used a technique called Maya abdominal massage to treat many conditions of the pelvic organs, including painful periods.

After studying Mayan traditional healing in Central America for more than thirty years, Dr. Rosita Arvigo was the first person to bring these healing techniques to North America. She is a native of Chicago who has a degree in Naprapathic medicine and now practices in Belize. Naprapathy is a system of manipulation that is known for treating the damage to the body's ligaments including those in the joints, along the spine, and in the pelvis. (One of her books, *Sastun: My Apprenticeship with a Maya Healer* [HarperSanFrancisco, 1994], tells the story of her training under her mentor, renowned Belize shaman Don Elijio Panti.)

The technique involves a gentle massage of the muscles and ligaments in the pelvic region and realignment of any pelvic organs that have shifted position (such as in a tilted or prolapsed uterus). When these organs are not properly aligned, the flow of blood, lymph, nerve, and Qi (roughly translated as "life-force") is disrupted, which then compromises the function of other pelvic organs. In addition to irregular or painful periods, Dr. Arvigo explains, other conditions such as endometriosis, bladder and yeast infections, miscarriage, infertility, ovarian cysts, uterine fibroids, uterine bleeding, and low back pain can result. Maya abdominal massage practitioners report that this technique reduces adhesions from old surgeries, endometriosis, fibroid tumors, and ovarian cysts and that proper pelvic alignment is essential for normal pregnancy, labor, and delivery. (For more information, including a directory of certified practitioners of Maya abdominal massage, visit www.arvigomassage.com.)

Women's Stories

Jane: Healing Menstrual Cramps. Jane first came to see me at the age of twenty-six. She had had years of very, very painful periods, starting shortly after she began menstruating at age thirteen. She described the cramping as occurring before her actual period started and continuing after the bleeding had ended. She was worried that something might be seriously affecting her reproductive organs, such as endometriosis or an ovarian cyst.

Jane had tried birth control pills for about a month several years before, but she had stopped because she didn't like the way she felt on them. She also had tried Anaprox, a nonsteroidal anti-inflammatory medication similar to Motrin that is now available over the counter as Aleve. It had helped her somewhat, but she was still quite incapacitated. In addition to her cramps, she complained of heavy bleeding (going through one tampon per hour on the second day), premenstrual irritability, acne, bloating, tender breasts, and vaginal itching before her period. Neither of Jane's two sisters had menstrual cramps or other gynecological problems. Jane's diet was based on dairy foods, such as cottage cheese, ice cream, and yogurt, all of which she ate frequently.

Jane was an elementary-school teacher and was not very pleased with her work. She said that she had always wanted to move to Idaho but felt guilty about doing that because her parents didn't want her to move so far away. Her parents felt that it was very selfish of Jane to want to pursue her own interests. They felt that she should stay near them, continue in the security of teaching, marry, and have children. Jane's childhood desire to please her parents now came into direct conflict with her own need for personal growth. She came to see that staying near her parents and ignoring her own needs would only result in illness for herself. I pointed out that she was in a classic codependent dilemma and that she needed to come to terms with this in order to heal fully. In addition to meeting the expectations of her parents, the stress of doing work she no longer found fulfilling was weighing her down.

Jane had a completely normal pelvic exam, with no sign of a cyst, tenderness, or anything else suggestive of reproductive disease. I recommended the following course of action:

~ Apply castor oil packs to the lower abdomen two times per week. (A good alternative is taking warm baths for twenty to thirty minutes; add a few drops of rose oil, an aromatherapy treatment known for its soothing effects.)

~ Stop eating all dairy foods and red meat.

~ Take a multiple vitamin two or three times per day.

~ Begin plans to move to Idaho.

~ Do some reading on codependency.

When Jane returned to my office three months later, her cramps had markedly improved. She said that she was shocked by the difference she had felt after stopping dairy foods and red meat. Her bleeding had lightened considerably. She realized that her diet really had a large effect on her cramps, and she said that the castor oil packs "felt great." When she was using these, she took the time to tune in to herself and her needs, and she thought of living out her dreams instead of being stuck in old patterns that didn't serve her. She read some books on codependency and came to see that she had been trained to be a "people pleaser" since childhood. She realized that she had to learn how to please herself if she hoped to find her life satisfying. She had outgrown being the good little girl in the family.

After three months, Jane's periods were much easier and she had been able to decrease her Anaprox dose considerably, as she changed her diet and decreased her stress level. Most impressive of all, she made plans to move to Idaho and would not start the next school year in a job and place that she didn't like. Though the prospect of moving into the unknown was frightening to her, it was also exhilarating. If she hadn't made plans to live her own life separately from her parents, I believe that her health would eventually have been at risk because of her "niceness." By using her body's wisdom, Jane healed not only her menstrual cramps but also her life.

PREMENSTRUAL SYNDROME (PMS)

No modern disorder points to the need to rethink our ideas about menstruation and reclaim the wisdom of our cycles more directly than the common malady known as premenstrual syndrome, or PMS. Having treated hundreds of women with PMS, I know that such a rethinking is needed to get to the root causes of PMS. Dietary change, exercise, vitamins, and progesterone therapy are all useful in treating PMS, and I initially recommend them for many women. But in persistent cases of PMS, a deeper imbalance exists that lifestyle changes alone won't help. As studies have confirmed, unresolved emotional problems may disrupt the menstrual rhythm and the normal hormonal milieu.[34]

At least 60 percent of all women suffer from PMS. It is most likely to occur in women in their thirties, though it can occur as early as adolescence and as late as the premenopausal years. PMS has been known since ancient times, but it was popularized in the 1980s by an article in *Family Circle* magazine, which articulated the monthly suffering of millions of women. The media picked up on this, and within a few months PMS became a nationally known problem and a household word.[35] It also became a hot topic with feminists, who argued that the diagnosis would be used against women. Doctors worried that it would become a "wastebasket" diagnosis that women or their families would use as an excuse when no one could figure out what was really going on. Meanwhile, scores of women finally had a name for their monthly suffering and sought medical help for it.

The demand created by women and the media for treatment of

PMS had become such that by the mid-1980s, PMS was a lecture topic at many major OB/GYN specialty meetings, and research began appearing in the journals. Just as the desire for natural childbirth forced doctors to reform their patriarchal approach to obstetrical practice, women's desire to understand PMS influenced the practice of medicine and helped move it toward a more enlightened attitude toward the female body.

Diagnosis

A wide variety of symptoms can be present with PMS. In making the diagnosis, it doesn't matter what specific symptoms a woman has premenstrually. *What is important is the cyclic fashion in which they occur.* Women who chart their symptoms for three months or more often see a pattern and are able to predict when in their cycle their symptoms are likely to start. Most women will have at least three days during the month when they are entirely free from the symptoms listed here, except in very severe cases. In the second half of the menstrual cycle many underlying conditions are exacerbated, such as glaucoma, arthritis, and depression. Exacerbation of underlying conditions is not defined as PMS, though it is related to PMS. There are more than one hundred known symptoms of PMS.[36] Every one of these symptoms is related to cellular inflammation, resulting from a complex interaction of emotional, physical, and genetic factors.

PMS SYMPTOMS

- abdominal bloating
- abdominal cramping
- accident proneness
- acne
- aggression
- alcohol intolerance
- anxiety
- asthma
- back pain
- breast swelling and pain
- bruising
- confusion
- coordination difficulties
- depression
- edema
- emotional lability
- exacerbation of preexisting conditions (arthritis, ulcers, lupus, etc.)
- eye difficulties
- fainting
- fatigue

~ food binges

~ headache

~ heart palpitations (heart pounding)

~ hemorrhoids

~ herpes

~ hives

~ insomnia (sleeplessness)

~ irritability

~ joint swelling and pain

~ lethargy

~ migraine

~ nausea

~ rage

~ salt craving

~ seizures

~ sex drive changes

~ sinus problems

~ sore throat

~ styes

~ suicidal thoughts

~ sweet cravings

~ urinary difficulties

~ withdrawal from others

If nothing is done to interrupt PMS, it often gets worse over time. In the early stages of PMS, women describe symptoms that arise a few days before their menstrual period and then stop abruptly when the bleeding starts. Then the symptoms gradually begin to appear one to two weeks before the onset of menses. Some women experience a cluster of symptoms at ovulation, followed by a symptom-free week—then a recurrence of the symptoms a week before menses. Over time, a woman may have only two or three days of the month that are symptom-free. Eventually, no discernible pattern of "good" days and "bad" days is left: she feels as if she has PMS virtually all the time.

Some women equate menstrual cramps and PMS, but PMS is different from menstrual cramps (dysmenorrhea). This difference is not always clearly stated in writings on PMS. Many women with PMS have completely pain-free periods. Many women with severe cramping have *no* premenstrual distress. Menstrual cramps are caused by uterine contractions and cramping that results from excess prostaglandin F2 alpha, a hormone produced as the lining of the uterus breaks down during the menstrual cycle. Prostaglandins and other inflammatory chemicals are also involved in PMS symptoms. For that reason, dietary change, vitamin and mineral supplements, and antiprostaglandin medication (usually nonsteroidal anti-inflammatory drugs such as Advil) are often useful both for cramps and for PMS.[37]

Though some doctors are still looking for a "biochemical lesion" that causes PMS and hundreds of scientific papers have been published on the topic, no one has been able to find such a lesion or a magic-bullet drug to cure it. A reductionistic approach—looking for the chemical "cause" and "cure"—simply doesn't work because the causes of PMS are multifactorial and must be approached holistically. The effects of the mind, emotions, diet, light, exercise, relationships, heredity, and childhood traumas must all be taken into account when treating PMS. All combine to create the end result of cellular inflammation, which manifests in many different ways.

All of the following events result in hormonal changes in the body. PMS is apt to be initiated or exacerbated by these changes unless treatment is initiated.

EVENTS ASSOCIATED WITH PMS ONSET

- Onset of menses or the year or two before menopause
- Coming off birth control pills
- After a time of no periods (amenorrhea)
- The birth of a child or the termination of a pregnancy
- Pregnancies complicated by toxemia
- Tubal ligation, especially as done in the 1970s, in which a greater portion of the fallopian tube was destroyed by unipolar electrocautery, a method of burning the tubes that is no longer used
- Unusual trauma, such as a death in the family
- Decreased light associated with autumn and winter and also lack of exposure to natural, full-spectrum light.

A variety of nutritional factors contribute to PMS. Studies have shown that women with PMS tend to have the following nutritional and physiological characteristics.

FACTORS CONTRIBUTING TO PMS

- High consumption of dairy products[38]

- Excessive consumption of caffeine, in the form of soft drinks, coffee, or chocolate[39]

~ Excessive consumption of foods that raise blood sugar too quickly, resulting in elevated insulin levels and subsequent cellular inflammation

~ A relatively high blood level of estrogen, resulting either from overproduction from dietary and body fat or from the decreased breakdown of estrogen in the liver. High estrogen levels are associated with deficiencies of the vitamin B complex, especially B_6 and B_{12}. The liver requires these vitamins in order to break down and inactivate estrogen.[40]

~ A relatively low blood level of progesterone, the hormone that works to balance excess estrogen. This decreased level is felt to be secondary either to lack of production or to excessive breakdown to this hormone in the body.[41] Studies in this area are inconsistent.

~ A diet that leads to increased levels of the hormone prostaglandin F2 alpha and also contributes to high levels of estrogen in conjunction with low levels of progesterone.[42] Vegetarians with a low-fat, high-fiber diet are known to excrete two to three times more estrogen in their feces than nonvegetarians. They also have 50 percent lower blood plasma levels of unconjugated estrogens (a type of metabolized estrogen) than women who eat the standard American diet, and as a result they have a decreased incidence of PMS.[43] (Note: It has been my experience that vegetarians tend to eat more fruits and vegetables and fewer trans-fatty acids than do nonvegetarians. Evidence is mounting that meat is not the culprit we once thought it was as long as it is consumed in moderate amounts and accompanied by an abundant intake of green leafy vegetables, whole grains, fruits, and other whole foods—and as long as one's diet doesn't contain excessive amounts of high-glycemic-index foods or those that contain trans-fatty acids.)

~ Excessive body weight, which increases the chances of excessive levels of estrogen and PMS.[44] Body fat manufactures estrone (one of the estrogens) and is also associated with an increase in inflammatory chemicals.

~ Low levels of vitamins C and E and selenium. As with the B vitamins, the liver also requires these substances to metabolize estrogen properly.[45]

~ A deficiency of magnesium, which is very common.[46] Chocolate cravings have been linked to low magnesium levels. The liver needs magnesium, along with B vitamins, to metabolize estrogen optimally.

~ Lack of exercise

SAD and PMS: Shedding Light on the Link

Many women with PMS notice that their symptoms get worse in the fall, when the days get shorter. Many of the symptoms associated with PMS are precisely the same as those associated with the form of depression known as seasonal affective disorder (SAD). Light acts as a nutrient in the body. When it hits the retina, it directly influences the entire neuroendocrine system via the hypothalamus and the pineal gland. In one study, patients with PMS responded significantly to treatment with bright light. Their weight gain, depression, carbohydrate craving, social withdrawal, fatigue, and irritability were reversed with two hours of full-spectrum bright light in the evening.[47] This is not surprising, because both natural light and carbohydrate consumption increase serotonin levels, which ease depression. Living under artificial light much of the time, without regular exposure to natural light, not only can profoundly affect the regularity of the menstrual cycle, but can also create PMS.[48]

The link between PMS and SAD is a profound example of how women's wisdom is simultaneously encoded in both the cycle of the seasons and our monthly cycles. Figure 4 (page 108) illustrates how the phases of the moon are linked to the phases of the menstrual cycle. In figure 6 (page 135), I've added the seasons to this diagram, so that one can clearly see that the time of the monthly cycle when PMS is most common parallels the calendrical period when SAD occurs. The natural tendency to turn inward during the premenstrual time of our monthly cycle is reflected in the natural tendency to turn inward during the autumn of the year. All of nature reflects this wisdom back to us. In fall and winter, the trees send their energy down into their roots, where profound activity and revitalization go on even though it is not obvious to us. The early luteal phase of the menstrual cycle, following ovulation, is when our energies go deep into our roots so that we can take stock and then prepare for the next cycle of outer growth in the world. Because our culture doesn't understand this cyclic wisdom, we have been taught to be afraid of both the times in our cycles and the seasons of year when wisdom demands that we go into darkness, withdraw, and take stock of our lives.

We have been taught to be suspicious of these natural energies—and too many women see them as a weakness that needs to be overridden and ignored. Heaven forbid we should follow our body's wisdom and take a break from getting it all done!

The second half of the menstrual cycle and autumn are times when the tide is out and everything that you don't want to see on the muddy bottom of the bay is uncovered for all to see. Women need to learn to pay attention to the information available to them at these times of the month and of the year. Think of this information as compost that you'll be using to create new growth in your life once the light comes back.

Treatment

Many women are given symptomatic treatments for PMS that over the long run don't work. Treating a woman's bloating with diuretics, her headaches with painkillers, and her anxiety with Valium often serves to create new side effects from the drugs themselves and ignores the underlying imbalances that lead to PMS in the first place. In the past, psychotherapy was often prescribed for women with PMS. Although it may provide insights about stress, it ignores the nutritional and biochemical aspects of this disorder. Many women with PMS are now given drugs that increase serotonin levels, such as Prozac. Studies have shown that these can be very helpful for alleviating symptoms of PMS in severe cases. These medications are best taken in low doses only during the luteal phase of the cycle.[49] But if they are not used with the insight that PMS is part of a much bigger imbalance, they do not help a woman truly learn from, and create health through, her PMS. And besides, after a couple years, they stop working and, worse, may deplete the body's own ability to make serotonin.

PROGRAM FOR PMS RELIEF

~ *A dietary approach.* See diet suggestions for dysmenorrhea, page 121, and also chapter 17.

~ *A multivitamin-mineral supplement.* It should contain 400 to 800 mg of magnesium (magnesium deficiency is common in PMS) and 50 to 100 mg of most of the B complex. All women should take this daily all month long, not just premenstrually.[50]

~ *Elimination of refined sugar, refined flour products, and trans-fatty acids.*[51]

~ *Elimination of caffeine.* As I've learned through the years, just getting off caffeine, even if consumption has been as little as one cup of coffee or one can of cola per day, can have a dramatic effect on PMS for some women.

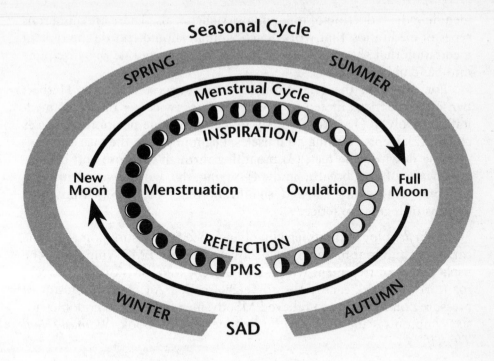

FIGURE 6: SAD AND PMS

PMS is to the monthly cycle as SAD is to the annual cycle. Both conditions respond to the same treatment while asking us to deepen our connection to our cyclic wisdom.

~ *Enough essential fatty acids.* Essential fatty acids are found in raw nuts and seeds, cold-water fish such as salmon and sardines, and many plants. Sesame oil is excellent, and so are sunflower, safflower, and walnut oils. You can also use supplements, which are widely available at pharmacies and natural food stores. Generally, 500 mg of fish oil three or four times per day is adequate. Flaxseed oil can also help: 500 mg four times per day. (See diet suggestions for dysmenorrhea, page 121.) The optimal metabolism of essential fatty acids in the body require adequate levels of magnesium, vitamin C, zinc, vitamin B_3, and vitamin B_6. (See chapter 17.)

~ *Stress reduction and energy medicine.* Women who practice meditation or other methods of deep relaxation are able to alleviate many of their PMS symptoms. Relaxation of all kinds decreases cortisol and epinephrine levels in the blood and helps to balance your biochemistry, including the reduction of inflammatory chemicals. There are numerous types of meditation that work. Each woman should choose the type of meditation that she feels most drawn to and incorporate this discipline into her daily routine.

For example, the relaxation response suggested by Dr. Herbert Benson is practiced fifteen to twenty minutes twice per day. This meditation involves: (1) sitting quietly in a comfortable position with eyes closed; (2) deeply relaxing all muscles, beginning with the face and progressing down to the feet; (3) breathing through the nose and becoming aware of the breath; and (4) saying the word *one* silently on exhaling. One study showed significant relief of PMS within three months of regular practice.[52]

~ *Reflexology.* Treatment involving specific pressure points on the ear, hand, and foot has also been shown to relieve PMS symptoms. The usual length of treatment with a trained reflexologist is once per week, for thirty minutes each time, for eight weeks. An entire program of pressure point therapy to relieve PMS, dysmenorrhea, and endometriosis symptoms can be found in Jeanne Blum's book *Woman Heal Thyself.*[53]

~ *At least twenty minutes of aerobic-type exercise three times a week.*[54] Brisk walking is all that is necessary. Such conditioning exercise decreases many premenstrual symptoms. It also increases levels of endorphins (naturally occurring morphinelike substances that help the body deal with depression and physical pain). It is estimated that half of all depression cases can be helped through exercise alone. (See chapter 18.)

~ *Full-spectrum light.* Expose yourself to full-spectrum light for two hours each evening or each morning (2,500 to 10,000 lux; a lux is a measure of light intensity) from either natural light or a full-spectrum light source.[55] A cloudy day in northern Europe provides 10,000 lux. A sunny day near the equator provides 80,000 lux. (See Resources for sources of full-spectrum lights.)

~ *Natural progesterone therapy when indicated.* Natural progesterone, in combination with lifestyle changes, often produces profound improvement in PMS symptoms.[56] In their capacity as neurotransmitters, estrogen and progesterone clearly affect mood. Estrogen, if unopposed by progesterone, tends to irritate the nervous system. Progesterone, on the other hand, is associated with tranquility and is a central nervous system relaxant. It binds to the same receptors in the brain as Valium and has a soothing and relaxing effect.[57]

I recommend natural progesterone for women who have moderate to severe PMS that doesn't respond to simple lifestyle changes and who often describe a Jekyll-and-Hyde personality change premenstrually. Natural progesterone also works well for women whose major premenstrual symptom is a migraine-type headache. These headaches often start with the gradual change in estrogen and progesterone levels that tends to occur in the years leading up to menopause.

Natural progesterone is not the same thing as the synthetic progesterones (progestins), such as medroxyprogesterone acetate (Provera) and norethindrone, which is commonly used in birth control pills. There are no serious side effects with natural progesterone at the usual doses. Sometimes it might cause intermenstrual spotting or delay the period. This usually resolves itself in one to two months. Extremely high doses—much higher than I recommend—have been associated with euphoria and occasional dizziness in rare cases. Oral natural progesterone is available by prescription from your doctor. It is also available in the form of skin creams. Note that while natural progesterone is synthesized from wild Mexican yams, creams that contain only yam extract, though helpful for some women, are not the same as those that contain adequate amounts of natural progesterone. Not all pharmacies carry natural progesterone and not all physicians know where to get it.

For application to the skin, you can use one of several natural progesterone creams available over the counter, or have your doctor prescribe one for you from a pharmacy that specializes in individualized prescriptions. I have recommended a 2-percent progesterone cream such as Emerita for many years. (See Resources for a list of brand names.) These 2-percent creams contain at least 375 mg of natural progesterone per ounce. One-quarter to one-half teaspoon applied to the skin once or twice per day has been shown to result in physiological levels of progesterone that match those found in the normal luteal phase.[58]

General instructions are to apply one-quarter teaspoon (approximately 20 mg) on the soft areas of skin (breasts, abdomen, neck, face, inner arms, or hands) in the morning and again in the evening. Alternate the sites with each application; apply on days fourteen through twenty-eight of your menstrual cycle for at least three months. The precise timing and dosage will vary from woman to woman, however. It is important to get the progesterone into your system *before* you normally experience your mood change. You need to apply the cream a day or two before ovulation or a day or two *before* your symptoms usually start. For some women, this will be on day twenty-one; for others, day twelve or thirteen. Continue through the first day of menstrual bleeding (day one of the cycle). This will often prevent symptoms or greatly alleviate them. Waiting until you are symptomatic to start treatment often doesn't work. Increase or decrease the dosage depending on the severity of the symptoms; most women have to experiment to find a level that works for them. You may safely use natural progesterone for more than two weeks of your cycle provided that you interrupt use in each cycle for at least twelve hours.

Synthetic progestins, as opposed to natural progesterone, have many known side effects, such as bloating, headache, and weight gain. Unfortunately, many woman are told that synthetic progestin is the same as natural progesterone. But synthetic progestins can actually increase PMS symptoms, because taking a synthetic progestin decreases the body's natural progesterone levels.

Women who do well on progesterone are often those who experience a rapid change in mood that begins after ovulation and ends just as the menstrual flow starts. They describe feeling fine and then within several hours having a "black cloud" come over them.[59] When their periods start, they feel as though "a light has gone on." These women are describing a biochemical change in their bodyminds that is very real and not just "in their heads."

The possible relative imbalance between estrogen, progesterone, and other hormones that is associated with PMS appears to be a dynamic, changing phenomenon that currently cannot be documented with existing laboratory tests. A subtle hormonal imbalance is also associated with irregular periods and emotional stress. Emotional stress increases levels of the hormone ACTH, often resulting in anovulatory cycles (cycles in which an egg is not released) characterized by inadequate levels of progesterone.[60]

The use of natural progesterone over time helps rebalance the estrogen-progesterone ratio. Using natural progesterone produces a gradual improvement of symptoms with each cycle. Many women are able to decrease or eliminate their dosages over time once their symptoms have been completely relieved (though progesterone has many beneficial effects, and some may want to stay on it even after PMS symptoms are gone). It is much more effective, however, to start out with dosages that are on the high end of usual and stay with these for several months.

Ultimately, when women are willing to look at the emotional issues behind their PMS, they are eventually able to change their internal hormonal status *without* outside hormones. The process of healing our emotional and psychological stresses *results in biochemical changes* in our bodies.

Women's Stories

Gwendolyn: transforming premenstrual rage. Gwendolyn was thirty-six when she first came to see me. She was tall, thin, dramatic, and articulate, with a great sense of humor, but her PMS was so bad that she routinely flew into rages and became manic. In one high-energy premenstrual manic phase, she stayed up all night painting her kitchen and then, without any rest, put in a full day of work. This was followed by several days of depression and fatigue so severe that she was unable to get out of bed. At one point her family was so concerned about this behavior that they considered removing her children from her care and called me for my advice. Her PMS and severe mood swings had begun early in her teenage years and were often accompanied by self-destructive behavior that led her into some dangerous situations. During one of these times, she was gang-raped. On another occasion, she became pregnant and later got an abortion. Because of the severity of Gwendolyn's symptoms, I initially prescribed high-dose progesterone therapy. Eventually, however, Gwendolyn healed her PMS as she addressed the imbalances in her life.

As she recovered, she told me, "In my premenstrual times, every ounce of anger, bitterness, and sense of betrayal erupted—often at such a rate that it became increasingly difficult to stay in my marriage and to continue to care for my autistic daughter and two younger children."

By the time of her first visit with me, Gwendolyn had divorced and was meditating regularly and eating a whole-foods, macrobiotic type of diet, which was helping her to some extent. She was exercising regularly and taking the appropriate food supplements. These dietary and lifestyle practices are often enough to cure PMS in its mild stages. Despite these adjustments, however, she still went through an emotional hell each month. She had so much unfinished emotional business in her life that her premenstrual wisdom was forcing her to look even deeper at the imbalances in her life.

By the time Gwendolyn began her progesterone treatment, many aspects of her life were totally out of control. She came to see that the emotional crash that she experienced premenstrually each month actually was forcing her to peel off all the layers of denial in her life. And looking back, she came to see that this process was essential for her healing. A significant factor in her healing was joining a twelve-step program known as Sex and Love Addicts Anonymous (SLAA). She realized that she had a history of moving from one abusive relationship to the next, never finding the "right" man but always obsessing about whomever she was with. When her artist boyfriend expressed his need to leave the relationship, Gwendolyn was premenstrual and flew into a rage, during which she beat him physically with a vengeance that both surprised and scared her. She realized that she had a significant relationship problem and went into counseling to explore and heal her abuse issues. She learned how a sex and love addiction is often the result of childhood sexual abuse, and she began to connect an early abuse experience and the rape with her current self-destructive behavior. She began to appreciate that her premenstrual rages were those of an unhealed child and that they needed to be addressed now that she was an adult. Meanwhile, she continued to meditate, exercise, eat well, go to counseling, and attend twelve-step meetings.

Through supporting her physical body with natural progesterone, good nutrition, and the regular deep rest of meditation, Gwendolyn developed the inner strength necessary to "handle all that had to erupt and clear out of my body." During her office visits, no matter how bad she felt, I repeatedly reminded her to stay with what she was feeling, that anger and rage were okay and a natural part of the healing process. She needed to feel her anger, even pound a pillow if necessary. But instead of attacking a person with her anger, she needed to respect it as a message telling her something she needed to know. As her healing process continued, she found that underneath her premenstrual rage and anger, the wisdom and the truth lay waiting. By feeling her anger and staying with it, she discovered tears and a profound sense of abandonment left over from the abuses. "The feelings of abandonment are overwhelming sometimes," she told me. "But if I allow the sadness to come, in the end I come out stronger." After nine months of progesterone therapy, Gwendolyn was able to cut way back on her dosages. At that time, she said, "I continue on the progesterone only two days a month and only because of mild irritability. I hit an occasional emotional wall, but the difference now is that I am able to cope much better knowing where it is all coming from. I believe that when a woman has PMS, the physical, emotional, and spiritual all have to be addressed so that a human being can feel whole again."

It has been a number of years since Gwendolyn first began to listen to and understand her menstrual wisdom through learning to trust and transform her rage. When I last spoke with her, she was doing better than ever. She said that if she had to describe her life in one word, it would be *empowerment*. She's taking care of old business, making amends to those she's hurt, and telling the truth to those who have hurt her. She is thrilled that "the talents I was born with are flourishing: my voice, music, and art. I believe that we all have these talents. But we aren't made to feel that we have anything worthwhile." She wrote me a note that said, "When I become angry at all, I give myself quiet space, go within, and ask myself, 'What is it that you're afraid of or what pain are you trying to escape?' I almost always get an answer that I can then work with."

PMS and Codependence

There is a strong correlation between PMS and growing up in an alcoholic family system, in which the parents or grandparents were alcoholic. The correlation between PMS and giving your life away to meet other people's needs—relationship addiction—is very high. In many families in which the men have a tendency to become alcoholics, the females tend to develop PMS. Children of alcoholics have a 40 percent chance of becoming alcoholic, not only because they have a genetic predisposition toward it but because they've learned that alcohol is the way to deaden their emotions. This behavior is frequently passed on to them, along with genes that predispose them to drinking. Women in alcoholic families or with alcoholic partners develop PMS as a result of cutting off their feelings. I've worked with countless women who have decided to break the chain of PMS experience by generations of women in their families. (Hypoglycemia [low blood sugar] and a resulting tendency toward sugar craving are also very common in women from alcoholic families who have PMS. This condition tends to be much worse premenstrually and can be easily treated with the dietary recommendations I've already covered.)

Leslie, a forty-nine-year-old homemaker and former teacher with PMS, came to see me with severe premenstrual mood swings, sugar cravings, and fatigue. As I read through her history, I noted that her husband was an alcoholic and that she was in a teaching position that she hated. She had had an alcoholic mother and sister and had never addressed any of these family issues. During the initial visit, I counseled her about supporting her body during the menstrual cycle through nutrition and exercise, and stressed that she wouldn't "cure" her premenstrual discomfort until she was willing to look at the messages it was sending her about her own family situation. I could tell that she wasn't ready to hear this information, and she did not return for a follow-up.

Seven years later, however, Leslie made an appointment. She told me, "When I was in to see you in 1985, you told me that I needed to check out my codependence and that my PMS and decreased energy were related to that. I left thinking, 'Dr. Northrup's a nice woman, but she doesn't know what she's talking about, and in fact I think she's crazy. How could codependence and PMS be related?' But now I realize the connection between what was happening in my life and my PMS. I finally realized that my husband has been verbally abusive for years. I am in the middle of a divorce, and I see now that I had totally 'de-selfed' myself."

Leslie told me that she had joined a twelve-step group and was picking up the pieces of her life and learning about the effects of living with verbal abuse and alcoholism for so many years. Leslie's feelings are no longer deadened. She's becoming her own person and determining what she will and will not accept about her family's behavior. She no longer has PMS most months, but when she does, she pays attention to it, slows down, and makes the necessary adjustments in her life, so that she gets her needs met.

IRREGULAR PERIODS

After nearly thirty years as a physician, I continue to be amazed by how clearly menstrual cycles and bleeding are connected to the contexts of our lives. Abnormal uterine bleeding is nearly always connected to family issues in some way. As Caroline Myss says, blood is family—always. One woman told me that she and her two sisters, who were living in different parts of the country, skipped periods in the same month when a fourth sister had a miscarriage, although they didn't realize it until they talked at their next get-together. One of my patients, age fifty-five, who had her last menstrual period at the age of fifty-two and went through a classic menopause with hot flashes and lab tests confirming "change of life," nevertheless got a completely normal period right after her mother died. When a menopausal woman develops postmenopausal bleeding, I always ask her what is going on with her and her family. She will often tell me that an emotionally significant family event preceded the bleeding. I had my final menstrual period on the day my youngest child left home for college. I hadn't had any bleeding for eleven months prior to this.

Menstrual blood, especially when it comes at an unscheduled time, is a message. It carries wisdom of some kind. Myss points out that most bleeding problems originate from an imbalance in our system: too much emotion and not enough mental, intellectual energy to balance it. She notes that bleeding abnormalities are exacerbated when a woman internalizes confusing signals from her family or society about her own sexual pleasure and sexual needs. A woman may, for example, desire sexual pleasure but feel guilty about it or be unable to ask directly for what she desires. She may not be consciously aware of this inner conflict.

Most practicing physicians have seen the profound effect that the psyche can have on the menstrual cycle. Way back in 1949, S. Zuckerman recognized that emotional disturbances could disorganize menstrual rhythm, accelerate uterine bleeding, and also influence the time of ovulation. Diffuse networks of nerves connecting the brain with the ovaries (called preganglionic autonomic pathways) may mediate this connection between emotions and uterine and ovarian function.[61] We also know that our thoughts and beliefs are likewise mediated throughout the body by neurotransmitters, the chemicals that the brain makes when it thinks.

What Are Regular Periods?

Before I examine the subject of menstrual period irregularity, it's necessary to explain what is normal. Women are sometimes taught that their periods are irregular if they do not occur every twenty-eight days. I consider periods *regular* when they occur roughly every twenty-four to thirty-five days. Having a period every twenty-eight days like clockwork happens for some women but not all. Thousands of women who don't fit the every-twenty-eight-day pattern are under the impression that their periods are irregular, when in fact they are completely normal.

Period regularity is determined by a complex interaction between the brain (hypothalamus, pituitary gland, and temporal lobes), the ovaries, and the uterus. Period patterns can change with changes in seasons, lighting conditions, diet, or travel, or during times of family stress. Irregular and anovulatory menstrual cycles are associated with premature bone loss. Often women can tell when they have ovulated because they have a clear discharge twelve to sixteen days from the first day of their last menstrual period. (This is discussed in more detail in chapter 11). Cycles in which a woman has ovulated are also characterized by what is called premenstrual *molimina*.

Molimina is a group of "symptoms" resulting from normal cyclic hormonal changes in the body. These include a slight premenstrual redistribution of body fluid, often experienced as "bloating" or slightly tender breasts, slight abdominal cramping, and mood changes associated with being in a more reflective, less active state. Women who don't ovulate usually don't have these changes and will often get a period "out of the blue," without having any idea that one is due. Periods in which there is no ovulation tend to be more irregular.

EXCESSIVE BUILDUP OF THE UTERINE LINING (ENDOMETRIAL HYPERPLASIA, CYSTIC AND ADENOMATOUS HYPERPLASIA)

In some women with irregular periods, a biopsy of the inside of the uterus (endometrial biopsy) reveals a condition in which the normal lining of the uterus has been replaced by an overgrowth of glandular tissue. Under the microscope, the endometrial glands look as if they are piled on top of each other and packed too closely. This overgrowth results from overstimulation of the uterine lining by estrogen without the balance of progesterone. It is known as cystic and adenomatous hyperplasia (meaning too many glands) of the endometrium.[62] (It is not to be confused with endometriosis, which will be discussed at length in chapter 6.) Hyperplasia results when a woman's ovaries haven't produced eggs regularly. Instead of a uniform thickening and then sloughing off of the uterine lining (the endometrium), caused by the hormones associated with regular ovulation, the endometrium gets out of sync. Some parts of the lining "think" it's day seven, while others think it's day twenty-eight. This results in irregular and intermittent bleeding.

Cystic and adenomatous hyperplasia or simple endometrial hyperplasia are not considered dangerous unless abnormal cells are present in the biopsy of the uterine lining. Finding some simple endometrial hyperplasia on the biopsy is fairly normal and is not a case for alarm if it happens only once or twice. Many women in their forties and fifties skip an ovulation every now and then as their ovaries undergo the changes leading up to menopause. When a woman's periods become irregular, she does not necessarily require a uterine biopsy, though this decision must be made on a case-by-case basis depending on her history and examination findings.

Treatment

Please note that for this and other conditions, I will be discussing the treatments that are most commonly prescribed in the United States. These treatments do not address the issues underlying symptoms. The underlying issues and what a woman can learn from them are covered in the individual stories at the end of this chapter.

Many cases of simple endometrial hyperplasia go away on their own. However, a very small percentile of women with this condition have atypical cells on their biopsies. Endometrial hyperplasia needs to be monitored and followed to be sure it is going away rather than progressing. Women with chronic anovulation over many years do have a statistically higher incidence of uterine cancer. Gynecologists are trained to treat everybody as though there were a potential cancer risk. Therefore initial conventional treatment of endometrial hyperplasia consists of giving a synthetic progestin hormone such as Provera or Aygestin for one to three months and then repeating the endometrial biopsy to make sure that the condition has cleared. I often recommend natural progesterone for this purpose, especially in those women who have adverse side effects from synthetic progestin. (See page 137 for the difference between synthetic and natural progesterone.) Physicians vary widely on how much of the drug they give and for how long they give it. Prescribing a progestin drug is sometimes called a "medical D&C" (dilation and curettage of the uterine lining), because it causes the endometrial lining to slough off in a uniform manner all at once and helps the uterus get rid of the tissue buildup. Natural progesterone, on the other hand, has the ability to down-regulate estrogen receptors, meaning that it reduces the cells' sensitivity to estrogen; this often clears up benign endometrial hyperplasia.

Some women with persistent endometrial hyperplasia do not respond to treatment with progestin or progesterone and may require a surgical D&C in the operating room. In extremely rare instances, they may need a hysterectomy if this condition does not go away or if it progresses to produce abnormal cells.

DYSFUNCTIONAL UTERINE BLEEDING (DUB)

Skipping periods more than just occasionally, frequent bleeding between periods, or spotting between periods is known as dysfunctional uterine bleeding, or DUB. (See also the section on polycystic ovaries

[PCO] and anovulation, in chapter 7.) Women who have had cesarean sections may occasionally have abnormal bleeding patterns because of disruptions of the uterine lining caused by the scar on the uterus. Many abnormal patterns are hypothalamic in origin, meaning that they are related to the complex interaction between the brain, ovaries, and uterus. Severe anxiety and depression change neurotransmitter levels in the brain and can affect hypothalamic function. Dysfunctional uterine bleeding is often associated with anovulatory cycles and too much estrogen relative to progesterone. It is also related to the hormonal imbalance that results from elevated cortisol and insulin levels, which change the way estrogen is metabolized. Though I've been trained to look for endocrine abnormalities—such as thyroid problems or pituitary problems—that can cause menstrual abnormalities, I rarely find anything wrong by using standard blood tests and a physical exam. Because DUB can also be related to high prolactin levels caused by pituitary tumors, I always order a blood test for this hormone as well. However, prolactin hormone levels that are too high, a condition known as hyperprolactinemia, is not common.

A diagnosis of DUB is made on the basis of history, blood tests that check pituitary and thyroid hormone levels, and sometimes a biopsy from inside the uterus to see if the uterine lining shows signs of anovulation or abnormal cells.

Conventional Treatment

The conventional treatment of DUB consists of giving hormones such as birth control pills to regulate the periods. This common treatment is now given even up until menopause in women who don't smoke. Birth control pills do result in reliable periods every month, and taking them may be the first choice for women whose lives are too busy to change their diets, take supplements, or exercise. But pills don't heal anything—they simply mask the underlying issues in the body or put an imbalance "to sleep" for a while. Nevertheless, like most gynecologists, I have prescribed birth control pills for many women, both for contraception and for DUB, because taking the pill is the easiest way for a woman to eliminate her symptoms without doing the work of changing aspects of her life that are contributing to the problem.

Women with DUB who are in their forties and older are statistically at greater risk for endometrial hyperplasia, and most physicians will do an endometrial biopsy before they initiate hormonal treatment. Progestin hormone (synthetic progesterone such as Provera or

Aygestin) is often the treatment of choice, both to clear up the hyper-plasia if it is present and to stop the abnormal bleeding. I recommend natural progesterone for the same purpose (Crinone or Prochieve vaginal gel or Prometrium capsules). If a woman is skipping periods and wants to get pregnant, the fertility drug Clomid, which tricks the brain and ovaries into ovulation, will often be prescribed.[63]

A subgroup of women with DUB are overweight. They don't ovulate regularly, in part because their body fat produces too much estrogen. The estrogen overstimulates the uterine lining and can result in anovulation. These women sometimes have a condition known as polycystic ovary syndrome, in which their ovaries develop a thickened outer wall, just under which many unreleased, partially stimulated eggs form cysts. On ultrasound examinations, the ovaries show up as being enlarged and having multiple small cysts in them. (Interestingly, medical intuitives report exactly the same appearance when they do readings on these women.) Studies have shown that the risk of menstrual irregularities is two to three times greater in obese women than in women of average body size.[64] Dietary change to decrease excess body fat can help lower estrogen levels. These women also have elevated androgen levels, which contribute to their problems. Androgens are a group of hormones that include testosterone and are produced in the ovaries, the adrenal glands, and body fat.

As with PMS and menstrual cramps, unabated stress, a diet high in refined foods and low in nutrients, and a lack of exposure to natural light can *all* result in DUB. Many of my patients with DUB have been helped by lifestyle and dietary changes alone. Some make these changes in addition to hormonal treatment.

Alternative Treatment Program

My treatment plan often includes one or more of the following:

~ *Dietary improvement.* (See chapter 17 and the diet recommended for menstrual cramps on page 122.)

~ *Multivitamin-mineral supplements and essential fatty acids.* These help metabolize excess estrogen and androgens and decrease cellular inflammation. (See information on essential fatty acids on page 123.)

~ *Natural progesterone.* This can be taken orally or transdermally. The dosage depends on the symptoms; usually it is 50 to 200 mg orally on a daily basis from midcycle to the onset of menses (usually days fourteen to twenty-eight of the cycle), for at least three months. (For mild cases, use 2-percent progesterone cream, one-quarter to one-half teaspoon once or twice per day on the same schedule.) Natural progesterone can also be given vaginally for thirty days or more, depending on the patient.

~ *Castor oil packs.* These are applied to the lower abdomen at least three times per week for sixty minutes each time. This regimen should be followed for at least three months and then can be tapered down to once a week. Packs should not be used while you are bleeding heavily.

Castor oil, also known as palma Christi (the palm of Christ), has been used for healing for hundreds of years. Castor oil packs are a treatment that the medical intuitive Edgar Cayce often prescribed for many different conditions. I was introduced to them by Dr. Gladys McGarey, who has used them in her general practice of medicine for over forty years. They are made by saturating a piece of wool or cotton flannel, folded so that it is four thicknesses, with cold-pressed castor oil. The oil-saturated flannel is then placed directly on the skin of the lower abdomen and covered with a piece of plastic, such as a plastic bag. Heat, in the form of a hot water bottle or heating pad, is then applied over the pack and the plastic. A blanket or towel can be placed over the heat source to keep everything in place. I prefer a non-electric heat source and often recommend a hot water bottle as a Fomentek bag. (See Resources for everything you need to do a castor oil pack.) The patient then reclines with this on her lower abdomen for sixty minutes. During this treatment, I ask her to pay attention to thoughts, images, and feelings that arise and make note of them in a journal. Preliminary studies on castor oil packs done at the George Washington University School of Medicine indicate that they improve immune system functioning.

~ *Light therapy.* Determine what the first day of your last period was, as nearly as possible. (You may need to guess.) From days fourteen to seventeen of your cycle, sleep with a 100-watt lightbulb in a common bedside-table lamp that has a shade that disperses light onto the ceiling and wall but is minimally disturbing to sleep, on the floor next to your bed. Do this for six months. In one study of two thousand women, more than 50 percent regulated their previously irregular periods to a regular cycle of twenty-nine days by doing this.[65]

~ *Acupuncture and herbs.* Acupuncture and herbs can help DUB and many other gynecological problems. But just as there are many emotional settings and energy dysfunctions that may set the scene for a woman's menstrual disorders, there are many appropriate and specific oriental herbal and acupuncture treatments that may be prescribed. When a woman seeks acupuncture and oriental herbal treatment for her menstrual disorder, she may receive one of numerous diagnoses, including (but not limited to) deficient blood of the heart, spleen, or liver; deficient *chi*; stagnant blood; and stagnant *chi*. Depending upon her history or physical symptoms, as well as her physical examination, specific acupuncture points and/or herbs will be selected that are appropriate for her condition. Each woman who is drawn to this approach must find an appropriately trained practitioner of oriental medicine with whom she feels safe.

~ *Medication and stress reduction.* Any modality that decreases stress can help menstrual period regulation because of the profound link between emotional or psychological stress and biochemical imbalance.

Women's Stories

Deborah: breaking family ties. Deborah was seventeen when she left her family to go to college. She described her family as "lower middle class and not oriented to a college education." In fact, Deborah was the first person from her family ever to leave home for any reason except to marry. Her family was not supportive of her living away from home, and they wanted her to visit every weekend.

During her first year in college, Deborah met many people who were interesting and exciting to her, and a whole new world of intellectual challenge and career possibilities began opening up for her. She was happier and felt more fulfilled than at any other time in her life. Unfortunately, her mother, fearing that she would lose Deborah, began to call her on the phone every evening, telling her that she was a failure and that she would never succeed at anything if she stayed in college. She threatened to call the dean of the college and have Deborah's scholarships rescinded so that she would have no choice but to come home.

Deborah became depressed, and her periods became irregular for the first time since menarche. They came two or three times per month, or not at all for two or three months at a time. To feel better about herself, she began to run as a form of exercise. At first, this made her feel physically stronger, more independent, and more in control of her body—which seemed to be out of control for the first time in her life. But the exercise didn't help her irregular periods. In fact, it contributed to long periods of amenorrhea (no periods at all). She saw a gynecologist, who told her that her pelvic exam was completely normal. The reason for her problem, he said, was that she was "fooling around with too many guys." Since she was not involved with any men at this time, she was not helped by this physician and avoided gynecologists for the next eleven years.

Deborah did, however, consult with an acupuncturist, who prescribed Chinese herbs for her in addition to acupuncture. These treatments helped regulate her periods within two months, but she discovered that her periods went right back to their abnormal pattern as soon as she stopped her acupuncture and herb treatments, and she found that she had to deal with the source of her depression, which returned when she had to stop running because of an injury. She came to see that her relationship with her mother was the source of her problems, and she eventually moved out of state to break her mother's control over her life.

When I first saw Deborah, she was recovering from an addiction to exercise and from her relationship with her mother. She had begun psychotherapy and was exploring these issues. I recommended an intensive workshop to learn to get in touch with her feelings, a whole-foods diet, natural progesterone creams, and a calcium-magnesium supplement. Over the next six months, her periods became regular, every twenty-eight to twenty-nine days, and she was no longer depressed. She finished college and completed her Ph.D. She has broken the original family ties that were at the root of her problem, and her life is becoming balanced on all levels.

Donna: dysfunctional family and dysfunctional bleeding. Donna, a forty-two-year-old professor, came into my office with a six-month history of irregular periods—bleeding for two weeks, then nothing for six weeks, then a few days of spotting, and so on. She also had bouts of severe anxiety and depression that lasted for three weeks straight, at just about the time the irregularity started. An endometrial biopsy revealed cystic and adenomatous hyperplasia, an abnormality associated with anovulation (failure to ovulate).

Donna's mother had also gone through abnormal periods and mood swings in her forties but had decided that it was all her hormones, and she was just going to have to live with it. Donna is quite sure that her mother had unresolved issues with her own father, since Donna remembers her grandfather as someone who was very scary to be around when she was a child.

Donna told me that she'd been having some dreams about and memories of sexual abuse by her uncles. "I've been terrified that if I tell anyone what happened or what I think happened, God will get me," she told me. "Can I force myself to deal with this stuff any faster?" Like many women, she was under the impression that merely having the facts—who, what, where, and when—would help her deal with her discomfort and get on with her life once and for all. But that's not the way healing our lives works. We have to let healing work its way through us gently, gradually, and respectfully.

Donna's upbringing had led her to claim, "Everything in life is my fault. I keep thinking that I must be crazy and must be making this stuff up." I reassured her that in this culture women have been labeled crazy for centuries for telling the truth and that what she was going through was quite normal, given her history. She decided to do some work with an incest survivors' group to help her break through her own and her family's denial. After several months of work, she had another endometrial biopsy—to check for abnormal cells—and it was perfectly normal, as were her pituitary hormones. Her periods had gradually become more regular.

Dealing with her emotional trauma was what actually "cured" Donna's period problems. Her periods, through their irregularity, had communicated to her a bodily wisdom. Her menstrual blood turned her attention to the healing that was required in her relationship with her family, her bloodline.

Darlene: irregular periods since menarche. I first saw Darlene, a teacher, as a patient when she was thirty years old. She was married, had no children, and had a very long history of dysfunctional uterine bleeding since puberty. She experienced long stretches of time with no periods, followed by bleeding almost continuously for a month at a time, then spotting infrequently. Darlene had ongoing anxiety issues and had panic attacks if she had to leave the house for a long period of time. Her marriage was a source of unhappiness to her rather than comfort. She was generally anxious, had trouble sleeping, and had frequent headaches.

Darlene's upbringing had been stressful. Her father and at least one grandfather were alcoholics—although, she said, there was a lot of family denial around this. Her mother, her maternal grandmother, and her cousin had had lifelong problems with irregular bleeding that led to hysterectomies. Her aunt and another cousin had uterine cancer and also had hysterectomies.

Darlene originally came to my office for a fertility workup. Because of her bleeding pattern, we did an endometrial biopsy, which showed endometrial hyperplasia. For treatment of this condition, she was placed on large doses of synthetic progestin. In contrast to most women on this therapy, however, her bleeding didn't stop. A repeat biopsy after the progestin treatment again showed the abnormality of cystic and adenomatous hyperplasia. The next step would be a surgical dilation and curettage (D&C) to be certain that she didn't have uterine cancer.

But Darlene was terrified of the procedure and begged me for an alternative. Because of her strong reaction, I compromised and recommended castor oil packs on her lower abdomen three or four times a week to help restore her immune system. I knew this would give her a chance to reflect at least three times per week on her condition and any messages it might hold for her. We agreed that if this didn't change her cells, we would go ahead with the D&C.

Two weeks later, I did another endometrial biopsy. The tissue was normal endometrium, consistent with the first phase of her menstrual cycle. Darlene was ecstatic and cried with relief. She then went on to have a completely normal period. In the ensuing months her periods were normal, too, and have remained that way. During these months she changed her biochemistry through biofeedback, which she practiced for her insomnia, headaches, and intense anxiety. Realizing that her marriage had not been healthy for her, she separated from her husband, began divorce proceedings, and entered into a love affair where her sexual needs were addressed and that turned out to be deeply healing for her.

Three years later, when Darlene came in for her annual exam, she told me that she was developing a feeling of power around her menstrual cycle that was new and very exciting for her. "My breasts get bigger," she said, "I feel powerful, and I walk around like I know the secrets of the universe. I think my family has been terrified of my power for years. I can remember feeling it even when I was a little girl. Although having this power seems new, it also seems like something I've known for a long time." Darlene has reclaimed her connection to the universal feminine and her sexuality. By doing so, she has broken a cycle of irregular bleeding that was generations deep within her family.

HEAVY PERIODS (MENORRHAGIA)

Some women bleed so heavily during their periods that they routinely bleed through one or two tampons and a pad worn at the same time. Their blood may even soak through their clothing. Some are unable to leave the house during certain days of their periods because the bleeding is so heavy. One of my patients decided to have a hysterectomy after she bled through her clothes into the upholstery of her airplane seat on two different business trips to Europe.

This kind of heavy bleeding is called menorrhagia. Women with menorrhagia have periods at regular intervals, but the periods are heavy. Over time, menorrhagia may lead to anemia (a low red-blood-cell count) if a woman doesn't get enough iron in her diet or if her body can't replace the blood she loses each month. Menorrhagia can be cause by fibroids, endometriosis, or adenomyosis. Rarely, it is associated with a thyroid problem. Some women bleed heavily for no obvious reason.

Chronically heavy periods can be related to chronic stress over second-chakra issues, including creativity, relationships, money, and control of others. One of my patients who sometimes had very heavy periods noted that her periods became heavy when she was upset and needed to weep. "When I bleed like that," she said, "I feel like it's the lower part of my body weeping for the losses I have suffered in my life." When she took the time to pay attention to the different problems she was having and let herself feel her disappointments and pain, her periods were normal. Another patient, who had bad cramps every month and bled profusely, began to think of the uterine pain as related to her strong need for creative space in her own life. She began to set aside one hour a day to do sculpture. Each time she did, she got in touch with the sheer joy of creating for its own sake, and her pelvic pain and bleeding gradually lessened each month.

Adenomyosis, a common cause of pain and heavy bleeding, is a condition in which the glands that normally grow in only the lining of the uterus—the endometrium—grow deeply into the walls of the uterus. (Sometimes called "internal endometriosis," adenomyosis is often present along with fibroids and/or endometriosis, but not always.) This condition can result in bleeding into the uterine wall with each menstrual period. The uterine wall becomes spongy and engorged with blood, producing a condition in which the normal uterine muscles can't contract normally to decrease the bleeding.

A diagnosis of adenomyosis is usually suspected from a woman's history and from a characteristic boggy-feeling uterus on pelvic examination. A definitive diagnosis can be made, however, only by magnetic resonance imaging (MRI) or by a biopsy of the uterine wall, which entails surgically removing a piece of the uterus or the entire uterus.

Treatment

As for all the conditions mentioned in this section, modalities that change the electromagnetic field around the body and unblock the energy in the pelvis can have a beneficial effect on menorrhagia. Acupuncture, meditation, homeopathy, and massage are among these modalities.

~ *Dietary change.* Whether or not a woman's bleeding is caused by adenomyosis, she often responds well to a diet that balances her hormones, decreases the effects of excess insulin, and reduces excessive circulating estrogen and androgen.

~ *Supplements.* For heavy menstrual periods, particularly during perimenopause, try the following daily: vitamin E, 100 to 400 IU; and vitamin A, 5,000 to 10,000 IU.[66] Vitamin A appears to help regulate excessive estrogen levels; vitamin E prevents excessive clotting and helps maintain a more normal flow. Doses of vitamin A as high as 100,000 IU per day can be given if limited to three months—otherwise, there is a risk of toxicity. (Though 5,000–10,000 IU of vitamin A is well within the safe range, it's best not to use this if you're trying to get pregnant.) Vitamin C with bioflavonoids (500 mg per day) and vitamin A have also been shown to decrease menstrual blood loss.[67] I also recommend a good multivitamin-mineral supplement that has adequate levels of all the vitamins, since they tend to work synergistically. (See chapter 17 for dosage recommendations.)

Eliminating all conventionally produced dairy foods (even low-fat ones) for at least three months often helps as well.

~ *Medications.* Women whose menorrhagia does not respond to diet or who prefer other options can often be helped by a synthetic progestin to keep the bleeding under control. My usual regimen is 5 to 10 mg of Provera or Aygestin, taken once or twice per day during the last two weeks of each menstrual cycle. Birth control pills also can work well in many cases. Natural progesterone, either applied as a skin cream or taken orally or vaginally, can also be used. The dosage depends upon the severity of the problem: For oral progesterone, I recommend 100 mg four times per day for the most severe cases, 50 mg two times per day for milder cases, from days fourteen to twenty-eight of the cycle. For progesterone cream (400 mg/ounce), I suggest half a teaspoon twice per day on the soft areas of the skin—breasts, neck, face, abdomen, inner thighs, inner arms, or hands. Vaginal gels of micronized progesterone are also available. The usual starting dose is 45 mg, either daily or every other day on days fourteen through twenty-eight of your cycle. Following the diet outlined in chapter 17 often decreases or eliminates the need for the progestin or progesterone over time. Some women have used this treatment for months or even years as an alternative to hysterectomy.

Prostaglandin inhibitors, such as ibuprofen (Advil or Motrin), naproxen sodium (Aleve), or mefenamic acid (Ponstel), have also helped some women decrease menstrual bleeding.[68] These are best taken one or two times per day for three to four days before the menstrual cycle is due and continuing through the days of the period that are usually the heaviest.

~ *Surgery.* Endometrial ablation, in which the lining of the uterus is cauterized, is a surgical treatment for heavy bleeding in women whose menorrhagia has failed to respond to other treatments. This is an excellent alternative to hysterectomy and effectively controls heavy bleeding in more than 85 percent of cases. It can be done on an outpatient or overnight basis in the hospital.[69] Women who opt for this procedure must be carefully screened beforehand to make sure that their condition is likely to respond, because it doesn't work for all women. Hysterectomy is also an option.

HEALING OUR MENSTRUAL HISTORY:
PREPARING OUR DAUGHTERS

Many women, like those about whom you've read in this chapter, have turned around their painful menstrual experiences and begun to reclaim their rightful heritage: their bodily and menstrual wisdom. As a woman does this, she passes on to the next generation a more positive body image and relationship to the body. In this way, she frees herself and others from the patriarchal degradation of the feminine, and the possibility of healing all women's cycles is greatly enhanced.

For too long, young girls have been introduced to the menstrual cycle solely in terms of sexual intercourse and the possibility of getting pregnant inadvertently. Most girls are not emotionally prepared to grasp the fullness of their female sexuality until they know about and understand the workings of their own uterus, fallopian tubes, ovaries, and cyclic menstrual nature. Reclaiming menstrual wisdom involves women envisioning a new and more positive way of thinking and talking about the menstrual experience to ourselves, our daughters, and to the men in our families. And it involves educating ourselves and others about female sexuality. Many fathers have voiced unease about their daughters' puberty. Fathers seem to hold a very old and probably unexamined sense of needing to protect their daughters from other men and boys. If this protection really worked and helped women to feel secure in their female bodies, we could feel happy about it. Realistically, however, fathers simply cannot protect their daughters effectively, and girls and women cannot and must not continue to seek out men as their sole protectors and providers.

Many women have told me about the lack of support they felt from their own fathers when they reached menarche: "As soon as I got my period, things changed between us. He never hugged or cuddled me again. Our relationship was never the same." One woman with a uterine fibroid suddenly recalled her father yelling at her across the room when she was fourteen and all dressed up to go on a date, "You slut, you whore!" She hadn't remembered this for years. She said that it had felt as if his words went right into her body and stayed there, affecting the way she felt about herself as a woman for the next twenty years.

From birth, females are indoctrinated with the idea that our bodies are subject to the appropriating gaze of others, and to public comment and observation. We parade our little girls out for the gaze of others and often dress them up like small confections for pleasing others. One of my colleagues described how his thirteen-year-old daughter sat down at the dinner table and her older brother said, "I see we've had a visit from the breast fairy." He told this story amidst gales of laughter, but I imagine that his daughter didn't find it very amusing.

For many girls in this society, puberty has been a time of loss. When my older daughter was eleven and I was tucking her into bed one night, she told me that she was worried about something. She had a sore growth on her chest that was scaring her. She wanted me to check it. I did and found a small nipple budding on the left—the first sign of puberty. I told her that it was normal and that she had nothing to worry about. I congratulated her!

Later, unable to sleep, she came into my room and said, "Can we talk?" I said, "Of course," and asked what was troubling her. She burst into tears and said, "I don't want to grow up." I held her and told her that I remembered feeling the same way. I hadn't thought about it for years. But now, with her in my arms, perched on the brink of puberty, I remembered the deep sadness I had felt about growing up. I recalled never wanting to leave home and never wanting my life to change. We sat on my bed while I shared this with her and held her.

After a while, I asked her if she wanted to talk about this with her father, and she said yes. She asked, "Dad, were you ever sad about growing up?" He responded, "Not until the last few years." All of us laughed together at his reply. After a few more minutes of acknowledging my daughter's feelings about puberty, she thanked us and went happily off to bed. This experience was a great example for me of how our emotions, when we respect and express them, quite naturally move through the body and are released.

My daughter didn't bring up the subject again but knew that she could. When she got her period at the age of fourteen she was well prepared and enjoyed getting flowers from her father and a special doll and book from me. Our celebration of our daughter's coming of age could not have taken place if I hadn't appreciated the fact that at some deep, inarticulate level, she knew that moving from the innocence of girlhood to puberty was not an entirely happy prospect in a culture in which the female body is a commodity. As we work together to create new rites of passage for women, we must acknowledge that moving forward also means letting go and grieving over what we are losing.

Clearly we cannot take our daughters into a space where we have never been. We cannot provide healing for them in areas in which we're still deeply wounded ourselves. If we still carry generations of shame about the processes of our female bodies, we cannot hope to pass on to our daughters a genuine sense of love for our own bodies. But the minute we decide to address this whole area, think about it in new ways, and begin the process of reclaiming our menstrual wisdom, the entire map changes. We can begin to create new ceremonies and new rites of passage for ourselves and for our daughters while at this same time working through our old programming and pain.

The good news is that this is now happening all over the planet. In the United States, for example, a group of menstrual health advocates has founded the member-run Red Web Foundation, (www.redweb foundation.org), which is dedicated to supporting a positive societal view of girls' and women's bodies and menstrual cycles, first bleeding through last, and creating physical, emotional, and spiritual well-being. This foundation provides a wide range of resources for introducing girls to their first menstrual cycle in an empowering way as well as educating women of all ages about the positive aspects of their cycles.

The Red Web Foundation was inspired by the pioneering work of the late Tamara Slayton, founder of the Menstrual Health Foundation. Tamara taught me that most girls are not emotionally prepared for a full-fledged understanding of their sexuality until they have first connected their own creativity cycles with their menstrual cycles. To that end, she often taught menstrual empowerment through doll-making and other creative arts. A recent issue of the Red Web newsletter, which reported on a wonderful modern-day coming-of-age ritual in England (see below), is a testimony to Tamara's original vision and how far it has come. Though there are dozens of ways to celebrate a girl's coming of age within her own family, there's nothing more powerful than doing this in a large group. When a girl is surrounded by her ever-important peer group for a coming-of-age celebration, her own hesitancy and embarrassment fall away and she feels embraced by the larger community in a powerful way. Just knowing that this sort of celebration is possible is very healing on all levels.

A MODERN DAY TRIBAL MENARCHE CEREMONY

The following account was written by Rachael O'Neill, a woman's health educator. I have included it here as an illustration of how women's wisdom is being consciously reclaimed all over the planet.

I was lucky to be involved in a huge menarche ceremony at Sacred Arts Camp in May 2005 in Dorset, UK, and I wanted to share the experience with you.

The menarche ceremony was for all young women who had begun bleeding over the course of the previous year. At the beginning of the week, each girl chose a "Moon Mother" who would attend the ceremony with her later in the week, help her get ready, share blood stories with her, and dream a "moon name" for the girl the night before the ritual. The girls then attended a menarche bracelet/necklace-making workshop. Using colored beads associated with different stages of the cycle: white (virgin phase: pre-ovulation), blue (mother phase: ovulation), red (transformer phase: bleeding), and black (enchantress phase: post bleeding). The girls decorated their creations with feathers, beautiful threads, and additional beads of gold and silver. While the jewelry was being made, I talked to the girls about old tribal traditions, moon lodges, and women's power of intuition. We followed with chanting beautiful women's songs.

All week the women of camp were meeting to arrange the ceremony, and the men were meeting for their part: they wrote a song and met to share stories about men's traditions and about honoring women. Their part in the ceremony was to "guard" the sacred ceremonial space by dressing as warriors and walking around the outside perimeter whilst drumming and chanting. The girls chose a Moon Father to make them a crown for the ceremony and he later came forward to represent all men of the community.

The ritual began with the decorating of a big-top tent which was draped in colorful clothes and had an entrance built from willow and flowers. Incense was lit and the space was prepared with singing and chanting. All women were invited to dress in colors matching their cycling phase (white, red, or black for pre-bleeding, menstruation, and menopause, accordingly).

Meanwhile the young women were getting ready with their Moon Moms, being anointed with sacred water and dressed in white with a white ribbon in their hair. The entrance to the big tent was guarded by the wise "Grandmother/Crones" who welcomed each girl. After singing "Merry Maidens," the girls left to change clothes, calling out their names, symbolizing leaving the "girl child" part of themselves behind. Every woman said three words to sum up her bleeding experience and the air filled with words such as "connection, pain, loss, renewal," and even... "I'm not pregnant!"

Amidst singing, the young women re-entered, dressed in beautiful red clothing and welcomed by songs. It was time for the ceremonial hair cutting where the hair with the white ribbon is cut away, symbolizing once again the letting go of childhood. I then anointed each girl with a red ochre crescent moon on her forehead, reminding her of her connection to the moon with its rhythm and flow. Each then drank black currant juice from the sacred goblet and received beautiful gifts from her Moon Mother as well as having her new "Moon Name" whispered in her ear. This was followed by an amazing Arabic dancer's performance.

The Grandmothers, who had been guarding the entrance this whole time, now stepped back to allow the men in, but not before challenging them with, "So you come in to this space with love and respect for your sisters?" To which, of course, they all answered, "YES!!" The Moon Fathers stepped forward and crowned the young women, as the men sang their gift song, which they had composed earlier. In return, our gift to the men for protecting our space was to tell them a blood mystery story. After that the female musicians played, joined by the male drummers, and another level of celebration began.

After the ritual, the girls left with their Moon Moms to ground their energies with chocolate cake ... Later on that full moon night, the women had a heavenly sweat lodge.

The whole experience was a roller coaster of emotions for me. I was so touched by the input of the men and boys, honored to take part, and overwhelmed by the support and love of this modern day "tribe."[70]

Most of us will not have the opportunity to participate in a menarche celebration with a large group. But we can still honor our daughter's first period with a special dinner, shopping trip, flowers, or special gift. It's also important to include their fathers. All of us have an innate need for ritual and recognition. I delivered a friend's daughter and saved her umbilical cord by wrapping it around a cardboard toilet paper tube and setting it inside a sunny window to dry. (If it's winter, you can do this in a slow oven.) The long, thin spiral of sinew that is left is a powerful symbol of the link that this child had with her mother. At the time, I had intended to present this cord to her at her own coming-of-age party but her mother and I fell out of touch with each other. And besides, I like having the card as a reminder of my obstetrical experiences. Some Native American tribes braided the umbilical cord into the mane of the child's first pony for protection. Many other cultures have special uses for the cord. My daughters were fascinated by this cord and wondered why I hadn't saved theirs. I told them that at the time I had never thought of it. I now wish I had. (An expanded section on coming of age appears in my book *Mother-Daughter Wisdom*, on pages 448–450.)

Of course menstrual empowerment doesn't end with a coming-of-age ceremony. Learning to embrace our bodies, our cycles, and our sexuality is an ongoing process. Many of today's teenage girls are precocious "fertile time bombs" because they have no knowledge of their own cycles and use sexuality and intercourse as a rite of passage.[71] I advocate teaching all teenage girls how to make love to themselves, so that they don't feel the need for teenage boys for an outlet! When we teach our young women respect for their bodies and for their cycles, and when we heal ourselves in these areas as well, we help break the cycles of abuse that have gone on for centuries.

After reading a newspaper article on Patricia Reis's work with the Goddess and women's bodies, Marge Rosenthal remembered that she had introduced the menstrual cycle to her daughter by creating a myth. In a letter to Reis she wrote, "When my daughter was four or five and I was premenstrual and searching for something positive about cramps, grouchiness, and all the other pleasures of being a woman, I created the Goddess Menses. She came out of a spontaneous situation: Mama grouchy—a kid wondering why, and me grasping for a believable answer.

"I told her that once a month the Goddess Menses visited a woman's body, and that she was a very mysterious goddess. Sometimes she sneaked in without us knowing, and sometimes she announced herself with powerful tuggings inside our bodies. I told her that when men bleed it is always a sign of illness or injury, but that the bleeding the goddess brought was a reaffirmation of life. A cleansing of our body. I told her that the goddess's arrival is a time of celebration, a time to buy flowers or something small and special, just for us women.

"I told her the grouchiness was because I wasn't listening to my body. Had I felt the tuggings, I would have known to be extra loving to myself (and perhaps taken a couple of aspirin!). As a result of my doing this, I saw all the positive value of creating our own goddesses. I created a little goddess to make positive association with the menstrual cycle. She is a high-spirited, energetic goddess who plays tricks with our bodies, arriving early or late, quiet or stormy, tagging or rolling over us, but once her presence is acknowledged she is very happy to quietly settle down and wait—until next time.

"As I approach menopause I will miss the goddess. It will be a time of her holding on to the youth we shared and me letting go to let the next spirit enter my body. I wonder what her name will be?"

Creating Health Through the Menstrual Cycle

Sitting quietly, ask yourself, "What is my personal truth about the menstrual cycle? How am I feeling about this information? What messages about menstruation and hormones have I learned from my family? What information have I handed down to the younger women in my life? What do I tell myself about my menstrual period? What can it teach me?" Regardless of where you are, be gentle with yourself.

For the next three months, keep a moon journal specifically for noticing the effects of your menstrual cycle on your life. Keep track of the phases of the moon. (These are often listed in the newspaper or in an almanac.) See if you notice any correlation between your cycle and the phases of the moon. See if you crave certain foods premenstrually. What are they? Would taking a long bath feel as good as eating that hot fudge sundae?

Give yourself time to tune in to and reclaim your cyclic nature.

Write a short journal entry every day. The rewards of doing this will be beyond measure. You'll feel connected to life in a whole new way, with increased respect for yourself and your magnificent hormones.

Celebrate the Goddess Menses in your own unique way, knowing that doing so will improve your life on all levels.

6

The Uterus

The oldest oracle in Greece, sacred to the Great Mother of earth, sea, and sky, was named Delphi, from *delphos,* meaning "womb."
—Barbara Walker,
The Women's Encyclopedia of Myths and Secrets

The uterus is located in the low center of the pelvis, in the middle of the pelvic bowl. Also known as the hara, this low-belly body center (which also includes the ovaries) is associated with power, passion, and creativity. This makes sense because the uterus is the vessel in which new life is nourished and brought to fruition. The uterus is connected to the vagina by the cervix and to the pelvic side walls by the broad and cardinal ligaments. The back portion of the bladder attaches to the lower front part of the uterus—the lower uterine segment. The fallopian tubes come off each side of the upper portion of the uterus, known as the fundus. The ovaries are located below the ends of the tubes, known as the fimbria. The fimbria look like delicate fern fronds. (See figure 7, page 164.)

The ovaries, tubes, and uterus are all part of the female hormonal system. Each of these structures is intimately connected to the others. The circulation of blood to the ovaries depends in part on the intact uterus. Following a hysterectomy, changes in the blood supply to the ovaries result in an earlier menopause in many women. The uterus itself is very sensitive to the effects of hormones. As the central organ in the pelvis, the uterus and its attachments to the pelvic side walls, the cardinal ligaments, are important, but underrated, components of the entire pelvic anatomy.

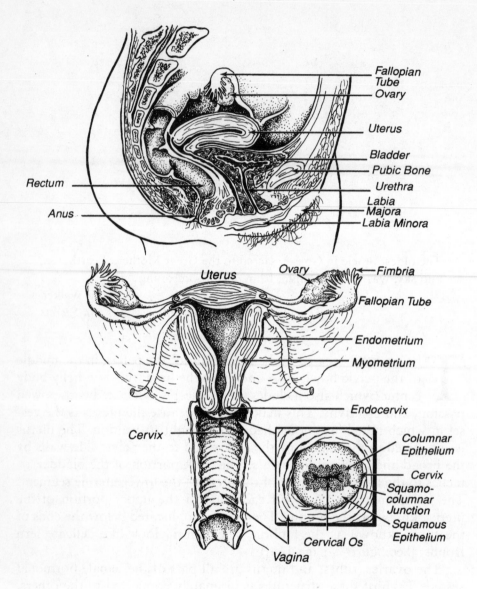

FIGURE 7: UTERUS, OVARIES, AND CERVIX WITH ANATOMIC LABELS

OUR CULTURAL INHERITANCE

The uterus has hardly been studied separate from its role in child-bearing, a fact that reflects this society's baseline cultural biases.[1] The uterus is seen as someone else's potential home and is valued when it can potentially play that role. After the uterus's childbearing function has been completed or when a woman chooses not to have a child, modern medicine considers the uterus to have no inherent value. The ovaries are usually viewed in much the same way because medical science believes that hormonal replacement from artificial sources can perform their functions as well as or even better than a woman's own ovaries. For centuries, women have been taught to view themselves in pretty much the same way—valuable as someone's mother or mate, with no inherent value of their own.

When I was in my residency training, one of our oncology fellows (a doctor doing specialty training in gynecological cancer) taught us, "There's no room in the tomb for the womb." Another slogan from my training was: "The uterus is for growing babies or for growing cancer." Occasionally, during my training, when one of our staff physician teachers removed a uterus that looked perfectly normal, we'd jokingly call the diagnosis CPU, a medicalized acronym for "chronic persistent uterus." These attitudes have pervaded conventional medicine for years, but now they are rapidly changing.

The possibility that the uterus might have any function other than childbearing or tumor production has only recently begun to be addressed in conventional OB/GYN training. Up until just a few years ago, if a woman with a fibroid wanted to keep her uterus even though she had no interest in childbearing, her medical team might have viewed her as overly emotional or sentimental, a bit superstitious, and not well educated about that organ. The general dismissive tone of some doctors was that if such a woman were more sophisticated, she would know that the uterus is useless to her except for childbearing.

For example, I once did a fibroid removal from the uterus of a forty-eight-year-old woman who didn't want a hysterectomy. The chief resident who assisted me said, "Why don't you just do a hysterectomy? They can have my uterus anytime they want. Now that I've had my children, it's only good for growing cancer." I told her she'd been brainwashed.

In truth, the uterus plays a role in hormonal regulation, sexual satisfaction, and also bowel and bladder function (see section later in this chapter on hysterectomy, pages 193–97). Its removal is not advisable unless absolutely necessary.

This undervaluing of the uterus by doctors and the public alike has contributed to the fact that, after cesarean section, hysterectomy is the second most commonly performed major surgical operation in the United States. In the 1980s about 60 percent of women had their uterus removed by age sixty-five.[2] The average age of a woman undergoing hysterectomy is 42.7 years, with the median age being 40.9. This figure has remained constant during the past two decades. The rate of hysterectomy varies by region of the country, with the South having the highest overall rate of this procedure and the Northeast the lowest. Hysterectomy is also performed more commonly on African-American women than on Caucasian women, and is performed more frequently by male gynecologists than by female gynecologists. The number of hysterectomies performed peaked in 1985, when 724,000 operations were reported. Since then the number has declined. In 1991, 544,000 hysterectomies were reported. In 2003, the CDC's Center for Health Statistics estimates that more than 615,000 women underwent a hysterectomy. More than one-fourth of American women will have this procedure by age sixty.[3] Women aged forty to forty-four have the highest rates of this surgery—but rates are rising more significantly in the slightly older group. In 1994, 8.9 out of every 1,000 women age forty-five to fifty-four had hysterectomies. By 1999, that figure rose to 10 in every 1,000.[4] Even though the overall hysterectomy rate has gone down since 1985, this surgery is still performed too often when other options are available. The incidence of hysterectomy for benign (noncancerous) conditions is five times higher in the U.S. than in Europe![5] The number of hysterectomies won't change significantly until women change their beliefs about their pelvic organs. Since our thoughts affect our bodies, the negative messages about the uterus that are reflected in the current statistics and which we internalize over a lifetime are associated with a large number of problems that women experience in this area.[6]

ENERGY ANATOMY

Though there are distinct differences between the energies of the ovaries and those of the uterus, many women have problems in both at the same time. For example, many women whose ovaries are affected by endometriosis also have fibroid tumors in the uterus. It is helpful, therefore, to discuss in general the overall nature of the emotional and psychological energy patterns that create health and disease in the pelvic organs.

The *internal* pelvic organs (ovaries, tubes, and uterus) are related to second-chakra issues. And second-chakra issues are always related to money, sex, and power. Thus the health of the pelvic organs depends upon a woman's feeling able, competent, or powerful to create both financial and emotional abundance and stability, and to express her creativity fully. She must be able to feel good about herself and about her relationships with other people in her life. Relationships that she finds stressful and limiting, and which she feels she has no control over, on the other hand, may adversely affect her internal pelvic organs. Thus, if a woman stays in an unhealthy relationship because she feels she cannot support herself economically or emotionally, her internal pelvic organs may be at increased risk for disease.

Disease is not created until a woman feels frustrated in her attempts to effect changes that she needs to make in her life. The likelihood and severity of disease in this area are related to how well the various other areas of her life are functioning. A supportive marriage and family life, for example, can partially compensate for a stressful job. A classic psychological pattern associated with physical problems in the pelvis is that of a woman who wants to break free from limiting behaviors in her relationships (with her husband or job, for example) but who cannot confront her fears about the independence that making that change would bring. Though she may perceive that *others* are limiting her ability to break free, her major conflict is actually within herself around her *own* fears. One of my patients developed a fibroid tumor of the uterus and an ovarian cyst when she was forty. I asked her if her need for creativity was being met, and she told me that she very much wanted to leave her job and begin a florist business. She'd been interested in flowers since childhood, but her parents always discouraged her interest, since they considered it "frivolous." She had dutifully gone along with their suggestion that she learn typing and secretarial skills instead. She eventually became an executive secretary in an accounting firm. Though this work was not satisfying to her, she stayed at her job because it provided her with a steady income and good benefits, and she was afraid of the risks of striking out on her own. As her fortieth birthday approached, she felt the need to pursue her childhood passion and had recurrent dreams about fields of flowers that she couldn't get to because they were fenced in by barbed wire. She came to see that through her ovarian cyst and fibroid uterus, her body's birthing center was trying to tell her something.

Another issue that affects a woman's pelvic organs is competition among her various needs. When her innermost needs for companionship and emotional support are in competition with her outer needs for success, autonomy, and tribal approval, this situation may manifest in her inner pelvic organs, the ovaries and the uterus. Our culture teaches us that we can't be both emotionally fulfilled and financially successful, and that our needs for them both are mutually exclusive; that as women, we can't have it all. Women are not usually taught to be competent in handling economic and financial assets because the patriarchal system depends on women being dependent. Since having money and status protects us and makes us feel safe, women have been taught that to find security they have to marry, and men have been taught that they have to provide women with money and social status. Success, in the dominator system, permits us to control others. These beliefs and the controlling behavior that results from them are a setup for pelvic problems.

The uterus is related energetically to a woman's innermost sense of self and her inner world. It is symbolic of her dreams and the selves to which she would like to give birth. Its state of health reflects her inner emotional reality and her belief in herself at the deepest level. The health of the uterus is at risk if a woman doesn't believe in herself, is excessively self-critical or is putting too much of her energy into a dead-end job or relationship.

Uterine energy is slower than ovarian energy. The biological gestation time for the fetus is nine lunar months, while the biological gestation time for an egg is only one lunar month. Think of the uterus as the soil, either symbolic or biological, in which the creative seeds from the ovaries grow over time.

Ovarian energy is more dynamic and quickly changing than that of the uterus. In the reproductive years, healthy ovaries release new seeds monthly in a dynamic way. When this dynamic ovarian energy needs to get our attention, the ovaries are capable of changing very quickly. A large ovarian cyst can grow in a matter of days under the right circumstances.

Ovarian health is directly related to the quality of a woman's relationships with the people and things outside herself. (See chapter 7.) Ovaries are at risk when women feel controlled or criticized by others or when they themselves control and criticize others.

CHRONIC PELVIC PAIN

Pelvic pain can occur in one pelvic organ such as an ovary, in several pelvic organs, or throughout the pelvis, even if all the pelvic organs have been removed. A certain percentage of women with chronic pelvic pain are not helped by surgery or medical treatment. Though hysterectomy can relieve chronic pelvic pain in some, almost one-quarter of those women who undergo hysterectomy for this condition fail to get pain relief.[7] Women who have chronic pelvic pain often have complex psychological and emotional histories. Studies have found that they are more likely to have sought treatment for unrelated somatic complaints, have a higher total number of sexual partners, and are significantly more likely to have experienced previous significant psychosexual trauma.[8] Their physical pain is also related to unfinished emotional pain in either past or current relationships with partners or with jobs, sexual abuse, emotional abuse, or rape (on any level). Emotional stress in a woman's personal or professional life that she perceives to be unresolvable is a big contributor to pelvic pain. Unresolved traumatic events from the past live in the energy system of the body, even after the pelvic organs have been removed surgically. I commonly see pelvic pain flare-ups in women who uncover incest memories, visit the place in which the incest occurred, or work at jobs that control them but in which they feel they must continue to work. I tell these women that, through their pain, the body is asking them to pay attention to it and take care of it. The body, in its wisdom, wants to bring their attention back to the physical site of their emotional pain so that they can begin the healing process.

In many cases of chronic pelvic pain, no physical cause can be found and therefore the medical profession does not take it seriously. But chronic pelvic pain that comes from unresolved emotional pain from the past is real—it is not just "in the head." Pain is patterned or stored physically and chemically in our nervous, immune, and endocrine systems; it is in the bodymind. It cannot simply be cut out surgically.

ENDOMETRIOSIS

Endometriosis is a mysterious but increasingly common condition. The tissue that forms the lining of the uterus, the endometrial lining, normally grows inside the uterine cavity (and is responsible for monthly menstrual cycles). In endometriosis, for some reason, this tissue grows in other areas of the pelvis and sometimes even outside the pelvis entirely. (There are documented cases of endometriosis in the lining of the lungs and even in the brain.) The most common site for endometriosis is in the pelvic organs, especially behind the uterus—but also on the pelvic side walls (which surround the internal organs in the pelvic cavity), and sometimes on the bowel.

Endometriosis is sometimes associated with infertility and pelvic pain, though not always. Since fibroids and endometriosis are often present in the same individuals at the same time, everything I say about fibroids often applies to endometriosis as well. Like fibroids, endometriosis is related to diet, immunity, hormone levels, and blocked pelvic energy.

Endometriosis is the illness of competition.[9] It comes about when a woman's emotional needs are competing with her functioning in the outside world. When a woman feels that her innermost emotional needs are in direct conflict with what the world is demanding of her, endometriosis is one of the ways in which her body tries to draw her attention to the problem.

Alycia's case illustrates this point well. When she first came to see me with pelvic pain and endometriosis, she related that she'd become pregnant in college and had had an abortion. Though she had felt torn over this decision, and though at some level she had really wanted to have the baby, she also felt compelled to finish college and go to law school. She told me that at some level she had never been able to resolve the conflict between her desire to have a baby and her competing desire to be creative in the outer world of law and business. It is this conflict that is so often associated with chronic endometriosis and pain. The conflict articulated by Alycia is almost archetypal, and I see it regularly. Women are now part of the traditionally male world of competition and business. And many do not get emotional support in their homes or personal lives. Others have abandoned the notion that they even have emotional requirements. A great many of the women I've seen who have endometriosis drive themselves relentlessly in the outer world, rarely resting, rarely tuning in to their innermost needs and deepest desires. It makes perfect sense that so many women would have this disease at this time in our history. One Jungian analyst has referred to endometriosis as "a blood sacrifice to the Goddess." It is our bodies trying not to let us forget our feminine nature, our need for self-nurturance, and our connection with other women.

Historically, endometriosis was called the "career woman's disease." Women who delayed childbearing were felt to be at greatest risk for it. In the recent past, many women with endometriosis were told that if they'd stay home and have babies, they would be okay. This is a controversial assertion, besides an offensive one, since some recent studies show that there is no difference in the incidence of endometriosis in women who have been pregnant and those who have not. Dr. David Redwine, an internationally known endometriosis expert, concludes that pregnancy offers no protection against endometriosis. What would protect against the disease would be business and personal environments that don't require a mental-emotional split. This split is why so many women are dropping out of the corporate world to work at home or start their own businesses. Regardless of what she chooses, a woman with endometriosis can work toward healing herself immediately, starting with a willingness to listen to her body.

Symptoms

Endometriosis is classically associated with pelvic pain, abnormal menstrual cycles, and infertility. These symptoms vary a great deal from woman to woman. Some women with advanced endometriosis have never had any symptoms at all and don't even know that they have the disease until their doctor diagnoses it. Others, with only minimal endometriosis, may nonetheless have debilitating pelvic pain and cramps almost continuously. Most women are somewhere in between these two extremes. The most common area for endometriosis to occur is behind the uterus in the area between the uterus and rectum, known as the cul-de-sac of Douglas. Endometriosis in this area can cause painful intercourse, rectal pressure, and pain with bowel movements, especially before a period.

Diagnosis

Endometriosis of the pelvic cavity can be diagnosed definitively only via laparoscopy, though I often suspect it in women whose symptoms are consistent with endometriosis, such as a history of pelvic pain and intermenstrual spotting. In a few rare cases, it can be seen during a pelvic exam if endometrial lesions are present on the cervix, vagina, or vulva. Unfortunately, studies show that the average woman with endometriosis goes to about five doctors before the diagnosis is made because many other medical conditions, such as irritable bowel syndrome, mimic endometriosis.

Some authorities believe that you can find endometriosis in anyone if you look hard enough.[10] I agree with this. I've found endometriosis in a surprising number of completely asymptomatic women at the time of laparoscopic tubal ligation. Neither they nor I would have suspected it.

What I'd like to know is the incidence of endometriosis in women who have no problems. I believe that all women probably have embryonic cells in their pelvic cavities that could grow into endometrial tissue. But if all of us have the potential for endometriosis, why do some women develop symptoms while others do not? Until further research clarifies this, the answers lie within the individual woman. It is up to her to decipher what her symptoms are trying to tell her and to take steps to change the factors that favor the growth of endometriosis.

Common Concerns

Why do so many women have endometriosis? When I was in training, we didn't see nearly as much endometriosis as we're seeing now. There are a number of reasons for the perceived increase in the disease. First, with the advent of laparoscopy, we are diagnosing it more frequently. The patient is in and out of the hospital on the same day. The ease of looking into the pelvis without doing major surgery results in laparoscopy being offered rather routinely to patients who have pelvic pain.

Another factor in the apparent increase in incidence of endometriosis is that women today are delaying childbearing and having more menstrual cycles than in the past. When they do have children, they are having fewer of them. Since endometriosis is a hormone-dependent disorder, when the body has relatively high circulating estrogen levels without a break for pregnancy and nursing, this would favor its manifestation.

Is endometriosis hereditary? Endometriosis often runs in families, so there is some hereditary link. I've seen patients whose sisters and mothers all had it. But having a sister with endometriosis does not guarantee that you'll have it, too, especially if you live your lives in different ways. The genetic potential for endometriosis does not have to manifest unless your environment and health habits promote it. The standard nutrient-poor American diet, which favors cellular inflammation and hormone imbalance in susceptible individuals, contributes to endometriosis and is often the type eaten by families who have endometriosis. In my clinical experience, intake of conventionally produced dairy foods and a refined-food diet are especially associated with exacerbating the pain of endometriosis.

Will endometriosis interfere with my fertility? Many endometriosis patients are fertile women whose main problem is pain. Endometriosis does not cause infertility, but it is felt to be a major contributing factor. Currently, 40 to 50 percent of women who have a laparoscopy to determine the cause of their problems with infertility are found to have endometriosis.[11] Many women with endometriosis have the massive pelvic scarring usually associated with infertility. Dr. David Redwine says, "Studying the disease among predominantly infertile women only serves to confuse the issue."[12] Whatever is causing the endometriosis symptoms may also be responsible for the infertility, but one doesn't cause the other.[13]

So what causes endometriosis? Medical theories about endometriosis abound, but no one really knows what it is and why so many women seem to have it now. The classic theory is that endometriosis results from retrograde menstruation, or menstruating backward, so that some of the menstrual blood and tissue that line the uterus go back up the fallopian tubes, then implant in the pelvic tissue and begin to grow.[14] Since retrograde menstruation probably occurs in every menstruating woman at some point, this doesn't explain why some women get the disease and others don't. Another theory is that pelvic tissues spontaneously convert to endometrial tissue, possibly due to irritation or hormonal activity from environmental toxins such as dioxin, which can have estrogenlike activity.

The pain associated with endometriosis clearly results from an increased production of inflammatory chemicals such as cytokines and prostaglandins that are produced by the endometriosis lesions. Endometriosis lesions are also stimulated in part by the hormones of the menstrual cycle, and the pain is worse at ovulation and during the premenstrual and menstrual times of the cycle. Since endometrial lesions are the same as the tissue inside the uterus, it is understandable that when a woman bleeds with her menstrual cycle, her endometriosis implants bleed microscopically inside her body, too. Some experts feel that the endometrial lesions also secrete some kind of chemical that results in bleeding from surrounding capillaries in the peritoneum (the Saran Wrap–like lining of the pelvic cavity, where endometriosis is found). Over time, this recurrent monthly bleeding into the pelvic cavity is believed to cause painful cysts and adhesions that tend to flare up under the right circumstances.

The theory that makes the most sense to me is that endometriosis is a congenital condition that is present at birth.[15] According to this theory, endometriosis arises from embryonic female genital tissue that never made it to the inside of the uterus during development. This helps explain why endometriosis can run in families and why some girls have severe pelvic pain from endometriosis *as soon as* they start their periods. Yet in this theory all females have the capacity to develop endometriosis if embryonic cells in their pelvis get stimulated by the right set of circumstances.

Though most gynecologists have been taught that endometriosis is a progressive disease that gets worse over time, some studies, including Dr. Redwine's, show that endometriosis doesn't spread or get worse over time (though its appearance changes) and won't recur if all of it is removed surgically or if the conditions which stimulate it are no longer present.

When performing laparoscopies to diagnose the cause of pelvic pain, many gynecologists miss the diagnosis of endometriosis in its early stages because they were taught to look only for the characteristic black "powder burn" lesions. In fact, endometrial lesions come in a range of colors: clear, white, yellow, blue, and red. Many of these early lesions are very subtle and difficult to see without the proper equipment.[16]

The color of endometrial lesions may be related to blood leaking from nearby capillaries. Over time, the lesions progress from clear to black, depending upon the amount of scarring present. The older the woman with endometriosis, the greater her chances of having "classic" endometriosis with black "powder burn" lesions and "chocolate" cysts of the ovaries. (Endometriosis in the ovaries can result in large ovarian cysts filled with old blood. When these are operated on, the contents of the cysts look just like chocolate syrup.)

The Neuroendocrine-Immune Connection

The intimate interactions between our thoughts, emotions, and immunity hold the key to interpreting the message that endometriosis has for the individual woman as well as helping her heal it. Studies on the immune systems of women with symptomatic endometriosis show that these women often have antibodies against their own tissue, called autoantibodies. This means that at some deep level, the mind of their pelvis is rejecting aspects of itself.

The autoantibodies interfere with various processes of human reproduction, including sperm function, fertilization, and normal progression of pregnancy. Their presence may explain the association between infertility and endometriosis in those women who have both problems at the same time. Endometriosis has been clearly associated with decreased egg fertilization, decreased success rates for in vitro fertilization ("test tube" fertilization), and increased miscarriages. The clinical experience of therapist Niravi Payne with women with infertility and endometriosis shows clearly that at an unconscious level, these women may have an ambivalence about becoming pregnant. Their minds may desire it, while their hearts aren't sure. The presence of these abnormal autoantibodies in patients with endometriosis holds the key to understanding many characteristics of the disease that scientists have been unable to explain when they have looked at it as a structural problem only, as if it were a tumor to be removed.[17]

Making antibodies against the body's own tissue is characteristic of other autoimmune diseases that stymie conventional medical science and that cannot be "cured" in the conventional sense. The immune system is highly sensitive, and our survival depends upon its ability to recognize and distinguish self from nonself. A new body of research is documenting the intimate link between a healthy immune system and a healthy bacterial ecosystem in the places in our bodies that interface with the environment. These include the vagina, the mouth, the lungs, and also the entire surface of the gut. When the bacterial ecosystem balance is lost, then immune system functioning suffers. It is well documented, for example, that antibiotic usage destroys healthy bacteria in all those areas, leading to an overgrowth of yeast and mold. This yeast and mold have been shown to trigger allergic responses in the lungs when they are exposed to mold spores, which is one of the reasons why there is so much more asthma and allergies in children now than in the past. Children are put on too many antibiotics and there is an ever-increasing use of household disinfectants.[18] The immune system imbalance that results could help explain the immune components of endometriosis. When a woman stops taking antibiotics, gets on a good probiotic to replenish her bowel and vaginal flora (normal bacterial life in this area), takes immune-enhancing supplements such as vitamin D (1,000 IU per day), and also follows a diet that halts cellular inflammation, the endometriosis pain often disappears in a few weeks.

Treatment

Women with symptomatic endometriosis do best with a comprehensive treatment program that fully supports their immune systems while they remain open to finding out what they need to change about their lives. My patients have healed endometriosis symptoms through a variety of treatments. Most important, many of them have come to a greater understanding of what they need to learn for true healing, not just masking of their physical symptoms.

Hormones. The most common treatment for endometriosis, once diagnosed, is hormonal therapy, in the form of birth control pills, synthetic progestin, danazol (Danocrine), or the GnRH (gonadotropin-releasing hormones) agonists, such as Synarel and Lupron. These drugs act on the pituitary gland to make a woman temporarily menopausal, thereby allowing the endometriosis to regress by stopping its cyclic hormonal stimulation.

All of these hormonal therapies change the amount of estrogen and other hormones in the system, so that endometriosis is not activated. When hormone levels are decreased, symptoms often disappear and the disease itself becomes inactive. Danazol and the GnRH agonists are also used to decrease the amount of endometriosis prior to surgery—in some cases, so that surgical removal is easier. The problem with these approaches is that they don't really cure the disease; they simply shut down the hormonal stimulation of it for a while. In addition, some women do not tolerate well the side effects of these treatments. Danazol is expensive—it costs about a dollar a dose—and it can have masculinizing side effects, such as hair growth and voice deepening. Most women gain some weight while they are on it. GnRH agonist therapy results in hot flashes, thinning of the vaginal tissue, and bone loss. Yet other women badly need these hormonal treatments as a respite from pain, even though the pain often recurs once the drug is discontinued.

I once saw a patient who had been on Synarel (a GnRH agonist) all summer. "It was so wonderful to go camping, water-skiing, and hang gliding and not have to worry about the pain," she told me. "I felt just wonderful. I know I can't stay on it forever, but I sure felt great." She had been off it for two weeks when I saw her, and her pain was beginning to recur. As we talked about her options, she said that when she was having the pain before she went on the drug, she would often get complete pain relief from a massage. She was surprised by that, but she felt that massage was too expensive and that dietary change was too difficult due to her schedule. Yet Synarel cost nearly $400 per month at that time.[19] Once she thought it all through, however, she decided to try to change her schedule to eat better, and she became willing to try a few nondrug approaches for a trial period of three months. She knew that surgery was an option. When I last saw her, she was doing well with lifestyle changes.

Even though the menopausal symptoms associated with GnRH agonists are reversible once the drug is stopped, this type of therapy, if used longer than a few months, is not appropriate for everyone. I'd be particularly wary of using it in anyone who has had a problem with irregular periods or central nervous system disorders, since it has been associated with memory problems in some. The lifestyle of a patient who may need it is characterized by a very high-pressure job, long work hours, a lot of travel, almost no time to herself, and lack of desire or ability to change her career. Using drugs in this type of situation makes it easier for the woman to continue activities that may nonetheless be harming her at some level. I worry about her using the medication, but I also trust her process, knowing that she will learn something from whatever option she chooses. I also trust that what brought her to the doctor will eventually open her to learning about her body. The body is innately self-healing, and when there's a genuine desire to be well, the patient almost always finds the modality that suits her best.

Natural progesterone often works very well to relieve endometriosis symptoms and is my first line of treatment following dietary improvement. The usual way is to use a 2-percent progesterone cream such as Emerita, one-quarter to one-half teaspoon on the skin twice a day. (See page 136.) Natural progesterone helps counteract endometriosis by decreasing the effects of estrogen on the endometrial lesions. Natural progesterone is free from side effects and is very well tolerated. Use it on days ten to twenty-eight of each cycle; some women may need to use it daily. Sometimes the dose of progesterone needs to be increased beyond what is available in 2-percent progesterone cream. In these cases, a prescription transdermal cream can be compounded by a formulary pharmacist. (See Resources for how to locate one in your area.) Natural progesterone capsules taken orally are another choice; the usual dosage is 50 to 200 mg per day, taken on days ten to twenty-eight of each cycle. Progesterone vaginal gels are also available by prescription.

Surgery. Many women with severe endometriosis, having tried hormones and pain medication for years, often end up at a very young age with complete hysterectomies, including removal of their ovaries. I regard this treatment as a last resort after trying other more benign alternatives.

More conservative surgery that removes only the endometriosis and preserves the pelvic organs can be very helpful. More and more gynecologists are skilled at this pelviscopic surgery and have learned how to remove endometriosis without missing any lesions. If any endometriosis is left behind after this conservative surgery, the pain is likely to recur. Pelviscopic surgery, done correctly, has a pain recurrence rate of only about 10 percent. In these women, the pain is frequently associated not with endometriosis but with fibroids, adhesions, or adenomyosis. (See chapter 5.) A woman who intends to undergo surgery for endometrial pain must go to someone who is skilled in this form of treatment. (See Resources.)

Energy medicine. Anything that improves immune system functioning and increases the flow of energy in the body is apt to help endometriosis. Ask yourself the following questions and answer them honestly:

~ What are my emotional needs?

~ What would I like to see happen in my job or my life that would nourish me fully?

~ Am I caught up in competition of any sort in my life? Am I willing to make changes?

~ Am I getting enough rest?

~ Do I believe that I have the power to change the conditions of my life? Affirm this power regularly by saying this affirmation out loud in the mirror twice per day for a month: "The healing power that created the universe is now working in and through me, creating quickly and easily the perfect outcome—the perfect result."

Apply a castor oil pack to your lower abdomen at least three times per week for one hour each time, except during times of heavy bleeding. (See page 148 for instructions.) Pay attention to all thoughts, images, and feelings that arise. Consider a course of acupuncture in conjunction with Chinese herbs. (See chapter 5.) Get a total body massage at least once every other week for two months. Notice how you feel after the massage. Also consider finding a physical therapist trained in the Wurn Technique, a noninvasive, nonsurgical type of deep tissue massage that can be very helpful in treating endometriosis and pelvic pain. (For more information, contact Clear Passage Therapies at 866-222-9437 or visit www.clearpassage.com.)

Dietary change. Endometriosis is an estrogen-sensitive disease and symptoms are increased by estrogen. They are also exacerbated by an excess of inflammatory chemicals, such as prostaglandin F2 alpha, the same hormone associated with menstrual cramps. Women with endometriosis who have significant pain have been found to have higher levels of cellular inflammation in their endometrial cysts than those who don't.[20] Dietary goals are to reduce excess estrogen production in the body and reduce cellular inflammation. The symptom relief that follows is often dramatic.

DIETARY APPROACH

~ Take essential fatty acids daily: 500 to 2,000 mg per day. Sources: ground flaxseed, wild salmon, fish oil, ground hemp seed, flaxseed oil, macadamia nuts, macadamia nut oil.

~ Eliminate partially hydrogenated fats (trans-fats).

~ Take a comprehensive multivitamin-mineral supplement that is rich in B complex, zinc, selenium, vitamin E, and magnesium—you need about 50 to 100 mg of each of the B vitamins and 300 to 800 mg of magnesium. Dian Mills, a nutritionist in London and a former trustee of the British Endometriosis Society, reported a double-blind study of dietary supplements that resulted in a 98-percent improvement in symptoms over those not on the supplement. The supplements used were thiamine, riboflavin, and pyridoxine, 100 mg each; zinc citrate, 20 mg: and magnesium aminochelate, 300 mg.[21]

~ Eliminate red meat, dairy foods, and egg yolks for at least two weeks. Then reintroduce and see if symptoms recur.

~ Eliminate caffeine. (See chapter 17 for full dietary discussion.)

One of my patients had had endometriosis for many years. She had unsuccessfully tried Danocrine and surgical treatments. But after she eliminated dairy products from her diet, she became free of endometriosis symptoms and has remained so for ten years. Recently, she conceived her first child without difficulty, even though another doctor told her that she probably wouldn't be able to get pregnant.

Foods that have been shown to modulate estrogen levels are the cruciferous vegetables, such as kale, collard greens, mustard greens, broccoli, cabbage, and turnips. Try for one or two servings of these daily (or take a supplement containing Indole-3-Carbinol, the active ingredient in these vegetables). (See Resources.) Soy foods can also help. Use tofu, tempeh, soy sauce, and miso regularly or supplement with soy powder made from whole soybeans. Also, a diet high in fiber can decrease total circulating estrogens. Try for 25 grams per day in the form of whole grains, beans, brown rice, vegetables, and fruits. Note: Most dry cereals contain far too much refined carbohydrates to justify their fiber content. Stick with oatmeal and shredded wheat.

With nutritional approaches, it's important to give them at least two to three months to achieve optimal results.

Women's Stories

Doris: learning from endometriosis. Doris was forty-one when she first came to see me. She was a highly successful professional who spent lots of time traveling and working but had little time for herself and her personal, emotional needs. She had heavy periods that got worse at night and sometimes would soak through the sheets. She complained of fluid retention, bloating, and severe menstrual cramps. Her uterus was enlarged to ten-to-twelve-week-pregnancy size from fibroids. She had a history of infertility, several miscarriages, and an abortion. A laparoscopy by another physician had confirmed the presence of endometriosis as well as fibroids, and he felt that these were associated with her miscarriages. Her gynecologist had suggested a hysterectomy because he said that her periods would continue to be difficult and that she would eventually end up with the surgery anyway. She was not happy with this diagnosis, however, and came to see me about her alternatives.

When I first saw her, she had a great deal of tenderness behind her uterus, which is very common in women with endometriosis. I asked her questions about her lifestyle, diet, miscarriages, abortion, exercise, and stress levels. I agreed that surgery was not something we needed to consider right then and suggested several alternative treatments. Among them were eliminating dairy products from her diet, applying castor oil packs to her lower abdomen, taking vitamin supplements, and reading about perfectionism, addiction, and whole foods. From what Doris had told me about herself, I felt that she needed to heal her feelings about her miscarriages and her abortion. She decided to follow my suggestions. To unlock her feelings about her fertility, she decided to write letters to the unborn potential beings who had been in her body. As she wrote me later, "Obviously they were still there in some form in my mind and had taken form as fibroids and maybe endometriosis in my body. The most incredible experience occurred after I wrote the letters. I had been remembering my dreams with great regularity through visualization techniques. One night in a dream, I was fully aware of my body, and I dreamed that thousands of white doves were flying out of my uterus. An unbelievable feeling of lightness came over me, and I awoke crying with joy."

Three months after Doris's dream experience, I examined her and found that many of her fibroids were gone and so was all of her uterine tenderness. The remaining fibroids seemed to have solidified into a smooth mass that was definitely smaller and smoother than it had been at the time of her earlier examination. Doris found that when she takes care of herself and follows her diet, gets exercise, and does some things just for herself, she feels fine and has no pelvic symptoms of any kind. Though her fibroids didn't disappear entirely, they didn't grow for years. The last time I saw her she had no tenderness on examination, a testimony to the fact that her endometriosis became very inactive.

Doris used the wisdom of her body to heal some very painful experiences about which she had not allowed herself to grieve. She was willing to risk completely changing the way she saw herself in the world, a change that often needs to be made if women are to heal at the deepest level. This often involves examining with microscopic honesty how we really feel about being female while also affirming our worth and our inherent goodness. It also may involve cutting way back on our worldly activities and creating a healthful balance between our inner and outer selves.

FIBROID TUMORS

Fibroids are benign tumors of the uterus. They grow in various locations on and within the uterine wall itself or in the uterine cavity. (See figure 8.) Standard medical practice to gauge the size of a fibroid is to compare the size of a uterus with a fibroid with the size of the uterus at

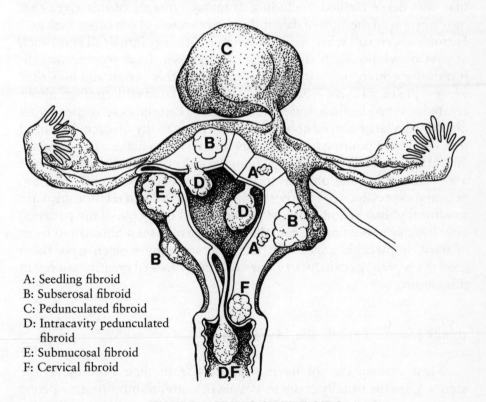

A: Seedling fibroid
B: Subserosal fibroid
C: Pedunculated fibroid
D: Intracavity pedunculated
   fibroid
E: Submucosal fibroid
F: Cervical fibroid

FIGURE 8: TYPES OF FIBROIDS

various stages of pregnancy. Thus, a woman will be told that she has a fourteen-week-size fibroid if her uterus is as big as it would be if she were fourteen weeks pregnant. Fibroids are made from hard, white gristly tissue that has a whorl-like pattern. They are present in 20 to 50 percent of all women. One of my patients, who watched her fibroid removal via a mirror, later said, "The appearance of the fibroid surprised me. I expected it to be messy-looking. A fibroid looks like a piece of high-density polyethylene plastic, the stuff cutting boards are made of."

Fibroids are responsible for as many as 33 percent of all gynecological hospital admissions, and they are the number one reason for hysterectomy in this country for women aged forty-five to fifty-four.[22] They are three to nine times more common in black women than in Caucasians. Many women with fibroids are unaware that they have them until they are discovered during a routine pelvic examination. No one knows, from a conventional medical standpoint, what causes fibroids.

Caroline Myss teaches that fibroid tumors represent our creativity that was never birthed, including "fantasy" images of ourselves that have never seen the light of day and creative secrets of our other "selves." Fibroids also result when we are flowing life-energy into dead ends, such as jobs or relationships that we have outgrown. I ask women with fibroids to meditate on their relationships with other people and how they express their creativity. Fibroids are often associated with conflicts about creativity, reproduction, and relationships.[23] I certainly can relate having developed a large fibroid about five years prior to my divorce. I realized that I had been pouring lots of energy into trying to make a dead-end relationship work! In our rapidly changing culture, where women's roles are in flux, it is quite obvious to me that conflicts about child-rearing, personal expressions of creativity, and changing roles in relationships are a cultural phenomenon, not just an individual one. One of my patients, after looking at her fibroid, said that it was easy to see a fibroid as a form of hard, implacable anger. The fact that so many women have these growths is perhaps evidence of our collective blocked creative energy in this culture.

Symptoms

Most women do not have symptoms from their fibroids. These uterine growths usually come to a woman's attention on routine pelvic examination. Whether a fibroid is symptomatic has to do with its size and location within the uterus. Those that are located in the muscle wall of the uterus just under the surface (subserosal) may not be symp-tomatic. But those growing into the uterine lining itself (submucosal) often cause heavy or irregular bleeding. Some fibroids are attached to the inside or even the outside of the uterus by a thin stalk. These are known as pedunculated fibroids. If they are on the outside of the uterus, they are sometimes confused with ovarian tumors. I've had two patients who "delivered" pedunculated six-centimeter fibroids through the cervical opening. I simply removed these fibroids by suturing and then severing the stalk. Neither of these women had any further prob-lems.

Women who have both fibroids and endometriosis may experience menstrual cramps, pelvic pain, or both. Most fibroids can be treated conservatively by letting them be and having an examination every six months to a year or so to monitor their growth.

Bleeding. Some women with fibroids have extremely heavy periods, re-sulting in anemia, fatigue, and even an inability to leave the house dur-ing the heaviest days. If the fibroids are growing quickly, if a woman's hormones are in flux (which is common around the time of meno-pause), or if she's been under a great deal of stress, she can even develop hemorrhaging from uterine fibroids. Some women grow so accustomed to their large monthly blood loss that they don't even realize how a normal flow would feel. Some even become severely anemic without knowing it.

Fibroid tumors can cause a lot of bleeding because the uterus is en-dowed with a very rich blood supply. If the fibroid is submucosal, lo-cated just under the uterine lining, the body has an especially difficult time with the usual mechanism that stops menstrual flow. Menstrual flow is stopped, in part, by muscular contraction of the uterus, and fi-broids may interfere with this mechanism. An endometrial biopsy (tak-ing a sample of tissue from inside the uterus) or sometimes a D&C is necessary in cases of abnormal bleeding to be certain that the bleeding is caused by fibroids and not cancer (though cancer is rarely found). This is especially true for those women who have bleeding at irregular intervals throughout the month.

Fibroid degeneration. A fibroid may start to degenerate, following its rapid growth. This can happen, for instance, during a particularly stressful or emotionally demanding time, during pregnancy, or during the year or so before menopause. Fibroid degeneration can occur when the fibroid outgrows its blood supply. When this happens, the center of the fibroid is deprived of oxygen from the blood, and the nerves deep inside this tissue register a lack of oxygen as pain, in the same way that frostbitten toes do. The pain can be a nuisance, but the condition is not usually dangerous. The degeneration in the center of the fibroid often causes some shrinkage in fibroid size, and on occasion a fibroid shrinks or disappears. The pain usually goes away after a week or so as the nerves adjust.

Pelvic pressure and urinary frequency. Sometimes the position of a fibroid causes symptoms because the fibroid pushes into another organ, such as the rectum or the bladder. Pressure or a sense of fullness in the rectum, lower back, or abdomen may result. If the fibroid is in the front of the uterus and relatively low, the pressure on the bladder can decrease the bladder's ability to hold urine, resulting in urinary frequency (having to void in frequent small amounts). These symptoms are annoying but are not harmful to the body in general. I've never seen an organ contiguous to a benign fibroid that was harmed by the fibroid. An occasional very large fibroid can partially block the ureter (the tube going from the kidney to the bladder) when a woman is lying down. Neither urologists nor gynecologists know for certain whether this situation can eventually cause kidney problems. I have never seen this happen or even heard of it! Most women with fibroids large enough to cause urethral pressure prefer surgery simply because they don't like looking pregnant. Several of my patients, however, have done very well without surgery, and their kidneys are fine. One of these women, who had a very large fibroid uterus for at least ten years, and whose ureter had occasionally shown some blockage from fibroids, began to experience rapid shrinking of her fibroids as she went through menopause. This is common.

Common Concerns

What if I have a fibroid? When fibroids are felt for the first time, I recommend a pelvic ultrasound to measure them and to check out the status of the ovaries. Sometimes it's impossible on a pelvic exam to tell the difference between an ovarian growth and a fibroid on the uterus.

Can fibroids be cancerous? Fibroids are almost never cancerous. Less than one in a thousand turns into a uterine sarcoma, a very rare type of cancer of the uterine muscle. The only way to tell for sure, however, is to take them out and look at them under the microscope. Since the mortality rate for hysterectomy itself is one in a thousand, the risk of surgery is actually greater than the risk of the fibroid being malignant.

The most common problem with fibroids is their tendency to grow and to cause bleeding. But, as with many women I've worked with, if the underlying energy patterns, life questions, conflicts, and emotional issues associated with the fibroids are addressed and changed, the fibroids usually do not grow or cause problems.

Are fibroids genetic? Fibroids can run in families. One of my fibroid patients told me that every female in her family for three generations had fibroids. She is planning to be the first woman in her tribe to get to menopause with her uterus intact. She has changed her diet and now is completely free from symptoms.

Just as in a strong family history of alcoholism, in a strong family history of fibroids the individual woman is up against a family belief system, from which it is very difficult to break free. I once read an article about familial ovarian cancer entitled "My Mother, My Cells," in which the author articulated her difficulty with inheriting a tendency toward a disease that terrified her and over which she felt she had no control.

In this country, we tend to think of a genetic predisposition as an inevitable "sentence" that we *will* get the disease. However, environmental factors play a huge role in whether that predisposition ever gets expressed. For example, some individuals with the gene for cystic fibrosis manage to keep the disease under control and live well into their fifties. This was unheard of several decades ago. And many women with very strong family histories of breast cancer never get the disease.

Some women who have strong family histories of fibroids, ovarian cysts, or endometriosis have developed these conditions themselves but have healed from them. One patient summarized a necessary part of this healing when she said, "I've finally realized that I am not my mother. I don't have to live out her life in my body." In families in which there is a genetic disease, we should study those members who *don't* get the disease. Most likely they are the individuals who broke the family mold, the ones who did not live out family expectations on a cellular or other level.

Will my fibroids interfere with pregnancy? During pregnancy, hormone levels are very high and preexisting fibroids can grow rapidly. If they begin to degenerate, fibroids can sometimes cause uterine contractions that can result in premature delivery. This doesn't happen with all fibroids, however. I've seen women with large fourteen-week-size fibroids get pregnant, carry to term, and go through normal labor and delivery without *any* problem.

One twenty-nine-year-old woman came to me already twelve weeks pregnant with a large fibroid in the posterior portion of her uterus. The pregnancy had been unplanned, but she was thrilled about it. Her doctor had told her to have an abortion and then have the fibroid removed before conceiving again. He told her that the fibroid would probably cause the early delivery of a baby who would be so premature that it wouldn't live. She was very upset about her dilemma and needed a physician who was willing to go along with the pregnancy, knowing that there might be a problem while being open to the possibility that all could go well. Her pregnancy proceeded normally, going to full term without pain, bleeding, or premature labor. She delivered a seven-pound, three-ounce girl after an eight-hour labor. Her fibroid had shrunk to an eight-week size by the time of her six-week postpartum checkup.

Fibroids can result in miscarriage or even infertility, particularly if they've distorted the uterine cavity enough. Whether there are problems seems to depend on the location of the fibroid within the uterus and how close it is to the developing baby and placenta. An ultrasound or hysterosalpingogram (an X-ray study in which dye is injected into the uterus and tubes) can give you some idea of fibroid location before pregnancy, as can an MRI (magnetic resonance imaging).

Some pregnant women have fibroids that start degenerating. They end up in the hospital to be watched closely while they rest in bed on pain medication. Generally, fibroids don't hurt the developing baby unless they cause so much uterine irritability that the uterus starts contracting and premature labor results. There are no guarantees against developing problems with fibroids during pregnancy because the entire uterus grows, including the fibroid wall. The farther away from the uterine cavity the fibroid is located, the less likely that a woman will have problems. Some doctors are willing to take a wait-and-see attitude about fibroids and pregnancy, suggesting that a woman try to get pregnant and see what happens. Others will suggest that she have the fibroids removed before attempting pregnancy.

Will the fibroids grow? Will they go away? Many women with fibroids are told that hysterectomy should be performed when their fibroids are relatively small so that a more risky and complicated hysterectomy in the future, should the fibroids grow, will not be necessary. Studies have shown that there is little or no justification for this.[24] Fibroids do grow sometimes, but not always. They tend to grow quite briskly during the years just before menopause, when hormonal levels fluctuate widely, then shrink dramatically after menopause. One of my perimenopausal, or "almost menopausal," patients, age forty-nine, whom I followed for more than twenty years, could easily feel her fibroids through her abdominal wall by pressing down with her fingers. She said that her fibroids grew up to her belly button just before her period and shrunk down to just above her pubic bone within three days after her period was over! Fibroids often change size during each menstrual cycle, reaching their peak during ovulation and just before the menstrual period begins. They can also grow during periods of stress. Fibroids can be followed by a physician or other qualified health care provider with an exam every six months to a year. There's no reason to rush into surgery, unless you have repeated episodes of severe bleeding that cannot be controlled with hormonal treatments or other measures.

Sometimes fibroids go away completely. I recently met a religious woman who had been scheduled for hysterectomy because of fibroids. She prayed about them daily. Six weeks later, when she went back to her doctor, the fibroids were gone and she didn't require the surgery.

One of my patients, a forty-three-year-old musician and sound healer named Persis, first came to see me with a fibroid the size of a four-to-five-month pregnancy. After two years of a strict diet, reflective inner work, massages, and therapeutic sound, her very large fibroid uterus returned almost to normal.[25] I rarely see fibroids shrink as much as hers did. This shrinkage was not because of menopause. She is still having normal periods. Here is her story:

"In the summer of 1988, I was diagnosed with endometriosis and a grapefruit-size fibroid tumor. The preceding years had been filled with increasingly excruciating pain that left me almost blacking out while driving. I had gotten used to being in pain for two weeks, then recovering from the exhaustion in the next two weeks, and had become terrified of getting my period.

"The doctor I was seeing at the time told me about all the alternatives for correcting the problem. His favorite was hysterectomy—'At your age you don't need your uterus anyway,' he said. Then there was hormone therapy to stop the periods for one to two years: 'Your voice will drop, and you will lose your sexual desire.' And the last offer he made was that I could continue with the pain and bleeding until menopause.

"Since I wanted to keep my body whole, didn't particularly like the idea of giving up my womanhood to hormone therapy, and couldn't tolerate the pain, I looked for other treatment. I made a commitment to my life. I accepted the responsibility for taking care of myself. I accepted the loving help of others. I began a very strict regimen of macrobiotic diet, sitz baths, exercise, and meditation. Looking back, I don't know how I fit all that into my busy life. I do know that I am a changed person.

"I also began gently to search out the reasons behind my 'woman's troubles.' I accepted my codependent nature and began opening up to the pain of my childhood and young adulthood. The pain in my belly was a culmination of a lifetime of pains. I knew just cutting it out wouldn't 'fix' all the other pains in my life.

"I now have little pain and feel extraordinarily well. I am and always will be in process throughout my life. Through meditation and sound healing on myself, I have renewed my inner faith. I accept my life and my ability to heal myself as well as to help others heal. As I do for others, I do for myself."

If I undergo fibroid removal treatment, will the fibroids grow back?
The answer to this question must be individualized. In general, a woman who is within five years of menopause when she has her fibroids treated is not likely to have them grow back, because her estrogen levels will be decreasing naturally. If the underlying energy pattern, emotional issues, or hormonal levels associated with the fibroids haven't changed, then other so-called seedling fibroids can start to grow. Women who change their diets dramatically, however, decrease the likelihood that the fibroids will return. Most of my patients' fibroids did not grow back or worsen. This is probably because of the law of attraction. Women who resonate with my approach are highly motivated to take responsibility for their own healing. I recommend dietary change, bodywork, homeopathy, and other alternative methods, even for those women who choose fibroid removal as their treatment. Surgery or fibroid ablation alone will not change the fundamental pattern in their bodies that encouraged the fibroids to grow. It is vital to listen to what our bodies are trying to teach us and affirm our ability to be whole.

Treatment

At no point is it appropriate for a doctor to make dictatorial treatment recommendations about what any woman should do with her uterus. There is no right and wrong. Instead, it's best to offer women ways to think about their uterus, ovaries, and body, so that when they need to make a decision about hormones, drugs, surgery, or fibroid ablation, they'll know what their personal truth is regarding those organs. More treatments for fibroids are now available than ever before. Once a woman has gathered the facts about treatment choices, she can tune in to her own inner guidance to decide which is the best for her.

For many women, just knowing that they have a choice in the matter is a huge relief. Some women interpret surgery, for example, as further abuse, when they have not freely chosen to undergo it. Incest survivors sometimes tell me that the very thought of an invasive procedure in their body, particularly of a gynecological nature, feels just like rape. Obviously, alternative modes of treatment should be tried in these cases, rather than allowing the abuse cycle to once again be ignited.

The following section illustrates different treatment approaches to problems in the uterus. There is no one right way to treat uterine problems. Each of these women mentioned in this section needed help for fairly straightforward and common symptoms, and each chose a different treatment. Only one woman wanted a hysterectomy. Each woman was able to arrange treatment that respected her individual choice. Medical technology, when consciously used in an individualized treatment, can be a major aid in healing women's lives. To claim that hysterectomy is always the wrong or inferior choice is as dualistic and harmful as claiming that all natural remedies are quackery. I do not address the specific psychological and emotional issues connected with "blocked energy in the pelvis" for any of these cases. Not all women are open or ready to explore their deep issues, and I respect their choice to wait for the right time.

Conservative: watch and wait. If a woman's fibroids aren't causing her any problems, I recommend a pelvic exam every six months to a year, depending upon her situation. I also recommend a sonogram (ultrasound) initially to be sure that the problem is a fibroid and not an ovarian cyst or tumor. Sonograms can measure fibroid size and check the ovaries. Conservative treatment is sometimes called "benign neglect" or the "tincture of time." Very often it's the best therapy.

Hormone therapy: synthetic progestin or natural progesterone. To women whose primary symptom is bleeding, I suggest synthetic progestin or natural progesterone as a treatment, to keep the lining of the uterus from building up too much. In many cases this therapy works very well to control bleeding and is much more benign than major abdominal surgery. Progesterone or progestin is an option for women who are unable to change their diets or whose symptoms aren't allevi-ated by dietary changes. Some women become depressed while they are on synthetic progestin; others feel bloated or premenstrual or get headaches. Bioidentical (or natural) progesterone is generally free of these side effects and is my first choice. Since each woman's life situa-tion is different, her medical treatment needs to be individualized.

GnRH agonist. GnRH (gonadotropin-releasing hormone) agonists such as Lupron and Synarel are synthetic hormones that cause the pituitary gland to shut down the function of the ovaries. After about one month on these drugs, a woman's body becomes artificially menopausal. Her es-trogen levels fall very low, and her periods cease. The cyclic stimulation of her fibroid tissue ceases, and in most cases the fibroids shrink in size. GnRH agonists are used in select cases to shrink fibroids before surgery or to shrink them enough so that surgery is not necessary. Some physi-cians use these drugs to keep a woman's fibroids asymptomatic until she reaches menopausal age, at which point the fibroids naturally shrink. In this way, she can avoid surgery. It takes about three months to get the maximum effect from these drugs, but most women only need to be on them for two months in order to get significant shrinking for a myomec-tomy. Not everyone gets the same result because not all fibroids are cre-ated equal.[26]

As I mentioned earlier, GnRH agonists are very expensive, and they are not recommended for use longer than six months. Once use of the drug has stopped, the fibroids grow back quite rapidly unless a woman becomes naturally menopausal during the time she is on the drug.

Many women are understandably hesitant to use such synthetic hormones. Baby-boom-generation women remember that diethylstilbes-trol (DES) was enthusiastically used for more than thirty years to pre-vent miscarriage. In 1971, the drug was withdrawn after it was linked to certain rare vaginal cancers and other genital tract abnormalities in some of the female (and even male) offspring of the women who used it. Having said that, it is clear that GnRH agonists do have a place in the treatment of fibroids. They can be used to shrink fibroids while ad-ministering enough "add back" hormones to lessen their menopausal side effects without compromising their effectiveness. This approach can save some women from undergoing perimenopausal hysterec-tomies.

Endometrial ablation. Christine had heavy periods for years—she had to use two super tampons at a time, as well as a pad. Sometimes these needed to be changed every half hour during day two of her period, making it very difficult for her to travel or even leave the house to grocery shop. The minimal dietary changes she made had not worked. Further testing revealed that she had multiple, very small fibroids in the uterine wall.

Christine very much wanted to avoid hysterectomy, so we tried synthetic progestin therapy for the last two weeks of each month for three months.[27] Even though this treatment almost always decreases bleeding, it didn't work in her case. A D&C also failed to alleviate her bleeding. I referred her for a procedure called endometrial ablation using hysteroscopy. Hysteroscopy is a surgical technique in which the lining of the uterus can be visualized and operated on by passing a scope through the cervix from the vagina. Various techniques are available, including cautery and laser. The technique used depends on the patient's condition and the choice of the surgeon. Submucosal fibroids can sometimes be removed this way by surgeons skilled in this technique. This procedure, done under anesthesia in the operating room, cauterizes and obliterates the endometrial lining—the part of the uterus that bleeds every month. When it works, menstrual periods cease or become very light. For Christine, the procedure worked beautifully. Instead of recuperating for a month from the removal of her uterus, she went into the hospital the day of her surgery and left the next. Though this type of surgery isn't appropriate for everyone, it is a great option for some. It cannot be done in some cases, depending upon the position of the fibroids.[28]

Fibroid embolization. Uterine artery embolization (UAE) involves injecting a substance such as polyvinyl alcohol particles into the uterine artery, blocking the fibroid's blood supply and shrinking the fibroid. Interventional radiologists specifically trained in this technique thread a catheter into the femoral vein of the thigh to reach the uterine arteries. The patient is usually conscious during the procedure (although sedated and in no pain) and usually spends one night in the hospital afterward. Most women resume normal activities within seven to ten days.

The results are encouraging. The Society of Interventional Radiology reports that 85 to 90 percent of women who have this procedure experience significant or total relief of their symptoms, including heavy or irregular bleeding, pain, uterine enlargement, and symptoms like increased urinary frequency that relate to the size of the fibroid. Recurrence within ten years of the procedure is rare, although long-term follow-up data aren't yet available. The complication rate is low, especially when compared to that of myomectomy or hysterectomy. Even so, some serious complications do exist, including renal failure or an allergic reaction to the clotting agent.[29]

One of my OB/GYN colleagues had the procedure done and was very happy with her result. Given that she has spent her career doing lots of hysterectomies and myomectomies, this speaks volumes in my mind. If this procedure appeals to you, seek out the advice of a specialist at a center where UAE is frequently done, or call the Society of Interventional Radiology at 800-488-7284 or visit their website, www.scvir.org.

EXABLATE: ultrasound treatment for fibroids. In the fall of 2004, the FDA approved a new device that combines MRI imaging to map out uterine fibroids followed by high-intensity focused ultrasound that heats up and destroys fibroid tissue. Fibroid tissue is very well suited to this treatment because the blood vessels in fibroids help the body dissipate the excess heat that is generated. The procedure is called ExAblate and is done on an outpatient basis. It is noninvasive, leaving the uterus and ovaries intact. It involves lying on your abdomen in an MRI tube for up to three hours while ultrasound heats up and destroys the uterine tissue. Side effects may include blisters on the abdominal skin, cramping, nausea, and some pain that is amenable to over-the-counter pain medication.

Studies show that the treatment successfully reduces fibroid symptoms in about 70 percent of women, but 20 percent will require additional surgery within a year. The FDA reports that though the ExAblate treatment successfully reduces symptoms in the majority of women who undergo the procedure, those symptoms will return in some women. And so will the fibroids. This is why I recommend that *all* women suffering from fibroids also do their best to employ the kind of lifestyle changes mentioned above that change the metabolism of hormones to reduce fibroid symptoms naturally. Still, I feel that ExAblate is a major step forward and a very exciting use of technology. If it had been available when I had my fibroid (mine was very large), I would have strongly considered this treatment. Note: ExAblate should not be used by those who want to get pregnant because we don't yet have enough data to determine what happens to the uterine wall and uterine lining following the procedure. For more information about ExAblate, you can call 866-392-2528 or check out the InSightec website, the company that developed the technology, at www.uterine-fibroids.org.

Myomectomy (surgical removal of fibroids). Mycomectomy is a surgical procedure in which the fibroid tumors are removed, but the uterus is repaired and left in place. Advances in surgical techniques over the past ten years have made this a very nice option for women who want to keep their pelvic organs intact or have children.

Many of my patients elected to have myomectomies even after they'd eliminated all of their symptoms with dietary changes. The presence of the fibroid can still cause an enlarged abdomen that affects how they look and feel about themselves. (I felt the same way.) More and more myomectomies are being done through the laparoscope (a telescopic instrument that is inserted through the abdominal wall into the pelvic cavity, thus making a large abdominal incision necessary). Typically this procedure is reserved for fibroids that are six centimeters or smaller, but that depends upon the surgeon. Many physicians prescribe a GnRH agonist to shrink the fibroid(s) first so that the surgery will be easier. The smaller the fibroid, the better the chance that it can be removed through the laparoscope.

Gloria was forty-five when she first came to see me. She had borne two children, and her husband had had a vasectomy. Gloria had a large fibroid that was pressing on her bladder, causing urinary frequency that kept her up at night. Her periods were regular, and she had no pain. Her gynecologist had recommended a hysterectomy, but this choice felt entirely too drastic to her. Instead, she opted for a myomectomy. Today I would have offered her the choices of uterine artery embolization or ExAblate. At the time, her gynecologist wouldn't do this procedure "because of her age," an ageist attitude on his part. Like many conventionally trained gynecologists, this one felt that Gloria's uterus was useless, since she was over forty and didn't want more children. The myomectomy that Gloria ultimately had completely relieved her urinary symptoms, and she started sleeping through the night. She is very glad to have kept her uterus.

When the position or size of a fibroid makes childbearing an issue, myomectomy is a good choice. (Neither ExAblate nor uterine artery embolization is recommended for women who want further children. We don't yet know how these procedures affect fertility.) Before they undergo myomectomy, some women are told that once they are in surgery the surgeon may find it necessary to turn the procedure into a hysterectomy. I never saw a single case in which this was necessary, either in my own experience or in the experience of those patients whom I referred out for the procedure. In general, myomectomies are best done by those gynecologists who have specialty training in infertility surgery. This type of surgery focuses on repairing the pelvis, not on removing organs.

Hysterectomy. Hysterectomy is probably the option most commonly offered to American women who have fibroids. This option is often chosen when a woman has been bleeding for months or even years, is anemic from the blood loss, has an abdomen that looks pregnant, can't leave home for fear of bleeding through her clothes, and has urinary frequency from a fibroid pushing on her bladder.

Studies have shown that a hysterectomy can improve the quality of a woman's life if she is given the choice of options other than surgery.[30] If, however, a woman has surgery for which she isn't really ready, without adequately exploring the alternatives, the results can be devastating. Over the years, I've come to see that women who give their options a great deal of consideration before deciding on surgery are much happier with the outcome. (On how to prepare for surgery and the recovery process, see chapter 16.) Unfortunately, there's often a tendency in medicine to create a crisis situation and rush in. Sometimes a woman who has had a single frightening episode of bleeding with a fibroid will be told to have a hysterectomy as soon as possible. Because of her fear and the sense of being pushed by her doctor or family, she will often go along, when she could have waited. The women who often regret their decisions later, I believe, are the ones who did not feel that they had any choice except surgery, usually hysterectomy. Before embarking upon any course of treatment, a woman should allow herself the time to gather all necessary information and weigh all her options.

Fran, a teacher with one daughter, came to see me when she was forty-two. Over the previous six months, she had developed bleeding between periods, increasing cramps, and some pain during intercourse. When I examined her, I found that she had a fibroid the size of a large grapefruit (about eleven centimeters in diameter). I had known Fran for many years before this, and I had delivered her daughter. She traveled to many different schools during the course of her teaching day and had always found it difficult to maintain a healthy diet. She was significantly overweight and married to a man who hated his job and was somewhat depressed. Given her life situation, her treatment choice was hysterectomy with preservation of her ovaries. She knew that although I could remove the fibroid and leave the uterus intact, this would not guarantee that she'd be rid of her cramps and irregular bleeding.

Fran wasn't interested in taking the time to pursue alternative treatment modes, nor was she interested in learning about what her fibroids might be saying to her. The idea of being free from periods, cramps, and the fear of pregnancy was very appealing to her. She had her surgery without complications and returned to her normal routine within one month. She has never had second thoughts or regrets. Fran is a good example of a woman who knew she had options and was very clear about her choice.

SEXUAL RESPONSE. About half of women who have their ovaries surgically removed (most often accompanying hysterectomy), no matter their age, will develop testosterone deficiency rather suddenly due to the total loss of ovarian testosterone production and the subsequent reduction in adrenal androgens.[31] In general, the incidence of sexual dysfunction following hysterectomy is anywhere between 10 and 40 percent of women. In studies conducted in the United Kingdom, for example, 33 to 46 percent of women reported a decreased sexual response after a hysterectomy-oophorectomy (removal of the uterus and the ovaries).[32] But the Maine Women's Health Study, done in 1994, failed to show a rate that high.[33] And some women actually report *increased* sexual response after hysterectomy. For example, Dutch researchers reported that among women who underwent hysterectomies for reasons other than cancer, post-surgical sexual pleasure increased. The results held true regardless of the type of hysterectomy. Of the women studied who were not sexually active before surgery, 53 percent became sexually active after the procedure.[34] Doctors haven't paid nearly enough attention to the connection between hysterectomy and sexual response and have regarded changes in sexual response or loss of interest in sex following hysterectomy as psychogenic only, or "all in the head." Though the brain is clearly the biggest sex organ in the body, it is also true that hysterectomy can and does affect pelvic nerves and blood supply, which are important for sexual response. One of my patients came to me for a second opinion when her doctor asked her why she was so attached to her ovaries (he wanted to remove them at the time of her hysterectomy). To put it into perspective for him, she asked him why he was so attached to his testicles. As most women know, the mind and the body are a unity. Quite simply, if a woman feels positively connected to her sexual organs, then their removal can affect her sex life for both biological and psychological reasons.

We now know that there is a physiological basis for decreased sexual response in *some* women following hysterectomy-oophorectomy. For example, the androgenic hormone loss associated with the removal of the ovaries is a factor in loss of libido following surgery. Even if the ovaries are left intact, some women experience orgasm differently after hysterectomy, probably because the cervix and uterus act as a trigger point for orgasm. These women feel the deep, rhythmic contractions of the uterus as a very satisfying part of orgasm. Once the uterus is gone, they sometimes experience the loss as a change, an actual decrease in orgasmic depth. Women who experience orgasm mainly through clitoral stimulation may not have this same experience. In a review article of sexual functioning following cervical cancer treatment, a group of European sex researchers concluded that there was considerable vaginal and urinary nerve disruption following surgical treatment for cervical cancer. It is unknown to what extent pelvic surgery for benign disease might be cutting nerves important for female orgasm. Though the nerve pathways for female orgasm haven't been well worked out, animal studies provide some clues. In 1986, British primate researcher Dr. Alan F. Dixson studied the genital sensory feedback in marmosets (small monkeys) and showed that two separate sensory pathways existed in the female: one that was fired by either clitoral or labial stimulation and a separate neural pathway for vaginal and cervical stimulation. On the other hand, for women who have experienced pain with intercourse for years or who have had pelvic pain from uterine or ovarian problems, a hysterectomy can greatly enhance the quality of their sexual experience and the overall quality of their life.

Women who suffer from loss of sexual desire or general loss of energy following hysterectomy should have their estrogen, testosterone, and DHEA levels checked and then use natural hormones to restore their levels to normal. In my experience, the best replacement consists of natural testosterone in a skin cream base. The usual dose is 1 to 2 mg every day or every other day. This must be prescribed by a health care practitioner and prepared by a formulary pharmacist. Some women, but not all, are helped by DHEA; the usual dose is 5 to 10 mg once or twice per day. A few women feel best on 25 to 50 mg per day.

MENOPAUSE. Removal of the uterus alone does not necessarily result in menopausal hormone levels in a woman who is still ovulating. It always results in cessation of menstruation. Even if the ovaries remain, however, their blood supply will be altered. This changes the hormonal milieu of the body and may result in menopausal symptoms and an earlier menopause. In one study this occurred in about 50 percent of the sample.[35] (Many women report hot flashes for several months following hysterectomy, even when the ovaries are left in place. The same thing can happen after removal of an ovary alone, with no other surgery. It sometimes takes a while for an ovary to recover function postoperatively or for one ovary to take over the function of two.) There is some evidence that women who have had hysterectomies have an earlier onset of osteoporosis than other women, even when the ovaries are left in. And clearly, anything that impairs ovarian function in any way can result in decreased libido.

URINARY PROBLEMS. Women who have had hysterectomies are more likely to develop stress urinary incontinence later in life. The reason for this is that the nerves innervating the bladder are very close to the uterus. Some of the nerve fibers may be damaged during hysterectomy.[36]

HEART DISEASE. Some studies have shown an adverse cardiovascular effect from ovarian removal prior to a woman's natural menopause (the average age of natural menopause is fifty-two). Since the ovaries continue to contribute hormones even after menopause, it is possible that there are adverse effects from ovarian removal even after menopause.[37]

After menopause: nature's hormonal treatment. Fibroids often shrink dramatically once a woman reaches menopause (usually between fifty and fifty-two). Women with fibroids frequently experience symptoms only when they are in their mid- to late forties, the age when hysterectomy is most often performed. If a woman prefers it, hysterectomy can be avoided by keeping the fibroids manageable until they naturally shrink during menopause. This can usually be accomplished by a combination of dietary change, progesterone therapy, stress reduction, exercise, and watchful waiting.

Bea, a single teacher with no children, first came to see me in 1984 with a fibroid uterus and a history of heavy bleeding for twelve to eighteen hours each menstrual cycle. Because of anemia from the blood loss, she was taking iron. Her fibroid was submucosal, the type that impinges on the endometrial lining and is often associated with heavy bleeding. She had started a macrobiotic healing diet but continued to bleed rather heavily each month. She took iron, maintaining a blood count that was slightly but not seriously low. When I first saw her, her uterus had been twelve-to-fourteen-week size. Within six months it was down to an eight-to-ten-week size, which I attributed to her diet. Several months after starting the diet, she began weekly shiatsu massage treatments. She felt that the shiatsu was more beneficial than the diet.[38] Over the next eight years, depending on how well she was following her diet, Bea's uterine size varied from ten-week to twenty-week size, which occurred just before menopause. I repeatedly reminded Bea that she could choose myomectomy or hysterectomy (the options available at that time), but she was simply not comfortable about having surgery. During the three to four years just prior to her menopause, a time when estrogen levels swing up and down in an irregular fashion, Bea required progestin therapy to control her heavy bleeding. Occasionally, her bleeding was so heavy that it frightened her family. Despite that, she avoided surgery and gradually entered menopause. Her fibroid began to shrink quite rapidly—from twenty-week size down to fourteen-week size in only one week! Throughout the decade that I followed Bea, she stayed with her dietary approach and remained firm in her decision to avoid surgery.[39] She moved into menopause and grieved the loss of her periods.

After menopause, any hormone replacement therapy may theoretically cause a woman's fibroids to grow again, but the low levels of hormones used in such therapy generally do not cause problems.

Dietary change. Dietary change is the mainstay of my treatment approach for women interested in alternatives to drugs and surgery. Since the uterus is estrogen-sensitive, anything that changes circulating estrogen levels can affect it (and fibroids and endometriosis). There is ample evidence that a diet high in partially hydrogenated and saturated fats, high in refined carbohydrates and sugar (that raise blood and insulin quickly), and low in fiber can increase circulating estrogens. The standard American diet is precisely the diet that puts a woman at risk for fibroid tumors as well as endometriosis, breast cancer, and obesity.

A woman who changes from a highly refined, nutrient-poor diet (high in prepackaged foods, cookies, white bread, French fries, candy, and pasta) to a diet rich in fruits, vegetables, and other whole foods will be amazed by how fast this approach decreases bleeding, lessens bloating, and even decreases the size of her fibroids. Many women are eager to try this approach first, knowing that they can have surgery later if the regimen does not work out.

I usually suggest a three-month trial of a high-fiber, whole-food diet that eliminates refined sugar and flour products and dairy foods. A diet used to treat fibroids must be quite strict for a while, to decrease circulating estrogens. The lipotropic factors methionine, choline, and inositol (1,000 mg of each per day) are available as dietary supplements; when these are used along with vitamin B, excess estrogen levels can often be lowered and symptoms alleviated. I advocate a multivitamin-mineral supplement that contains at least 600 mg of magnesium and the same levels of B complex and other nutrients that I've already mentioned on pages 178–179. (See chapter 17 for levels of nutrients to look for in a multivitamin.)

The vast majority of women who treat their fibroids through diet get rid of their pain and heavy bleeding within three to six months of beginning this diet. A whole-food diet puts the fibroid to sleep, so to speak, but doesn't cure the problem. The energy blockages in the pelvis must also be worked with and released. In fact, I've seen women on very strict macrobiotic diets whose fibroids have actually grown. These women usually had unresolved childhood issues, such as incest, or were married to abusive partners.

Freeing blocked energy. These therapies can be very healing when done by a person who is a well-trained and gifted healer.

TCM (Traditional Chinese Medicine and acupuncture), acupressure, polarity therapy, and massage often work very well for fibroid symptoms, though the fibroids don't always shrink with these therapies.

Although I have not been trained in it, I wholeheartedly embrace homeopathic medicine, which addresses the vibratory nature of life at its deepest levels. Practitioners report that fibroids shrink or disappear and symptoms can be alleviated with the right homeopathic remedy. Homeopathic medicine is a type of natural medicine that was very popular at the turn of the century. In fact, the very first placebo-controlled, double-blind clinical trials were designed by homeopaths to prove the efficacy of homeopathic remedies, which must be individually prescribed.

The Chinese acupuncture literature indicates that it often takes a hundred or more daily treatments to eliminate large fibroids. Daily treatments require a major commitment from both the patient and the practitioner. I've seen smaller ones shrink with weekly acupuncture appointments.

A relatively new therapy known as NAET (Nambudripad Allergy Elimination Technique) has been used to treat fibroids and a wide variety of other illnesses as well. NAET was developed by Devi Nambudripad, an acupuncturist and chiropractor who had very severe allergies herself. It is based on the premise that allergies (and other illnesses such as fibroids) are the result of allergic and emotional reactions that are originally programmed in both the brain and body simultaneously. Using a process known as kinesiology (muscle testing), the NAET practitioner pinpoints the offending allergens and the accompanying emotional pattern. Then, using specific acupuncture or acupuncture points, these patterns are cleared from the body. The philosophical basis for this technique makes a great deal of sense, and I recommend it if used by a well-trained practitioner. (See Resources.)

Almost every community in the United States and abroad has holistically oriented practitioners. In the past they often were not well integrated with the orthodox medical community; fortunately this is changing as women who have become well educated about safe and effective alternatives to drugs and surgery are demanding them.

HEALING PROGRAM FOR FIBROIDS

~ Whole-food diet that keeps insulin and blood sugar stable: no dairy foods for at least three months, plenty of leafy green vegetables, soy products, and cruciferous vegetables

~ Supplements: a comprehensive multivitamin-mineral combination containing B complex, plus lipotropic factors methionine, choline, and inositol, approximately 500 to 1,000 mg of each per day (see supplement recommendations in chapter 17)

~ 2-percent progesterone cream: one-quarter to one-half teaspoon once or twice a day during the two to three weeks before the period is due, to block the overproduction of estrogen

~ Aerobic-type exercise: twenty minutes three times per week

~ Massage, tai chi, meditation, acupuncture: to increase energy flow to the pelvis

~ Castor oil packs to the lower abdomen: three times per week at minimum, with attention to thoughts, images, and feelings that arise during the treatment; an alternative is a warm bath with rose oil aromatherapy drops in the water

~ Journal: Write down everything that you'd like to create in your life. See how much enthusiasm and energy you can muster simply by imagining what it would be like to let your creative talents or secret selves manifest fully. Note where you have any blocks to this process. They will usually be identifiable as "yes, but" statements, such as "Yes, I'd love to sew beautiful clothing regularly, but there's no way I can get the time." You will soon be able to identify the limiting beliefs that are blocking your creativity.

~ Go through the steps in chapter 15 of this book.

Try this program for at least three months, then make adjustments as necessary. Each woman's needs are different, and you must therefore individualize this program. See what you can learn about your body and its responses to this new regimen. Listen to your body's messages.

Women's Stories

Fibroids, like other disorders, don't just come out of nowhere and land on your uterus. When you become willing to be in relationship with your uterus by letting its messages speak to you, you have taken the first steps toward healing, instead of just masking or eliminating symptoms. After you get in touch with the messages from your uterus, you can choose the treatment that works best for you, whether it's surgery, diet, acupuncture, or a combination of these.

Many women can correlate the onset of their fibroids with the onset of verbal abuse from their mates, job stress, or other problems in their relationships with the outside world. Inner work is often very useful for finding new ways to deal with these hurtful or limiting situations.

Shirley: fibroids and creativity. Shirley, a nurse in her mid-forties, had been experiencing irregular periods and heavy menstrual flow when she was diagnosed with a small fibroid at the time of her annual exam. Shirley had been in treatment for an eating disorder and codependency a year before this. When I diagnosed her fibroids, she was in the midst of a career change, trying to decide whether to leave a stifling but lucrative management job.

I suggested she go on a whole-food diet and supplementation program and use castor oil packs. I also asked her to think about what she really wanted to do, what she would find truly satisfying. As she thought about it, she realized that her creativity had been stifled at work. She asked her body what it was telling her and to reveal it to her in dreams or meditations. Several months later, she told me, "I learned to surround myself with healing energy and love through the use of castor oil packs, meditation, and therapy."

She used Reiki treatments, a type of energy treatment similar to therapeutic touch, involving healing with the hands. Two weeks after her office visit with me, she reported, "I had a vision of the masseuse lifting a bowling-ball-shaped apparition from my abdomen. She had me draw it, and I drew what looked like a burr that you would find on your socks in the woods. It had exactly forty-five spikes on it. [Shirley was forty-five years old.] My apparition, the burr, represented me and how I cling to things in an unhealthy way. It symbolized clinging to work and people through whom I try to find fulfillment. From my dreams and meditation, I learned that my uterine growth was a physical manifestation of my own stifled creativity that could never be expressed fully through depending upon others. Through my emotional and physical healing process, my fibroid reduced in size, and I was led to a more creative, satisfying job in direct patient care." Her follow-up exam three months later showed that her uterus was much smaller, and I could find no fibroid.

Marsha: unsupportive relationships. Marsha, a massage therapist from out of state, first came to see me in 1986, when she was forty-one years old, to get a second opinion about her fibroids. Though her uterus was only moderately enlarged, to the size of a twelve-week pregnancy, and she was having no symptoms, she had been told that she should have a hysterectomy. Her mother had also had fibroids and had had a hysterectomy. Marsha wanted to avoid surgery. Marsha had mistreated herself for years by overeating and getting involved in harmful relationships with abusive men. She had three abortions and no children. When she came for her first visit, she had already started a macrobiotic diet to keep her fibroids from growing.

Since everything else was normal on ultrasound testing, I affirmed Marsha's choice to treat her fibroids with dietary changes and suggested that she visit her gynecologist back home every six months. Given her insight into her own patterns of behavior, I felt she should work with alternatives to surgery. She followed the treatment plan in her home area.

Four years later, she returned to see me because she had had several episodes of very heavy bleeding and her gynecologist had strongly suggested surgery. Marsha, who was in the twelve-step program Sex and Love Addicts Anonymous, told me that she had just gotten out of a very unhealthy, addictive four-year relationship. She was still completely consumed by the relationship, even though both of them had agreed that it was over. She told me that she had begun to appreciate that "all the anger I've felt toward my old boyfriend has been a way to avoid doing my work on myself, my emotions, and my past." Now she began to take responsibility for her life and her situation and to get on with self-healing. Through her recovery work, she was finding that every relationship she'd ever been in since her childhood, with an alcoholic father, had been dysfunctional. She admitted that she was very good at creating drama in her life to fill the void of deadened feelings within herself and to compensate for her lack of connection with her own body.

Marsha was just starting to realize the profound connection between her relationship and her sense of self, and how they manifested in her body. She knew that not all the aspects of her fibroid were related specifically to food, but yet she used food to cover up her emotions. Her recovery, one day at a time, has gradually put her in touch with her inner wisdom. When I saw her for a checkup in 1992, her fibroid size was stable and she was having regular periods. She had entered a stage of healing that is sometimes necessary for many women, though not all: she felt the need to withdraw from men for a time and be mostly with women. Each time I saw her, she was more centered, more positive, and stronger. She realized that her fibroids were a signal, calling her back to herself and her own life.

Louise: children and loss. Louise is a woman who is willing to assume partnership in her health care and who is not afraid to express her views. A producer for a radio station, she came to see me for a second surgical opinion regarding her fibroid uterus. Her fibroid had developed shortly after her second daughter had decided to leave home for boarding school. After her visit to me, Louise wrote the following letter to her gynecologist, who had suggested a hysterectomy.

> Dear Dr.———,
> On your recommendation I went to a second opinion for hysterectomy because of my uterine fibroids. Let me tell the story behind my process, in hopes that you can incorporate a broader, less conventional approach to other women who present with fibroids in the future.
> First, I was struck by how powerless I felt by your recommendation for surgery. Suddenly, I began to think of myself as sick, diseased. But my heart was telling me, "No, there's nothing the matter with you!" So I followed my heart's voice. I got my hands on everything I could read about fibroids, especially books and articles presenting alternatives to surgery.[40] I have learned how many unnecessary hysterectomies are performed each year in this country, and I learned of the significant, often long-term postoperative problems.
> Even the small amount of research I did on the function of the uterus, especially postmenopausally, suggests that it is integral to overall good health. Chemical hormones cannot substitute for the magnificent functioning of the female organs.
> So I became determined to keep my uterus—and not just for physical reasons. You didn't ask me anything about my feelings, about my family or lifestyle, or about how a hysterectomy might affect all that.
> My two beautiful daughters have both left home within a

year's time. My nineteen-year-old is in her second year of college, and my fifteen-year-old has gone away to private school in Vermont, at *her* insistence. Though I am supportive of them, at the same time it is a major life adjustment for a mother to have them both leave home so close in time. My children are gone, the off-spring of my uterus, and then you tell me I should have my uterus removed as well. No, thank you. I'll hold on to it for the time be-ing and, I expect, always. If I had a life-threatening disease of the uterus, I might feel differently.

All of this may sound bizarre to you, but I firmly believe that we contribute to illness in our bodies. The flip side is that we can contribute to healing our bodies as well. I urge you to take a little extra time with your patients to hear their full story. If I had not questioned what you were telling me, I might have been one of those unnecessary hysterectomies. It would have been a conven-ience, perhaps, to be rid of the heavy periods, but it would have been at such a cost—in dollars, lost work, and long-term hormone replacement therapy, and in long-term psychological damage.

Please give your patients all the options, and the time to con-sider them.

Sincerely,

Louise T.

Louise's gynecologist is not unusual. We doctors are not trained to listen to our patients' feelings about what their diseases mean to them. Dr. Larry Dossey, in his book *Meaning and Medicine*, tells the story of Frank, a patient with chest pain whom he admitted to the coronary intensive care unit. Frank was able to change his heart rate at will by thinking about what his chest pain *meant* to him. He told Dr. Dossey that if he let the pain mean a heart attack, he immediately got anxious thinking about his damaged heart, clogged vessels, the loss of his job, and the possibility of another heart attack. But if he let the chest pain mean just a muscle ache or indigestion, he felt relieved and his heart rate came down. Dossey discovered that Frank's heart monitor acted as a "meaning meter." The same is true for fibroids.

When I saw Louise seven months after her initial visit to me, she had taken a job in another state, at a radio station where her work was truly appreciated. She had realized the degree of loss associated with her daughters' leaving home and had taken the time to grieve that. While she was interviewing in the new city, she had realized that her relationship with her husband had been unfulfilling for years—that they had really stayed together only for the children. She saw it clearly and began plans for a divorce, which was accomplished mutually. She then met a new lover, something she had never dreamed would happen and hadn't been seeking. This relationship proved very sensual and meaningful to her. She had changed her diet significantly and stopped eating dairy foods. When I examined her, the fibroid was almost completely gone. She had basically changed her entire first- and second-chakra energy.

Paula: fibroids and abortion. I occasionally see women whose fibroids appear to be related to an abortion or abortions. When I say "related" I don't mean "caused by." Abortion, in study after study, has not been associated with adverse physical effects on the body. The problems that women have after abortion, if any, are related to the *meaning* of abortion in their lives, and in the society in which they live.

Paula came to see me for an annual exam at the age of thirty-six. She had had three abortions when she was in her teens and her twenties and had no children. I do not know the circumstances of her abortions except that she was matter-of-fact about them. She developed fibroids in her early thirties and had suffered from pelvic pain for at least five years. When I saw her, she was feeling well and healthy and felt that her well-being was related to the following story: "I was having increasing problems with bleeding between my periods and pelvic pain. Not happy with the prospect of surgery or hormones, I went to a Native American healer. He told me that I had to release the spirits of the beings who had been with me before my abortions. He performed a releasing ritual with me in which I literally saw and felt white wings flying out of my lower pelvis and away. I cried for hours with grief and relief. After that my periods went back to normal, and I've never had a day of pain since."

Paula's story is a dramatic example of the power of emotional release for healing. Though I could still feel an enlarged fibroid uterus of about eight-week size in her, this was not a problem that required more than regular checkups. She told me that it was a relief to be able to tell her story to a doctor, since she was certain that most doctors would laugh at her and think she was nuts. That, of course, is why doctors rarely hear these stories of wonder and healing from their patients. The stories are common, and yet they are kept secret because they are too often discounted or patronized by medical professionals.

*   *   *

True healing, not just curing our body or soothing our mental anxiety, involves transformation of our energy field and consciousness. In the women I've just described, the healing came in part because each woman created meaning from the messages and symptoms her uterus was sending her about how she was using her creative power in the world. And then she took the next step. She affirmed her innate wholeness and followed an action plan to manifest it in the here and now. You can do the same!

7

The Ovaries

From an energy medicine standpoint, ovaries are the female equivalent of male testicles. They can be thought of as "female balls"
because they represent exactly the same thing in the world. When
a man goes out into the world to perform acts of difficulty or courage
that require manipulating the external world of things or people, he's
said to "have balls." For a female, going out into the world, particularly a male-oriented world, also "takes balls," but she must use her
ovarian energy. She should not try to imitate a man, because her ovaries
and their energy field can be adversely affected by an overly masculine
relationship with the outside world. To maintain health, she needs to
understand how to use her "balls" in a life-enhancing way.

Our ovarian wisdom represents our deepest creativity, that which
waits to be born from within us, that which can be born only through
us, our unique creative potential—especially as it relates to what we
create in the world outside of ourselves. Biologically, when a woman
ovulates, the egg attracts the sperm to it by sending out a signal to the
sperm. The egg simply waits for the sperm to arrive; it does not go actively seeking sperm. The resulting biological creation, a baby, has its
own life and consciousness connected to, but also separate from, that
of its mother. Although its growth and development are influenced profoundly by the mother, they are at the same time separate from her. She
cannot use her will to force her baby to develop faster; nor can she use

her will to determine when her child will be born. And once the child is born, she must acknowledge that her creation has and always will have a life and personality of its own, even though it was created from her own flesh and blood.

Similarly, all of the creations that come from deep within us, from our ovarian wisdom—whether they be babies, books, or works of art—have a life of their own that we have a responsibility to initiate and allow but ultimately not to control. Just so, our deepest creativity cannot be forced. It must be allowed the time and space to grow and develop in tune with its own internal rhythm. Like biological mothers, we as women must be open to the uniqueness of our creations and their own energies and impulses, without trying to force them into predetermined forms. Our ability to *yield* to our creativity, to acknowledge that we cannot control it with our intellect, is the key to understanding ovarian power. We must *allow* this power to come through us.

Society tries to overly control creativity through the imposition of deadlines (note the connotation of the word—sometimes the time factor literally kills our creativity), quotas, and productivity ratings. One of my colleagues, who has always maintained very healthy ovaries, used to do scientific research as a research assistant in laboratories. The lab director would always tell her exactly what he wanted her to produce. Once, for example, he wanted her to manufacture an artificial cell called a liposome. Whenever she tried to create this cell model by running the experimental design according to his predetermined directions, using her will and intellect to try to force and control the setup, the attempt failed and the artificial cell was nonfunctional. She felt miserable. She then looked beyond the lab director's specific demand and asked herself, "What do I want to know in this situation? How can I find out more about an aspect of life by doing this experiment? What can this teach me about cells in general?" At these times she connected with the broadest possibilities inherent in the experiment, which she described as like "touching the hand of God." Invariably, in the liposome experiment and in others, she would design an experiment that yielded far more information than had been originally expected of her. The end result was never exactly what the lab director had asked for, but it was usually far more valuable and enriching. In the liposome experiment, my colleague ended up creating not only an artificial cell model but an experimental design that could potentially be used to produce a vaccine against a serious disease. A by-product of this was that the lab director was always thrilled with her results and eventually learned to allow her to design her own experiments without interference. Her scientific work was brilliant. By remaining true to her deepest creative wisdom, her end results benefited everyone concerned. This is feminine creativity at its finest. We can do this in our own lives and jobs by always considering how one task is connected to others and by remembering our interconnections and how one act can give birth to or build bridges to others.

ANATOMY

Ovaries are the small, oblong, pearl-colored organs that lie just below the fallopian tubes on each side of the uterus. Ovaries produce eggs. A woman has the greatest number of eggs in her ovaries that she'll ever have—about twenty million—when she is a twenty-week fetus inside her mother. Although the number of eggs starts to decrease from that point on, all females continue to have far more eggs than they ever need. Though it has long been believed that the mammalian ovary loses the ability to create new eggs after fetal life, new research in mice has established the existence of cells that replenish new eggs throughout a female's reproductive life.[1] Some results of this research hint at the existence of egg stem cells in adult women as well. In commenting on this research, Roger G. Gosden, Ph.D., Sc. D., who was at the time the scientific director of the Jones Institute for Reproductive Medicine at Eastern Virginia Medical School in Norfolk, where the research was done, said, "The mind boggles at the implications. The ability to make more eggs would be a revolution in women's health. In theory, it would allow you to have better control over the timing of menopause, to grow more eggs for one's own fertility treatment, to prevent premature menopause, to recover fertility after chemotherapy, and on and on." Though these findings are preliminary, they allow us to think about our ovaries and our eggs in a whole new, more positive way!

Ovaries produce eggs about once a month, from about age fourteen or fifteen onward—sometimes earlier, sometimes later. After a girl's first period, it takes two or three years for ovulation to get going regularly, just as at menopause, it takes a number of years for ovulation to cease altogether. Because ovulation always produces a small cyst in the ovary, it's very common for ovaries to have small cystic areas in them that are either the result of newly developing eggs or ovulations that have already occurred. As the egg begins to develop each month, a nourishing fluid-filled area forms around it, so that it is encapsulated or walled off from the rest of the ovary. This fluid-filled area, known as a cyst, is physiologically and completely normal, a fact that many women don't appreciate. At ovulation, when the egg is released and picked up by the fallopian tube, the cyst actually bursts as part of the ovulatory process, and the surrounding fluid, known as the liquor folliculi, is released into the pelvic cavity along with the egg.

After ovulation, in the space where the egg used to be, a second small cystic area, known as the corpus luteum, develops and begins to secrete progesterone. The corpus luteum eventually gets reabsorbed by the ovary. Frequently the process of egg development begins and a small cyst forms, but ovulation doesn't occur in that particular site. In this case, a small cyst will be left in that area of the ovary for a while. Because of this monthly process of egg development and cyst formation, it is perfectly normal for a woman to have small fluid-filled ovarian cysts at almost any time throughout her reproductive life. In fact, ovaries almost always have small cysts in them.

Whenever a woman gets a pelvic ultrasound for chronic pelvic pain, a fibroid, or any other reason, her ovaries are also scanned and these cysts show. Small one-to-three-centimeter cysts are almost always normal, because producing small physiological cysts that come and go is part of what normal ovaries do. They gestate little eggs, little cysts—or in energy medicine terms, young ideas ripe with potential.

Ovaries also produce hormones—including estrogen, progesterone, and androgens—throughout the life-cycle, though the amounts they produce change (not necessarily declining), depending upon a woman's age. Androgens, the hormone type associated with libido, were thought in the past to be produced almost entirely by the adrenals, which are the endocrine glands located at the top of the kidneys. In the last two decades, however, various studies have established that both pre-menopausal and postmenopausal ovaries produce a significant quantity of androgens, perhaps as much as 50 percent of the body's supply.[2]

It has been commonly thought that ovaries become essentially non-functional after a woman stops having periods, but the role of the ovary in the second half of life is now being reevaluated. We now know that the normal ovary should not be surgically removed because it maintains its ability to produce steroid hormones for several decades after menopause.[3] Parts of the ovaries do start to decrease in size when a woman is in her thirties, and they do lose mass more rapidly after age forty-five on average, but they are *not* the inert fibrous tissue masses they've been thought to be.

As women age, only part of our ovaries regresses, the part known as the *theca*. The theca is the outermost covering of the ovary where the eggs grow and develop and where physiological cysts form. In midlife the theca regresses, but the innermost part of the ovary, known as the inner stroma, becomes quite active for the first time in our lives.[4] In other words, as one function is winding down, another one is starting up. This process deserves much more study than it has heretofore received. In the second half of life, women's ovaries still produce significant amounts of a hormone known as androstenedione, a type of androgen. This substance is often converted to estrone (a type of estrogen) in our body fat deposits. Studies have shown that our ovaries can produce progesterone and estradiol even after menopause. These hormones are significant in preventing osteoporosis and heart disease and also in maintaining energy and libido.[5]

Up until fairly recently, menopause has been studied mostly as a "deficiency disease." Because of this cultural attitude toward menopause, scientists have studied this natural process only to find what is lacking. If we were to design studies of postmenopausal women in which the ovary was viewed as active and useful, we would find out more and more about the ovary's role in maintaining normal balance in our bodies as time goes on. The truth is that our ovaries are dynamic organs that are part of our body's wisdom throughout life, not something useless or potentially harmful to us when we are over forty!

Some ancient traditions have supported this view. In Taoist cultures the ovaries are thought to contain large amounts of the life-force that constantly produces sexual energy. Special "ovarian breathing" exercises can be learned to release the life-force energy produced by the ovaries and "store" it to revitalize other organs of the body, while the person achieves a higher state of consciousness. Ovarian sexual energy is thus transformed into *chi* (life-force energy) and *shen* (sheer spiritual energy).[6] In the fascinating book *The Sexual Teachings of the White Tigress* (Destiny Books, 2005), author Hsi Lai presents teachings from Japan that suggest that women can maintain their sexual attractiveness far into old age by consciously working with this energy.

When a woman does not heed her innermost creative wisdom because of her fears or insecurities about the world outside herself, ovarian problems can arise. They may arise in situations in which she perceives herself as being controlled by or criticized by forces outside herself. Financial or physical threats in the outer world affect the ovaries, particularly if a woman believes that she has no way to alleviate the threats. Thus, a woman who is abandoned by her mate or feels stressed on the job may develop ovarian problems if she feels that she has no means of escape from her situation and that the "outer" world is preventing her from changing. Just as life stresses may cause uterine problems, they may also cause ovarian problems. Uterine and ovarian problems are often intimately related, but there are also differences. The primary energy involved in uterine problems is a woman's perception in her innermost self that she can't or shouldn't or doesn't deserve to free herself from a limiting situation or create solutions that can support her. The uterus is very intimately linked with the third chakra and self-esteem. Uterine problems result when a woman's personal and emotional insecurities keep her from expressing her creativity fully. In these cases, she believes that she herself lacks the inner resources to do so; in other words, she is doing it to herself.

Ovarian problems, on the other hand, result from a woman's perception that people and circumstances *outside of herself* are preventing her from being true to herself and living from her center: they are doing it to her. An additional energy affects only the ovaries and not the uterus—the energy of vengeance and resentment, or the desire to get even. The second-chakra area is the part of the body where we traditionally wear weapons, such as guns, knives, and wallets. When a woman uses her emotional weaponry to indulge in being highly critical or wanting to get even, it is her ovaries that are at risk, not her uterus.

Benign ovarian growths differ from cancer only in the degree of emotional energy involved. Cancer in a woman's ovarian area is also related to an extreme need for male authority or approval, as she gives her own emotional needs last priority.

Note: this so-called male approval may come not from an outside source but from a critical "male" thought pattern she has internalized and which causes her to drive herself relentlessly. I once saw an outstanding example of this. I was exercising in a hotel gym where the woman beside me on another elliptical trainer was talking incessantly on her cell phone. This went on for thirty minutes, rendering her unable to use her arms or her breath to get the full benefit of the workout. When she was finally finished, she limped—yes, limped—out of the gym, still on the phone. She hadn't bothered to stretch or cool down. And her limp (on her right leg; the right represents the male side) suggested that she had perfected the art of ignoring her body and need for balance completely. Though I had no way of knowing what the health of this woman's ovaries was like, it was very clear to me that if her behavior in the gym was any indication of the overall balance of her life, she was heading for a health crisis (or at least an orthopedic injury that would force her to get off her feet!).

A woman at risk for ovarian cancer may feel that she doesn't have enough power, financial or otherwise, to move or to change even an abusive situation. In contrast to cervical cancer, which may incubate for years, ovarian cancer usually develops rather quickly due to a precipitating psychosocial trauma, such as a mate announcing that he or she is leaving.[7]

A friend of mind developed an ovarian cyst when she began to realize that her job was not good for her and that her relationship with her husband was not mutually supportive. During the same time period, her husband began having an affair. Dealing with her cyst helped her to realize that there were real problems in her day-to-day life that she had to deal with. Her body was concretizing her emotional dissatisfactions and, in its wisdom, drawing her attention to her need to care for herself.

One of my patients, Beverly, had a long history of endometriosis, and her right ovary had been removed because of a benign growth four years before I met her. When she first came to see me, she was complaining of intermittent pain associated with her left ovary. She was worried that she might have to have this ovary removed as well, but she did not want to do this. She was only thirty-two and didn't want to be on hormones to replace her body's own supply. She was ready to work toward the deepest level of inner healing. On ultrasound, her remaining ovary had some small cysts in it consistent with endometriosis of the ovary. Medical intuitive Caroline Myss did a reading that revealed that Beverly had a lifelong history of truncating her own creative needs in order to meet the demands of her family, who lived close by. She also hated her high-powered executive job, which took up about seventy hours of her time per week.

Caroline told Beverly that she would not get well until she allowed herself at least one hour a day of creative time just for her. During this time, she was to release all expectations of productivity. She should simply allow her creativity to flow in whatever way it needed to. Beverly had always enjoyed working with fabric and was accomplished at needlecraft. She began to sit each day and create small, very magical-appearing dolls that, she said, "seemed to have a life of their own." She told me that the dolls themselves dictated to her how they would look and what they would wear. When she first brought a few into my office, I was enchanted by them and purchased two for my daughters for Christmas. As she allowed herself this creative time, her pelvic pain eventually disappeared. It returned intermittently when she got caught up in the demands of the external world at the expense of her own creative work. Her ovary, through its persistent voice, became a personal barometer for her of how well she was allowing her innate creativity to flow. She has begun to change her entire approach to life. The dolls that are being birthed through her continue to evolve and change as well.

OVARIAN CYSTS

We women are meant to express our creative natures throughout our lives. Our creations will change and evolve as we ourselves grow and develop. Our ovaries, too, are always changing, forming, and re-absorbing those small physiological cysts. As long as we express the creative flow deep within us, our ovaries remain normal. When our creative energy is blocked in some way, abnormally large cysts may occur and persist. Energy blockages that create ovarian cysts may result from stress. Such stress is not necessarily negative; for example, a woman may have a job that she loves but may sometimes simply neglect her need for rest. A cyst may be the result.

The left side of the body represents the female, receptive, yin side, while the right side is the more analytic, action-oriented yang, male side. And amazingly, these differences are reflected in the differing connections of each ovary in the brain.[8] Most of the ovarian cysts I've seen are on the left side—symbolic, I feel, of the wounded feminine in this culture. Many women try to imitate male ways of being in the world that don't always fit their inner needs. When I had my first intuitive medical reading with Caroline Myss, she told me that if I had stayed in my former medical group, I would have developed a nonphysiological ovarian cyst within the next year that probably would have required surgery. It had already been forming in my body's energy field! When I heard this, I realized that my inner guidance and decision to leave that practice proactively had averted a health crisis!

In premenopausal women in general, cysts that are less than four centimeters in diameter are considered normal. An ovarian cyst is called a *functional cyst* when it arises as part of the ovulation process. A cyst larger than four centimeters may be watched for a few months to see if it goes away. An abnormal cyst may contain fluid, blood, and cellular debris under the surface covering the ovary or within the body of the ovary itself.

Symptomatic Functional Ovarian Cysts

Follicular cysts. Many ovarian cysts that grow bigger than four centimeters and persist after two or three menstrual cycles are actually functional. Such cysts form when the follicle, the physiological cyst in which the egg develops, fails to grow and discharge the egg in the normal way. When this happens, the ovarian follicle may continue to grow beyond the time when ovulation should have taken place. It sometimes grows as big as seven or eight centimeters in diameter and can be painful. These cysts are described on ultrasound as unilocular and thin-walled, meaning that they consist of just a single collection of fluid contained within a thin membrane. They usually go away on their own, but some persist and require surgery. Although some physicians prescribe birth control pills to stop the ovulation process and allow the cyst to regress, the newer low-dose-estrogen birth control pills do not contain enough hormone to shut down the ovary and influence the cyst.

Luteal cysts. Another type of functional cyst is known as the corpus luteum. A corpus luteum, or luteal cyst, forms when the mature egg is discharged from its follicle at ovulation. This process is sometimes accompanied by a small amount of bleeding into the ovulation site on the capsule of the ovary—and sometimes into the pelvic cavity as well—at the time when the egg erupts from the ovary.

Some ovarian cysts are completely asymptomatic, while others cause pain. The pain can be sharp and knifelike if, for example, the cyst bursts and spills its contents into the pelvic cavity. Or the pain can be dull and aching if the condition is more chronic, as in many cases of endometriosis of the ovary. A small pain sometimes accompanies ovulation, caused by the release of blood into the pelvic cavity. It is known as *mittelschmerz* (middle pain). Bleeding into a cyst cavity or the pelvic cavity often causes pain because it stretches the ovarian capsule (the tissue on the surface of the ovary). This pain can last from a few minutes to a few days. If the bleeding continues into the cyst wall for longer than a few hours, the corpus luteum becomes known as a *corpus hemorrhagicum,* which simply means "a body that bleeds." Bleeding from a corpus hemorrhagicum can last for several hours or even days and sometimes mimics an ectopic (tubal) pregnancy. It may be accompanied by vaginal bleeding. Hemorrhagic cysts usually go away on their own, but they can cause several days of pain. Very occasionally, the bleeding doesn't stop and surgical intervention, usually through the laparoscope, becomes necessary. Most often, this procedure stops the bleeding and removal of the ovary isn't necessary.

Most functional ovarian cysts are diagnosed by a pelvic examination, followed by an ultrasound evaluation. Both ovaries are examined and compared to be sure that it is an ovarian cyst and not something else, such as a fibroid, that is being felt.

Neither type of functional ovarian cyst—follicular or luteal—leads to cancer. Some women have symptoms from them repeatedly while others have them only once in a lifetime. The important point to keep in mind is that these cysts can arise in only a matter of days or hours because our bodies are able to produce ovarian cysts rapidly. They can also go away rapidly.

Benign neoplastic cysts. Because ovaries contain cells that are capable of growing into complete human beings, they also contain cells that are capable of growing into a wide variety of cysts and growths, reflecting our enormous creative potential. When our creative expression is frustrated, this creative energy calls our attention to it through our body and physically manifests itself in the ovary rather than moving through us smoothly into the outer world. Conventional medical training teaches that the cause of ovarian cysts is not known unless they are of the "functional" variety and related to ovulation.

Benign, nonfunctional ovarian cysts occur when those cells of the ovary that are not associated with ovulation begin reproducing. The term *neoplastic* is often used in discussing these and other growths, both benign and malignant. *Neoplasia* means "new growth."

Other cysts. Besides follicular, luteal, hemorrhagic, and benign neoplastic cysts, some ovarian cysts are solid in character and don't go away after two or three menstrual cycles. This kind of cyst is assumed to be an ovarian growth arising from something other than ovulation. They require further investigation and treatment via surgery, because until a doctor has surgically removed tissue and examined it under the microscope, it is not certain whether the cyst is benign. I've occasionally had patients with ovarian cysts that were present on pelvic exam and visible with ultrasound for many years but that did not change in any way or cause any symptoms. These women knew that they were taking a risk, in the conventional sense, by not having surgery. Some were willing to take that risk and live with their ovaries untouched and undiagnosed for years. Though this approach is not advocated by my training, I also respect the decisions of well-informed adults to avoid surgery after all the options have been thoroughly explained.

POLYCYSTIC OVARIES (PCO)

Many women have a condition known as polycystic ovaries. So-called polycystic ovaries are a sign of hormonal malfunction. PCO is a complex disorder because it is so affected by a woman's emotions, thoughts, diet, and personal history.

Doctors used to call PCO "polycystic ovarian disease," but currently PCO is considered not a disease, but a sign of an underlying imbalance. It is the end result of a complex series of subtle hormonal interactions. A few cases are genetic and therefore run in families, but most cases have no known genetic link. Conventional medicine cannot explain why or how PCO occurs, but we do know that it is strongly associated with excess body fat. About 50 percent of women with PCO have excess body fat. Women with a high waist-to-hip ratio (apple-shaped figures) are more likely to experience ovarian dysfunction.[9]

The major problems associated with polycystic ovaries are that the woman's ovaries do not produce eggs, and her body produces too many hormones known as androgens. As a result, her periods may cease or become very irregular. Androgens occur naturally in both men and women, but in women with PCO they are present at higher levels than normal, often because of high levels of circulating insulin.[10] And high circulating insulin is a direct result of a refined food diet that raises blood sugar too quickly. This is a crucial link for women to understand because high insulin levels are associated with so many other diseases. High blood insulin levels increase circulating androgen levels, as well as a higher risk for obesity, diabetes, heart disease, hypertension, and hirsutism (excess facial hair).[11] Chronically high levels of androgens also prevent normal cyclic egg development in the ovary, blocking the growth and development of eggs before they reach full maturity. When a woman's normal hormonal cycle is blocked by chronic androgen overproduction, neither she nor her ovaries will experience the natural cyclic changes associated with normal ovarian function. Her hormonal levels remain static. Thus, a woman's ovaries contain many small cysts from underdeveloped eggs. On ultrasound, the ovaries look enlarged, with multiple small cysts just below the entire surface of the ovaries (hence the name "polycystic ovaries"). Dietary change often produces amazingly fast improvements. (See chapter 17 on nutrition.)

The Mind/Body Connection in Amenorrhea

Whenever a woman has a problem with something as complex as the ovulation process, we know that there may be a problem with the regulatory mechanism of the menstrual cycle in the brain. The hypothalamus is affected by emotional and psychological factors, such as stress and repressed pain from the past, which can cause menstrual cycle dysfunction. Because most causes of amenorrhea are hypothalamic in nature, which means they are somehow associated with alterations in the fine-tuning of brain neuropeptide levels that are poorly understood, it is possible that the hypothalamus may have something to do with PCO. In women with PCO, the normal cyclic release of hypothalamic hormones from the brain is altered. It is not known whether this change is the result of the ovarian problem or the cause of it. It is well documented that the stress hormone cortisol also increases insulin levels. So both diet and emotional or other stresses can and do affect ovarian function.

Stresses that have been found to suppress ovarian and menstrual cycle functioning include negative feelings about being female and also feeling subordinate or inferior. I have found that when a woman has grown up being told that women are inferior, on some level she wants no part of being or becoming a woman. In some women, these negative feelings may work in the body to cause it to stop ovulating and become more "androgynous."[12] In fact, studies in female monkeys have shown that those who are in a position of social subordination will often undergo ovulation difficulties.[13]

Studies have also shown that women who don't ovulate may be tense, anxious, more dependent, and less productive mentally compared to ovulatory women. They may also have suppressed rage at their mothers. Some feel guilt and fear about their need for parental care and protection and also fear losing this protection. As they grow up, this can manifest as amenorrhea—an attempt to "halt" becoming fully mature women.[14]

Treatment of PCO

Since standard medicine doesn't know the cause of most cases of PCO, treatment is aimed at quelling the symptoms only. Therefore, most women are currently placed on birth control pills, antiandrogenic drugs such as spironolactone, aromatase inhibitors that change the way hormones are metabolized, insulin-lowering drugs such as metformin, and/or progestin to create cyclic menstrual periods. These treatments do not address lack of ovulation or the hormonal status of the brain, though they can be helpful. Birth control pills and progestin also prevent excess hormonal stimulation of the uterine lining. These agents, therefore, decrease the risk of uterine cancer, which may result from years of buildup of the uterine lining if a woman doesn't have her period. Though birth control pills and other hormonal therapies do prevent some of the risks and symptoms associated with PCO, they only partially mask the problem and never address the baseline cause.

In those women who desire pregnancy, ovulation can sometimes be included with drugs. The most common one is clomiphene citrate (Clomid).

A woman with PCO can help restore cyclic ovulatory function through the following:

⁓ Look carefully at any negative childhood messages you may have internalized about being a fertile woman. Commit to bringing these messages to consciousness so that they no longer control your body and your ovaries. One of my patients who had been diagnosed with PCO three years before I first saw her realized that she had internalized feeling bad about herself as a woman because of being raped by her father. She unconsciously blamed her mother for not protecting her and so saw women as powerless. When she became aware of these messages, got off birth control pills (for PCO), and began to celebrate her female nature, her periods and her ovulations reestablished themselves in about six months. (She also needed to hear from me that PCO did not need to be a lifelong, chronic condition for her.) One of the fastest ways to uncover and transform old negative messages is by affirming new, healthier ones. Paste the following affirmation on your bathroom mirror or other obvious place and say it out loud looking into your own eyes every morning and every night for at least thirty days: "I now give thanks for my fertility and my femininity. I am completely safe to be all of who I am."

⁓ Reestablish cyclic emotional flow. Allow yourself a full range of emotional responses to the events in your life. Try recording these in a journal to discover the natural rhythm of your emotions and moods. Are they related to the seasons, the time of day, and other cycles? Keep track of the phases of the moon on a calendar and in your date book. It is well known that the menstrual cycle is affected by the cyclic waxing and waning of the moon. If you live near the ocean, keep track of the tides. As already mentioned, simply paying attention to environmental cues including the light, the moon, and the tides may regulate a woman's menstrual cycle and fertility.[15]

⁓ Reestablish cyclic ovulatory flow through connecting with light and nature. Get out in natural light as much as possible. Natural light affects the hypothalamus and pituitary gland and thus affects ovulation. Sleep with the light on for three days each month. (See page 136.)

It might even be helpful to purchase a source of full-spectrum light and have it in your home—especially during the fall and winter months. (See Resources for sources.)

~ Nourish your body fully via a nutrient-rich whole-food diet that balances insulin/glucagons and decreases cellular inflammation. (The diet recommended for PMS, endometriosis, and fibroids does this.) Loss of excess body fat increases insulin sensitivity and normalizes insulin secretion, which results in normalization of blood sugar and a reduction in excess androgens. Women who are adult-onset diabetics often greatly improve their health by this approach.[16] (I highly recommend the USANA Reset program for this purpose. See chapter 17 on nutrition.)

~ Take a good multivitamin-mineral supplement. A dietary approach that nourishes the body fully will also help a woman attune herself to her spiritual, intuitive side. This helps reestablish emotional flow and can often help normalize a woman's hormonal levels and alleviate PCO.

~ Use 2-percent progesterone cream as directed in the section on PMS to help alleviate symptoms of estrogen excess.

Women's Stories

The following stories illustrate how several of my patients have used their ovarian cysts to change and improve their lives. These stories show women waking up to the messages their bodies were sending them and then changing their lives. The message to all of us is particularly clear: to see the ways in which we participate in the dominator system and allow ourselves to be swayed by outside authorities rather than following our inner guidance. And then to appreciate how we can change our point of attraction by changing our perception and redirecting our thoughts.

Gail: crystallized overdrive. Gail has been a friend of mine for years. In 1989, she first consulted me about a persistent ovarian cyst, and eventually, when she was in her late thirties, it required surgery. Here is her story.

"In 1984, during a routine gynecological exam, a woman doctor found a large ovarian cyst on my left side. This sleek doctor in New York's SoHo district announced to me that this was dangerous and that

I should have surgery to remove it as quickly as possible. I should then expect to be completely laid up for about four to six weeks, she said. She, of course, would be glad to perform the surgery. All of this transpired in about fifteen minutes.

"I was terrified, completely blown away. At the time I didn't know enough about myself to know why I was so scared by this information. As was my pattern in those days, I covered the terror by increasing my activity and going into high gear. This was supremely easy for me to do in 1984, as I was directing a massive global peace initiative that had me traveling to several different continents a month. Besides covering my feelings by going into action, I had a strong intuitive sense that this ovarian cyst was neither as urgent nor as serious as this doctor seemed to think. I did not have the surgery.

"Several years went past, and I didn't really think about the cyst too much. I was in warrior overdrive, changing the world and lots of people's lives while ignoring my own. Though much of this activity was positive and deeply meaningful to me, I was out of balance in my life.

"In late 1987 my father died. Though he was well into his eighties and had led a full life, I had had no idea of the impact this would have on me. I experienced a kind of spiritual crisis. Through what I consider pure grace, a friend recommended a therapist who might help me. My journey with this wonderful man changed my life. With consummate skill and rare gentleness, he empowered me to recognize and heal much about myself that I had been afraid to look at. A pattern that was enormously important to my healing was my understanding that I had betrayed my feminine/mother and sided with my masculine/father. For much of my life this had resulted in my absolute allegiance to doing over being, thinking over feeling, and the outer world over the inner world. For me, this was a deeply personal betrayal, as well as a symbol of the collective societal betrayal of the feminine that has so profoundly wounded our culture.

"I began to experience my ovarian cyst as a physical manifestation of the warrior/masculine part of my personality that caused me to be so driven all the time. I called it 'crystallized overdrive.' I had betrayed my deep feminine side to such a degree that this warrior cyst was literally taking up much of the room in the feminine creative center of my body. It had grown to the size of a large grapefruit.

"Though I began to have more spiritual and emotional clarity about my cyst, I still struggled with how to deal with it on the physical level. I never felt it—I had absolutely no pain. Rather, it had a kind of looming presence, reminding me that something in me was out of balance."

In the fall of 1991 Gail came to see me. Her most recent ultrasounds showed that the cyst had begun to grow again and that the inside was changing, becoming more solid and dense. When a cyst becomes more solid, it means that its fluid parts are being replaced by more cells and growth within it. It was becoming more substantial. I felt that she had watched it long enough and that these changes signified the potential for the cells to become precancerous. (If an individual does not heed the body's wisdom that is announced by a bodily growth, the growth often needs to speak louder and more clearly. Thus, it may grow more quickly and become symptomatic. Nonphysiological ovarian cysts have the capacity to become large very quickly, depending upon the circumstances.) Gail was also starting to get some pressure on her bladder. I suggested surgery, since I felt that the persistent and now-changing cyst was a drain on her energy. As we have seen, unhealthy tissue literally "drains" the molecules needed for cellular metabolism from adjacent healthy tissue. (See chapter 4.)

A consultation with Caroline Myss confirmed my suspicions. She said that the cyst was now "waking up" and becoming active. It had the capacity to undergo rapid growth under the right circumstances. She felt that it should come out within three months. She confirmed that the growth had developed because of Gail's conflict between her personal inner needs and the demands of her outer world. Myss also said that the energy difference between Gail and her husband was at its most extreme ever; Gail felt drawn toward the quiet, reflective archetypal feminine, just as her husband (her partner in work as well as marriage) was reaching his peak in recognition and activity in the outer world. This was recognition in which Gail could share if she wished. She felt acutely the competition between this drawing inward toward the core of her being and the demands of success in the outer world, for which she had worked for years. If she didn't participate in this worldly success, the culture would judge that she was now "throwing it all away." Despite this conflict between her inner and outer worlds, Gail's ovarian wisdom was drawing her more inward than ever before in her life. This is a classic example of the type of competition in energy and body language that hits women in their ovaries.

Gail agreed to have the surgery, performed by me, whom she trusted. As part of her preparation, she worked with a spiritual studies group. The process included a kind of guided meditation in which she experienced her surgery in archetypal images, her warrior/masculine aspect standing behind her hospital bed protecting her emerging mystic/feminine aspect. As she remembered it, "The warrior reached to stroke gently the mystic's forehead. At the conclusion of the surgery my mystic held the cyst and handed it to the warrior. The warrior took the cyst and bowed deeply to the mystic. This was a profound image for me. I knew at that moment that through this surgery something very old, at my very essence, would come into balance.

"In partnership with this mythic changing of the guard, another friend led me through a meditation several days before my surgery. I had a dialogue with my cyst. I visualized it as being like the inside of a golf ball. I told it I was ready to release its 'crystallized overdrive.' I was ready to balance my outer warrior side and my inner reflective mystical side. I truly yearned for this as a healing for me.

"During this second meditation, I gave Chris [Northrup] permission to cut open my body and remove the cyst. I meditated about the removal of the cyst. I experienced vast space in my body, the turquoise color of the Caribbean Sea healing and cleansing me. Into that infinite turquoise, the female lineage of my family appeared—a long line of sister, mother, grandmother, and on and on back. They acknowledged me for reclaiming my feminine self for myself and for them."

With these healing images instilled in her mind and heart, Gail created a medicine pouch of items of significance to her. It included some crystals that had been given to her, some special stones from a beach she loved, pictures of her mother and grandmother, and some childhood toys. She packed her bag and left for Maine, to have her surgery at the hospital where I performed surgery. As she later said, "My husband and two of my dearest friends were with me before and after my surgery. Their presence created a calm, loving, and joyful center from which my surgery/initiation could unfold.

"The surgery went smoothly and gracefully. Chris removed the benign cyst that had replaced my left ovary. She reported to me that I had a gorgeous and healthy uterus and right tube and ovary. When she showed my dear friends the cyst she had removed, one of my friends said that it looked like the bulging red muscles in the neck of a runner who is overexerting. Overdrive itself.

"I felt only a small amount of pain from the surgery and only mild effects from the anesthesia. I left the hospital after two days with an enormously positive feeling about my adventure there. My body then began the miraculous process of healing itself.

"I am enjoying my time of healing retreat. It's too soon to understand all of what has changed and transpired in me. What I do know is that I have faced one of my scariest dragons, and for that I am a fuller, richer person. I know that I can ask for support when I am afraid, and I know that I am loved and cared for by many dear ones. I know that I have shifted and balanced an ancient partnership within myself where the warrior waltzes with the mystic."

In many cases of large, complex ovarian cysts like Gail's, the healthy ovarian tissue is replaced almost entirely by that of the cyst, and there is almost no way to distinguish healthy from unhealthy tissue. Therefore, the entire ovary requires removal.[17] Gail continues to do well, however. The very way in which she approached her cyst, her hospitalization, and her postoperative care are good examples of allowing more feminine, intuitive, nurturing energy into her life, part of the lesson she learned from her left ovary.

Mary Jane: married to the job. Mary Jane is a molecular biologist who has spent her entire career working in male-dominated institutions. When she was in high school, she wanted to take physics and advanced mathematics, but her father, a physics professor, told her that she should take typing instead, because it would be much more useful to her. Like many men of his generation, he felt that his daughter would only get married and have children and that higher education would be wasted on her. Ironically, Mary Jane eventually went on to get an advanced degree in science, and she published many more research papers than her father. Though she was once married and has one child, her marriage was unsatisfying to her almost from the beginning. She divorced, and then became married to her job.

Mary Jane had been a patient of mine for a few years, always traveling from out of state to my office in Maine for her annual exam. At one of these exams, I felt a seven-centimeter left ovarian cyst, which was confirmed by ultrasound. Because she was very open to working with the symptoms in her body in a conscious way, I told her that this manifestation was there to teach her something about second-chakra issues, specifically her relationships and her creativity. I told her to talk with her ovary and see what it was telling her. My plan was to reevaluate her in three months or less.

An intuitive reading by Caroline Myss revealed that the cyst was filled with anger, the anger of violation. It also had "cancer energy." This isn't the same as physical cancer but is moving toward it, and Caroline felt the cyst would have to be removed soon. Although there was no cancer now, the angry energy in the cyst was very strong.

After Myss's intuitive reading, Mary Jane started a dialogue with her ovary. As she discovered, "I found that it was filled with anger, a sense of abandonment, and also jealousy. But there was love there as well. Though I had felt this love on occasion, I couldn't express it. I had needed a place to put all of this—it went into my ovary."

Mary Jane took a leave of absence from work. She had decided to have the surgery because of Myss's warning. I affirmed her decision and told her that she should not look at surgery as a giving-up on her self-healing capabilities. Surgery can be a very healing choice, and it would allow her to move forward quickly with healing her life on all levels. Mary Jane's personal healing issues would mean working to heal her relationship with her father and her work.

Mary Jane had her surgery and all went well. The cyst was benign. During her immediate postoperative period, she went through a process of deep grieving and let go of the unattainable vision of the relationship with her father that she had always wanted but could not have. She realized that her longing for paternal approval that never came had set up a lifelong pattern of unsatisfactory relationships with men that also affected her work and work relationships. She realized that she had to release her father from her expectations and demands. She realized that she had used her research as a method to win the approval of her peers, not simply for the joy of scientific discovery. Four weeks later, at the time of her checkup, she was doing beautifully—grateful to her ovary for showing her a truth about her life that was not obvious to her intellect. Mary Jane used her ovarian growth as a transformational journey that reconnected her body's wisdom and joy in her life's work.

Conny: truncated creativity and need for outer approval. Conny was thirty-eight when she developed a six-centimeter benign left ovarian cyst. It was removed surgically, leaving some normal left ovarian tissue behind. During the time she was developing this cyst, she had been trying to decide whether to have a child. At the time of her surgery we had discussed how she could best maximize her cyst experience for change and growth. She knew that her job was stifling her. She very much wanted to pursue making pottery and was, in fact, very good at it—she was always able to sell what she had time to make. But her job had great "benefits." I told her to check out whether it was worthwhile to kill herself for her "benefits."

A year after her surgery, Conny was back in my office, reexperiencing the pain in her left side that had been there when she had the ovarian cyst. This time there was no cyst, but the pain was the same. She found that as soon as she arrived at work, the pain started, and it was getting worse. Her body was speaking loudly to her this time. She had already had one surgery. The conditions leading to the cyst in the first place—the energy pattern in her body—hadn't really changed.

Conny understood her dilemma intellectually, and she knew that something had to change. But somewhere deep inside, whenever she thought about leaving work to pursue her creative instincts, she heard her father's voice in her head saying, "You're a fool to leave your job security. Making art is not a job. That's a hobby. That's what you do when you've finished your work." She'd been carrying this belief from her father since childhood. Her job represented his approval in her life. She thus allowed forces outside herself to control her inherent creativity. Meanwhile she was denying the anger and rage associated with this situation.

I asked Conny to consider what she would do if she were given six months to live. She gave it a great deal of thought. Finally, exhausted, depressed, and in pain, she took a three-month leave of absence from work with the blessings of her company in order to sort out her priorities. The pain went away almost immediately, her energy returned, and her artistic side began blossoming. Her challenge was to balance her creative needs with her job.

When she first returned to work after her leave, her company put her in a different location, one in which she didn't have to deal directly with the public. Instead, she worked behind the scenes processing paperwork and invoices. This change fit her needs only temporarily. It was not satisfying work, and she was still allowing many aspects of her life to be controlled by her need for approval from her parents and her bosses. Within three months of a completely normal pelvic exam, she developed a very large precancerous tumor of the left ovary. It was growing so fast that she noticed a bulge in her abdominal wall that hadn't been there the week before. At surgery, the tumor was found to be a "borderline tumor"—halfway between benign and malignant. The tumor growth at the time of surgery appeared confined to the left ovary only, and after consultation with a gynecological oncologist, only the left ovary was removed—leaving Conny with a normal uterus and a normal right ovary. (Borderline ovarian tumors often grow so slowly that it's possible to remove only the abnormality, leaving a woman's other pelvic organs—and physical fertility—intact.)

However, she knew at a deep cellular level that her creativity was desperate for expression and that her body would not settle for anything less than her complete yielding to her innermost wisdom. She quit her job and spent as much time as she could making pots. She eventually planned to return to school to study holistic medicine. When I last saw her, the veil of depression that had surrounded her for the previous three years had lifted. She was blossoming into the fullness of her creative self. Her relationship with her parents had never been better. She was making peace with the fact that they might never understand her creative needs fully, but that didn't mean she couldn't have a relationship with them. She also learned that she could not hold her parents responsible for the years when she chose to curtail her creativity. She regarded her ovarian message as a "kick in the pants" that she really needed. She was grateful.

OVARIAN CANCER

Many American gynecologists are trained to remove the ovaries after the age of forty if a woman has pelvic surgery of any kind. The reason for this is to prevent ovarian cancer. Yet ovarian cancer affects only one in eighty women in the United States. This means that thousands of women throughout the country are having normal organs removed to prevent a condition that will actually affect very few of them. Thousands will be deprived of the essential benefits that these hormone-producing organs provide. In fact, premature removal of the ovaries is associated with increased risk for osteoporosis and heart disease, as well as a host of menopausal symptoms, including decreased skin thickness, which results in a more aged appearance and possible increased susceptibility to bruising and injury.[18] Other problems include decreased sex drive and decreased sexual attention. The research of Winnifred Cutler, Ph.D., has shown that hysterectomy with ovarian removal decreases or eliminates a woman's ability to produce sex-attractant pheromones, rendering her less attractive to appropriate partners.[19] The good news is that the use of commercially available pheromones reverses this. (See chapter 8, "Reclaiming the Erotic.")

Medicine in this culture, however, focuses on ovarian removal for its potential cancer-prevention benefits and downplays any adverse factors possibly associated with it. Removal of the ovaries to prevent ovarian cancer is based on the assumptions that (1) prophylactic removal of the ovaries during hysterectomy is associated with a lower incidence of ovarian cancer, and (2) a woman's own hormones can be easily replaced with hormone medication. But studies have shown that neither of these assumptions is always true.[20]

In the absence of ovarian disease, the ovaries are best left in place unless a very clear genetic risk has been identified: that is, a woman has one or more first-degree female relatives who have had ovarian cancer. (See Resources for information on genetic counseling.) Neither synthetic nor

bioidentical hormones can match the complex mix of androgens, progesterone, and estrogen that the normal ovary produces. When the actual
drug-taking behavior of patients is considered, including their lapses in
taking medication and other erratic factors that impede a drug's absorption and performance, retaining the ovaries results in longer survival.[21]

We need another approach to prevent the needless sacrifice of our
ovaries. Understanding ovarian wisdom and energy holds the key to
this approach. Ovarian cancer may result from the energy of unexpressed rage or resentment, encoded in the second-chakra area of the
body. A woman may not be consciously aware of this encoding. But
this energy may be present in a woman whose mate or boss is always
angry with her and who may be otherwise abusive. A woman can be in
an abusive partnership with her work or even with herself, and it may
affect the ovaries in the same way. A woman who continues this pattern because of her fear of physical, emotional, or financial abandonment does not believe in her own inner ability to change her
circumstances. She is out of touch with her innate power, and sometimes her body will try to get her attention via the ovaries, especially if
she feels resentment or anger or blames others for her circumstances.
(Remember that the uterus has a more passive energy than the ovaries.)

Though other choices may be available to her, such a woman consciously believes that she is being *forced against her will* to keep her life
as it is. She is being controlled unconsciously by the pattern of behavior I discussed in chapter 4 as the rape archetype. If the woman continues to participate in an abusive relationship in which she is continually
violated either emotionally or physically (or in which she continually
violates or abuses herself), she is, in energy terms, being raped. Neither
she nor her abusive partner or abusive work situation recognizes her inherent dignity and inner creative power, and so her dignity, too, is
raped. Such a woman often feels paralyzed by her rage—an energy that,
if it were recognized and expressed, could help her create change.
Another part of her paralysis is the belief that her job, husband, or
other external source has control over her. Finally, her emotional
wound may not have been validated or witnessed on some level and in
some way. Yet in most abusive situations in which women feel powerless, a husband, boss, or other external authority rarely assumes any responsibility for their part in the continued abuse—they, too, are unable
to validate the wounding. To deal with this, women in these situations
often blame themselves or absorb their own anger and rage deep within
themselves. They are often afraid that if they were to let their feelings
be known, they would be abandoned. Such women can begin to listen

to their bodies' wisdom, and their inner guidance systems can help them create the changes needed in their lives.

The Golden Handcuff Syndrome

Ovarian cancer is linked epidemiologically with high socioeconomic status. Women of higher socioeconomic status often suffer from the "golden handcuff" syndrome—that is, a situation in which a woman is unhappy with her marriage or work and even despises her husband or job, yet that same husband or job provides her with the financial wherewithal to take expensive vacations, live in a beautiful home, and belong to a fancy country club. Fearing that she would lose all these "benefits" if she left her situation, the woman stays—meanwhile stuffing her emotions into her body and feeling miserable and trapped on some level.

I've seen several women with ovarian cancer whose husbands have accompanied them into the office. The energy of criticism coming from these men has been palpable. I recall feeling suddenly vulnerable, guarded, and defensive in their presence. Though they said nothing, I was sure that they were silently criticizing everything about me and my office. One man shook my hand at the end of the visit without looking at me! When this man and his wife left, I said to my nurse, "How could any woman live with that energy day in and day out? I felt battered simply being in his presence."

There is such a wide variety of types of ovarian cancer that a full discussion of them all is beyond the scope of this book. Basically ovarian cancer occurs when some kind of ovarian cell begins to grow abnormal tissue. Ovarian cancer can grow very rapidly. Almost every gynecologist I know has had the experience of seeing a woman with a normal pelvic exam who three to six months later had a pelvis full of ovarian cancer that had spread rapidly and widely.

Possible Contributors

Conventional medicine doesn't know what causes ovarian cancer, though epidemiologically it's linked to a high-fat diet and the consumption of dairy foods. These environmental factors can clog the system, once the energy blockages in the second chakra are already present, and swing the body's cells into disease. Studies have shown that ovarian

cancer patients consume 7 percent more animal fat in the form of butter, whole milk, and red meat than do healthy controls, and they eat
more yogurt, cottage cheeses, and ice cream.[22] The higher the socioeconomic status and the richer the food, the higher the rate of ovarian
cancer.

Ovarian cancer incidence is known to be highest in those countries
with the highest consumption of dairy foods (Sweden, Denmark, and
Switzerland) and the lowest in those countries with low dairy intake
(Japan, Hong Kong, and Singapore).[23] Galactose, a sugar produced
during the digestion of dairy products, has been associated with ovarian cancer. Cottage cheese and yogurt appear to be the *worst* culprits
in the production of this ovarian toxin because in these foods the dairy
sugars are "predigested" into galactose as the end product. The body
doesn't even need to accomplish this step. Meanwhile, women who are
lactose-intolerant and therefore cannot tolerate dairy products are at a
lower risk for ovarian cancer.[24]

Several studies have linked the most common types of ovarian cancer, known as epithelial cancer, with the use of talcum powder applied
either to the external genitalia or to sanitary pads. The talc can migrate
into the pelvic cavity via the cervix and vagina, and then out the fallopian tubes.[25] Talc, and possibly other substances, might act as an irritant to the covering of the ovary and thus be a risk factor for ovarian
cancer. It has been shown experimentally, for example, that carbon particles applied to the vulvar area can migrate into the pelvic cavity via
the pelvic organs in a rather short period of time.[26] Other factors linked
to ovarian cancer:

⁓ A variety of toxins that poison the oocytes (the eggs of the
ovary) may increase a woman's risk of having ovarian cancer.

⁓ Radiation, mumps, virus, polycyclic hydrocarbons (which are
present in cigarette smoke, caffeine, and tannic acid).

⁓ High levels of gonadotropins. Though not all studies support this,
it has been hypothesized that the reason birth control pills lower the risk
of ovarian cancer is because they lower gonadotropin levels and thus decrease ovarian stimulation.[27] Conversely, fertility drugs increase gonadotropin levels, which has been hypothesized as the reason that these
drugs have been associated with ovarian cancer.[28]

⁓ Chronically high levels of the androgen androstenedione. The
researchers who discovered this link failed to show any association
between high gonadotropin levels and ovarian cancer, but found a
relatively strong link between androgens and ovarian cancer.[29]

Androgens are increased by chronically high insulin levels from diet and/or chronic stress.

Several studies have demonstrated a significant reduction in ovarian cancer risk, up to 37 percent, following either tubal ligation or hysterectomy.[30] The explanation for this might be, in part, because after either of these procedures, the passageway from the external genital organs to the inner pelvic cavity is permanently blocked.

What these data suggest is that women who are concerned about ovarian cancer might consider avoiding or decreasing their consumption of dairy foods, especially yogurt and cottage cheese, after the age of thirty-five, when gonadotropin levels normally tend to rise. The data do not suggest that all women over forty should go on oral contraceptives, since these, too, have side effects and risks.

Diagnosis

One of the biggest problems with diagnosing ovarian cancer in the early stages is that there are very few symptoms. Vague abdominal complaints such as indigestion are often cited. Unfortunately, a number of other problems can cause such pains, too.

Ovarian cancer is most often diagnosed in the late stages, but by then it is far less curable. We still do not have any well-tested screening methods to diagnose ovarian cancer in the early stages, let alone prevent it. In fact, the U.S. Preventive Services Task Force and Canadian Task Force on the Periodic Health Examination report that even just defining "high risk" is not yet possible (although women with hereditary cancer syndromes should see a specialist).[31]

Genetic or molecular biomarkers like BRCA1 may indicate if a woman has a particularly high risk of ovarian cancer, yet their use as a screening tool is still experimental and currently limited to research purposes.[32]

Hundreds of women are now asking for sonogram screening and the blood test known as Ca-125, which checks for tumor antigens—proteins that are shed from the surface of cancer cells. Unfortunately, neither test can give a guaranteed yes-or-no answer to the question "Do I have ovarian cancer?"[33]

A high Ca-125 reading in an otherwise normal woman creates a great deal of anxiety and fear—yet it doesn't necessarily mean ovarian cancer. Endometriosis, fibroids, liver disease, and other unknown factors can also give high readings. At the same time, if a woman's Ca-125 level is normal, it doesn't guarantee that she doesn't have ovarian cancer. (In women who've had their ovaries removed, 10 percent can go on to develop a form of cancer that originates in the peritoneal lining of the pelvis. Although this type of cancer does not originate in the ovary itself, it looks and acts just like ovarian cancer!) Research shows using Ca-125 for routine screening (with or without ultrasound) increases life expectancy an average of less than one day per woman screened.[34] In short, Ca-125 tests are for the most part neither reliable nor cost-effective at this time.

Ultrasound doesn't give a definitive answer, either. One study estimates that using ultrasound screening in one hundred thousand women over the age of forty-five would uncover forty cases of ovarian cancer—along with 5,398 false-positive results.[35]

No one can guarantee that everything is all right until laparoscopic surgery is performed and the pelvis is explored, a procedure requiring general anesthesia. Even among women generally considered at high risk who have laparotomies, relatively few cancers are diagnosed as a result. In one study of 805 high-risk women, thirty-nine laparotomies uncovered only one case of ovarian cancer (plus eight other benign tumors).[36]

Clearly, when it comes to ovarian cancer, current screening methods are not the answer to saving lives. A very real dilemma for women and their doctors, this type of cancer requires an entirely different diagnostic approach from the one we have used for the last forty years. As one of our medical center's gynecological cancer specialists recently stated at a conference, "Everything seems to succeed initially, but nothing works long term. Wake me up when it's over." The interface between the immune system, the emotions, nutrition, and genetics in ovarian cancer deserves further exploration in new and creative ways.

Familial Ovarian Cancer

A woman who has a sister, mother, maternal first cousin, maternal aunt, or other first-degree female relative with ovarian cancer has a higher-than-average risk of getting the disease herself. Familial ovarian cancer was brought to general public awareness by the Gilda Radner story.[37] Some women who have a very strong family history of ovarian cancer (20 to 30 percent chance of getting the disease) opt for prophylactic oophorectomy. Prophylactic removal of the ovaries after childbearing is over is often recommended for these women. Yet even in women who have family histories of ovarian cancer, prophylactic ovar-

ian removal does not necessarily prevent the disease. Even after prophylactic removal, cancers indistinguishable from ovarian cancer can still
occur from cells in the lining of the pelvic cavity.[38]

I've noticed that women who have seen a close friend die of ovarian
cancer are more inclined to have their ovaries removed because of fear.
Though this might be unscientific, I find that most of our major life decisions are based on our emotional realities and not on statistics.

When a disease runs in families, we need to realize that we're not
dealing solely with a simple matter of genetics. Attitudes also run in families. It would be very interesting to study only those females in families
with a history of ovarian cancer who did not get the disease. Most likely,
these would be the women who have broken the family mold and left
their tribe, on both an energetic level and a physical level.

Oophorectomy During Other Pelvic Surgery

When a woman chooses to have a hysterectomy, to remove a fibroid uterus or for any other benign condition, she must also decide
whether to remove the ovaries, too. I ask each individual woman before surgery how high her fear level of ovarian cancer is, and I ask her
to check out how she feels about her ovaries. I tell her that it's not possible to discern the condition of the ovaries until the surgeon visualizes
them directly during surgery. If there's a problem at that time, they may
need to be removed.

If the patient decides to preserve the ovaries, she must defer to her
surgeon's judgment if the ovaries look abnormal during surgery. It's
best to find a doctor who is "ovary friendly." The ultimate decision
about what to do with the ovaries must be left to the patient following
informed consent. There are many factors, conscious and unconscious,
that come into play when each of us makes major decisions about our
bodies.

As you might imagine, the women who are drawn to my approach
usually choose to keep their ovaries during hysterectomy because—like
me—they value their female organs. Though my training led me to believe that ovaries should be removed as early as age thirty-five, I'm well
past that age now, and I value my ovaries as a part of my body that will
continue to function and support me as long as I live. I know that they
are part of my inner guidance system and they will let me know if adjustments are required for their health.

Most gynecologists train in large university centers that, because of
their specialty nature, treat more women with ovarian cancer in a week

than the average practicing gynecologist sees in a decade. Thus, gynecologists tend to see more ovarian cancer in their training years than
they ever see again. This creates a biased attitude against the ovaries.
An ovarian cancer death is difficult to watch and difficult to treat. It
can be associated with pain, recurrent bowel obstruction, huge
amounts of fluid collecting in the abdomen, and a variety of other extremely uncomfortable symptoms. A doctor who has seen someone die
of ovarian cancer is apt to be prejudiced in his or her relationship to
ovaries from that point on, even though the vast majority of women
will not get ovarian cancer.

One of the hospitals in which I worked in the past is the major referral center for our state. The GYN pathologist at that time said,
"I'm scared to death of ovarian cancer. I'm having my wife have her
ovaries removed when she's forty, and I even think she should have
her breasts removed prophylactically." He was not completely serious
about this recommendation, but this physician spent his days doing
autopsies on women from all over the Northeast who had died of
breast and ovarian cancer. He saw the devastation of these diseases as
a daily part of his work. He cut into huge tumors and received surgical specimens in which a woman's uterus, tubes, ovaries, and even
vagina, bladder, and rectum had been replaced by tumor. He saw the
devastation of breast tumors that had eroded into the chest wall. It is
little wonder that he felt the way he did, and it is no wonder that routine ovarian removal at the time of hysterectomy is still advocated so
strongly!

Conventional Treatment

When diagnosed at advanced stages, ovarian cancer is considered a
difficult disease to treat. Conventional treatment is surgical, sometimes
followed by chemotherapy and radiation, depending upon how far it
has spread. The diagnosis itself is usually made definitively at the time
of surgery for some kind of pelvic growth. Despite advances in treatment and attempts at early diagnosis, long-term survival has been statistically unfavorable with less than 46 percent of Caucasian patients
surviving five years.[39] Without looking in the abdomen and taking a
biopsy, there is no way to tell whether an ovarian growth is benign or
malignant.

If an ovarian growth is malignant, treatment usually consists of removing the ovaries, tubes, uterus, omentum (the apron of fat covering
the bowel), and any tumor that has spread into the pelvis. This is fol-

lowed by chemotherapy. A new treatment for advanced ovarian cancer has recently been shown to improve survival by an average of sixteen months. This treatment involves pumping two generic cancer drugs, paclitaxel and cisplatin, directly into the abdominal cavity of women suffering from ovarian cancer who meet certain medical criteria. This new treatment, though not a cure, is clearly a major breakthrough. In fact, it's considered so significant that the National Cancer Institute issued a clinical announcement early in 2006 to encourage doctors to use the abdominal treatment or refer their patients to medical centers that do it.[40] For further information, go to the NCI website http://ctep.cancer.gov/highlights/ovarian.html or call 800-4-CANCER. In the very early stages of ovarian cancer, surgery can be curative. Let me hasten to add, in addition, that there have been well-documented cases of so-called spontaneous remission even in advanced cases of ovarian cancer.[41] That means there's always hope.

Women's Stories

One of my patients who died of ovarian cancer healed her life and her emotional issues more in her last month of life than in all her prior years. She had gone through extensive surgery and had also followed a dietary approach to her problem. She had done all the "right" things. But still her tumors grew. A physical cure was not part of her healing, though her healing came in the course of her search for a physical cure.

A doctor friend of mine who was working with her for her pain took her through a process of meditation during deep relaxation in which he asked her body to tell him what was feeding her tumors. She replied, "Fear and sadness." He then asked her to remember and reexperience a time when she did not have this fear and sadness. She went back to a time when she was a twelve-week fetus in her mother's uterus. Her mother had tried to abort her with a red and white pill. In her final days she was able to bring this information to consciousness and share it with her mother, who herself was in need of healing around this incident from many years before. My patient died in her mother's arms, free from pain, and finally free from a lifelong burden.

CARING FOR YOUR UTERUS AND OVARIES, OR PELVIC SPACE

~ Know that the inherent creativity symbolized by your ovaries is always present for you, regardless of whether they are still physically present in your body.

⌐ Find a creative endeavor that makes time stand still for you. Immerse yourself in something so absorbing that you forget to eat. If you don't know what that is, ask your Higher Power to guide you to it. What you are seeking is also seeking you!

⌐ Make time each day to do something of creative value that has meaning for you. Let it come through you. This could be as simple as organizing your underwear drawer beautifully!

⌐ Write down a list of your past creations. Notice how many of them have a life of their own now.

⌐ Consciously let them go and allow yourself to move on into even greater creativity.

⌐ If you're still hanging on to and trying to control someone or something you've created, see what it feels like to let go and trust.

⌐ Know that your creative power is sorely needed in the outer world now. This power can serve you and others very well when you access it fully and don't try to control or force it. Acknowledge your ovarian power—your female balls.

8

Reclaiming the Erotic

If you cannot face directly into your sexuality,
You will never discover your true spirituality.
Your earthly spirit leads to discovering your heavenly spirit.
Look at what created you to discover what will immortalize you.
  —Hsi Lai, *The Sexual Teachings of the White Tigress*

When I speak of the erotic, I speak of it as an assertion of the lifeforce of women; of that creative energy empowered, the knowledge and use of which we are now reclaiming in our language, our history, our dancing, our loving, our work, our lives.

  —Audre Lorde

WE ARE SEXUAL BEINGS

Appreciating and embracing our sexuality is important for maintaining or regaining our health. We are hardwired from birth for sexual pleasure. It is our birthright. Humans are the only primates whose sexual desire and functioning are not necessarily related to the reproductive cycle. Women's sexuality is involved in giving and receiving sexual pleasure, as well as reproduction. In fact, the clitoris is the only human organ whose sole function is to generate sexual pleasure. And though the clitoris (with its 8,000 nerve endings) is clearly the most erogenous part of the female body, our experience of sexuality is not necessarily determined by our genitalia; nor is it limited to the external genitalia, any more than male sexuality is defined solely by the penis. In fact, it is well documented that women who have spinal cord injuries and can't feel anything below the waist are still capable of having orgasms. This is because the brain can receive signals of sexual response through pathways other than the spinal cord. Dr. Gina Ogden, a well-known sexuality researcher and author of the ground-breaking book *The Heart and Soul of Sex* (Trumpeter Books, 2006), has found that some women can reach orgasm just from thinking about things that are erotically stimulating to them.[1]

Sexuality is an organic, normal, physical, and emotional function of human life and we are capable of sexual function and pleasure for our entire lives. Women's vaginas have a cyclic sexual response of lubrication about every fifteen minutes throughout the sleep cycle, while men get erections. During sexual arousal the female clitoris becomes engorged with blood and becomes very sensitive, the vagina elongates, and the innermost third of the vagina balloons out, lifting the uterus and cervix. If intercourse occurs after full female sexual response, this changed shape in the vagina helps bring sperm to the cervix, facilitating conception. But sexual expression and pleasure don't require intercourse.

Most women experience pain during intercourse if penetration occurs before their arousal has been sufficient to lift and move the uterus and cervix out of the way. In these cases, the ovaries may be hit during repeated thrusting, resulting in pain. This generally doesn't occur when a couple allows enough time for full female sexual arousal prior to actual intercourse. The key to pleasurable sex for heterosexual couples is the knowledge that it takes the average woman about thirty minutes of lovemaking before reaching orgasm. The average man can have an orgasm only five to ten minutes after lovemaking begins!

During sexual arousal, the vagina produces lubrication from a number of sources. The glands (Bartholin's and Skene's glands) at the junction of the vulva and the vaginal opening (the introitus) secrete fluid. The walls of the vagina itself produce a fluid known as transudate during sexual stimulation. Some women experience a gush of fluid from their vaginas during orgasm, called female ejaculate. The female ejaculate is actually made up of different fluids from different parts of the urogenital system, including a female "prostatic" gland.[2] This fluid has also been called *amrita,* or divine nectar. A number of my patients mistake this female ejaculation for loss of urine at the time of orgasm, but this fluid is not urine, even though it does come in part through the urethra. This fluid release, which may amount to a cupful or more at a time and may occur more than once during lovemaking, is a normal component of female sexual response. Knowing its true nature is very reassuring for women.

Caroline and Charles Muir, a couple who have popularized the ancient link between sexuality and spirituality, say that this nectar is often produced when an area deep inside the vagina, known as the "sacred spot," is activated (usually through gentle and compassionate lovemaking), though direct stimulation of this spot is not always necessary for production.[3] Release of the amrita may occur even without an orgasm, such as when a woman "loses it" during laughter, joy, or love. In such a case, the woman is not "losing it"—she is actually *becoming* the energy of joy or love and, far from losing anything, is *gaining* the essence of these ecstatic feelings.[4] Though every woman has the potential for experiencing this outpouring of her divine nectar, she can do so only by learning to surrender herself to deep happiness—which may or may not be sexual.

The Muirs teach that the "sacred spot," deep inside the vagina and well hidden, is often the place where women store all their personal hurts and pain about sexuality. For many women, arousal of this spot for the first few times is often associated with pain or unpleasant memories. A woman and her partner who understand this will proceed slowly with their lovemaking, and persevere, and the pain will begin to heal on all levels. Healing in this way can awaken a woman to joy that she has never before known.

Elizabeth, a forty-seven-year-old accountant who was beginning to go through menopause, came in for a checkup and told me the following: "Over Thanksgiving vacation, I met a wonderful man through a mutual friend. We were immediately attracted to each other and began a relationship. When he made love to me for the first time, it was such a beautiful thing. But at one point, when he was stimulating me deep in my vagina, I had a flashback to my sexual abuse. I began to shake and to cry. I couldn't seem to help it, and I was worried that he'd think he'd done something wrong. But he just held me and told me that everything was all right and that he was there for me. Now when we make love, I still sometimes find myself getting upset, but it doesn't last nearly as long and I feel safer each time. My pleasure also increases. I had no idea that being with a man could be this wonderful. He was gentle and caring and took his time. I am so grateful." The sexual attentions of a caring man often go a long way toward helping a woman achieve her true sexual potential.

Ironically, new research is showing that oral contraceptives, the effectiveness of which has long made women feel freer to have sex without worrying about pregnancy, might actually contribute to long-term sexual dysfunction because the pill lowers testosterone levels—even after women discontinue taking it. (See the section on oral contraceptives in chapter 11, "Our Fertility," for more information.)

THE G-SPOT: MYTH OR MAGIC?

The G-spot (or Gräfenberg spot, named after Ernst Gräfenberg—the gynecologist who first described it in Western medical literature) is a nickel-sized area of erectile tissue located about two inches inside the vaginal opening on the anterior (or front, stomach-side) wall, about halfway between the pubic bone and the cervix. When stimulated, this area swells and can trigger orgasm (or even multiple orgasms, sometimes involving female ejaculation). The tissue that makes up the G-spot is analogous to the prostate gland in men.

When *The G Spot and Other Recent Discoveries About Human Sexuality* by Alice Kahn Ladas, Beverly Whipple, and John D. Perry was published in 1982 (by Holt, Rinehart, and Winston), it became the first popular book to describe the G-spot and talk about how to find it, although ancient Indian and Chinese texts had also covered it long ago. Although the subject has been controversial (the *American Journal of Obstetrics and Gynecology* dubbed the G-spot "a modern myth"),[5] studies do exist backing up Ladas, Whipple, and Perry's claims.[6]

To find your G-spot, it's best to start after you're fairly aroused because this tissue deep in the vaginal wall is easier to find if it is already swollen, which happens with sexual stimulation. Use plenty of lubricant, and you also might want to trim your nails so you won't scratch yourself. (By the way, diaphragm users may find the diaphragm can interfere with this sensation in some women, so you might want to experiment before you insert the diaphragm.)

If you're exploring on your own, it's easier if you're upright (on your knees is ideal) rather than lying down. If you and your partner are exploring, you can lie on your belly with your hips slightly elevated or on your back. Insert one or two fingers or have your partner insert his fingers about two inches (usually up to the knuckles) into your vagina, palm facing up. The fingers should then press lightly on the front wall of the vagina, looking for a slightly swollen spot. Experiment with a few different ways of stroking and different amounts of pressure. Some women prefer a tapping motion. Others prefer pulling the fingers in and out of the vagina, while curving them as if making the "come here" gesture during the out motion. Keep up the stimulation. The area will continue to swell (to about the size of a walnut) and become spongy. It may feel slightly ribbed, sort of like corduroy.

Because the G-spot is located along the urethra and near the neck of the bladder, women often feel the urge to urinate when this spot is stimulated. If you're worried about leaking as you are exploring, know that you probably won't and that the urge will pass. (You can urinate before you start, if you want to re-assure yourself that your bladder is empty.)

Just as with any kind of sex, the most important thing is to relax and take your time. Maintain a curious attitude, rather than being performance-oriented. Don't have any goal other than to have fun and see what happens. If you're at all worried that you're too old for this sort of thing, remember that some experts believe that women in their forties and beyond get more pleasure from G-spot stimulation than younger women because their lower estrogen levels make the vaginal lining thinner, which makes the G-spot more prominent when stimulated. Have fun with this.

Regardless of where a woman begins to reclaim and explore her sexuality, it's helpful to know that female sexuality, by its very nature, is a total sensory experience involving the whole body (not just the genitals). (The same is true for men, by the way—but most aren't as aware of this as most women.) A woman's sexuality may include actual genital contact with someone, or it may not. She does not need a partner or a significant one-to-one relationship to be in touch with her sexuality. She may not even require orgasm or physical touching. Each woman's bodily wisdom dictates what is right for her sexually. In today's society the prevalence of sex and relationship addiction, the lack of self-esteem, and the fear of abandonment all seem to impede women's ability to listen to their body's wisdom and messages. Sometimes what a woman desires sexually may be far removed from what our culture considers normal for women—it may even mimic what is considered culturally normal for a man.

OUR CULTURAL INHERITANCE

The functioning of our sexual organs and our sexual response are determined in large part by our cultural conditioning concerning sexuality.

To understand female sexual response and the workings of the organs involved in it, we must also understand women's cultural inheritance. In this society, sexuality is closely linked with body image and self-esteem. There's a saying, "Men and women will never be equal until a woman can be bald and have a potbelly and still be considered good-looking." Women are brought up to feel that they deserve sexual pleasure only if they look a certain way or weigh a certain amount. Not only that, there's also the fear of getting pregnant. There is reason to believe that in ancient prepatriarchal times, women knew how to control their fertility naturally and understood the importance of sexual pleasure as a natural part of human experience. Many couples who follow natural family planning as a method of birth control become acutely attuned to each other's fertility and sexual cycles. Not only does this method afford them the means to plan or avoid conception when they desire, they often find that their intimacy and pleasure increase as well.

The culture also believes in the "big bang" theory of heterosexual pleasure, which holds that the thrusting of the penis into the vagina is the most important part of sexuality. Though this is true for some women, it is not true for others. It's only one aspect of sexuality and pleasure, and women who do not enjoy it or who don't reach orgasm through it, need not feel abnormal in any way. For some women, penis-in-vagina intercourse—the kind that we're taught is the "real" thing—is not particularly satisfying. Therefore, many women fake orgasm to make their male partners feel that they are good lovers. This is a shame and robs both members of the couple of true pleasure and intimacy.

In her 1980 survey of 486 women, Naura Hayden found the following:

- ~ 310 said they faked orgasm every time they had intercourse.

- ~ 124 said they faked orgasm most of the time they had intercourse.

- ~ 52 said they faked orgasm some of the time they had intercourse.[7]

These statistics are now changing because our culture is awakening to the differences between male and female sexuality and also recognizing the importance of female sexual satisfaction. Research demonstrates that clitoral, vaginal, and uterine stimulation, or a combination of these, leads to orgasm.[8] Only 25 percent of women regularly reach orgasm through intercourse.

It is not uncommon for *frequency of intercourse* to be the sole measure by which the quality of a sexual relationship is judged—especially in medical circles.[9] It is clear, however, that many other factors determine actual relationship quality besides the number of times per week that a couple has intercourse.

Nor is the quality of a person's sex life determined by the number of sexual partners he or she has or has had. An unhealthy, potentially destructive sex life is one in which a woman bases her sexual relationships on working out her emotional needs using another person's body. Some women medicate their fears of loneliness and abandonment by having sex with people they do not love or respect, using sex addictively. Women in these unhealthy sexual relationships often had childhoods associated with sexual abuse, either subtle or blatant.

The cultural imperative that judges a woman's worth by her attachment to a man and by her sexual attractiveness to men—all men—runs very deep. And as a result, far too many women turn themselves into pretzels trying to become what they think men want. What we're not taught is that we're far more attractive to men if we first figure out what we want! Far too many women have internalized the culturally sanctioned sexual habits and needs of men as their own, when in fact male sexuality and sexual needs are probably more different and varied than we've all been led to believe.[10] Even in lesbian relationships, a woman's partner or who she is sleeping with can be used to define a woman's worth. One of my lesbian friends told me that because of her engineering degree, she is considered a "good catch" with "good income potential." In the lesbian community in her western city, she says, there is a phrase, "You are who you sleep with."

Clearly many women believe that it is their duty to fulfill their partner's sexual desires and frequently ignore their own erotic or physical needs. They may engage in sexual behavior from which they receive very little more than an unwanted pregnancy, discomfort, or various diseases. A study on dyspareunia (painful sexual intercourse), for example, found that of 324 women surveyed, only 39 percent had never had it, while 27.5 percent had suffered from it at some point in their lives. Fully 33.5 percent (105 women) still had painful intercourse at the time of the study at least some of the time, while 25 percent of them had the problem virtually all the time. Yet the frequency of intercourse among all of the groups of women was virtually the same! The study also found that most of the women had never discussed the problem with their health care practitioner. This means that a very large number of women are suffering during sex and not saying anything about it. Since the transmission of sexually acquired diseases in women is increased by any break in the integrity of the vaginal mucosa, dyspareunia is not only painful, it can also put a woman at risk from the trauma to her tissues.[11]

In addition to enduring pain, some women put their very lives at risk when they have sex. In November 1991, when the news came out that Magic Johnson had AIDS, an article in *Time* magazine pointed out, "Sex and sports have almost become synonymous." The article reported that "Wilt Chamberlain boasts having slept with 20,000 women—an average of 1.4 per day for 40 years." It quoted another basketball player: "After I arrived in L.A. in 1979, I did my best to accommodate as many women as I could—most of them through unprotected sex."[12]

In wondering what kind of woman would have a one-night stand with a man—even one who is famous—the article informed us that "for women, many of whom don't have meaningful work, the only way to identify themselves is to say whom they have slept with."[13] In their own eyes, these women weren't *nobody* any longer: they had had sex with a sports star. Even though this man didn't care for them at all or even remember them, they had achieved some perverse kind of status by letting their bodies be used in this way. One need only listen to the lyrics of popular rap songs to see that this attitude is still too common.

Many women are so invested in their sexual relationship at the expense of themselves that they repeatedly put themselves at risk for pregnancy or sexually transmitted diseases rather than jeopardize the relationship. A teenage girl wrote a letter to Ann Landers in which she complained that all her boyfriend wanted to do was have sex. He barely even talked to her anymore, and they no longer did much of anything together except have sex. She was afraid to say anything to him, however, for fear of losing him!

I lectured at a local private high school several years ago on prochoice issues. Afterward, several young men came up to me and told me that the girls they were having sex with didn't even ask them to use condoms—in fact, they had even told these boys, "It's okay—you don't have to use anything." These girls (they were upper-middle-class, mostly white students at a private school) perceived discussing contraception with their boyfriends as putting their social worth at stake. Some of today's middle-school girls are providing oral sex as a way to win the attention of boys. Women have been socialized for centuries to put their physical bodies at risk in order to sustain interpersonal relationships that really don't support them or their well-being. Though some studies show that condom use has increased, it is still true that no contraception is used by many teenagers, despite the fact that by age nineteen 85 percent of boys and 77 percent of girls have had sexual intercourse.[14] A report from the National Campaign to Prevent Teen Pregnancy in 2005 revealed that about 44 percent of boys and 55 percent of girls reported they used condoms inconsistently, and an additional 8.6 percent of boys and 17.8 percent of girls didn't use them at all.[15]

Women who have experienced rape and incest have even greater trouble than nonabused women in establishing fulfilling sexual relationships that are free of abusive elements and victimized behavior. Many of these women have never had a sexual encounter that was supportive and pleasurable.

Patricia Reis, a therapist who worked at our office for a number of years, counseled one of my patients, Lydia, for several years concerning her chronic vaginitis. Reis learned that Lydia's husband liked oral sex a great deal and rented numerous pornographic movies to try to stimulate her to perform oral sex. Lydia had been raped as a teenager. During the rape she had had to perform oral sex on her assailant. She recalled that the odor and the trauma of the event were so bad that the thought of oral sex had disgusted her ever since. Fortunately for her, after two years of therapy she was finally able to tell her husband firmly that oral sex was not something she could cooperate with willingly at that point. She had felt used by him sexually for years and needed to distance herself from this kind of sex for a while and reestablish comfort with her own sexual desires before she would be ready to consider the possibility of lovingly providing oral sex.

Whenever people use sex to diminish, control, or harm others, it does not contribute to the health of either participant. Many women have experienced the controlling attitudes and negative effects of certain religions on female sexuality. The tenets of the Roman Catholic and other Christian churches degrade sexuality—a normal human function—and subordinate it to reproduction. The consequences of such repression are seen in the problems women have in expressing their sexuality as well as in the sexual deviancy of some church representatives, e.g., priests who have sexually abused children.

Most Western religions seldom perceive female sexuality and motherhood as component parts of the same whole.[16] Christian churches have, for instance, a very long history of separating motherhood and sexuality, resulting in a virgin/whore split in our psyches that has caused much distress for many women. Barbara Walker, who has researched this history and its purpose extensively, writes, "The impossible virgin mother was everyman's longed-for resolution of Oedipal conflicts: pure maternity, never distracted from her devotion by sexual desires... Theologians in effect severed the two halves of the pagan

Goddess whose realistic femininity combined abundant sexuality and maternity. One half was labeled harlot and temptress, the other a female ascetic even in motherhood.... Churchmen often presented the doctrine of the virgin birth as 'ennobling' to women, since they viewed women's natural sexuality as degrading."[17] Elizabeth Cady Stanton, one of the most famous early feminists, wrote the following at the end of the nineteenth century: "I think the doctrine of the Virgin birth as something higher, sweeter, nobler than ordinary motherhood, is a slur on all the natural motherhood of the world... Out of this doctrine, and that which is akin to it, have sprung all the monasteries and nuns of the world, which have disgraced and distorted and demoralized manhood and womanhood for a thousand years. I place beside this false, monkish, unnatural claim... my mother, who was as holy in her motherhood as was Mary herself."[18]

FINDING OUR TRUE SEXUALITY

Our task as women is to distinguish our own personal truths about our sexuality from the distortions that we've inherited from the culture. Our first step in defining our sexuality from the inside out is to consider ourselves as sex *subjects* rather than sex *objects*. This is a revolutionary paradigm shift that can change your life. It starts with the absolute knowing that it is possible to have all the pleasure and fun you have ever wanted in life with or without a man. You don't need a man to be happy. This requires reversing the programming of the last five thousand years and realizing that our own pleasure and happiness must become a priority and guiding principle in our lives. It's the only way we have anything of value to share with another. When we reclaim our own sexuality and experience on our own terms, the whole world changes. When we learn how to turn ourselves on to life, instead of waiting for a Prince Charming to come along and do it for us, then we hold the reins of revolution in our own hands. Clearly the old myths no longer work.

Understanding our sexuality on our own terms—and then taking the time to learn about what gives us pleasure—takes courage and faith because of the degree to which our culture worships suffering. But when you have the courage to do this, your world changes. And so does your sex life. There is a quiet revolution going on as women discover sexual pleasure on their own terms and then teach it to the men in their lives. I heard the following story from one of my newsletter subscribers. "For years my sex life has been influenced by my belief that men's sexual needs come first. Though I can reach orgasm most of the time, I have really focused on my husband, not myself. To tell you the truth, sex had become pretty ordinary in my marriage. I used to joke that my husband and I were in a same-sex marriage. The same sex over and over again. Then a friend gave me the book *It's My Pleasure* by Maria and Maya Rodale and I started to think more and more about pleasure and how to add it to my life. By the law of attraction, I was also drawn to Steve and Vera Bodansky's *Extended Massive Orgasm.* (See page 253.) I work as a biofeedback therapist and I know that the Bodanskys are on to something important about the human nervous system. I know from my work that it is possible to train our nervous systems in such a way that our perception of pain changes. It stands to reason that we are also capable of more pleasure than we've been led to believe. Anyway, wanting to see what was possible, I followed the directions in the Bodanskys' book about experiencing more pleasure with my body. I started with the palms of my hands, just feeling them fully. Then I moved on to my inner wrists, my thighs, my feet, and finally my genitals. Once I became more and more comfortable with my own body, I decided to introduce my husband to a new world of sensual pleasure. I encouraged him and thanked him every time he got it right. This has made him feel like a hero and it has transformed our lives. I have always believed, intellectually at least, that if we're going to be happier and healthier we have to start with ourselves. Now I have absolutely proved to myself how true this is—both in the bedroom and outside!"

Until you make this paradigm shift and plan to have more pleasure in your life, your sex life probably won't be what it could be. In fact, it may well be a source of discord and resentment for either you or your partner. How many women, for example, are really ready for physical lovemaking at the end of a day of work, just before they go to sleep? I've seen countless women in my practice who feel that something must be wrong with them because they don't want to have sex at night. When my kids were still home and I had worked a full day, I certainly didn't want to. For me, afternoons are much better. (I'll admit, it can take some planning.)

Frankly, nothing kills the libido faster than a day of work, then coming home to do housework, then cleaning up after dinner and doing the other attendant family tasks. For most women, their desire to make love is directly related to the quality of their connection with their partner. Ideas are sexy for women and men alike because sex is a form of nonverbal communication—good communication and good sex are directly linked. And you can't do it well or be fully engaged in it, mind and body—and you probably shouldn't—when you are exhausted.

Everything a woman's partner said or didn't say during the day affects her desire to be sexual with that person. But once a woman learns how to take charge of her own pleasure and then teach her mate how to do this, she has the power to transform her sex life. For both men and women, attentiveness and tenderness are part of lovemaking, whether or not intercourse happens. So many women have asked me, "Why can't I kiss or hug my partner without it always having to lead to the bedroom?" Tragically, too many men have learned to separate sexual function from the other aspects of the relationship. Too many take a caress or a hug as a signal that it's time to have sex. What most men don't realize is that a whole world of enhanced pleasure is available to them when they slow down and learn how to really feel. Most have no idea how much of a turn-on a sensual kiss can be. But giving and receiving more pleasure takes practice and intent. Lovemaking also needs to extend way beyond genital contact.

A world of health and pleasure is possible between men and women (or women and women or men and men) when both of them are fully engaged with each other—body, mind, and spirit. Too often this gets lost when women have sex because of a sense of obligation and not out of pure free will, just for the pleasure of it. Making love to get somewhere or achieve a goal other than pleasure is ultimately counterproductive because it automatically shuts down our feelings. Sex therapists often teach couples a technique known as sensate focus in which their assignment is to spend fifteen to twenty minutes simply touching their partner for their own pleasure only. They have to avoid intercourse and just stay focused on the sensuality of the moment. And guess what? If they really stay present with the exercise, they find themselves far more aroused than they would have been otherwise. That's because nothing in the world is a bigger turn-on than another person who is taking pleasure in you!

So if a woman believes that it is her duty as a wife to have sex with her husband even when she's tired or doesn't want to, simply complying with his needs while ignoring her own, she is not creating health in her life or following her own inner guidance. Some women watch and enjoy the occasional "dirty" movie and learn about sex that way; they feel that this is part of their sexual freedom. Other women who enjoy sex fully find that watching "porno" movies diminishes their sexual desire completely. They feel degraded by the way in which sex is portrayed there. One of my former patients, who was a lesbian in a new relationship at the time and had always enjoyed a healthy and robust sex life, was asked by her new lover to make love while watching a pornographic movie. My patient was open to trying this new experience, but she found that her body was revolted both by the movie and by the entire evening's activities. There is no wrong or right in such a situation. A woman will need to let her body decide.

The original meaning of the word *virgin* had nothing to do with sexuality. It referred instead to a woman who was whole and complete unto herself, belonging to no man.[19] It's time for all of us women to reestablish our virginity in that sense.

WOMEN'S SEXUALITY AND NATURE

For many women, myself included, sexuality is profoundly connected to nature. One of my friends recalled that when she went out the door of the church one Sunday morning in spring, the warm, earthy smell of a newly plowed field nearby awakened her senses. She remembered the combination of the smell and the sunshine as very erotic.[20] This makes sense—the brain pathways for the sense of smell are very close to those associated with arousal and sexuality. Another woman, a lesbian, said that she always thinks of the Grand Canyon when she's making love. A third described swimming with dolphins as the most erotic experience of her life.[21] Sunbathing is also associated with sexual arousal for many men and women. In ancient Greece, men used to run on the beach naked to expose their testicles to the sun. Modern studies have shown that this increases their testosterone level. It is likely that in women sunlight increases the level of androgen, the testosteronelike hormone associated with sexual desire.

The ocean and waves are erotic images for many people. Before patriarchal societies became dominant, fertility, sexuality, and nature were celebrated together as aspects of the same energy and the same phenomena. The pagan festival of Beltane in the spring celebrated human sexuality and the earth's fertility at the same time. (This festival is beautifully described in the book *The Mists of Avalon,* by Marion Zimmer Bradley.) Most of the Christian holidays were originally Earth-based festivals, celebrating the cycles of Earth's fertility. To women who live in cities or other places where their contact with the natural world is minimal, the subtle erotic forces connected with the Earth are not perceptible. Barraged by artificial light and noise for much of the day, they are prevented from tuning in to the smells, rhythms, and feeling of the natural Earth.

Ancient Taoist practices, still taught today, view sexual energy as life-energy. When it is consciously directed during meditation, this energy can help rebuild organs within the body. Sexual energy is one of our most powerful energies for creating health. By using sexual energy consciously, whether we are in a relationship or not, we can tap in to a true source of youth and vitality. Using certain techniques combined with loving and conscious intent, we can learn to direct orgasm upward through the body so that every organ benefits from this rejuvenating experience, not just the genitals.[22] (See www.jadegoddess.com.)

Although it takes time to learn these techniques, every woman's health can benefit from developing pelvic floor muscles (PFM) including the strong pubococcygeous (PC) muscle, one of the major muscles of contraction during female orgasm. Women who have healthy, strong pelvic muscles are less prone to vaginal problems and urinary stress incontinence, and they tend to have more fulfilling sexual functioning with better pelvic blood flow, better vaginal lubrication, and stronger orgasms. There are a number of ways to condition and strengthen your pelvic floor muscles including Kegel exercises or using special devices for resistance training (see page 330). For women who have experienced sexual or other pelvic trauma, I highly recommend seeing a physical therapist who specializes in pelvic floor rehabilitation.

The human experiences that provide us with the greatest ecstasy and the greatest pain are sex, love, and religion. In her book *Sacred Pleasure,* Riane Eisler writes, "Candles, music, flowers, and wine— these we all know are the stuff of romance, of sex, and of love. But candles, flowers, music, and wine are also the stuff of religious ritual, of our most sacred rites. Why is there this striking, though seldom noted, commonality? Is it just accidental that passion is the word we use for both sexual and mystical experiences? Or is there here some long-forgotten but still powerful connection? Could it be that the yearning of so many women and men for sex as something beautiful and magical is our long-repressed impulse toward a more spiritual, and at the same time more intensely passionate, way of expressing sex and love?"[23]

How to Strengthen Your Pelvic Floor for Better Sex

Kegel exercises involve strengthening and toning the pelvic floor muscles, particularly the pubococcygeous (PC) muscle (the same muscle you use to stop the stream of urine). I recommend the following set of Kegel exercises:

Slow clenches: Squeeze your PC muscle and hold it for a slow count of three. Relax for a count of five, then repeat. Over a few weeks, gradually work up to holding for a count of 10. Make sure you keep your belly and thighs relaxed.

Quick contractions/flutters: Squeeze your PC muscle quickly and release—one contraction per second. Work up to 10 flutters.

Do five of these sets three to five times per day, with ten repetitions per set. After a week, add five reps to each exercise, for a total of 15 reps per set. Add five the following week until you are doing 20 reps per set, all the time continue doing three to five sets per day. Results are noticeable in six to eight weeks—and those results include better sex, including stronger orgasms and better lubrication. The exercises need to be performed regularly to keep up the beneficial effect. Other methods are available to strengthen the pelvic floor including vaginal weights. For more on pelvic floor strengthening, see chapter 9, page 330.

One reason sex, love, and religion cause so much pain is that our dominator culture has brainwashed us into believing that it is holy to suffer and sinful to experience pleasure. If we get "too happy" or feel "too good" we've been taught to wait for the boom to drop! And because our beliefs shame our reality, that's exactly what happens. That's why we have phrases like "No good deed goes unpunished." But it's natural for humans to seek out joy and pleasure. We're born that way and then get talked out of it. So instead, our culture trains us to seek the experience of ecstasy through addictive means such as food, cigarettes, alcohol, drugs, or even sadomasochistic sexual practices, which actually serve, over time, to further numb us!

Sexual energy, or *eros,* is life-force that permeates all of creation and is part of the joyfulness of life creation. It is exactly the opposite of *thanatos*—the force leading to death. For too long, our culture has dwelt on thanatos, without a balance from eros. It has taught us to fear, denigrate, and suppress our own eroticism, instead of using our erotic feelings as a sure sign that we are healing in the direction of a healthy and fulfilled life.

It is important to understand that the human capacity for ecstasy is a normal part of who we are and that the ecstatic sensual experience can be a spiritual one. We can experience the uplifting ecstatic energy through art, through intense feelings of love, and during the experiences, such as those we feel in religious worship or meditation, in which we partake of an ecstatic energy that can be erotic in nature. Only by recognizing that ecstasy and spirituality are part of human nature can we generate ways to provide and experience ecstasy and connections with one another that are nondestructive and nonaddictive. We must feed our souls as well as our bodies.

Program for Consciously Reclaiming the Erotic in Your Life

Before you get to the steps below, I want to stress that every man and woman I know has been, to one degree or another, adversely affected by our culture's view of sex and the way it exploits and objectifies both men and women. Almost no women look the way our culture's sex symbols look. Most of us don't accept and love our bodies fully. Many women have been sexually abused in some way. Others have endured very hurtful comments from partners that have damaged their self-esteem. Men have also been harmed by our culture's view of dominator sex. Many feel inadequate and worry about being acceptable to women.

Men thrive in truly loving, sensual relationships as much as women. And they long for love and sex in the same package, too. In the end, both men and women are looking for unconditional love and acceptance as well as sensual pleasure. Most long to find all of that in one beloved partner. Most men and women have never learned how to be good lovers. Most really want to know how to please their partners and get it right.

Staying overly long in a place of wounding and blaming men, women, your family, or your culture doesn't do anyone any good. If we are to heal our relationship with our sexuality and enjoy the sexual pleasure that is our birthright, we have to start with ourselves. Right now. Whether you are single or in a relationship, whether gay or straight. When you change yourself and your relationship to your sexuality, then your outer experience of sexual relationships with others will change as well. One final thing: remember that sex, money, and power are all second-chakra issues. In the past thirty years, the vast majority of women have entered the workforce and have the ability to earn their own incomes. This has been a necessary step toward true partnership between men and women. A woman who earns her own money and knows how to survive on her own—without a man—is generally in a far stronger position when it comes to reclaiming her sexuality on her own terms, compared to those who are financially dependent on a man for support. Relationships, including sexual ones, work best when both members of the couple feel as though they could leave if they needed to. (At the same time, it's lovely to have a man pay for dinner and open the car door for you sometimes.) With that caveat, the following steps will get you started in creating a more fulfilling sex life.

1. **Consciously decide to become a sex subject and feel sexy.** Start affirming yourself as sexy. I don't care how old you are or what you look like. Trust me. This is an inside job. Say the following out loud to yourself at least twice a day: "I am a sexy, irresistible woman." Make up your own affirmations. Begin to experience the power of your own sexuality. Steve and Vera Bodansky teach that a woman's desire is an enormously powerful force for creating a more pleasurable life. I agree. When a woman feels sexy and consciously knows how to turn herself on by feeling sexy and exuding sexuality (just to please herself), she sends out a signal to the world that changes what and who she attracts.

Here's another suggestion. In her playful book *Life Magic: The 7 Keys to Unlocking Your Magical Life* (Miramax, 2005), gifted clairvoyant Laura Bushnell recommends the following: Imagine that a person you consider very sexy (e.g., Sophia Loren, Salma Hayek—your choice) is pressed against your left side (the feminine receptive side). Breathe in her essence for about two minutes, imagining her sexy qualities permeating your body. Do this twice per day for about six weeks. You will notice a change. Consciously decide to do things that make you feel sexy. Wear sexy underwear under your business suit. Take more sensual baths. Read sexy romance novels. Fantasize more. (I know this is difficult when you have little kids and are working full-time. But like all good things, you have to consciously decide to have a good sex life.)

2. **Focus on sex more.** If you want your sex life to improve, you have to spend time thinking about sex. Though it is true that our culture is obsessed with sex and uses it to sell everything, few people

actually make it a priority in their lives. We become voyeurs, not direct participants. It's time for that to change. Developing the capacity for sexual pleasure is a skill that can be learned like any other skill. The more you practice, the better you become. It starts with conscious intent. The more you decide to think about sex, the more sexually aroused you'll become. Libido will naturally increase. Commit to exploring your own sensuality and sexuality. Spend time caressing your skin and noticing what feels good. Experiment with different kinds of pressure. The more sensual you feel about yourself, the more attractive you will become to others. Get a mirror and get to know your genitals. Spend time touching them and learning exactly what feels the most pleasurable.

3. **Get fit and healthy.** A sexy person is a healthy person. Take a good multivitamin and do aerobic exercise three times a week for twenty minutes. You can't be at your sexual best without good blood flow to the pelvis, and exercise and the right nutrients help with this. Do your Kegels regularly, too.

4. **Know thyself.** Get to know your body, including your clitoris. The clitoris is the key to sexual satisfaction for the vast majority of women, though there are many other areas of the body that are erogenous, such as the lips and the nipples. In general, the part of the clitoris that is on the upper left quadrant is the most sensitive. Using a lubricant such as K-Y Jelly or Crème de la Femme, try stroking this area, noticing the pleasurable sensations. The opening of the vagina also has many pleasurable areas. You can't take another person where you yourself have never been. And you can't expect another person to know how to please you if you can't please yourself. So commit to self-pleasuring yourself twice per week in order to learn exactly what kinds of strokes you like. Then you can teach your partner. Use a vibrator or your hands. Whatever works best for you. All vibrators are not the same. I recommend one called the Eroscillator, which works on the principle of gentle oscillating back and forth instead of the usual overall vibration of a vibrator. It comes with a number of different attachments and is very effective at helping women reach orgasm as well as learn what parts of their bodies are most sensitive. Couples can use it, too. (For more information, see www.eroscillator.com.)

In her book *Five Minutes to Orgasm Every Time You Make Love: Female Orgasm Made Simple* (JPS Publications, 2000), author D. Claire Hutchins makes the point that the most sexually satisfied women are those who know what to do to please themselves—and then do it even with a partner, including stimulating her own clitoris so that she reaches orgasm every time. Taking responsiblity for one's own pleasure takes the onus off the man to "make it happen" for his partner. It's as much of a burden for a guy to feel that it's his job to bring a woman to orgasm as it would be for a woman to believe that it is her job to bring a guy to orgasm. (Can you imagine the pressure of that!)

Noting that both men and women take about the same amount of time to reach orgasm through self-pleasuring (about four minutes), Hutchins explodes the myth that it always takes women much longer than men to reach orgasm. The reason it takes longer for women during sex (thirty minutes as opposed to about ten minutes for men) is because women are socialized to be more inhibited in bed than males. We worry far more about how we look. And if we don't look like *Playboy* centerfolds, we're not sure we deserve sexual pleasure or attention. Note that most men who have potbellies or who are bald don't worry at all about deserving a good sex life!

Hutchins also points out that a missing link for many women is using some good fantasies to turn them on. Interestingly, studies have shown that women are as aroused by visually erotic material as men are. But we've been led to believe that we're not supposed to be. Remember, a fantasy doesn't hurt anyone. It's not something you would actually do. But if the thought of having sex with a gorgeous stranger in an elevator (or whatever does it for you) works, then use it! When you use your imagination to turn yourself on, your body will respond in kind because of the power of the mind/body connection. Frankly, one of the very best fantasies for every woman is to imagine herself as sexy and irresistible. Here's a fantasy affirmation that really helps: "I love the pleasure that my body gives me and I always reach orgasm quickly and easily!"

In addition to fantasy, I also recommend using the woman-on-top position for intercourse so that the clitoris is maximally stimulated. Just as a man knows exactly how to move during intercourse to get maximal pleasure from the sensations, a woman on top can do exactly the same thing. And if she needs extra help, she can also use her finger (or a vibrator) to give her clitoris extra stimulation while in the on-top position.

5. Consciously increase your capacity for pleasure. Understand that we humans are capable of far more pleasure than we've been led to believe. It's now common knowledge, for example, that women are multiorgasmic. What most people don't know is that men can be, too! It is possible for couples to help each other reprogram their central nervous systems for extended orgasms, including multiple orgasms in men who can learn to orgasm without ejaculation, thus maintaining their erections. For a program that a man can do himself without a partner, see *How to Make Love All Night (And Drive a Woman Wild)* (HarperCollins, 1994) by Barbara Keesling, Ph.D.

Extended Sexual Orgasm (ESO) is a technique designed to enhance orgasmic pleasure at least far longer than the usual sixty seconds. Learning ESO requires time and commitment to giving and receiving pleasure. Pleasure is given with the hands. And you have to practice. But given the amount of time we think about and talk about sex, and also given the health-giving benefits of sexual pleasure, increased sexual enjoyment is a goal worth striving for. For more information about ESO, I recommend *Extended Massive Orgasm: How You Can Give and Receive Intense Sexual Pleasure* (Hunter House, 2000) by Steve Bodansky and Vera Bodansky. This book has the best instructions I've ever read for getting out of your head and feeling more sensations in your body. So it's helpful even for those who don't have partners yet. I also like *Hot Monogamy* (Dutton, 1994) by Patricia Love and Jo Robinson, and also *The Passion Prescription: 10 Weeks to Your Best Sex—Ever!* (Hyperion, 2006) by Laura Berman, Ph.D.

6. Help your partner become a good lover. Whether or not ESO is of interest to you, please realize that neither men nor women (nor monkeys for that matter) are born knowing how to be good lovers. You have to learn. Men are often under a great deal of pressure to perform. They've been taught that it's their job to bring a woman to orgasm. But this is difficult if a woman doesn't know what pleases her and can't talk about what she wants. Please remember that his ability to really please a woman makes a man feel really good about himself. Most men will want to please you if you continually give them feedback about what they're doing RIGHT! Make an effort to learn more about sex. Get videos (for a very thorough couples' guide to erotic videos, visit www.clitical.com/sensual-senses/porn-for-couples), read books. Talk about it—this can be very erotic! A very good resource is the links page of Candida Royalle's website (www.royalle.com). Her book is called *How to Tell a Naked Man What to Do* (Fireside, 2004). I also love Olivia St. Claire's book *227 Ways to Unleash the Sex Goddess Within* (Harmony Books, 1996).

Steve and Vera Bodansky point out that most women are angry with men at some level because we women have been second-class citizens for so long. And though this anger is justified, the problem with it in an individual relationship is that it interferes with your ability to experience sensual pleasure. The way around this is to decide that you'd rather have pleasure than be angry. Learn how to discharge your anger effectively without blame. (See part 3: Women's Wisdom Program for Vibrant Health and Healing.) Though this isn't easy, please make every effort to leave your resentments at the bedroom door. Schedule time to make love. Let your partner know when he's doing it right. Most men (assuming that your partner is a man) are performance oriented. They like to know they're doing it right. When you let them know when they are doing it right, they will go out of their way to do it right every time. When they are able to give you pleasure, they feel good about themselves. And women who know their own bodies and who feel good about themselves are in the best position to train a man to be a good lover.

In the process, lose the goal orientation. Nothing is more elusive than the orgasm that you are "trying" to get to. And nothing is less sensual than the goal orientation of today's hurried couple. The problem with this approach is that it leads to very routine sex and also limits the erotic potential of any couple. It's okay to have a "quickie" now and then. But make sure you have some uninterrupted afternoons or evenings when the only goal is to explore each other and not try to reach a finish line. Remember, orgasm doesn't have to be the ultimate goal. For most women, the intimacy and sense of closeness is equally (or even more) valuable.

In fact, once you know how to have an orgasm, you don't have to worry about it. Now you're free to lose yourself in the sensation of your partner's skin, scent, kisses, etc. This is what's really missing from many couples' lovemaking. And it's why lack of desire is so common. We literally have to train ourselves to stay in the moment and bask in the delicious sensation of being touched or kissed, without any other goal in mind. It's like being seventeen again—when you weren't ready for intercourse and spent hours and hours necking and petting instead. The amount of desire and fulfillment you can build up is wonderful.

7. Give nature a hand, if necessary. It is very well documented that humans secrete sexual attractant pheromones in their sweat. These are particularly potent in women at ovulation, which, when women lived together under natural light, tended to occur at the full moon. One example of the power of pheromones is their effect on mosquitoes. It's also well documented that the biting activity of female mosquitoes increases five hundred times at the full moon. At ovulation, women are also more likely to be bitten by mosquitoes, and blondes are more likely to be bitten than brunettes.[24] According to the research of Winnifred Cutler,

Ph.D., and others, external application of specially formulated
pheromones can mimic the sexual attractant properties of naturally
occurring pheromones, thus rendering the wearer more attractive to
potential sexual partners. In her research on women who had had hysterectomies and who were using pheromones, the researchers stopped
the study because it was so obvious that the women who were using
the pheromones were attracting more attention than the control
group.[25]

We're just beginning to appreciate this new and exciting area of human biology. For example, there is evidence that when the hormone
oxytocin used as a nasal spray is given to people, they become more
trusting.[26] Oxytocin is the bonding hormone and is produced in the
body in large amounts during childbirth and breast-feeding and in lesser
amounts during pleasurable social interactions and also during sex.

Pheromones are a different class of hormones than oxytocin, but
I use the example simply to document the powerful effect that small
molecules can have on our brains and behavior. Given that scent is
the most remembered sense and that smells go right into the most
primal areas of our brains, affecting all bodily functions, I wouldn't
hesitate to give pheromones a try. After all, everyone has had the experience of having a certain smell bring back potent memories from
childhood. Though commercially available pheromones are generally odorless, they are often mixed with cologne or perfume or used
on the skin just as they are. Pheromones are available from
Winnifred Cutler's Athena Institute (see www.athenainstitute.com)
and also from www.love-scent.com. Remember, though—the biggest
"pheromone" will always be your ability to turn yourself on
through appreciating yourself while focusing attention on someone
else!

8. Get creative. Don't be afraid to try new things, step out of the
box a little and expand your ideas about who you are. Adding some
spice keeps your sex life exciting, and a little creativity can go a long
way. For example, a colleague of mine takes turns reading erotic fiction out loud with her boyfriend in bed. "The book we're reading,
part of the Herotica series of women's erotic fiction, has almost seventy stories, so if one doesn't appeal we just flip to one that does. I
love these stories because they're written for women, which is better
for couples than the male-oriented material out there (much of
which is a turn-off for me)." She finds that reading such stories out
loud works because it's far less intimidating to speak someone else's
words than to come up with her own.

She's also experimented with using a silk scarf as a blindfold. "It doesn't have to be kinky," she says. "It just heightens your senses (when you're the one who is wearing it) and builds anticipation in a major way. When we did this the first time, in front of a wonderful fire on a cold winter night, my boyfriend gave me a fabulous massage with essential oils. What we did wasn't necessarily so amazing, but using the blindfold dialed up the excitement so it felt pretty amazing. A side benefit is that this also fosters trust, because the person being blindfolded is trusting his or her partner, and the partner is honored by being the recipient of that trust."

Another idea she's tried is listening to a specially engineered CD designed to tweak brain waves that heighten sexual pleasure. The CD, called *Ecstasy*, was developed by Brain Sync. (See www.brainsync.com.) "It doesn't much matter to me if it is really doing something or if it's the placebo effect," she says. "It's fun, and that's what counts. The only drawback: you have to take care not to get tangled up in the headphone cords!"

Of course, every woman needs to find what works for her, and the variations are endless. I personally like the erotic literature edited by Lonnie Barbach, such as *Erotic Interludes* (Plume, 1995).

CIRCUMCISION AND SEXUALITY: THE CRUCIAL LINK

If we are to reclaim the erotic in our lives and move toward a partnership society in which the sexuality of males and females is celebrated equally, we must be willing to look at our participation in practices that are as harmful to the sexuality of men as they are to women. In other words, women aren't the only ones who have suffered sexually in our dominator society. Routine male infant circumcision done within the first three days of life and often without anesthesia is a form of massive, societally approved male sexual abuse that removes a very important erotic tissue in men. Few people would argue that routine female circumcision—the removal of the clitoris and labia—is completely unacceptable. In fact, the United Nations has issued a decree against it. Happily the rate of male circumcision continues to fall in the U.S.

Uncircumcised Is the Norm. The vast majority of the world's men, including most Europeans and Scandinavians, are uncircumcised. And before 1900, circumcision was virtually nonexistent in the United States as well—except for Jewish and Muslim people, who've been performing circumcisions for hundreds of years for religious reasons. Believe it or not, circumcision was introduced in English-speaking countries in the late 1800s to control or prevent masturbation, similar to the way that female circumcision was promoted and continues to be advocated in some Muslim and African countries to control women's sexuality.[27] As the absurdity of this position became apparent, new justifications, such as the prevention of cervical and penile cancers, received the blessing of the medical establishment. But these are justifications that science has been unable to support. Nor is there any scientific proof that circumcision prevents sexually transmitted diseases.

The Pleasures of Natural Sex

The male foreskin, one of the most richly innervated and hyperelastic pieces of tissue in the male body, is there for a reason. In her well-researched book, *Sex as Nature Intended It* (Turning Point Press, 2001), author Kristen O'Hara documents why the design of an intact penis not only ensures maximal sexual sensation for the male but also satisfies the female need for clitoral stimulation at the same time. Most American women have not personally experienced the sensation of sex with an uncircumcised man because the majority of men in this country, especially those born before 1980, have been circumcised. But O'Hara's long-ago affair with an uncircumcised man was the spark that touched off years of research, the result of which is her eye-opening book. Consider the following:

~ The primary pleasure zones of the natural (uncircumcised) penis are located in the upper penis, which includes the penis head, the foreskin's inner lining, and the frenulum—the hinge of skin that connects the foreskin to the head of the penis. When a male is circumcised, some of the most erotically sensitive areas of the penis are removed: the foreskin that normally covers the head of the penis (the glans) and some or all of the frenulum.

~ The frenulum contains high concentrations of nerve endings that are sensitive to fine touch. The glans was designed by nature to be covered all the time except during sexual activity. Upon erection, both foreskin layers unfold onto the upper penile shaft, leaving the highly innervated frenulum, glans, and inner lining exposed and readied for sexual activity. This is one of the reasons why the penile tip is the focus of sexual excitement.

~ New scientific evidence shows that highly erogenous tissue equivalent to the female clitoris is located in the core of the penis, beneath the corona (the hooklike head of the penis) and coronal tip. This sensitive tissue extends all the way down the length of the penile shaft to the pubic mound, and onto the pelvic bone in a manner analogous to the anatomy of the female clitoris. Though the penis contains nerves that are sexually excited by pressure, its tip contains the greatest density of these nerves and is therefore the most sexually responsive part, just as the tip of the clitoris is the most sensitive part in the female. And like the tip of the female clitoris, the tip of the penis is sexually stimulated by the pleasurable sensations created by the massaging actions of the movement of the foreskin upon it during intercourse.[28] During intercourse, these exquisitely sensitive nerves of the upper penis both excite a man sexually and control the rhythm of penile thrusting. "When the natural penis thrusts inward, the vaginal walls brush against the erotically sensitive nerves of the glans, the foreskin's inner lining, and the frenulum, causing these nerves to fire off sensations of pleasure," writes O'Hara. "The inward thrust of the penis keeps these pleasure sensations ongoing, but after these nerves have fired, the penis senses a reduction in pleasurable feelings, so it stops its inward thrust and begins its outward stroke in search of stronger sensations. During the outward stroke, the foreskin's outer layer slides forward to cloak the nerves of its inner lining, while the inner lining itself covers the frenulum," she continues. "Once covered, these nerves are allowed to rest from stimulation until the next inward thrust. As the foreskin moves forward on the shaft, it bunches up behind the coronal ridge, and may sometimes roll forward over the corona, depending upon the length of the stroke. This applies pressure to the interior tissue of the corona and coronal ridge where nerves that are excited by pressure send a wave of sexual excitement throughout the upper penis. The natural penis receives pleasure sensations from one set of sensory nerves on the inward thrust and a different set of nerves on the outward stroke. It can maintain a continuous stream of highly pleasurable sensations by maintaining the right rhythm." And intriguingly, because the area of sexual sensation is so localized in the tip, the penis only has to travel a short distance to excite one set of nerves or another. In other words, it doesn't have to withdraw very far to receive pleasure on the outward stroke. This allows the penis to stay deep inside the vagina, keeping the man's pubic mound in close and frequent contact with a woman's clitoral area, which increases her pleasure and a sense of closeness. Most women really enjoy the sense of melting into their mates that this position enhances.

Ms. O'Hara surveyed approximately one hundred and fifty women—enough to make her study statistically reliable. Here's how one survey respondent described sex with an uncircumcised partner: "Sex with a natural partner has been to me like the gentle rhythm of a peaceful but powerful ocean—waves build, then subside and soothe. It felt so natural, as if it were filling a deep need within me, not necessarily for the act of sex, but more in order to experience the rhythm of a man and woman as they were created to respond to each other."

The Sexual Consequences of Male Circumcision. After circumcision, the exposed head of the penis thickens like a callus and becomes less sensitive.[29] Men who have been circumcised later in life and who therefore know the difference report a decrease in their sexual sensations.

Also, because erotically sensitive areas of the penis have been removed, the circumcised penis must thrust more vigorously with a much longer stroke in order to reach orgasm through stimulating the less sensitive penile shaft. In her study of women who have had sexual experiences with both natural and circumcised men, O'Hara notes that respondents overwhelmingly concurred that the mechanics of coitus were different for the two groups of men. Seventy-three percent of the women reported that circumcised men tended to thrust harder, using elongated strokes, while uncircumcised men tended to thrust more gently, to have shorter strokes, and to maintain more contact between the mons pubis and clitoris.

What If You're with a Circumcised Man? As with the millions of women who've suffered from genital mutilation, it's important for all of us to acknowledge the damage that has been done by circumcision on the body, mind, and spirit of men—even though men "don't remember the procedure." Believe me, their bodies do! Obviously, despite this wound, men are capable of a great deal of sexual pleasure. And though I've no doubt that nature designed our genitalia to facilitate the kind of physical intimacy so many women crave, it's important to know that it's possible to experience deeply satisfying sex with any kind of penis when you have true intimacy with and respect for each other.

Women's Stories

Once we have named the societal inheritance that no longer serves us, we must let go of thoughts and behavior that are not in our best interest. For many women, this is a lifelong process.

Sarah: allergic to partner's semen. Sarah was fifty-eight years old when she came to see me for vaginal dryness and irritation. They were made much worse every time she had intercourse, after which she would experience burning and irritation. She was in a very satisfying and loving relationship, but she was troubled by her body's response to sex. Physically, her vagina looked fine, without any obvious signs of thinning or irritation. She was also on hormone replacement. I prescribed some vitamin E suppositories to help soothe her vaginal tissue and asked her to think about what was going on in her sexual relationship that her body might interpret as a "boundary violation" of some kind. When she came back, she said, "I think I've got it. When my partner and I first started having sex, he was having trouble with impotence, and I had to spend a good deal of time and effort stimulating his erections. But I unconsciously became the one who gave him a phallus—the one who had to 'get it up.' Though this is okay once in a while, I'm a very feminine woman and my body didn't like this role. Now that the two of us have talked it out, I find that my allergic reaction doesn't happen anymore."

Over the years, I've treated many women who seemed to be allergic to their husband's semen. Since the immune system in the vagina is beautifully set up to keep our bodies healthy, I've found that when this is happening, there is almost always something deeper going on. Once again, it's the body's wisdom, giving voice.

Elaine: old memories locked inside. Elaine first came to see me when she was in her early thirties. She had a very long history of pelvic pain, particularly in the vaginal area. For her entire adult life she'd had painful intercourse (dyspareunia). Several treatments that she had undergone to remove the painful areas of tissue in the vagina had been unsuccessful.

Elaine also had problems in other areas of her life. She found herself troubled by mood swings and had a recurring pattern of relationships that started out as sexually intense followed by breakups that were painful both emotionally and physically. In her mid-twenties and early thirties she used recreational drugs, such as marijuana, with her sexual partners to enhance their relationship sexually.

Standard medical care, a macrobiotic diet, and the practice of yoga improved Elaine's health a great deal but provided her with little relief from the pain. In addition, she had been in and out of therapy since the age of sixteen, but it provided no relief from her problems. Even though she couldn't remember much of her childhood, she wondered if she had a history of abuse.

She divorced her husband simply because they didn't get along. After a few years she found herself in a new relationship, but once again the same thing happened: her pelvic pain worsened and she developed recurrent urinary tract infection and outbreaks of herpes. After one episode she came to my office very upset, saying, "I don't know what's happening. I'm on overwhelm. I don't know why this keeps happening to me. And if I don't know what's happening to me, I can't fix it. I don't even know what to eat. Am I too acid or too alkaline? Have I had too much juice? When am I going to have a healthy sex life? When will I feel normal in this area?" And on and on her intellect went, circling, circling, obsessing and obsessing.

I asked Elaine to stay with the despair she was feeling and not instantly jump to the what-should-I-do-to-fix-it mode. She had already been on medication for the urinary tract infection and the herpes; over the next few weeks, she let herself feel the depth of her despair completely. Then she experienced a memory of being in the womb when her mother was pregnant with her. No technique, meditation, or therapy was required for her body to give her this information. It arose spontaneously, as it often does when a woman is searching for meaning as to why her life is the way it is. She experienced the feeling of her father's penis pressing against the amniotic sac through the wall of the uterus, and she felt clearly and viscerally her mother's disgust and "just get this over with" indifference. Elaine concluded that she had been "victimized" in some way by that experience—that her mother's sexual revulsion was responsible for her own current sexual, emotional, and physical problems. Elaine also found that she had a very difficult time feeling her own individual feelings. She couldn't distinguish them from those of the other individuals in her life.

Within days of experiencing this memory and allowing herself to feel the accompanying emotions, Elaine's pelvic pain and vaginal pain with intercourse lessened. Unfortunately they returned after a few months. Her initial hopes that she had found the source of her lifelong emotional, physical, and sexual problems were dashed. It became apparent to both of us that Elaine had some core beliefs encoded in her brain and body that were holding her immobile in her life. These included the belief that she was unlovable at some level and that she would never experience her birthright—a healthy sexual relationship—because her mother had somehow damaged her. Although it is true that Elaine experienced childhood trauma, it is also possible to learn to handle the painful emotions and feelings that often accompany childhood trauma and set the stage for so many difficulties in adult relationships, as well as emotional and physical health problems. It was at this point that I referred Elaine to a relatively new form of cognitive behavioral treatment know as DBT (dialectic behavioral therapy). Elaine went for a year and learned many skills for handling her emotional and physical pain, and I am happy to report that she has been in a stable and fulfilling sexual relationship for some time now. When Elaine feels a compulsion to have sex or feels that she can't say no to sex she doesn't want, or when she feels pushed in other areas of her life, she uses her skills to name the emotion she is experiencing, describes the *function* of the emotion she is experiencing, and comes up with a strategy to take care of her emotional needs herself without having to rely on an outside source. Though each person's timing for this process is different, I have found that DBT skills training is a highly effective and practical solution to many of the problems resulting from a history of trauma and abuse. (See chapter 15, step 8.)

Only when we are in touch with our sexuality on our own terms can we hope to share it with someone else in a meaningful relationship. A wise woman once said to me, "If you can't give *yourself* the tenderness, the love, and the caresses that you want another to provide for you, you'll never find them anywhere else." This statement is so true. I have seen it happen many times with my own patients—as soon as a woman learns to provide these things to herself and for herself, her personal life and her relationships almost invariably improve.[30]

Karen: healer in celibacy. Karen was thirty-five when she first came to see me, with a history of having difficulty reaching orgasm. Her pelvic exam was completely normal. While she was a child and teenager, her father, a very successful businessman, had rarely been home. Like so many women, Karen grew up without the affirmative physical presence of a loving father. She told me that she had come to associate the notion of a loving relationship from a man with emotional and physical distance. She had found herself in several consecutive relationships with men who traveled a great deal and often canceled dates with her at the last minute. Each time this happened, she felt emotionally abandoned and angry that she could never count on them. Finally she went to a "Living in Process" intensive with a trainee of Anne Wilson Schaef's and began to name and confront her own part in attracting addictive relationships.

"Looking back," Karen said later, "it's no wonder that I was never able to experience any sexual pleasure when I made love. A part of me always held back—not able to surrender to the experience. Though I had sex, I faked liking it and only did it to please my partner at the time. Opening myself up to the possibility of feeling real love and passion would mean having to feel the same things that I had felt as a little girl—disappointment, vulnerability, and a sense of abandonment from the first male relationship in my life. I wasn't conscious of any of this, of course. But after hitting the despair I felt about my continual bad relationships, I knew I needed help. At the intensive, I went through several deep processes in which I felt what it was that I had been running from all of my life—the pain and despair of my childhood. Now I am in recovery, going to twelve-step meetings, and I've recently started a friendly, nonsexual relationship with a man who lives nearby and rarely travels. Initially, I wasn't attracted to him. In fact, I found him boring. He never 'hooked' me in the same way as the others had, and so I don't feel the same fascination and obsession for him as I have for others.

"As I live my life one day at a time and pay attention to receiving the small sensual gifts of life, I know that my relationship with myself is healing and that a loving relationship with a man is a possibility. But first I need a loving and sensual relationship with myself. I've decided that a period of celibacy is in order for me now. I feel more alive than

I have in years. Every day I notice how good the breeze feels on my face and how loving the warmth of the sun feels on my skin. I go to the beach and watch the waves every chance I get. I pay attention to sunsets and how beautiful the moon looks in the sky. I chart my menstrual cycles and notice that I feel increased sexual desire at ovulation. I am free now to feel it but not to act on it. It is simply part of how I am reclaiming my own bodily, sensual wisdom."

RETHINKING SEXUALITY: CONCLUDING THOUGHTS

⁓ As women, we need to consider becoming "virgin" again by being true to our deepest selves. We must do and be what is true for us—not to please someone else but because it is our truth.

⁓ We need to acknowledge that we all have access to the life-force—the erotic, ecstatic energy of our being. It is part of being human.

⁓ We need to imagine what our sexuality would be like if we thought of it as holy and sacred, a gift from the same source that created the ocean, the waves, and the stars.

⁓ We, each of us, need to try to reconnect without sexuality simply as the expression of this creative life-force.

⁓ We need to learn how to experience and then direct our sexual energy (with or without actually having sex) for our greatest possible pleasure and good. Secondarily, we need to imagine how we can use it to benefit other people in our lives as well.

⁓ We need to think about new attitudes toward being sexual. Allow your life to change by completely embracing your innate sexuality without guilt, shame, or fear. Doesn't that feel better?

9

Vulva, Vagina, Cervix, and Lower Urinary Tract

This...is dedicated with tenderness and respect to the blameless vulva.
—*Possessing the Secret of Joy*, by Alice Walker, from which this quotation comes, names and bears witness to the extreme suffering of tens of millions of women around the world whose external genitalia have been cut off and who have otherwise been mutilated in girlhood because of the dictates of their patriarchal cultures. This practice still goes on, even in some areas of the United States.

As an essential gateway to life, the vagina, vulva, and cervix should be celebrated, not maligned, mutilated, or considered shameful in any way. After all, this is the area of the body through which the seeds of human life are planted and later harvested through birth. It is also the area associated with the most exquisite pleasure that women are capable of experiencing.

More than 80 percent of the human immune system cells are at the mucosal openings in the body, including the vulva, vagina, cervix, and urethral openings. When this area is intact and healthy, it affords effective protection against sexually transmitted disease, including AIDS. Keeping the genitals healthy is also essential for optimal fertility, sexual functioning, and elimination. The very first step that a woman must take to achieve this is to lovingly accept this area of her body!

OUR CULTURAL INHERITANCE

It's crucial that we tell the truth about the cultural programming that makes the lower genital areas so problematic for so many women. Writing about the link between sex, brutality, and male human nature, Riane Eisler, author of *Sacred Pleasure* (HarperSan Francisco, 1995) and codirector of the Institute for Partnership Studies, writes, "On the one hand, the association of sex and violent domination is said not to exist except in the case of just a few perverts. On the other hand, this same association is said to be not only normal but inevitable—just part of human, or more specifically male, nature." She quotes Robert Stoller, the author of *Sexual Excitement: The Dynamics of Erotic Life* (Pantheon Books, 1979): "Putting aside the obvious effects that result from direct stimulation of erotic bodily parts, it is hostility—the desire, overt or hidden, to harm another person—that generates and enhances sexual excitement." It was Stoller's contention that "harm and suffering" are central to sexual excitement, and that the debasement and "fetishization" (dehumanization and objectification) of the "sexual object," and even the use of sex in a "search for revenge," are normal.[1] Our culture's fascination with sadomasochistic sexual imagery and practices stems from this antipleasure programming. But this needn't be the case.

Western culture has considered the genital area "dirty" and defiles it by this attitude. Every function associated with the genitals—birthing, bleeding, sex, and elimination—is *highly* charged emotionally and psychologically. Since childhood, most of us have picked up the idea that this part of our body is different from other parts: it is taboo, dirty, and unworthy. Over the years, many patients of all ages and backgrounds have asked me during their pelvic exams, "How can you do this job? It's so disgusting." One woman recalled visiting her college health service to be treated for a yeast infection and being told by a young male M.D., "the female genitalia are like a cesspool." The most common reason that women douche, moreover, is their mistaken belief, handed down from mother to daughter, that this area of the body is offensive and requires special cleaning. It is now well documented that douching is not necessary and can even be harmful (it can irritate tissues, making them more susceptible to infection). The practice is on the decline. Still the promotion and sale of feminine hygiene deodorants and deodorant-impregnated tampons and sanitary pads give women the impression that the vagina in its natural state is unacceptable, that it must be sanitized and deodorized.

The very word *vagina* comes from Latin and originally meant "sheath for a sword"—or the sheath for a penis, an example of a woman's body being defined only in reference to men.[2] In prehistoric egalitarian societies, vulvas and pubic triangles were frequently drawn or inscribed on cave walls to symbolize a sacred place, a gateway to life. And as already mentioned, sexuality and spirituality were appreciated as intimately connected, an idea that is now reawakening in our culture.

Given our collective history, then, it is little wonder that the entry points to the female body are associated with problems for so many women. Problems in the vulva, vagina, cervix, and lower urinary tract are primarily associated with a woman's feelings of violation in her one-on-one relationship with another individual or in her job. Given the substantial number of immune cells at the mucosal surfaces, such as our vagina, urethra, cervix, and bladder, and given that the function of these cells is highly influenced by stress hormones such as cortisol, it is not difficult to see how a perception of violation and the subsequent biological cascade of hormones that results in response to this perception might well impair optimal function in this area of the body.

Indeed, it has now been well documented that psychosocial stress increases both the prevalence and incidence of bacterial vaginosis (BV), a type of vaginal infection caused by an imbalance in the normal vaginal bacterial environment. BV raises the risk of postoperative infections, HIV shedding and acquisition, and premature labor in pregnant women. BV is difficult to eradicate and often recurs. Though it is also associated with douching, oral sex, and multiple sexual partners, psychosocial stress has now been found to be an independent risk factor for it, probably because of the adverse effect of stress hormones on the immune function of the vaginal mucosa.[3]

The inability to say no to a boundary violation can lead to increased susceptibility to infection secondary to decreased levels of immunoglobulin type A or immunoglobulin type M. Think of it this way: any perception of invasion in one's emotional life can result in increased permeability of one's immune system boundary both on the surface areas of the body and internally. This is especially true in those women with a history of psychosexual trauma in early life. A woman who has been in a sexually active love relationship and is rejected may perceive her rejection as a violation, and vulvar or vaginal problems can result. If she can't feel and release her anger over this, she may develop recurrent urinary symptoms. Incest memories, sexual violation, and guilt feelings about sexuality can also result in repeated episodes of vaginitis.

A woman who has a health problem in the vagina, vulva, or cervix may be involved in a situation in which she is being used sexually or in a job without her complete conscious cooperation and consent. Or she may be feeling forced to do something against her consent or to act in a sexual way about which her emotions are divided. In such a situation her body is likely to respond with problems that we associate with sexual violation. These physical problems can appear if, for instance, she is using sex to obtain financial, physical, or emotional security or to manipulate another person, rather than to bring mutual pleasure. Feelings of being used or raped are associated with chronic vaginitis, chronic vulvar pain, recurrent venereal warts, recurrent herpes, cervical cancer, and associated abnormal Pap smears (cervical dysplasia).

Women with episodic urinary symptoms often find that the episodes are accompanied by anger or feeling "pissed off." Getting a urinary tract infection (UTI) may be the body's way of releasing anger. Women with recurrent UTIs should pay attention to what happened in their lives and relationships twenty-four to forty-eight hours before the onset of the symptoms. With practice, we can often become aware of the offending situation and take steps to change either the situation or our response to it. When the anger becomes more chronic and less available on a conscious level, the symptoms may take the form of continual urinary urgency and frequency.

Studies have shown that women with chronic bladder infections have more free-floating anxiety and more obsessive personality traits and tend to experience emotions only through their bodily symptoms (somatoform disorder) compared to women without this problem. In one study, in fact, women with chronic cystitis had scores comparable to those of psychiatric patients for levels of obsessionality. They were also prone to emotional states that were not balanced by their intellect.[4] Several researchers have found that women who feel the need to urinate frequently but who don't have infections are more anxious and neurotic than those without the problem. It has also been found that symptoms of anxiety correlate with urinary urgency (feeling as if she can't make it to the bathroom in time), needing to get up at night to urinate, and frequent urination.[5] Many women can relate to urinary frequency around exam time at school or when trying to get to sleep at night while worried about something.

Chronic vulvar problems such as pain and itching are associated with stress from anxiety and irritation related to being controlled either by a partner or by a situation that in energy terms is equivalent to a partner. An example would be a woman who feels so "married" to a job that totally controls her that, unconsciously, she is not free to experience her life on her own terms. Medical intuitive Caroline Myss suggests that we might think of this external control as a modern-day "chastity belt." A woman's mate may control her either by forcing her to have sex or by withholding sexual activity that she desires.

Ruth came to see me with a history of recurrent vaginitis and urinary tract infections that had not responded to the usual treatments, such as antifungal creams and antibiotics. Her husband wanted sex every night, and she believed that filling his sexual needs was part of her "job." She did love him, but she was often too tired to make love in the evening and his desires irritated her. Nevertheless, she forced herself to do it, even as her unconscious resentment grew. Like many women, Ruth equated having a lot of sex with having a "satisfactory" sex life. At first she denied to me that her sex life had any problems. I pointed out to Ruth that when she had sex that she didn't want, the normal lubrication associated with female sexual desire was not present, and this, coupled with the friction of intercourse, set the scene for vaginal and urethral irritation and inflammation. (It is very clear that when women engage in any sex that is traumatic to their tissues, infection and inflammation can result.) When tissue trauma is combined with a lack of receptivity and a feeling of not being able to refuse, then the immune system will be affected adversely, making healing from the trauma that much more difficult. Eventually, as part of her treatment, Ruth sought help through therapy and learned how to express her needs in a positive way that enhanced her marriage.

The sexual imperative of our culture—that desirable women serve men sexually—is largely what gets women into trouble in the first place; in other words, into sexual situations that don't serve their needs and that are in fact harmful. Many women are conflicted between needing to be loved and needing sexual pleasure, on the one hand, and wanting to say no to intercourse, on the other. Gynecological problems in the vulva, vagina, and cervix are often related to a woman's inability to say no to entry into this area of her body when she wants to but doesn't believe she should. These problems are quite literally related to allowing herself to "get screwed." One of my patients developed chronic vaginitis, for example, when her college (illegally) refused to award her credit for courses that she had completed. At first, she decided that she had no choice but to accept their mistreatment because she didn't want to "make waves." Despite many external remedies of vulvovaginitis, however, she did not get better until she appealed her college's decision about her credits and then refused to back down. She was eventually awarded the credits due her, and her vaginitis cleared up.

Besides frustration and anger, another emotion that generally tends to affect our health adversely is guilt. When our guilt is centered on our sexuality, it can become associated with problems specific to our entry points. The sexual revolution of the 1960s and 1970s broke down some of our culture's puritanical views about sexuality, but a sexually repressed culture cannot be healed just by taking off its clothes. Now it is even more important for women to be clear about their sexuality and their choice of sexual partners. It is especially important that women consciously use their freedom to understand what their bodies really want and not be led by the blandishments of partners who equate freedom with irresponsible behavior.

Scientific research supports the premise that certain emotional factors are associated with chronic urinary, vaginal, vulvar, or cervical problems, including cervical cancer.[6] One study showed that, compared to women with other types of cancer, women with cervical cancer are more likely to have sexual ambivalence, lower incidence of orgasm during sexual intercourse, and a dislike of sexual intercourse amounting to an actual aversion. They have more marital conflict, as evidenced by the increased incidence of divorce, desertion, or separation.[7] Another study was done on women who had severely abnormal Pap smears that required further evaluation to assess whether the woman had progressed to actual cervical cancer. The authors found that they could predict which women had progressed to cervical cancer based on the women's responses to their questions about recent stressful life events. If a husband or boyfriend had been unfaithful, was drinking, or was running around, for example, a woman with cervical cancer would always say something like, "I should have left him, but I couldn't because of the kids" or "I thought he needed me." When responding to the same situation in their own lives, the women without cervical cancer would say, "I can't trust him—he wants more than he gives." In this same study, if a family member got a major illness or died, the women with cervical cancer would say, "I should have worked harder and taken better care of him [or her]." The women without cervical cancer, on the other hand, were more realistic about the limits of their responsibility to others and about their ability to change the natural course of events.[8] One could argue that because these studies were done in the 1950s and 1960s, their conclusions are no longer valid. However, a 1988 study revealed the same thing—the cervical neoplasia and subsequent risk for invasive cancer were more likely to develop in those women who were passive in their relationships, avoided an active coping style, and were more socially conforming and appeasing when compared to a control group whose Pap smears were more benign.[9] A 1986 study showed that women scoring high on scales of helplessness, pessimism, and social alienation had a higher incidence of disease involving the cervix. These personality characteristics were measured before the diagnosis of cervical cancer was made, thus minimizing the possibility that it was the diagnosis of the cancer that caused the personality characteristics.[10] On the other hand, those women who were resilient, optimistic, and had active coping styles tended to have Pap smears that did not reflect abnormal and invasive cells.

Most women with chronic vaginal, urinary, or vulvar problems have had them for years. These problems are usually associated with unexpressed complaints about a situation in their lives that have been accumulating for an equally long period. Clinically, it is well known that treatment for chronic problems of this nature is often unsuccessful if the psychological and emotional aspects of the problem are ignored. Unfortunately, many such women have been to scores of doctors, looking in vain for the physical cure for their problem.

In energy terms, a woman sets the stage in her body for chronic vulvar, vaginal, or urinary problems when she *lacks the courage to change* the negative aspects of an unhealthy relationship. When Dr. Mona Lisa Schulz does an intuitive reading, she finds that women with these problems have often had boundary violations early in their childhoods. In adulthood, when a woman stays in a relationship with someone she doesn't respect or even like, because she is afraid to leave—for whatever reason, be it fears about financial or physical insecurity, about being single, or about her own dependence—she is participating in a prostitute archetype. If she continues to have sex with someone whom she doesn't respect or love, she is participating in an energy pattern that is associated with chronic vaginal, cervical, or vulvar problems.

ANATOMY

The vulva and the vagina form the outermost points of entry into the female genital system. The cervix and its opening, known as the cervical os (*os* is an anatomical word for "entrance" or "mouth"), forms the entryway into the uterus and inner pelvic organs—the tubes and ovaries. (See figure 7, page 164.) The vulva comprises the labia majora (outer lips) and labia minora (inner lips). The outer entrance from the vulva to the vagina is known as the *introitus*. The pubic hair on the vulva forms a protective barrier to the more delicate tissues of the vagina and the cervix. The vulvar skin contains apocrine sweat glands, identical to those under the arms. Apocrine sweat glands differ from regular sweat glands in that their secretions are triggered by emotional situations, not just by physical exertion. The vulva "sweats" more than any other part of the body.

The bladder is located just above the vagina, while the urethra, the structure that leads from the bladder to the outside, can be felt as the protruding tubelike ridge that runs down the top part of the vagina to just above the vaginal opening. The anus lies just below and in back of the vagina.

The vagina constitutes a passageway to the cervix, which is actually the lowermost part of the uterus (and is sometimes called the uterine cervix). The cervix protrudes into the uppermost part of the vagina and is covered by the same type of cells as the vaginal lining.

The Pap smear, a screening test for abnormal cervical cells, is taken from the opening in the center of the cervix, where the squamous cell covering of the outer cervix meets the inside of the cervical canal. (*Squamous* refers to a flattened type of epithelial cell that covers mucous membranes of the body—for example, inside the vulva, vagina, and mouth.) This area is known as the *squamocolumnar junction* (SCJ), a very dynamic location in which the mucus-producing endocervical gland cells are constantly changing into the tougher squamous cells. As a result, the normal secretions from the endocervix sometimes get trapped, causing mucus-filled cysts (Nabothian cysts). These feel like little bumps on the cervix and can sometimes grow to one or two centimeters in diameter. Though many women who feel these bumps think they have an abnormality, they are completely normal and don't require treatment.

In some women and most teenagers the SCJ is located way out on the outer part of the cervix, with the inner, redder-appearing cells of the endocervix extending outward onto the cervix. In the past many physicians have confused this normal anatomy with pathology, referring to this red glandular area out on the cervix as "cervical erosion" or "chronic cervicitis." Many women have had normal cervical tissue cauterized because of this misunderstanding.

At this time in our history, chronic vaginitis, sexually transmitted diseases such as venereal warts and herpes, and abnormal Pap smears (also considered a sexually transmitted disorder) are virtually epidemic. These disorders can affect the vulva, vagina, and cervix all at the same time. And because the urethra and bladder are contiguous to this area, they are often affected as well. Though these disorders are often blamed on certain viruses, countless women who do not develop symptoms also have these same viruses present in their bodies.

Gynecologists work right in the middle of women's most secret and painful issues. To be healers, they must recognize that a woman's sexual vulnerability often hovers around her gynecological exam. When a woman is diagnosed with a sexually transmitted disease or has an abnormal Pap smear, all her fears, beliefs, and misconceptions about her sexuality and body may well come up. It's vital for healers to be sensitive to these emotions and try to help their patients articulate their distress and grief, as well as their questions. If you do not think that your feelings about an exam or diagnosis are being treated with concern, tell your practitioner that your feelings are important to you and that you've learned to respect them as a necessary key to eventually understanding yourself better. Ask her or him for help and compassion during the pelvic exam. Though strong emotions may occur during a pelvic exam, don't expect your practitioner or yourself to know exactly why at the moment they first arise. Simply stay with what you are feeling, with the intent to heal the situation. Then relax and allow the healing to come, by turning the situation over to your inner guidance. Eventually, when you are ready, you will get the insight you need about the situation.

A pelvic examination is an ideal time to become acquainted with your lower genital tract in a positive and healthy way. Here's how: Ask your health care provider to push the back of the exam table into an upright position so that you can watch the entire exam. Ask him or her to explain to you exactly what they are examining and why. If you are nervous about the exam, request that your health care provider tell you what he or she is about to do—and get your permission before proceeding with each subsequent step of the exam.

A pelvic exam begins with close examination of the labia majora (the large outer lips) and then the labia minora (the small inner lips) of the vulva. The urethral opening and clitoris are also examined and so is the perineum—the area between the vagina and the anus. It's a good idea to ask for a mirror so that you can see these parts of your body and recognize exactly what "normal" looks like. After that, a warmed speculum is inserted into the vagina and opened so that the vaginal side walls and the cervix can be seen. (It should be routine for the doctor to use a warmed speculum. But when my daughters recently had their first pelvic exams by a female gynecologist in NYC, both the speculums and the doctor were very cold!) Many different speculum shapes and sizes are available—so this part of the exam should be comfortable. Your doctor can also show you what your cervix looks like and where the Pap smear is taken.

The part of the exam before the speculum is the perfect time to learn where your PC muscle is and how to contract it. Your health care provider can point out the muscle and then teach you exactly how to contract it. He or she will usually put one gloved finger in the vagina so you can tighten around it. Contracting and releasing the muscle several times before the speculum is inserted makes this part of the exam much more comfortable. After the speculum exam is completed and the Pap smear is taken from the cervix, the speculum will be removed and your doctor will do what's called a "bimanual" exam, meaning that he or she will insert one or two fingers in your vagina and, with the other hand, palpate your lower abdomen above the pubic bone in order to feel the uterus and ovaries. This will be followed by a rectovaginal exam with one finger in the vagina, and one in the rectum to feel the area behind the uterus. This part of the exam is simply not comfortable, though it doesn't cause pain.

It's perfectly acceptable for you to ask that the exam be stopped before it is complete. Some women with a history of trauma or adverse childhood programming about their genitals may find that going through a complete exam is too much for them until they get to know their practitioner better and feel more comfortable. This is fine. Many women feel uncomfortable during pelvic exams. But as you learn to accept and appreciate your lower genital tract, and also to contract and relax your PC muscle at will, you will be well on your way toward better GYN health and also sail through your pelvic exam!

HUMAN PAPILLOMA VIRUS (HPV)

Human papilloma virus (HPV) is a very common virus that can cause venereal warts and is associated with abnormal Pap smears. It has been estimated that 75 percent of women will have a genital HPV infection at some time in their lives.[11] For most, this viral infection will spontaneously clear from the immune system within six to eight months—without any symptoms at all. The vast majority of women who have been exposed to HPV do not develop any warts or cervical dysplasia. But in others HPV is associated with cervical cancer.

Certain high-risk subtypes of HPV DNA are associated with a higher risk of developing cervical cancer.[12] The DNA of HPV (the genetic material of the virus, used for identification) has been found in virtually all abnormal Pap smears and cervical cancer cells. However, the majority of women who have been exposed to even the most virulent strains of HPV do *not* get cervical dysplasia. HPV should be thought of as an important risk factor for cervical dysplasia but shouldn't be seen as the single cause of it.

We don't really know, in a conventional sense, who will develop abnormalities from the virus and who won't, unless we look at the factors that can contribute to decreased immunity. Abnormalities start to grow and cause damage only when the immune system has already been weakened in that area of the body and is unable to maintain the health of the tissue. The good news is that even though HPV is quite common in women under thirty, it usually clears up by itself in six to eight months. Because of this, the American College of Obstetricians and Gynecologists recommends HPV-DNA screening only in women age thirty and over. And this doesn't need to be done regularly. (See Pap smear recommendations on pages 294–95.)

Chronic stress and specific attitudes about sex actually change the blood flow to cervical tissue and affect its secretions. Studies suggest a link between stress and the subsequent development of disease in this area of the body.[13] Suppression of the immune system as a result of chronic emotional or other stress can lead to changes in immunity that allow increased virus production in the first place. The link between abnormal Pap smears and deficient immune system functioning is well known: women who have organ transplants and are on drugs that suppress the immune system (such as prednisone) have a much greater chance than normal of developing abnormal Pap smears. They also frequently have recurrent wart and herpes outbreaks. (Emotional reaction to the diagnosis of venereal warts can be similar to that of herpes. If you have concerns about either condition, please read through both sections.)

If our bodies are a hologram in which each part contains the whole (see chapter 2), then the HPV virus and the abnormal cells associated with the virus are two interrelated aspects of a greater whole that is not as yet entirely understood. For a variety of reasons, depressed immunity makes it much more likely that any HPV present on the cervix or in the vagina will attack already weakened cells. I think of the HPV virus as an opportunist at the scene, like buzzards around a dying calf. The virus doesn't "cause" cancer any more than the buzzards caused the calf to get sick. But once the calf is sick and dying, the buzzards start to hover. Most women who have the HPV virus don't go on to develop abnormal Pap smears or cervical cancer, because most viral activity and infections are halted by good immune functioning.

Symptoms

Most women with HPV have *no* symptoms. In those who do, the most common symptom is warty growths (condylomata acuminata) on the outside of the vulva that are painless but can be seen and felt. These can grow and multiply during pregnancy, when the hormones associated with pregnancy stimulate their growth. They often disappear on their own following delivery, when the hormones once again change. Warts can vary in appearance, from plaquelike growth to pointy, spiky lesions. Some women have only a few, while others have many all over the vulva. The virus can also cause warty growths on the tongue, the lips, and in the throat, though these sites are rare. Sometimes a woman has no obvious warts on the vulva but has them in the vagina or on its cervix. She may not be aware of these.

HPV infection is sometimes associated with chronic vulvar pain, chronic vaginitis, and chronic inflammation of the cervix (cervicitis). A vaginal discharge is usually not present, although it can be. Because some women have HPV infection in association with vaginal infections from yeast or from an imbalance in the vaginal flora known as bacterial vaginosis, it is not always possible to tell exactly what virus or bacteria is causing what symptom. Unless a woman has actual warty growths on her vulva or has chronic vulva or vaginal irritation associated with HPV, she won't know that she has it.

Diagnosis

Warty growths on the vulva, vagina, or cervix and abnormal cells on a Pap smear or cervical biopsy are usually associated with HPV. If these appearances are a first occurrence, a biopsy is taken and sent to the lab to confirm the diagnosis. Sometimes HPV is diagnosed by a colposcopy, an examination of the cervix and vagina through a magnifying lens, or a cervigram, a screening test in which a photograph of the cervix is made after applying dilute acetic acid (vinegar) to the tissue. When vinegar is applied to the vulva, cervix, or vagina and HPV is present in the tissue, the tissue often turns white. (This tissue is then called acetowhite epithelium, or white skin cells.) Biopsies of the white area often reveal HPV.

Common Concerns About HPV

Why do so many women have it? HPV has probably always been present in the human genitals. You can certainly find it on old slides of Pap smears from thirty years ago. Back then, HPV simply wasn't recognized or studied as much as it is today. Several factors have contributed to its more frequent diagnosis now. One is the advent of colposcopy, a diagnostic technique developed in the 1970s to evaluate abnormal Pap smears. A colposcopy may include biopsies of the vagina or cervix if any abnormal areas show up on examination. (See page 298 for more details.) As more cervical biopsy specimens were read and cervical abnormalities came to be diagnosed in their earlier stages, pathologists began to recognize the cellular changes associated with HPV more frequently.

The sexual revolution and multiple sexual partners have increased the number of women who have been exposed to the virus. Condoms don't always prevent the transmission of HPV (which is transmitted by physical contact) because the virus can exist in areas other than the penis, such as the scrotum; they do help, however. Even if a woman is monogamous, she can be exposed to warts depending upon the number of sexual partners that her partner has had. Factors implicated in HPV leading to abnormal growths include a depressed immune system from suboptimal nutrition, emotionally unhealthy relationships, excess alcohol, and cigarette smoking. Therefore, it's not simply the viruses from our past sexual partners that we bring to our current sexual partners. We also bring our current state of emotional health, which in part determines whether those viruses will become active.

How did I get this? Who gave it to me? This is one of the big questions for most women. The truth is that HPV, like the herpes virus, inserts itself into the DNA of the tissue it infects, and once it does this, it may lie dormant for years. That means theoretically that a virus a woman "caught" in 1985 may not express itself in any visible way until 2005. This also means that whoever "gave" it to her may well not have known that he or she even had it. I've seen monogamous couples in whom one partner has warts or herpes but the other does not, despite twenty or more years of sexual relationship without condoms.

In a culture that believes in cause and effect, HPV and herpes infections dash our illusion of control. Some people are "asymptomatic shedders"—that is, they potentially shed the virus to others without ever knowing that they have it—so no one can be 100 percent sure that they won't give it to another person once they've got it, if they even know.

What this means for women is the following: to the degree that a woman has guilt or self-loathing about her sexuality, she will worry or obsess about herpes and HPV infections. Countless women, most of them from strict male-dominated religious backgrounds, have gone into massive shame attacks when I made the diagnosis of herpes or warts. Somewhere inside, they believe that people who get herpes or HPV have done something wrong. I have seen many other women with these conditions become paralyzed with guilt and feel they will be tainted forever. They are terrified that they will pass on the virus to someone else. Because they already feel themselves to be unworthy, the herpes or HPV diagnosis pushes their self-esteem even lower, thus beginning a vicious cycle in the body that continues to depress the immune system and that can potentially result in continual outbreaks. Media stories linking HPV and herpes with cervical cancer make their state of mind even worse. Shame combined with fear is a very deadly combination for the immune system. (Later in this chapter, I will give some recommendations for dealing emotionally and mentally with these conditions and for boosting your immune system.)

Will HPV interfere with pregnancy? Vulvar warts are often stimulated to grow by the hormones associated with pregnancy. In rare instances, a woman's warts will cause bleeding at the time of delivery, especially if an episiotomy is made through an area of the vulva that is affected by warts. In general, however, warts do not interfere with pregnancy. They often disappear without treatment once a woman has delivered. A woman with HPV can theoretically transmit it to her baby at delivery, and some babies can theoretically get vocal cord papilloma (which can be treated with surgery) from HPV. This is very rare, however; I have never seen a case of it, and it is not a reason to do a cesarean section in a woman with HPV. The immune system of the baby protects it almost every time.

Treatment

Treatment is aimed at removing the visible warts and making sure that she isn't growing any of the abnormal or precancerous cells that are sometimes associated with the warts. Once the bulk of a wart is removed, the immune system can deal with and remove the remainder more easily. Removal or disappearance of a wart, however, doesn't necessarily prevent recurrence or the possibility of transmission.

It is controversial as to whether it's important for males to get treated for warts. Many doctors downplay the male role in HPV, and many men are infected without visible warts. Therefore, many men don't know that they have them, and no consistent effort is made to diagnose them.[14] The female cervix is a unique environment and appears to be more susceptible to virus-associated abnormalities than male penile or scrotal skin.

Laser treatment. Laser treatment, very popular for warts back in the 1990s, has not lived up to the medical profession's initial expectations. If a physician is highly skilled in the use of the laser, it can be a good way to remove persistent warts, but a few studies have shown that once warts have been lasered off the cervix or the vulva, they come back faster after laser treatment than after other treatments. Perhaps this is because the laser vaporizes tissue and spreads the wart virus into the surrounding areas. HPV on the mucous membranes of the vagina and cervix can be compared with the virus that causes the common cold in the respiratory tract. We would never think of using a laser to denude the surfaces of the trachea and bronchial tree of the cold virus. But using a laser to remove warts from the genital tract is really no different— we know that ultimately we can't eradicate the wart virus, any more than we can eradicate the common cold virus. Since there are many different strains of wart virus, as of cold virus, making a vaccine is impractical. I have not been impressed with the effectiveness of laser treatment over the long term and prefer other treatment.

Podophyllin. Podophyllin is a chemical resin derived from the mayapple. It interferes with cell division and therefore stops genital warts from growing. It can be effective in some people, but it is for use with external warts only, because it can have toxic effects on surrounding tissues whose cell division is normal. Podophyllin is used only on the wart itself and must be washed off within several hours.

Podofilox (Condylox) is a topical 0.5-percent antiviral treatment that a woman can apply herself to external warts after an initial treatment from her health care provider. This convenient treatment may decrease the number of office visits she must make for recurrent warts. This medication is related to podophyllin and is available by prescription.[15]

Aldara (imiquimod). This an immune response modifier that comes as a topical cream for use on HPV warts, among other things. It can take several weeks to work but is more effective than placebo. It can cause skin irritation.

Acids. Many doctors use trichloroacetic acid (TCA) to treat warts on the cervix, vagina, and vulva. This acid is very effective but doesn't "cure" the warts—it just burns away the visible ones. This acid must be applied in minute amounts and only to the warty areas themselves because it causes painful burns to healthy tissue. (It also can burn through clothing.) Even on warty areas, it can cause immediate stinging, followed later by ulceration of the skin. If the acid gets on any area other than the wart (and it often does), it takes from one to two weeks for the skin to heal. It also takes about that long for the ulceration of the wart to slough off. The treatment may need to be done more than once.

Cryocautery. Warts can be frozen with a cryocautery device in the office. Freezing a wart causes it to disappear over a one- to two-week period. I have found this treatment to be time-consuming and often painful for the patient. I don't use it.

Electrocautery. Removal of very large collections of warts is possible using electrocautery. In this treatment the wart is burned off by a heated electrical device. This procedure is usually done under anesthesia in the operating room. It is used only when all other methods haven't worked.

LEEP. Loop electrosurgical excision procedure (LEEP), also called large loop excision of transformation zone (LLETZ), can be used to remove warts and wart-affected tissue on the vulva, cervix, and vagina. It removes warts by electrocautery, using an electrically charged wire loop. It is also used to treat cervical dysplasia. It can be very beneficial. The problem is that a LEEP procedure on the cervix doubles the risk for premature rupture of the membranes during subsequent pregnancy. This increases the risk for prematurity.[16]

I've seen all manner of treatments "work" for warts. Warts on the hands, for instance, are known to disappear after a variety of treatments ranging from hypnosis to applying cold potato or even duct tape.[17] We just don't know what makes warts go away, even after thousands of years of observing that warts are responsive to suggestion and folk remedies.

Even though removal of warts doesn't really "cure" anything, it does help the body fight HPV. One reason for this is that treatment reduces the amount of virus that the warty growth sheds. Another reason is that the immune system is enhanced by the feeling that we're "doing something." We live in a very action-oriented culture, and Americans want to get things done. When we treat a wart and get rid of it, the patient at some level feels that it's been "taken care of." The immune system gets the message and continues to "take care of it."

Vaccine. In the summer of 2006, Merck Pharmaceuticals received FDA approval to market the first HPV vaccine, Gardisil, a genetically engineered drug that helps prevent the most common HPV infections which are implicated in cervical cancer. With the rapid approval of Gardisil, HPV and its link to cervical cancer suddenly became front-page news, with media ads marketing the virus to all young women. The CDC and many other groups quickly recommended vaccinating all women ages nine to twenty-six, and even beyond.

Overnight, women with virtually no risk for cervical cancer (the vast majority) were suddenly made to feel vulnerable, thus creating a huge market for a vaccine that most healthy women won't need and that is dangerous for some (visit the National Vaccine Information Center at www.909shot.com).

Here are the facts: There are an average of 9,710 new diagnoses of cervical cancer and 3,700 deaths from the disease in the United States each year, according to the CDC. Of these, 70 percent are related to HPV. That's about 6,790 cases. More than fourteen types of HPV are associated with cervical cancer. Gardisil protects against the four most common ones that are implicated in about 90 percent of HPV-associated cases. That further reduces the number of cervical cancer cases that might potentially be prevented to fewer than 6,000. Recall that 75 percent of all people have been exposed to HPV, but very few get cervical cancer. Those who develop cervical cancer typically have a weakened immune system. Even then, the vast majority of cervical cancer cases could be prevented with routine screening, safe-sex practices, and early treatment measures that are already in place. Though some women might benefit from this vaccine, you have to ask yourself: Who really benefits by vaccinating roughly 30 million girls and women with a vaccine that costs about $360 per dose, isn't always safe, and doesn't guarantee immunity for longer than five years?

Nutritional approach. Wart removal treatment can be enhanced with dietary change, supplements, and education about immune system functioning. Persistent warts are an indicator of immune system depression—that is their message. The expression of the warts is dependent to some degree on how well a woman takes care of herself. Studies have shown that foods high in antioxidants, such as vitamin C, folic acid, vitamin A, vitamin E, beta carotene, and selenium—or supplements containing these—help heal and prevent cervical dysplasia.[18] The antioxidant class known as the proanthocyanidins, found in pine bark and grape seed, have proven to be very helpful in some cases. (See section on cervical dysplasia for dose instructions, and see Resources for reliable sources.) Because of the connection between HPV, cervical dysplasia, and cervical cancer, I recommend that a woman with HPV take a good daily multivitamin-mineral supplement containing these nutrients and also follow a whole-food diet.

Energy medicine. Of course, none of us has complete control over whether a virus inserts itself into our DNA or whether it gets expressed once it has done that. Especially in persistent cases of warts or herpes, however, tuning in to oneself with love, forgiveness, good food, and a good multivitamin can work wonders to keep the warts or herpes from showing up again. I also suggest meditating on the following affirmation from Louise Hay daily: "I rejoice in my sexuality. It is normal and natural and perfect for me. My genitals are beautiful and normal and natural and perfect for me. I am good enough and beautiful enough exactly as I am, right here and right now. I appreciate the pleasure my body gives me. It is safe for me to enjoy my body. I choose the thoughts that allow me to love and approve of myself at all times. I love and appreciate my beautiful genitals!"[19]

HERPES

Herpes is a kind of virus that can cause small, painful ulcers on the vulva, in the vagina, or on the cervix. Herpes viruses can also cause cold sores. Herpes viruses are divided into several types. Type 1 (HSV-1), the kind that causes cold sores, tends to live "above the belt" but it can also cause genital herpes. In fact, herpes simplex Type 1 has now emerged as a major cause of genital herpes, particularly among college-age populations in which oral-genital contact is the biggest risk factor in up to 80 percent of new cases of genital HSV infections.

Type 2 tends to live "below the belt" and up until very recently has been the most common herpes virus associated with genital herpes. Type 2 can occasionally live "above the belt," too, and cause oral infections. Once a person has herpes, he or she has it for life. A herpes virus that is dormant (or latent) resides in the infected tissue around the lips (either genital or oral) or in the spinal nerves.

About 1.6 million new cases of genital herpes occur annually. A national survey in the early 1990s showed that about 22 percent of the general population in the U.S. shows evidence of HSV-2 on blood tests. This represents an increase of 30 percent from 1978.[20] The percentage of people with genital herpes is probably higher because this figure doesn't include those with HSV-1 exposure.

Both HSV-1 and HSV-2 have the same symptoms. The good news is the difference in prognosis. The frequency of genital reactivation is much less with HSV-1, which rarely recurs after the first year of infection.[21] In contrast, Type 2 (HSV-2) can continue to recur for many years.[22] This difference in prognosis is a good reason to have a blood test for the type of herpes if you suspect you have it.

Symptoms

As with HPV, most women who have been exposed to herpes never get sores and therefore have no reason to suspect that they have the virus. The latest studies show that between 75 and 90 percent of HSV-2 infected people aren't aware that they've ever had the infection. The same is probably true for those with HSV-1 genital herpes. Many women attribute their mild genital symptoms to something else, such as a yeast infection or irritation from panty hose. In fact, in one study of women at high risk for sexually transmitted diseases, 47 percent had evidence of the virus on testing, though only one-half of these had ever had any symptoms.[23] When the virus becomes active, however, it causes very characteristic small ulcers on the genital organs. The first episode of herpes outbreak that a person has (known as a primary herpes infection) can be extremely painful, resulting in a fever, systemic illness, swollen lymph nodes in the groin, genital pain, and even an inability to urinate secondary to pain and herpes infection in the bladder or urethra. Herpes virus can also cause urinary retention by temporarily paralyzing the motor nerves to the bladder. This is rare and also self-limiting. After a primary herpes outbreak, a person will almost never have symptoms this severe again, since the body produces antibodies to the herpes.

Subsequent outbreaks are known as secondary herpes. These usually start with a sensation of tingling in the affected area, prior to the outbreak of an actual sore. Some women will feel pain down their legs as well, because the herpes virus lives in the portion of the spinal nerves that innervate both the genitals and the inner thighs. Emotional factors, such as depression, anxiety, or hostility, may allow increased production of the herpes virus and subsequent chronic vaginal irritation.[24]

However, herpes tends to "burn itself out" after a number of years. That means that a person may get outbreaks frequently for a year or two, but they usually don't continue. One of my patients had only one outbreak. At the time of this outbreak she had found out her husband was having an affair. She eventually divorced him, is now in another relationship, and has *never* had a recurrence. Her immune system has kept the herpes virus inactive, even though her lifestyle includes behaviors that are often associated with immune system depression, like heavy smoking and the stress of constant dieting. In this woman's case, her immune system in the genital area is keeping her herpes in remission—further evidence that the immunity of our entry points is enhanced when our one-on-one relationships are going well.

Diagnosis

Given the high number of women (and men) who don't know they have herpes, the most accurate way to diagnose it is through blood testing. New serologic testing is available that detects the specific glycoproteins in the two different herpes strains. It is important to make sure you get a test that is glycoprotein-based because older, less accurate tests that are non-glycoprotein-based provide inaccurate results. A finger stick test known as a biokit HSV-2 can be done in a doctor's office. Other glycoprotein-specific assays can be drawn and sent to a reference lab.

If you have an active herpes sore, or have developed herpes for the first time, cultures can be taken by a health care practitioner. Cultures can also be taken even when you are asymptomatic to determine whether or not you are shedding virus.

Common Concerns About Herpes

Where did I get herpes? Can I give it to someone else? The answer to the first question is the same as for HPV: the virus can be dormant for years, so a person who has a primary outbreak may have "caught" it twenty or more years ago! I've seen first-time genital herpes outbreaks in eighty-five-year-old women who've been celibate and widowed for twenty years.

Most sexual transmission of HSV occurs when the virus is reactivated but asymptomatic among people with unrecognized infections. Recent studies indicate that virtually all HSV-2 seropositive persons shed the virus intermittently from mucosal surfaces.[25]

I have seen monogamous couples in which one member had herpes outbreaks while the other never got it, even though they did not use condoms during their many years of sexual relations. But it is generally recommended that people with herpes do use condoms to cut the risk of infecting someone else. Oral-genital contact can also spread the virus.

In general, herpes outbreaks are associated with the following stressors: anxiety and depression, lack of sleep, overexertion, and microabrasions of the vagina from sexual intercourse. These outbreaks can be greatly decreased or eliminated by following the nutritional and herbal advice below.

What are the risks of herpes if I'm pregnant? Neonatal herpes is the most severe complication of genital herpes and is caused by the newborn's contact with infected genital secretions at the time of labor. Herpes does not pose any risk for the baby during pregnancy itself unless a woman is first exposed to it when she is pregnant and the virus reaches high enough levels in the blood (known as viremia) and also crosses the placenta to infect the baby. Getting herpes for the very first time during the last four months of pregnancy carries the biggest risk for neonatal herpes because the mother's body hasn't yet had a chance to produce antibodies to the virus.

Though no one actually knows how many babies are exposed to herpes virus during labor, we do know that neonatal herpes occurs in up to 1 in 3,200 live births with an estimated incidence of 1,500 cases annually in the U.S.[26]

To give you an idea of how rare it is for a baby to actually get herpes, consider the fact that there are a little over four million births per year in the U.S. And given the large number of women with undiagnosed herpes infections at the time of labor, it's clear that the immune system of mothers offers protection most of the time! Here's the problem: when a newborn does get infected with herpes, it can cause disseminated or central nervous system disease about 50 percent of the time. Of these cases, up to 30 percent will die and up to 40 percent will have some kind of long-term neurological damage. And that's why it's important to do everything possible to minimize the risk of a baby getting infected with herpes during labor. This is why women with active herpes lesions who are in labor almost always deliver by C-section.

If you are pregnant or considering pregnancy. If you are considering getting pregnant, it's a good idea for both you and your partner to be tested for herpes. (About 2 percent of pregnant women will become infected during pregnancy.) If you know that your partner is seropositive for herpes and you aren't, then you can use condoms during intercourse or rubber dams during oral sex to prevent genital transmission.

Make every effort to remain as well nourished and healthy as possible during your pregnancy. Worrying for an entire pregnancy about having an active herpes sore at the time of labor may, in my view, increase the chances for an outbreak.

Follow the steps in this section on treatment to prevent an outbreak, such as taking supplements like garlic and a good multivitamin.

Note: Antivirals such as valacyclovir and acyclovir (see below) can be used in pregnancy for those with severe or recurrent lesions. No significant adverse effects have been found in newborns exposed to this drug.[27]

Herpes doesn't mean an automatic C-section. If you have a history of herpes but have no lesions during labor, then you can safely deliver vaginally. The major sites of entry of the virus into the newborn include the skin, so any procedure that damages the baby's skin could increase the risk of transmission. Among newborns exposed to herpes at delivery, studies have shown that 10 percent of those delivered with the use of fetal scalp electrode, vacuum, or forceps were infected, compared to only 2 percent of those who did not have invasive obstetrical procedures.[28]

Because the risk of transmitting the virus to the baby is so low even for HSV-2 seropostive women with active herpes lesions, some experts are suggesting that it's safe for these women to deliver vaginally.[29] After all, once you've been exposed to herpes, your body makes antibodies against herpes that cross the placenta and help protect the baby. Despite this evidence, however, the current standard of care in most centers is delivery by C-section for those who have active herpes lesions when they go into labor.

Treatment

Medication. A variety of antivirals (e.g., acyclovir [Zovirax] and valacyclovir [Valtrex]) are widely available antiherpes drugs. Acyclovir comes in both pill and ointment form, and some people take it on a long-term basis (for two to three years). When taken orally, this antiviral medication works like any antibiotic in the system. Within twenty-four hours of taking the pills, the virus is inactivated. The topical ointment for actual outbreaks takes a bit longer to work. Antivirals are available only by prescription and are particularly effective in primary (first-time) infections.

Though antivirals are very helpful in first-time outbreaks, I'm concerned that chronic use of them may result in resistant viral strains that will be even stronger and harder to treat later. This has happened with other disease-causing organisms over the fifty years that doctors have been prescribing antibiotics and antivirals. Routinely giving antibiotics or antivirals when they are not indicated and failing to look at other ways to support the immune system's own ability to fight germs has resulted in our current battle against "superbug" strains of tuberculosis, pneumonia, and staphylococcus. For that reason, I prefer an approach that bolsters a woman's inherent ability to keep the virus under control.

Nutritional and herbal treatments. Garlic is a highly effective remedy for herpes recurrence, and it has no known side effects. It also works for cold sores. Garlic has been shown to have a number of antiviral, antibacterial, and antifungal properties.[30] For women with recurrent herpes, I recommend the following: When the familiar tingling sensation starts, signaling that an outbreak is about to occur, take twelve capsules of deodorized garlic (available in health food stores) immediately.[31] Then take three capsules every four hours while you are awake, for the next three days. In almost every case, the herpes outbreak will be prevented. Take the deodorized variety of garlic, to prevent the bad breath that is the only downside to garlic's use. I generally recommend brands that contain allicin (such as Garlitrin 4000 and Kyolic, both widely available from most health food stores).

For women with a history of herpes who are planning a pregnancy or who are already pregnant, I recommend they take two garlic capsules every day. This can be increased to six to eight capsules per day if they are under more stress than usual. In my clinical experience, women who do this don't get herpes outbreaks.

Melissa extract (*Melissa officinalis*), also known as lemon balm, has been scientifically shown to have antiviral activity against herpes infections. It can prevent ulcers and speed healing if used at the onset of symptoms.[32] A cream form of this extract can be purchased at natural food stores under the brand name Herpalieve. It should be applied to the affected area two to four times daily for five to ten days.

Melaleuca oil, from the Australian tea tree, can be applied directly to the tingling area just prior to a herpes outbreak, using either a Q-tip or your finger. In most cases, this topical treatment will prevent an outbreak.[33]

Some people take zinc or vitamin C with bioflavonoids, while others apply zinc sulfate ointment, vitamin E ointment, or lithium succinate ointment to prevent or treat herpes outbreaks. Still other people use the amino acid lysine to prevent outbreaks. I would recommend these only if garlic, melissa extract, and melaleuca fail to prevent an outbreak.

⁓ Vitamin C, zinc, and bioflavonoids: 220 mg of vitamin C with bioflavonoids, and 100 mg of zinc. Each of these is taken three times a day with meals, at the onset of discomfort.

~ Lithium, zinc, or vitamin E ointments: These are applied within forty-eight hours of the onset of a herpes sore and are continued four times a day until the sore disappears.[34]

~ Lysine: Some women have very good success in preventing herpes outbreaks by taking the amino acid lysine as a food supplement, 400 mg three times per day. At the same time, the amino acid arginine is restricted in the diet, to maximize the lysine/arginine ratio. This suppresses symptoms and decreases the rate of recurrence. In addition to supplements, good foods for increasing dietary lysine are potatoes, brewer's yeast, fish, beans, and eggs. Foods high in arginine, which should be avoided, are chocolate, peanuts, and other nuts. If lysine therapy is used, cholesterol levels should be followed, as this therapy may stimulate the liver to manufacture cholesterol.[35]

~ Change your perception: Neither herpes nor genital warts need be a big deal. In the vast majority of cases your immune system will take care of them and they won't cause you or anyone else any harm. It's the perception that you are somehow bad or tainted if you get them that's the problem. You can "cure" this through affirming your genitals and your sexuality as something good. (See "I love my genitals" on page 285.) Here's an example from one of my newsletter subscribers who took my advice and subsequently healed her herpes—in both mind and body—simultaneously. Here's her story.

Dear. Dr. Northrup,
I went through a divorce five years ago after a monogamous marriage that lasted twenty-three years. It took me about four years to even have a date. I finally found a guy I really liked. We both got ourselves tested for AIDS before having sex. And neither of us had a history of anything else. So we had sex. It felt so good to be making love again with someone I like and trust. But four days later, I came down with herpes. At first I was horrified. I felt like such a fool. How could I have let this happen? My lover also felt so badly that he had "made me sick." But then I read your book and realized that my attitude and shame weren't helping my immunity a bit. So I took your advice. I started to eat better and take a good multivitamin every day. I also started to affirm the goodness of my own sexuality. I realized that I hadn't done anything wrong. I wasn't bad or tainted— and neither was my lover. The herpes sores healed in about ten days. And now my lovemaking is more pleasurable than ever. I found a guy who really cares, is a wonderful lover, and who affirms my beauty and desirability every day. Believe me, herpes was a small

price to pay. I'm certain that it will never recur now that I feel better about my genitals and my sexuality than ever before!

I applaud my reader for her courageous turnaround of a situation that is devastating to many women. And it is my fervent hope that she really never does get a recurrence!

CERVICITIS

True cervicitis is an inflammation of the cervix caused by the same infectious agents that cause vaginitis, such as trichomonas or yeast. Cervicitis and vaginitis are usually present at the same time, and treatment for them is the same. (See section on vaginitis, page 308.)

In some women, the mucus-secreting cells of the endocervix sometimes extend out onto the outer cervix (the exocervix). This is a normal anatomical variation and is not true cervicitis. Though these women sometimes experience a bit more vaginal discharge than usual, this only rarely requires treatment. In cases in which the discharge is truly a problem, cryocautery (freezing) of the cervix or LEEP cautery can be done. (See page 283.)

CERVICAL DYSPLASIA (ABNORMAL PAP SMEARS)

Cervical dysplasia is the name given to cellular abnormalities that arise in the endocervical canal or on the cervix itself: *dysplastic* simply means "abnormal." A Pap smear shows when the cells of the cervix are abnormal, and the cells are classified according to nationally agreed-upon standards. The terminology used for these abnormalities is *cervical intraepithelial neoplasia* (CIN), which means abnormal cells in the epithelial layer of cells covering the cervix, or *squamous intraepithelial lesions* (SIL), which means abnormal cells in the squamous layer covering the cervix, vagina, or vulva (SIL has replaced the term CIN in some medical centers). The pathologist who reads the Pap smear ranks these cells numerically, according to the degree of the cellular change. Thus CIN 1 or SIL 1 is considered mild, while CIN 3 or 4 or SIL 3 or 4 is severe.

When a Pap smear comes back as abnormal, I know that a woman is likely to immediately jump to the worst-case scenario: *"Oh, no, I have cancer!"* Prompt investigation of the abnormal Pap smear generally results in her being reassured. Most abnormal Pap smears *do not* mean cervical cancer, though a certain percentage of dysplasias will go on to become cervical cancer if they are not diagnosed and treated. Some CIN abnormalities, particularly the mild ones, will go away by themselves. This is because the majority of mild dysplasias are actually HPV infections that are self-limiting. Self-limiting infections are those that the body's immune system takes care of on its own.

Cervical dysplasias can result when a woman is conflicted about wanting to be all things to all people, such as the woman who is a mother, works full-time, and is worried that she does neither of these jobs well enough. I call this the treadmill dysfunction. Feeling as though we're on a treadmill certainly doesn't enhance our immune system functioning. A poor diet, environmental pollution, low self-esteem, and a bit of religious shame can also set the scene for cervical dysplasias.

Scientific studies have shown that there are emotional differences between women whose cervical dysplasia progresses and those whose dysplasia remains mild or goes away. Women whose dysplasia became more severe were those who were passive and pessimistic in stressful situations; they avoided and somatically acted out their anxiety. For instance, they tended to get physical symptoms, such as migraines, backache, and other disorders. Women whose dysplasia remained mild, on the other hand, were those who dealt with stress in a more optimistic and active fashion, effecting change in their lives by seeking creative solutions to their problems.[36]

Symptoms

Cervical dysplasias are not usually associated with symptoms, though some women who have had abnormal Pap smears have told me that they knew something was wrong because they felt a "burning" sensation in the cervical area. (Cervical cancer can be asymptomatic as well, but its symptoms usually include bleeding between periods, pelvic pain, foul discharge, and/or bleeding after intercourse.)

Pap Smear Screening

The Pap smear is the single most cost-effective disease screening test known to modern medicine. Ever since the Pap smear was introduced by George Papanicolaou, M.D., in the late 1940s, the incidence of invasive cervical cancer and the death rates from this disease have gone down dramatically. In fact, it is estimated that 70 percent of cervical cancer deaths are actually prevented because of this inexpensive and noninvasive test.

The results are so impressive that I've often joked about the need for a drive-through Pap test center that would make the test as easy to obtain as a McDonald's meal.[37]

A Pap smear is made by taking a sample of cells from the transformation zone in the squamocolumnar junction (SCJ) of the cervix, up inside the cervical opening. The cells are fixed onto a slide by spraying them or covering them with a cell-preserving chemical. A person trained in reading cellular abnormalities under a microscope then reads the sample.

The Pap smear is not perfect: cervical cancer has not yet been eradicated. About seven thousand women still die from this condition annually in the U.S.—and not all of them failed to get a regular Pap smear.

Abnormalities from the upper genital tract, the endometrium, the fallopian tubes, and occasionally the ovaries show up on Pap smears, but only rarely. The Pap smear screens for cervical abnormalities only. Many women don't understand this limitation in their health care practitioner's ability to diagnose problems.

The American College of Obstetricians and Gynecologists updated its Pap smear screening recommendations in 2003. Here are the recommendations:

~ *First Pap Smear:* About three years after first sexual intercourse or by age twenty-one, whichever comes first.

~ *Women Up to Age Thirty:* Annual Pap smears along with routine annual gynecological exams (for women eighteen and older or for sexually active teens younger than eighteen).

~ *Women Age Thirty and Older:* Three screening options:

  1. Women who have had three negative results on annual Pap smears can have subsequent Pap smears every two to three years (although an annual gynecological exam is still recommended).

  2. Annual Pap smears

  3. Pap smear with the addition of an HPV-DNA test. If both the Pap smear and the DNA test are negative, women can wait three years to have their next Pap smear (although annual gynecological exams are still recommended).

~ *Special Cases:*

  1. Women of any age who are immunocompromised, are infected with HIV, or were exposed in utero to DES should have annual Pap smears.

2. Most women who have not had abnormal cervical cell growth but who have had a hysterectomy with removal of the cervix for other reasons may discontinue routine Pap smears. However, even if they have had a hysterectomy, women who have had a history of abnormal cell growth (classified as CIN 2 or 3) should have annual Pap smears until they have three consecutive negative Paps; then they can discontinue routine Paps.

I'd recommend a yearly Pap smear if you have had any of the following:

- A history of multiple sexual partners or a male partner who has had multiple partners
- First intercourse at an early age
- A male sexual partner who has had a sexual partner with cervical cancer
- Infection with HIV (human immunodeficiency virus)
- Immunosuppression secondary to organ transplantation (e.g., kidney transplant)
- Smoking or regular use of alcohol, cocaine, or other similar substances
- A history of abnormal Pap smears, cervical cancer, or uterine, vaginal, or vulvar cancer
- Low socioeconomic status (the American College of Obstetricians and Gynecologists points out that this factor appears to be a surrogate for a number of closely related factors that often place these women at greater risk)

How reliable is the Pap smear? No test is 100 percent reliable, and the Pap smear is no different. Studies have shown that the false negative rate of the test runs from 5 to 50 percent, depending upon the practitioner and the lab used. Occasionally a Pap smear will come back negative even though abnormal cells are present. About two-thirds of these false negative smears are the result of errors made by the health care practitioner in the collecting of the cells (known as sampling errors). About one-third of false negatives are due to laboratory error. The laboratory error problem has now been addressed nationally through stricter government standards for quality assurance in labs that interpret Pap smears. There are also times when the abnormal cervical cells are located in areas of the cervix that simply can't be reached by a Pap smear. So even under ideal circumstances, when everything is done perfectly, some cervical cancers will not be picked up early with a routine Pap smear.

One way to ensure the best possible quality in your Pap smear result is to find out what kind of relationship your health care provider has with the laboratory where your Pap smears are sent. Ask your health care practitioner if she or he is able to personally call the pathologist overseeing the lab to go over abnormal or suspicious results that may require special attention. When the practitioner who takes your Pap smear and the pathologist who is responsible for signing off on Pap smear results can talk to each other about problem cases, the quality of your care will be improved. (See also the section on new technologies for testing cervical cells.)

What if your Pap smear isn't negative? Sometimes you'll get a Pap smear result that is scary or confusing. Here are the basic categories of Pap smear results and how to deal with them.

~ Sometimes a Pap smear will come back labeled "unsatisfactory for interpretation" or "limited." This is not a cause for alarm. It just means that there were not enough cells present on the slide to interpret the smear adequately or that the cells seen were normal but interpretation was limited due to the low number of cells. An "unsatisfactory" reading doesn't necessarily mean that your practitioner took a bad Pap smear or did it wrong. It just means that you need to get it repeated.

~ Another designation used on Pap smear reports is "limited interpretation secondary to inflammation." Sometimes a yeast, trichomonal, or bacterial infection will result in inflammation being present in the cells taken on a Pap smear. Inflammation is also sometimes associated with thinned cervical and vaginal tissue (called *atrophy*) that occurs after pregnancy, after menopause, or during other times of low estrogen. Inflamed cells on a Pap smear are almost never a cause for alarm. Just get your Pap smear repeated after getting the infection or atrophic tissue treated. In many cases, the inflammation simply clears up by itself without treatment, especially if you improve your diet and lifestyle when necessary.

~ A Pap smear category that is often very confusing for practitioners and patients alike is known as ASCUS (atypical squamous cells of undetermined significance), present in 10 percent of Pap smears. Most of the time when the Pap smear comes back with this designation, it means that the cells of the cervix are atypical-looking because of some kind of reaction—healing, inflammation, atrophy, and so on. In 75 percent of cases of ASCUS, no actual cervical disease is present. Current guidelines recommend a test known as a colposcopy. During a colposcopy, your cervix is looked at through a magnifying lens; areas of abnormality can be seen very clearly, biopsied for further investigation, and often removed immediately. I'd also recommend antioxidant supplements.

If you have inflammation present and your practitioner can find a cause, get it treated and then have your Pap repeated. ASCUS associated with atrophic changes in a postmenopausal woman will disappear with topical estrogen treatment or treatment that nourishes and replenishes vaginal mucosa. Remifemin, a standardized extract of black cohosh, has been shown to thicken vaginal tissues after four to six weeks, so this is a good choice for women who need to avoid estrogen. Estriol is another good choice. (See chapter 14.)

~ Sometimes ASCUS Pap smears are associated with what is called LGSIL (low-grade squamous intraepithelial lesion). When LGSIL is suspected you'll want to be sure to get close follow-up, with repeat Pap smears and HPV-DNA testing every four to six months until your results come back normal. Statistics have shown that up to 50 percent of these abnormalities go away on their own—which is very good news. In some cases, your health care practitioner may recommend (or you may prefer) further investigation of your cervix through a colposcopy.

~ Finally, if your Pap comes back as HGSIL (high-grade squamous intraepithelial lesion), your health care provider will schedule a colposcopy and directed biopsies of your cervix and possibly even a LEEP (loop electrosurgical excision procedure) to be absolutely certain about the extent of your abnormality. LEEP removes abnormal tissue from the cervix for diagnostic and treatment purposes while preserving normal cervical function. It can be done in the office and sometimes can be used instead of surgical cone biopsy, a treatment for precancerous changes in the cervix that must be done in the operating room under anesthesia. Either way, I'd recommend a diet high in folic acid and B complex (or supplements) to anyone whose cervical cells show any atypical changes that may or may not be precancerous.

Other Technologies for Testing Cervical Cells

In an unending quest for improved accuracy in picking up pathology—plus the belief that more information will save us—researchers developed technologies that give more information about cervical abnormalities than the Pap smear alone. Examples of this are PapNet screening, which uses a computerized reading of cervical cells to pick up abnormalities that a human screener my have missed; ThinPrep, which makes the Pap smear slide easier to read; and various systems to test for the presence of HPV virus. In the ThinPrep test, the cervical sample is immersed in a vial of liquid to keep the cells from drying out, then filtered to remove debris and placed on a slide. Studies performed by the manufacturer suggest that the ThinPrep test improves the detection of abnormal cells by 65 percent and reduces the number of less-than-adequate smears by 50 percent when compared with regular Pap smear techniques.[38] Having this information doesn't necessarily change the treatment. What these improved screening techniques have in common is that they increase the chance of finding abnormalities (some of which may not even be worth finding) and they also increase the expense of Pap smear by $20 to $40. These newer technologies have largely replaced the old Pap smear in many medical centers.

Colposcopy. Once a woman has an abnormal Pap smear, the next step is to further delineate the extent of the problem by a test known as colposcopy. In this test the cervix is observed through a magnifying lens, to check the blood vessels and tissue patterns. Biopsies are taken from the areas that appear abnormal, and these are sent to the lab. Special attention is paid to the SCJ, making sure that this entire region is seen. Sometimes the abnormal cervical cells extend up into the endocervix, where they cannot be seen or tested. In these cases, a cone biopsy (a biopsy of the internal cervix is the shape of a cone) or LEEP procedure (see page 283) is recommended to further test the tissue in the endocervix. This procedure is not only diagnostic but also often curative. Local anesthetic is available that can be sprayed on the cervix (or vagina) before the biopsies are taken, making this procedure virtually painless. Ask your doctor about it.

Common Concerns About Cervical Dysplasia

How did I get it? No one knows precisely why one woman develops cervical dysplasia and another doesn't. Like HPV, cervical dysplasia is related to the functioning of the immune system. In one study, women who were on immunosuppressive drugs for kidney transplants had a seven-times-greater chance of an abnormal Pap smear than did a control group of nonimmuno-suppressed patients. Smoking is a definite risk factor for cervical abnormalities leading to cervical cancer. Women with cervical abnormalities have been found to have lower levels of antioxidants and folic acid in their blood. There is a known link between birth control pills and certain kinds of cervical dysplasias.[39] This may be in part because the pill decreases blood levels of nutrients such as the B vitamins.

Can smoking affect my risk for cervical dysplasia? Many studies have documented the link between smoking and cervical dysplasia. Cotinine, a toxic by-product of tobacco, has been found in the cervical mucus of cigarette smokers. If you smoke, your mucosal immunity will be adversely affected in the cervical and vaginal areas.

Treatment

Women need to know that up to 50 percent of mild cervical abnormalities return to normal without treatment. A smaller percentage of the more severe abnormalities also regress. Follow-up Pap smears can help determine whether or not you need treatment.

When dysplasias don't regress on their own, the treatment goal is to eradicate all the abnormal tissue. Standard gynecological medicine has excellent tools to treat both cervical dysplasia and early cervical cancer. The cure rate by standard methods is over 90 percent. Everyone who has an abnormal Pap should follow the nutritional recommendations in chapter 17, "Nourishing Ourselves with Food."

Methods to destroy abnormal cervical tissue include laser, cryocautery, trichloroacetic acid, and LEEP. LEEP is used to diagnose and treat some cases of SIL that in the past required cone biopsy under anesthesia in the hospital. Some practitioners use laser in the same way. The cervix heals well after a LEEP procedure, but it does increase the risk for subsequent prematurity in pregnancy.

Regular follow-up with a Pap smear every three months for one year, and every six months thereafter, is necessary to be sure that the abnormality doesn't return. After several years of normal Pap smears at six-month intervals, many women can be tested yearly. This decision is made on an individual basis. As one of my colleagues says, "No one ever died from close follow-up." Women who have had moderate to severe cervical dysplasia are likely to get into trouble if the disease progresses, which is why more frequent screening seems appropriate.

Nutritional approach. Numerous studies have linked low levels of vitamins A and B complex with cervical dysplasia. Oral contraceptives can increase a woman's chances of having an abnormal Pap smear, though the data supporting this are not well known by gynecologists; the pill lowers B vitamin levels in the blood. In women whose diets are already low in nutrients, the pill can set up a slight deficiency state. High doses of folic acid have been used to reverse cervical dysplasias in women who developed them while on the pill. That's why every woman who is on the pill (or HRT) needs to take a good multivitamin rich in B complex and containing folic acid.

If you have a Pap in the LGSIL or another abnormal category, add 5 mg of folic acid to your diet every day with a good B complex vitamin and multivitamin-mineral. (The usual recommended intake of folic acid is 400 mcg per day, so this is a much higher dose.) Also add antioxidants to your diet. One of the best is from a group of plant substances known as proanthocyanidins, found in grape pips or pine bark. Popular brand names are Pycnogenol and Proflavanol. Initially, take 1 mg per pound of body weight, in two to three divided doses, daily for one week. Then decrease your dose to 20 mg two or three times per day. Anecdotally, I have seen many cases of mild to moderate cervical dysplasia greatly improved with a multivitamin-mineral supplement plus added antioxidants.[40] One more thing. If you smoke, stop!

Women's Stories

When a woman is willing to look at the stress points in her life, then combines this inner work with standard medical techniques, she is almost guaranteed a successful outcome. Three women's stories of their reactions to cervical and vulvar abnormalities and to cervical cancer, and their struggles to understand and deal with their emotional issues, follow.

Sylvia: a wake-up call. Sylvia was thirty-nine when she first came to see me. Two years earlier, she had been diagnosed with the beginning stages of cervical cancer and underwent a cone biopsy treatment. She had had normal Pap smears for two years, but a follow-up smear came back with the rating CIN 2. Following that diagnosis, as she was going out of the room, the nurse had remarked, "Too bad this is going to keep recurring every two years."

Sylvia later said that that remark finally galvanized her into action. She had always intended to get around to stopping cigarettes, alcohol, and caffeine, but this time she realized that it was a matter of life or death and that she had to clean up her act. She also said, "I realized, too, that it was time to stop hating my mother. I was a typical 'bad' girl until about a year ago. I then began doing healing visualizations and meditating. I realized through my healing work that I came from a family in which many generations of women have hated themselves. My sister-in-law died of lung cancer from smoking four packs per day, and at her funeral my mother was more abusive to me than I can ever remember. About two days after that, I was diagnosed with cervical cancer. I'm grateful, because I feel like I'm alive now and I hardly was before." Sylvia also told me that her sisters had all had hysterectomies and that one had had a breast removed for breast cancer. She said, "My mother has had her uterus removed, and she is a woman who is filled with self-loathing. Now suddenly I'm realizing that all of these women in my family just hate themselves and have done so for years."

Sylvia decided to break this pattern. To do so, she improved her diet, stopped smoking, and began to keep a journal in which she recorded any insights that arose about beliefs that no longer served her. She began to treat herself with more respect on every level. Her Pap smears have all remained normal since the abnormality was excised.

Faith: healing cervical and vulvar dyplasias. Faith, a woman in her early thirties, first came to see me in 1989. She was a nurse and was taking art classes. She had been diagnosed the year before with CIN 1 of the cervix, VIN 1 of the vulva (vulvar intraepithelial neoplasia), and VAIN 1 (vaginal intraepithelial neoplasia). All of these abnormalities were felt to be secondary to HPV infection and had been treated with laser a year before. Now the same abnormalities had returned. Faith's doctor had recommended laser treatment again, but she was reluctant to proceed. It had been quite painful, and there were no guarantees of success.

By the time Faith came to see me, she had already made some dietary improvements that she was enjoying. I explained to her the viral nature of the HPV infection and the subsequent cellular abnormalities, and I told her that she could improve her immune system by further improving her diet and by using the healing practices for a while. She understood the importance of careful follow-up.

Then I didn't hear from her again until three years later, when she came in for a consultation. She told me that within six months of her dietary changes and meditation practice, all her HPV abnormalities had gone away. Her doctor couldn't believe it. Her Pap smears had remained normal. But now she was contemplating entering a sexual relationship once again, and she was worried about the HPV. Would it flare up again? She had already done a great deal of inner work around her sexuality through reading and going to twelve-step groups, particularly Sex and Love Addicts Anonymous. She realized that she had had sex in the past when she didn't want it and had participated in it almost automatically, as a way to stave off her fears of abandonment. She had been brought up in a religion that made her feel guilty about her sexuality. Her brothers had been taught by her parents not to get anyone pregnant, while she had been taught that she wasn't supposed to be sexual at all—or at least, not until marriage. Having gone through a period of celibacy, she felt that she was once again ready to explore her sexuality with another person. At the time I saw her, she had developed a supportive and loving relationship with a man that did not yet include sex.

Faith and her potential lover had both had HIV tests that were negative. I suggested that he be checked for HPV and herpes, though both of us agreed that we wouldn't be sure this would help anything. I asked her to consider whether the relationship would be a source of nourishment and joy for her. When I last saw her, she was in the midst of deciding and didn't plan to proceed until she and her inner guidance were in complete agreement about her next steps.

Barbara: when surgery failed. Barbara was thirty-nine when I first saw her. Her story illustrates beautifully the connection between her past, her social situation, her body's "entry points," and her subsequent healing of them all.

The first time I saw Barbara, she was blond, petite, perfectly dressed, and had a smile on her face that looked permanently glued in place—a mask to cover what was going on underneath. Though she loved her work as a teacher, her body was giving her a lot of warning signals. Her mother had died at sixty-three of ovarian cancer. Her maternal grandmother had had the same disease. Over the previous nine years, she herself had had over fifteen different surgeries for early-stage cancer, first of the cervix and later of the vagina.

She said of her earlier history, "As time passed, subsequent doctors' reports continued to show precancerous cells. Biopsy after biopsy led to one surgery and then another. Laser treatments proved ineffective. Finally a total hysterectomy, with removal of the ovaries, was done nine years after the first signs of abnormal cells appeared. I was advised not to worry. There was still some normal tissue. I was grateful."

Barbara's hysterectomy was done when she was thirty-six, three years before she came to see me. At her first visit, we took a Pap smear of her vagina, which once again came back abnormal.[41] It was read a "mild dysplasia with koilocytotic changes" (this refers to specific changes in the nucleus of the cell, usually associated with an active HPV infection). She underwent a colposcopy and biopsies, which confirmed that she still had the abnormal cells in her vagina. Treatment consisted of removing the abnormal cells.

Because of the recurrent nature of Barbara's problem, we knew that there was nowhere for her to go but inward—to explore, if possible, why her body kept giving her the same message. We wanted to work with her to bolster her immune system and stop the process of disease that was resulting in more and more pieces of her vagina being surgically removed, frozen, or cauterized. All the treatments that she'd had so far—surgery, laser, cautery, and various medications—had failed to "cure" her problem.

As we took a deeper history, we found that Barbara's husband had been an alcoholic for the first fifteen years of their marriage. Much later, she found out that he had been having a series of affairs for years. As she put it, "He'd be holding my hand in the morning, and that of another woman in the afternoon. All the lies he told me were finally confirmed a few nights prior to when I asked him to leave, truths I had known in my heart. One affair after another, moments with prostitutes, encounters in large cities. He had previously denied this and more. The truth left me empty and alone." When she originally came to the center, Barbara had started to see a therapist and was in the process of piecing together her family history.

Barbara gradually began to put her life back together. She said, "I embarked on a journey that would eventually lead me to believe that I could make it on my own. Asking my husband to leave was the first well-thought-out decision I had made on my own. I was fully cognizant of the impact it would have on my life, and I had the courage to initiate and pursue a life outside of marriage. I missed the closeness and the union one feels in marriage. I missed the special person next to me and the knowledge that he would come home. He was my rock. He defined me. He owned me. He abused me. He left me. It hurt, and the pain has lightened, yet it will never fully go away." (This series of revelations on Barbara's part nicely illustrates the lifting of denial. As Anne Wilson Schaef once remarked, "It's hard to lose what you never had.")

Barbara kept a journal and told me that its pages revealed a frightened woman—a child, in many ways. She said that she feared tomorrow and that staying positive felt unnatural and uncomfortable to her. Aloneness and learning to live alone seemed insurmountable to her. Her one real joy was caring for her daughter, then eleven, and watching her grow.

Barbara started to do creative visualizations of her tissues as strong and healthy while also undergoing therapeutic touch treatments to help her move the "stuck" energy in her pelvis.[42] This modality helped her learn how to relax and become less stressed. She told me that up until that time, she had never thought about her sexuality, her breasts, or her vagina as free of disease, clear, healthy, and pink. "My body parts had always been dirty and not a part of me. They did not exist," she said.

She described her therapeutic touch sessions as follows: "Therapeutic touch began as I sat in the chair. I was asked to put my hands on my knees and to think about warm water and a clean healthy body. Trust this woman, I kept saying. Trust! For the first time—ever—my body felt free of anxiety. A true sense of peace prevailed, a high that was truly unexplainable. Empowered. They want me to become empowered. I should change my diet and continue to vision my life as it could be. Trust, I kept saying. This may work. This *will* work."

Barbara attended a conference with Dr. Bernie Siegel and Louise Hay and went through a guided imagery experience that focused on the highlights of her life. She said that during this experience, pictures and pain surfaced that caused a knot in her stomach that she thought would never go away. She also did some releasing rituals to try to let go of her past. One of these was to bury her wedding ring in a creek that flowed away from her home. She said the affirmation "I'm open to receive myself." She continued working with this theme repeatedly, returning to it over and over.

Despite all of this work, another Pap smear returned as abnormal six months after her first treatment. This time Barbara was treated with a chemotherapy cream called 5 FU for ten weeks. (This treatment is reserved for very resistant cases.) She decided at this point to work with her dreams and try to listen more deeply to her cells.

Around this time Barbara's father died, and another part of her past began to surface. A mentally ill woman had lived with Barbara's family ever since Barbara was born. Barbara noted that this woman, Kerry, had great power and controlled the entire family through manipulation. Barbara wondered if Kerry had been having a lesbian relationship with her mother all these years. Was that why Kerry had always come first in the eyes of Barbara's mother—first over her husband and children?

Barbara writes, "My dreams eventually revealed the horror that I had denied. Kerry had sexually abused me as a child. My anger at this was profound. She had violated me, and how I hated her for what she had done! She often told me that I was dirty. I can still feel her hands on my body. And then she would place me in the tub and tell me to wash all the dirt away. She made me scrub my vagina until it was raw. I felt ashamed and feared the loss of those who loved me.

"I'll never know where my parents were and why they did not protect me from the witch that had bound me for so many years. She can no longer hurt me. She is old now and suffering from the pain of her own cancer, a cancer that has bound her for many years now in a home. The family's codependency has been altered. My work with the twelve-step programs has confirmed my thoughts that we all must separate and become individuals and learn to live alone.

"I struggle to forgive her for taking my mother and father from me. She also took my freedom, my dignity, my sexuality. These attributes are returning, and I've begun to love myself. The shame has lessened and the guilt is dwindling. I have begun to recognize other Kerry figures in my life. I am drawn to them; I fear them; I now avoid them.

"In my search for peace and contentment, I continue to take three steps forward and two steps back in all phases of my being. I refuse to give up the fight. I have fulfilled my promise to see my daughter through college and to present her with a model that strives to validate her while validating others and their efforts."

Barbara is making peace with her losses—her loss of her mother and father, and her loss of her relationship with a brother who is alcoholic. She says that she is grieving the "loss of the dream that someone special will come into my life and rescue me from my aloneness." She is angry that it has taken her so long to realize that no one can save anyone, she says.

"Now I know that no one can get under my skin and do for me what I must do for myself. I have let my daughter go. I have released her from being my social support and comfort. The aloneness is a new reality that I no longer deny. I will look to embrace special times with others and special times with myself. For I now see myself as a person who does not have to change. I like me. I like the warm, loving woman who peeks her head out occasionally. I will work on showing her off more. I have some wonderful qualities that can be offered to the universe. I'll be there if you'll be there."

Barbara's body is now healthy. Her six-month checkups and Pap smears all returned to normal. She has become a vibrant, beautiful woman whose entire being radiates health. When she smiles, her smile comes right from her center. Her mask is gone. She is a healed woman.

The entry points of our bodies have been defiled and denied as part of us for too long. Though we often have much pain stored there, we can commit to listening to these forgotten parts of our bodies and reclaim them as sacred and worthy—as worthy as our minds, our hearts, and our dreams.

CERVICAL CANCER

I've seen several women who had the beginning stages of cancer on their Pap smears—microinvasive cervical cancer, confirmed by cone biopsy—who have refused hysterectomy, the recommended treatment. In those women who desire children, this choice is increasingly being supported—along with close follow-up. Depending on the situation, the prognosis can be very good.

Women's Stories

Constance: microinvasive cervical cancer. "Cancer I can cope with; it is men that perplex me," says Constance, who was diagnosed with cervical cancer. "I interpreted my cervical cancer as a signal to reassess my life. Although I meditated daily, did some exercise, and was generally aware about nutrition, I found my emotional life was out of control. In short, 'my woman,' a part of me that's very deep inside, was enraged at sexual rejection by my partner. He did not send me a clear message, he didn't just say, 'Let's be friends instead of lovers,' but instead gave me a mixed bag of approach and avoidance.

"Our relationship was of several years' standing. We had chosen to have a child together after my firstborn was in a fatal auto accident at age four. We had a daughter, but our relationship was not what I wanted or needed. My disappointment and rage ran deep and manifested themselves in the cells of my cervix.

"When I heard the results of my Pap smear and colposcopy, I stopped to reassess while I waited for my cone biopsy surgery to tell me how deeply the cancer had invaded and whether more surgery or other treatment would be necessary. I realized that the essence of my problem was a pattern of victimization by men, manifested in my body.

"In my immediate situation, the sexual rejection of me by my child's father, alternating with sweet nurturing and occasional lovemaking a few times per year, left me angry. This behavior paralleled how most men in my life had alternated nurturing with mistreatment. My past shows a pattern of classic codependency. My father had suddenly died when I was in first grade. He had been a warm, jovial man who loved children in general and me in particular. My brother, seven years my senior, had alternately accepted and rejected me as a sister. My mother's boyfriend and ersatz father figure had sexually abused me as a teenager, and my mother refused to believe me when I told her about it. My first husband, in spite of two degrees from Harvard University, physically and emotionally abused me and gambled compulsively. My second husband was an active alcoholic and was emotionally and verbally abusive.

"In the month between my abnormal Pap smear and the cone biopsy surgery, I became proactive regarding my health. I reached out to women friends and invited them to participate in my visualization of health. I scheduled extra visits with my spiritual teacher. I let go of my rage and desire to be intimate with my daughter's father. I repeatedly fed my unconscious and my soul with this little song/mantra:

> I am free, free, free to be me.
> My anger's gone.
> Forgiveness is on
> I don't want——.
> I don't need him either.
> I am free, free, free to be me.
> My woman's healed
> By a fine blue light.

"This song/mantra came to me spontaneously as I went deeply into my healing process. My goal was to stop wallowing in my martyrdom and my anger. This goal was only intellectual at first. I chanted and sang my song to get the information into my cells. A mantra is very portable. I had read about other people healing on a 'soul' level, and I realized that I had to do this, too. This would involve releasing my pain and letting in forgiveness.

"My song/mantra symbolized forgiveness for me. The biggest piece of my healing was forgiveness 'from the gut,' not just intellectually. This process was a slow wearing-away and letting-go that took several months.

"Once the cone surgery was completed, my surgeon said she personally called the pathologist to discuss my biopsy because the results showed such marginal abnormality—or at least, less than expected. Her interpretation was that I had sought medical intervention earlier than is the rule. My interpretation is that because I had let go of my rage, my woman had begun to heal.

"Choosing to be proactive regarding my cancer meant choosing to follow the path of rediscovering my authentic self, which I had started to lose after the death of my father. Instead of a knee-jerk 'yes' to others' requests, I am learning to say no and to say, 'I need some time to think things over. I'll get back to you.' Now I'm much more respectful and considerate of myself. I am cultivating a love relationship with my inner self."

Constance's Pap smears and exams have remained normal for more than five years.

VAGINAL INFECTION (VAGINITIS)

Almost all women normally have some kind of vaginal discharge. A yellowish or whitish stain on a woman's underwear at the end of the day, particularly if she has been wearing panty hose or pants, is almost inevitable. Many women don't know this and often think that they have some kind of infection, but it is quite normal and does not require a visit to a gynecologist. Vaginal discharges of some kind can begin the year before a girl gets her first period. Her gradually increasing estrogen levels stimulate the estrogen-sensitive cells of the vagina and cervix, resulting in an increased production of cervical mucus and increasing the cell turnover rate in the vagina.

A normal vaginal discharge comprises vaginal and cervical cells mixed with cervical mucus. When one looks through the microscope at a smear on the slide, one sees mostly normal vaginal squamous cells. Normal cell turnover of the lining of the vagina can increase when a woman is under stress, so that she will have an increased amount of discharge. But this discharge, too, will comprise normal cells.

Vaginal discharges differ at different times in the menstrual cycle. Many women notice an increase during the days surrounding ovulation; some feel that they have "wet" themselves. Ovulatory flow, or fertile flow, sometimes resembles egg white. Some women have premenstrual spotting of brown old blood. This in itself is not an abnormality.

Just about every woman, however, is susceptible to a vaginal infection at some point in her life. Both the vagina and the vulva are often involved in this infection. Hence, when I use the term *vaginitis*, understand that the more inclusive term would be *vulvovaginitis*.

Common organisms that produce infection under the right circumstances are chlamydia, Gardnerella, trichomonas, and yeast. The key concept here is "the right circumstances." The vagina, which normally maintains an acidic pH, is colonized by many different types of organisms, all of which work together to form a healthy vaginal ecosystem and functioning immunity. Even yeast and Gardnerella can live in the vagina normally.[43] When a woman is healthy, these organisms do not cause problems. Only when something in this area becomes imbalanced are these organisms associated with infection.

Almost every type of organism that can cause a vaginal infection when conditions are out of balance can also be found in women who have no symptoms. For instance, some women have trichomonas protozoans, a well-known sexually transmitted cause of vaginitis, present in their vaginas for years with no symptoms whatsoever. Others are incapacitated by the itching and burning the protozoans can cause.

Symptoms and Common Causes

Most vaginal infections make their presence known by a burning or itching sensation, sometimes accompanied by a change or increase in vaginal discharge.

Anything that disrupts the pH balance or bacterial balance of the normal vagina can result in an infection. The time you're most likely to get a vaginal infection is during or right around your menstrual period, when your mucosal immunity is at its lowest point in the monthly cycle. The pioneering work of Dr. Charles Wira on mucosal immunity has shown that immunoglobulins A and M are affected by the levels of estrogen and progesterone. These hormonal levels decrease just before the onset of a period, making you more vulnerable to infection. The immune system thus mirrors the emotional permeability of this time in the cycle.[44] Some women experience a similar sensitivity to infection after menopause, when both hormone levels and mucus production drop, but this is not inevitable.

Repeated intercourse over a short period of time. Semen is buffered alkaline fluid, with a pH of about 9. One episode of intercourse with ejaculation can increase the pH of the vagina for eight hours. When vaginal pH is higher than normal for long periods of time, the bacterial balance can be lost. Those organisms that are normally present only in small numbers can begin to grow and cause infectionlike symptoms. If a woman makes love with ejaculation of semen into the vagina three times in a twenty-four-hour period, her vagina will not return to its normal pH for that entire twenty-four-hour period. For some women, this is a setup for infection, particularly women who are in long-distance relationships and whose sex lives are sporadic and limited to increased activity over a few days. To prevent problems, you can douche within a few hours of intercourse with Summer's Eve Medicated Douche, which contains potassium iodide and lowers vaginal pH. Or use a vinegar douche—one tablespoon per quart of warm water.

Chronic vulvar dampness. The vulva sweats more than any other place in the body, especially when a woman is emotionally stressed. Thus, wearing restrictive, nonabsorbent, synthetic clothing close to the skin in the vulvar area can be a setup for chafing and subsequent infection. This is especially true if a woman exercises in this type of clothing. Riding a bike or a horse or using a rowing machine in such clothing can also cause vulvar irritation.

Chemical irritants. Some women develop vulvar irritation through chemical irritants found in scented, softened, and colored toilet paper; bubble baths; and sanitary tampons and pads that contain deodorants. All women should avoid using pads and tampons that contain deodorants. These tampons can produce vaginal ulcers, and the pads can cause vulvar irritation. No tampon should ever be left in for more than eight to twelve hours at a time. Other irritants can include chemicals in swimming pools and hot tubs, scented douches, and vulvar deodorant.

Emotional stress. Some women respond to a perceived boundary violation with a vaginal infection. Many yeast infections also occur premenstrually, when a woman's stress is more apt to manifest in symptoms—and when the hormonal milieu is more susceptible as well. They often clear up spontaneously once the period starts.

Antibiotics. After the introduction of broad-spectrum antibiotics in the 1940s and 1950s, the incidence of yeast vaginitis increased dramatically. Many women can date the onset of their vaginitis to their teen years, when they took antibiotics such as tetracycline to treat acne. Unfortunately, every time we take an antibiotic, we disrupt the natural balance of organisms in the vagina and bowel, and a yeast infection, either full-blown or chronic, can result. In the last decade, while the percentage of women over the age of eighteen has increased by only 13 percent, the number of antifungal prescriptions for women has increased by 53 percent.[45]

Birth control pills. Some women notice more yeast infections on the pill, which may be related to the type of progestin in the pill. Try switching pills or stopping the pill for three months and see if the yeast infections clear.

Diet. Many books have now been written on the connection between repeated courses of antibiotics, a refined-food diet, and excessive yeast growth in the vagina and bowel. Eating a lot of food made with refined sugar and flour can favor the overgrowth of vaginal yeast. Dairy products can also contribute to yeast vaginitis in some women because of their high lactose (milk sugar) content, which favors the overgrowth of yeast in the bowel and vagina. One of my patients developed recurrent yeast infections when she drank an instant-breakfast-type milk drink every morning. The high sugar content of this so-called healthy meal substitute threw off her body's ability to fight excess yeast growth.

Many conventionally trained physicians don't look at repeated courses of antibiotics and poor diet as factors in chronic vaginitis. Many women have seen ten or more doctors for their vaginitis and have had every conventional culture and biopsy done without uncovering a definitive cause. Once these women begin to support their bodies' natural healing abilities through emotional work, dietary improvement, and supplements, their vaginitis problems have often gone away.

Diagnosis

The vast majority of common vaginal infections can be diagnosed by looking at a sample of the vaginal secretion under a microscope and testing it for pH. Some infections, like chlamydia and herpes, require that a culture be sent to a laboratory for further testing.

Women with chronic vaginitis are suspected to have a condition known as intestinal dysbiosis, or an imbalance of bacteria in the bowel that is often accompanied by an overgrowth of yeast. Women with this condition often reintroduce yeast into their vaginas, even after repeated treatment. This is because yeast in the bowel reinfects the nearby vagina.[46] When intestinal dysbiosis is suspected, a special stool culture can be sent to a laboratory that specializes in proper diagnosis of intestinal dysbiosis.[47] Alternatively, simply changing your diet and adding probiotics and digestive enzymes is all that is usually necessary. (See Nutrition, next page.)

Treatment

Over-the-counter preparations. Many women can treat an occasional episode of vaginal burning or itching with one of the over-the-counter preparations that is now widely available, e.g., Monistat and Gyne-lotrimin. If you've tried an over-the-counter preparation for a week or so with no improvement of your symptoms, see a health care practitioner to be certain that you're not missing something. Once a diagnosis of a vaginal infection is made, the practitioner can prescribe the proper treatment.

Resistant cases of bacterial vaginitis can be treated with vaginal antibiotic creams available by prescription: Cleocin (clindamycin) vaginal cream or MetroGel (metronidazole) vaginal cream.

A trichomonas infection can be treated with Flagyl (the oral antibiotic metronidazole), available by prescription. The side effects from this treatment are nausea and an adverse reaction to alcohol drunk during the treatment period. If a woman has trichomonas and has a sexual partner, both partners must be treated. Otherwise, they may reinfect each other. A male has no symptoms but carries the trichomonas in his genital tract.

Evidence also suggests that some women have chronic yeast infection even after treatment because they are continually reinfected by their sexual partners.[48] In these cases, treatment of the partner is helpful.

Preventing recurrence. Avoiding the chemical irritants involved in vulvovaginal infections can be very helpful for susceptible women. Women with a history of repeated infections may choose to avoid using tampons for six months. Avoid panty hose when possible, or cut out the crotch. Oral sex has also been associated with an increased risk for yeast infection, as has consuming yeasted bread.

Douching. I don't recommend douching except for specific symptoms that you are treating or after repeated intercourse to prevent infection. Especially with commercial preparations, douching simply disrupts the normal bacterial flora of the vagina and may actually increase the risk of infection. It is not necessary to "clean" the vagina.

Nutrition. For women with recurrent yeast infections, I recommend a whole-food diet, in which all sugar and refined carbohydrates are eliminated, including all cookies, cakes, juices, soft drinks, and the like. I also suggest avoiding all antibiotics.

To eliminate yeast in the intestinal tract and rebalance intestinal flora, which will help avoid reintroducing yeast into the vagina, you can use a variety of supplements, such as acidophilus and bifida factor, both intestinal biocultures. One of the best is known by the brand name PB8; unlike other formulations, it doesn't require refrigeration. It is available in health food stores.

I recommend two other brands of probiotics—Gastro Flora and ProFlora—as well as Caren Full-Spectrum Plant Enzymes. Many other good brands are also available. Finally, decrease stress as a way to enhance your immune system functioning.

Psychological and Emotional Aspects

Some women with chronic vaginal infections fail to respond to any treatment. Some, too, are not open to trying any but the most conventional treatments, convinced that "there's a reason for this that you doctors are simply not finding—so do more tests." These situations present a very difficult dilemma for both the patient and the health care practitioner.

For a true cure of the problem, the emotional aspects of chronic vaginitis and vulvovaginitis must be looked at and worked through.[49] This is not to say that the problem is just in those women's heads. What might have begun in the head becomes physical. Studies have shown that many women with these infections have antibodies that work against their own immune and reproductive cells.[50] Dr. Mona Lisa Schulz once did a reading on one of my patients who had a chronic vaginal condition. The intuitive said, "She's got Doberman pinschers in there. You go near there, and you'll lose a limb." As it turned out, this woman had experienced incest as a child. She came to see that one of the decisions she had made in her early teens was that no one was ever going to get near her vagina again. Because she had not made this decision with her intellect, on a conscious level, it was manifested through her body.

Chronic vaginitis is a socially acceptable way for a woman to say no to sex. For some women, saying "No, I'm not interested in having sex with you tonight or the rest of the week" is not acceptable, given the mate they have chosen and the home in which they grew up. If they believe that sex is one of their duties, regardless of whether they derive pleasure from it, no matter how unconscious this belief may be, chronic vaginitis may well represent an out for them. But the immune system is never fooled.

Another common problem associated with chronic vaginal and vulvar infections is infidelity by the woman's partner. Even when a woman doesn't intellectually "know" that her husband is having an affair, her body may well be aware of it. I've seen several women in whom chronic vaginitis began at about the same time their mate started an affair. Of course, we might explain by saying that the husband was bringing something home to his wife in the form of germs, and that does happen. But in most of these women, I've been unable to find a physical cause for the vaginitis.

In a woman who has been in a monogamous relationship for years, a sudden onset of primary herpes, fever, general illness, genital sores, warts, or other obvious infections can be classic indicators of infidelity. For reasons already discussed, however, this is not always the case and is almost impossible to "prove." Women may also have vaginal problems exacerbated by guilt over affairs that *they* are having.

It's not uncommon for a spouse to lie if he is confronted about having an affair. Several of my patients, especially premenstrually, have had dreams that their husbands were lying to them. After years of questioning their own sanity, they've found out that the dreams had been correct—they had in fact been lied to. And guess what? A woman's body knows it, often long before her intellect accepts the information.

Joyce: vaginitis as a message. Joyce was fifty-three when she first came to see me. For almost twenty years she had had chronic vaginal infections that always returned after treatment. When I met her, she was bitter and angry over her recent divorce. Her husband of many years, a wealthy and charming alcoholic, had left her for one of her own friends. She felt abandoned and cast aside, even though further questioning revealed that her relationship with her husband hadn't been satisfying for a long time. His drinking and workaholism had been constant problems, and her sex life had been complicated by painful intercourse and frequent infections for almost twenty years.

Joyce's physical exam on this first visit was basically normal, though her vaginal tissues were thin and tender. As long as she wasn't having intercourse, she didn't have any vaginal infections or other discomforts, and no treatment was necessary. Over the next several years, I saw Joyce for her annual exams. Each year she was a little less bitter about her ex-husband and was slowly able to see how much better she felt without him. She then remarried. When she moved in with her new husband, she had a dream in which their house was part hospital and part school. This dream was very meaningful for her because it symbolized this new marriage as one in which both healing and learning would take place. She felt cared for for the first time in her life. She realized that she had never experienced true intimacy before her marriage to this man.

Her sex life with her new husband was wonderful, she reported. In fact, she had never dreamed that it could be so good. She has never had another vaginal infection, and her vaginal tissues are normal and healthy in every way. She has come to see that for years her body, through chronic vaginitis, was sending her a message about her prior relationship, before her intellect "got it." It is entirely possible to heal chronic vaginitis once the stage is set for healing.

Katherine: the body's wisdom. Katherine came in for her annual visit complaining that she had had several recurrent vaginal infections in the previous two months. But by the time of her visit, these infections had started to go away by themselves and she was already virtually free of the symptoms. She had recently ended a relationship that she'd been in for only two months. She said, "When he said to me, 'I want to keep you all to myself and keep you away from the world,' I knew I had to get out of there." After leaving this man, Katherine thought she would feel better—but instead she found herself bingeing on food a great deal.

As we talked, I suggested she look back over her life since her last visit a year earlier. She said that she had gotten out of a ten-year relationship with a drug addict and was in a group working on incest issues. When I asked her if she'd listened to Pia Mellody's tape on love addiction, something I'd suggested the year before, she replied, "I don't even dare to." We both laughed, and I reminded her how much progress she had made. As we were discussing the fact that the body gives us signals long before the intellect is willing to hear them, she said, "You know, I developed endometriosis in the second month of my relationship with that drug addict, and I knew at that time that it was probably caused by the stress of the relationship. But I didn't let my intuition speak to me."

Looking back, she was able to appreciate her body's wisdom, both in her long-term relationship and in the one she had just ended. I suggested to her that her vaginal symptoms—now going away— might have been telling her something.

A NOTE ON SEXUALLY TRANSMITTED DISEASES

Our current media-driven atmosphere often leads women to believe that it's both desirable and expected to have sex on the first or second date with a person who is almost a complete stranger. Simultaneously, we're all more aware than ever about the risks for contracting sexually transmitted diseases (STDs) of all kinds, including AIDS—a risk that increases with the number of sexual contacts that we (or our partners) have. This double message—sex is expected of you, but make sure you don't catch anything or infect someone else—has resulted in virtual sexual paralysis for some women, and outright risky behavior in others who are fortified mostly with denial. I've seen the unpleasant consequences of behavior at both ends of the spectrum. I've sat with women who reacted to a diagnosis of herpes as though their lives were over. And I've seen many others who've ended up with pelvic inflammatory disease and subsequent infertility—the result of sexually transmitted infections that did their damage before treatment was started. There is a better approach. For a sexually active person, there is no guaranteed way to avoid exposure to sexually transmitted diseases. Despite this, exposure in itself does not make developing a sexually transmitted disease inevitable. Even in the case of AIDS, the overall chance of contracting HIV from one act of intercourse with an infected person is about one in a thousand.[51] And even with repeated exposure to HIV, some people have not become seropositive.[52] Immune function depends in part upon how safe and secure you feel in the world throughout your life in general, or during a particular time. A large individual variation in immune status is common. This information is certainly not meant to suggest that a woman should ever neglect safe sexual practices and condom use. Instead, I present it as evidence that there's a great deal of potential within the human body for resilience and health. A woman's biggest defense against sexually transmitted diseases is self-respect, self-esteem, love and acceptance of one's sexuality and genitals, a functional immune system (which goes hand in hand with intact and healthy vaginal mucosa), and commonsense measures, such as the use of condoms and being discriminating about sex partners.

You have only two choices when dealing with STDs:

1. Gear up your illusion of control, become paralyzed by fear, make a vow of celibacy, and don't touch anyone—including yourself—down there. Sterilize everything in sight. (This doesn't work—the world is crawling with germs, and so are we all.)

2. Keep your vaginal mucosa healthy through the power of your thoughts, diet, emotions, and sexual practices; take a good multivitamin-mineral supplement; practice safe sex as best you can until you've made a monogamous commitment; accept yourself for who you are and what your natural talents are; and expand your understanding of what sexuality is and how your views of it affect you. Finally, always follow Dr. Frank Pittman's hard-and-fast rule of condom etiquette: "Bring it up before he gets it up."[53]

I believe that the only way we can get out of the STD dilemma is to learn to cherish our bodies and our sexuality. (See chapter 8 for information on how to do this.) We have to learn to be discriminating about what we put into them, and to think about and work with sexuality as a form of communication based on mutual respect and commitment, not as a way to hold on to a man or to fill an inner emptiness and be comforted. I understand that internalized oppression leads many women to carry unwanted pregnancies and put themselves at risk for sexually transmitted disease, but I also know that women must awaken from the effects of the oppression and learn how to control their fertility and sexuality on their own terms. The reality of AIDS and other STDs may help women change the age-old, gender-imbalanced relationship between sex and power and really take control of their own bodies and health. This is the first step toward true partnership in our sexual relationships. Try the following affirmation: "I now fully accept and respect my genitals. The more I send love and appreciation to this area of my body, the healthier my genitals become."

A Word About AIDS

I am not an authority on AIDS and I don't treat AIDS patients. I *am* often asked questions about it, and have sent many women for testing. Of the estimated 900,000 to 1 million people in the U.S. who are infected with HIV, about 25 to 33 percent of them don't know that they are infected, thus jeopardizing their own care and putting others at risk. Though the number of new cases of AIDS has been stable (at approximately 40,000) for the past several years, the incidence of HIV infection has increased in certain at-risk populations, including men who have sex with men, Blacks, Hispanics, and women—all of whom are disproportionately represented among people who are HIV positive, have AIDS, or both.[54]

Though it is a much more serious disease, AIDS is related to herpes and warts in that one of the modes of transmission is sexual contact. Because people can have HIV for years before it shows up as AIDS, there are potentially *no* safe sex partners until we have been monogamous with someone for at least eight to twelve months and both have negative HIV tests. (Even a negative HIV test is not a 100 percent guarantee, because you can have the virus when the test is taken but not yet have the antibody in the blood that is the basis for the HIV test.) The concept of the asymptomatic shedder that I mentioned in reference to herpes virus essentially applies, in my opinion, to almost *all* infectious diseases, especially the sexually transmitted ones.

I believe that the AIDS epidemic is a consequence of a large-scale breakdown in human immunity, resulting from such factors as chronic drug and alcohol abuse, relationships in which sex is the central focus, pollution of the environment, soil depletion, poor nutrition, and generations of sexual dysfunction and repression. AIDS has been called a metaphor for the breakdown of planetary immunity as a result of excessive dumping of toxins into the Earth's—and thus our own—lymphatic systems.[55] Long-term AIDS survivors and those who have reversed their HIV status to negative all have the same things in common. They have chosen to transform their lives and their immune systems through the healing power of nature and love.[56]

Fortunately, their numbers are increasing. Since antiretroviral therapies were introduced in 1996, there's been a marked reduction in the rates of illness and death due to HIV infection in the developed world. HIV is now considered a chronic disease, and life expectancy after diagnosis can be decades long. In a recent article on the subject in the *New England Journal of Medicine,* Scott Hammer, M.D., an HIV researcher, writes, "An otherwise healthy person with asymptomatic HIV infection and no coexisting illnesses, such as the woman described in the vignette (who was 25 years old and healthy and found to be HIV positive on an insurance physical), should be advised that decades of productive life, which can include intentional pregnancies if desired, are possible with proper care."[57]

I am also certain that the fact that HIV is no longer an automatic death sentence is immune system enhancing, in and of itself.

Back in 1992, at the annual meeting of the American Holistic Medical Association in Washington, D.C., a panel of long-term AIDS survivors and their doctor said that despite what the *New York Times* and the Centers for Disease Control led us to believe at that time, AIDS is not necessarily fatal. Dr. Laurence Bagley, an expert on natural therapies for AIDS, said that many people are HIV positive and are perfectly well—*until they find out.* When they're told that they are HIV positive and the disease is inevitably fatal, they almost immediately get sick.

In some cases the information itself, not the HIV virus, is what causes immune system depression. Obviously, the HIV virus does do damage, but its effects can be alleviated greatly through a program that includes dietary change, supplements, social support, and spiritual attunement.[58] In fact, a double-blind placebo-controlled study from the *New England Journal of Medicine* in 2004 showed that taking multivitamins delayed the progression of HIV significantly![59]

This past year I met a university professor who has been HIV positive since she was originally infected back in college in the 1980s. Though she has had occasional bouts when she's been really sick, for the most part, she remains healthy and functional. She told me that she finds hope and solace in the Buddhist approach of nonviolence and endeavoring to live in peaceful coexistence with the HIV virus instead of seeing it as "the enemy." It's certainly working.

CHRONIC VULVAR PAIN (VULVODYNIA)

Women with chronic vulvar pain and burning—known as burning vulva syndrome—have a condition known as vulvodynia or vulvar vestibulitis syndrome. Women with this condition experience searing pain at the opening of the vagina during intercourse and sometimes also have unrelenting pain and burning, stinging, or redness. There is acute tenderness to pressure in the ring of vestibular glands that are located just outside the vagina. This may preclude intercourse altogether. Because vulvodynia patients may have seen many doctors without finding a straightforward cause or cure, they often require a good deal of compassion. I've put together the best options I've found for this problem, but I must stress the importance of the mind/body connection for anyone who desires permanent relief from this condition. The same approach applies to those with interstitial cystitis. (See page 323.)

What Causes Vulvodynia?

Numerous studies have failed to isolate a cause for vulvar vestibulitis, but some believe that it could be triggered by vaginal yeast infections, gynecological surgery, or childbirth. It has also been associated with sexual abuse. Research has not been able to demonstrate that allergies, human papilloma virus, or bacterial overgrowth is the cause of vulvodynia. Under the microscope, the most frequent finding is a nonspecific inflammation in the vestibular gland.[60] Inflammation is, of course, associated with virtually all disorders, so this isn't particularly helpful. Surgical procedures such as laser vulvectomy or vulvar vestibular gland removal often fail to eradicate the pain, though these procedures have helped some.[61] What is interesting is that scientists have found that the glands in this area have associated nerve structures containing the neurotransmitters serotonin and chromogranin. This explains why treatments that work for nervous system and mood disorders sometimes also work for vulvodynia.[62] Anything that affects neurotransmitter levels in our cells can affect our health. And a wide variety of modalities ranging from biofeedback to antidepressant medication have been shown to alter serotonin levels.

I advise my patients to start with nutritional and mind/body approaches to this problem first, and then resort to the other treatments listed here only if necessary.

Nutritional Aspects of Vulvodynia

Some research has indicated that vulvodynia may be associated in some way with calcium oxalate in the urine.[63] The calcium oxalate is thought to be highly irritating to the skin of the vulva in affected women. Not all research bears this finding out. But whether vulvar irritation is caused by high levels of urinary calcium oxalate or simply abnormally high sensitivity to normal levels of calcium oxalate, the fact remains that many women are helped by following a low-oxalate diet and taking calcium citrate daily. Some doctors claim a 70 percent success rate with this approach. Following a low-oxalate diet can take three to six months to work. Foods rich in oxalate include rhubarb, celery, chocolate, strawberries, and spinach. (See Resources for references on low-oxalate foods and low-oxalate recipes.)

Taking calcium citrate also lowers oxalate levels. Citracal is a widely available brand that contains 200 mg calcium and 750 mg citrate per tablet. Take this or another brand with similar amounts at the rate of two tablets one hour before meals three times per day. Sometimes this alone is all that a woman will need to help relieve her vulvar pain and resume a more normal lifestyle.

I recommend that women with vulvodynia clean up their diets and start on a good multivitamin-mineral supplement in the doses recommended by their health care practitioner or in the nutrition chapter.

Add proanthocyanidins (antioxidant substances found in grape pips or pine bark, available at health food stores) at an initial dose of 1 mg per pound of body weight, divided into two to four doses daily, for two weeks. Then decrease to a maintenance dose of 20 to 60 mg per day. A comprehensive regimen of vitamins, minerals, and antioxidants has been shown to improve immune system functioning and help support cellular healing and regeneration throughout the body. This is probably why this regimen sometimes works to help women with vulvodynia.[64] A diet that decreases inflammation is also important. (See nutrition chapter.)

Psychological Aspects of Vulvodynia

Like all other conditions, vulvodynia has physical, emotional, and mental aspects. Failure to address all of these aspects of a problem simultaneously may lead to temporary relief only, while your inner guidance tries to find another way to get your attention. Research on the emotional aspects of vestibulitis has compared vulvodynia patients with a control group of women with other vulvar problems. Compared to the control group, women with vulvodynia were shown to be more psychologically distressed, more likely to have sexual dysfunction, and more likely to have increased awareness of completely normal sensations throughout their bodies. But instead of knowing that these are normal, they are more likely to believe they are symptoms of serious illness. For example, they may sense that their abdomen bloats a great deal after meals and fear that this indicates some major disease process. Small pink spots and other normal discolorations on the skin are believed to be cancerous, or they may think that hearing their heart beating in their ears at night indicates a brain tumor.[65] This is known as somatization.

As already mentioned, vestibulitis patients are more likely to have had a history of sexual or physical abuse than women with other vulvar problems.[66] Since it is well documented that women who've experienced sexual or physical abuse or assault often have difficulty negotiating healthy sexual relationships, it is not surprising that the vulvar area of the body might be where a woman's inner wisdom is trying to get her attention for healing. One approach to changing the nervous system's messages in this area is through biofeedback. Vaginal biofeedback—that is, learning how to progressively relax and rehabilitate the pelvic floor muscles—has been shown to decrease the subjective experience of pain in 83 percent of the women in one study who practiced this technique for sixteen weeks. The majority of these women were also able to resume intercourse by the end of the treatment period.[67] Kegel exercises can work in the same way, so a woman can try this at home. Many physical therapists are trained in pelvic floor rehabilitation. Those who work with stress urinary incontinence may be able to help with this as well.

Other Treatments

Antidepressant medication. Tricyclic antidepressants such as amitriptyline and desipramine have been shown to help some women because of the ability of these drugs to block the reuptake of the neurotransmitters serotonin and norepinephrine, which can affect the function of the vestibular glands themselves or the pudendal nerve. Some clinicians refer to the use of antidepressants in these cases as "giving the nerves a rest." Antidepressants such as Prozac have not been as well studied for this indication.

Treatment starts with the lowest dose possible, increasing it if necessary if there are no side effects. With amitriptyline, for example, begin with 10 mg each night for one week, then increase to 20 mg each night for the second week, then 30 mg each night for the third week. You and your physician will need to individualize the dose, but most women will respond at 30 to 75 mg per day.

Dr. Benson Horowitz, an authority on vulvar pain syndrome who sees many more women with this problem than the average doctor, notes that it takes about three weeks for these drugs to work, during which time most patients won't feel their best. With time, however, and a positive attitude on the part of the health care provider, antidepressants can be part of an overall regimen that helps women with chronic vulvar pain. If a woman uses these drugs, she should not discontinue them abruptly.[68] Generally, a woman with vulvodynia will need to stay on them until she is pain free for six months. Then she can begin the process of decreasing the dose very slowly by 10 to 25 mg each week.

NAET. Though vulvodynia has not been shown to be associated with allergy, clearly it is related to some immune response. It may respond well to the Nambudripad Allergy Elimination Technique, discussed earlier. (See page 199 or go to NAET's website at www.naet.com.)

Interferon. Interferon is an antiviral substance that stimulates the natural killer cells of the immune system. It is often helpful in certain cases of vulvodynia even though we don't understand how it works. However, in women with chronic vulvar symptoms, it is evident that something is "off" with the immune response in the mucosal system. So it makes some sense that a substance that affects mucosal immunity, such as interferon, might help. Some researchers believe that interferon works only in those women with evidence of HPV infection; others don't make that distinction.

Interferon is injected into the vestibular glands three times a week for four to six weeks. Relief has been reported in 40 to 80 percent of the cases, depending upon patient selection. Since studies suggest that HPV is not the cause of the vulvar pain, the success of this treatment is an interesting paradox that can't be easily explained. Interferon doesn't work well in women with no evidence of HPV.[69]

Surgical treatment. Surgical excision of the vestibular glands is successful in some women, but not all. I would recommend it only as a last resort, because this procedure doesn't address the underlying imbalance and often doesn't work.

Given all of the scientific evidence and treatment choices, it is clear that the optimal treatment for vulvodynia must address physical, emotional, and psychological aspects simultaneously. A symptom as persistent as chronic vulvar pain requires a great deal of trust in your inner wisdom, and a lot of compassion and patience.

INTERSTITIAL CYSTITIS
(PAINFUL BLADDER SYNDROME)

Interstitial cystitis has more in common with vulvodynia than with urinary tract infection. (See page 325.) Unlike a UTI, the symptoms are not the result of infection. Both vulvodynia and interstitial cystitis are chronic pain syndromes.

Interstitial cystitis is a condition most common in women between the ages of forty and sixty. It is characterized by disabling urinary frequency and urgency, painful urination, needing to get up at night to urinate, and occasional blood in the urine. Pain above the pubic bone as well as pelvic, urethral, vaginal, and perineal pain are also common; this pain is partially relieved by emptying the bladder.

Examination of the urine may reveal some blood cells but no bacteria or white cells. It is often present in women who also experience vulvar pain. Though the cause is unknown, many feel that it is, in part, an autoimmune disorder. There is a significant crossover between the population of women who experience vulvodynia and those who experience interstitial cystitis.

Diagnosis is made on the basis of the patient's history and also by a procedure known as cystoscopy, in which a lighted viewing instrument is placed in the bladder under anesthesia. There are some characteristic findings, such as hemorrhage under the bladder lining and cracking of the mucosal lining; a biopsy reveals evidence of inflammation.[70]

Treatment

Behavioral therapy. Biofeedback and behavioral therapy—both of which have definite benefits, with no side effects—have been reported to help many women with this problem.[71] Behavioral therapy consists of learning deep relaxation, meditation, or other techniques that boost the immune system and calm the nervous system, thus allowing the body to heal itself. (See section on relaxation response, page 136, for treatment of PMS.)

Nutritional therapy. Stop bladder irritants such as coffee (even decaf), cigarettes, and alcohol. Castor oil packs help immune system functioning: lie down with a castor oil pack over your lower abdomen three times per week or more, while saying—and really feeling—the affirmations suggested in the section on urinary tract infections, below. The same antioxidant therapy that has worked for vulvodynia patients may also help those with chronic interstitial cystitis. (See section on vulvadynia.)

NAET. My acupuncturist, Fern Tsao, reports good results with NAET, which I would personally recommend to anyone who is open to this approach.

Bladder distension. This diagnostic procedure is often also used as an initial therapy and involves filling the bladder with water and allowing it to expand while the patient is under general anesthesia. Although it isn't certain exactly why this works, it's possible that it increases capacity and also interferes with pain signals.

Bladder instillation. This procedure is also called a bladder wash or bladder bath, and it involves filling the bladder with a solution that the patient must then hold for about ten to fifteen minutes before voiding. Generally, women receive treatments once a week or once every other week for six to eight weeks.

Elmiron (pentosan polysulfate sodium). This pill (the first to be developed for IC) is taken three times a day. In clinical trials, it improved symptoms in 30 percent of patients—although it might take as long as four to six months to notice improvement.[72]

RECURRENT URINARY TRACT INFECTIONS

Most women will experience a few UTIs over their lifetime. The "honeymoon cystitis" our mothers were told about speaks to one of the primary causes of UTIs—the milking action of sexual activity, which, under the right conditions, causes bacteria from the vaginal or anal area to get into the bladder and urethra. The symptoms include burning on urination, blood in the urine, and fever. If a UTI goes untreated, the infection can ascend into the kidneys, which can be dangerous. This is why a woman who feels she may have a UTI should have a urine culture taken, and an antibiotic prescribed if it is positive for bacteria. This will cure the problem in the vast majority of cases without further treatment.

Many women, however, experience recurrent bladder infections, which are treated with repeated courses of antibiotics. This is a different story, and requires a different approach. Chronic use of antibiotics to treat recurrent UTIs doesn't address the underlying imbalance in the body that is leading to the infections, and antibiotics can also kill off helpful vaginal flora, resulting in yeast infections, diarrhea, and—unfortunately—recurrent urinary tract infection.

Treatment

Nutritional aspects. Start taking a good probiotic. Many are on the market, and most require refrigeration to keep the bacteria alive. PB8 is a brand that doesn't require refrigeration; it is available at natural food stores. Another way to help restore your vaginal flora if you've had repeated UTIs and multiple courses of antibiotics is to dip a stiff tampon (for example, OB is a good brand) in plain, organic yogurt and put it in your vagina. Change "yogurt tampons" every three or four hours. This will replenish the vaginal flora and decrease the risk of repeated infections associated with the yeast problem. You can also douche with yogurt or put a probiotic capsule directly in your vagina each night for a few nights.

Coffee, even decaf, can also have markedly adverse effects on your urinary tract and act as a bladder irritant, so if you currently drink it, stop.

Many women with UTIs are also helped by using cranberries, which contain an ingredient that helps keep bacteria from adhering to the walls of the bladder, thus helping prevent infection.[73] Cranberry juice also acidifies the urine, making it harder for bacteria to grow. Long a popular home remedy, drinking cranberry juice has been confirmed by scientific studies to eliminate bladder infections in a majority of the women tested.[74] Sugar-sweetened cranberry juice partially nullifies the benefits, so use the unsweetened variety. You can buy unsweetened cranberry juice concentrate and use 16 ounces of reconstituted juice daily to treat an infection. (Add a small amount of the herb stevia if you want to avoid saccharin or aspartame. Stevia has been used for decades as a noncaloric sweetener in many countries and is widely available in powder or liquid form in health food stores.) Use 8 ounces per day for prevention. Or you can look for cranberry juice in pill form; Cranactin is a popular brand.

The herb uva ursi contains a substance known as arbutin, which is a natural antibiotic that relieves bladder infection.[75] You can take the powdered solid extract (20 percent arbutin) as capsules, two capsules three times per day. Or take the tincture, one dropperful in a cup of water three times per day. Continue this treatment until symptoms disappear. Both capsules and tincture are available in health food stores.

Vitamin C can be very helpful to prevent reinfection. Take 1,000 to 2,000 mg every day, and if your infections are associated with sexual activity, take 1,000 mg before and 1,000 mg after sex. Drink plenty of fluids as well, and make sure you get up to urinate within one hour of having sex. Women who do this do not get as many infections after sex as those who wait for an hour or longer, probably because drinking fluid and then urinating prevents bacteria from adhering to the tissues and starting an infection.

Hormones. Menopausal and perimenopausal women often have thinning of the outer urethra from lack of estrogen in that area of the body, which results in burning with urination. This can be mistaken for a UTI. The condition can be treated well by putting an estrogen-based cream in the upper part of the vagina, right along the urethral ridge. I recommend estriol 0.5 mg vaginal cream. The usual dose is 1 gram (one-quarter teaspoon) once daily for one week, then twice or three times per week or as needed thereafter. This will restore your vaginal tissue to its normal thickness and the burning will stop.[76] Other forms of vaginal estrogen also work well, including Estrace and Vagifem. The small amount needed to re-estrogenize the urethra does not raise levels in the blood significantly and is considered safe by most doctors.

Sexual activity. UTIs are often associated with frequent or traumatic sex (sex that involves injury to the vaginal and vulvar tissues). For example, in couples who travel separately or live apart during the week, frequent intercourse during a weekend visit can irritate vaginal and urethral tissue. Treatment for this involves making the necessary adjustments in your sex life to decrease trauma. This may mean using a lubricant if you suffer from vaginal dryness. It may also mean rethinking any aspects of the relationship that are less than satisfactory.

Repeated bouts of infection and/or burning on urination can also be related to a woman's contraceptive method. If your diaphragm is too large, it can irritate your urethra during intercourse, causing bacteria to enter the urethral opening and migrate up to the bladder area. Also, the use of condoms or contraceptive creams that contain nonoxynol-9, a spermicide, can cause urethral irritation and burning on urination. It will go away when you stop using the offending agent.

Other treatments. Don't introduce bacteria into your urethral area. After using the toilet, make sure you wipe yourself from front to back, not the other way around.

Castor oil packs applied to your lower abdomen two or three times a week can work wonders in preventing UTIs, because they appear to improve immune system functioning. Acupuncture can also be very helpful.

Psychological aspects. As I've already stated, there are some very specific stresses that affect the bladder and urinary system that are often related to unacknowledged anger at someone or blaming someone—often of the opposite sex. So as you're drinking your cranberry juice, taking your uva ursi, or lying down with your castor oil pack, try the following affirmation: "I flow easily with my life. I easily release and let go of old concepts and ideas. They flow out of me easily and joyously. I am at peace with my thoughts and emotions."

Women's Stories

Chrissa: recurrent UTIs. Chrissa was thirty-two when she first came to see me for an annual exam. She was in relatively good health but had menstrual cramps, intermittent bouts of pelvic pain, and also recurrent UTIs, for which she'd been on repeated courses of antibiotics. She told me that every time she went on a short trip or vacation she worried that she might get a UTI and be unable to get an antibiotic prescription filled. She was also tired of the yeast infections she developed when taking antibiotics.

When I asked Chrissa what was going on in her life, she told me that her husband had a job that kept him on the road for about two weeks out of every four. His irregular schedule made her life difficult to plan. She was interested in starting a family, but he was ambivalent. When I asked about her sex life, she said, "It's full speed ahead when he's home, and I use a diaphragm and vaginal gel alternating with condoms." I asked if she tended to get a UTI after sex with her husband. She thought about it and realized that if she was going to get one, it was usually a day or two following sex.

I checked her diaphragm to make sure that it fit her properly and it did. I knew that Chrissa needed a strategy to prevent UTIs, so I suggested that she follow the nutritional and supplement program I've already outlined:

~ Decrease the refined sugar and flour products in her diet and switch to a whole-food approach.

~ Drink cranberry juice regularly.

~ Start taking a good multivitamin-mineral supplement.

~ Take 1 to 2 grams (1,000–2,000 mg) of vitamin C as soon after intercourse as possible. Take the same dose the next day.

~ Take a good probiotic the day before, the day of, and the day after intercourse.

I also asked her to observe her emotional "triggers." Specifically, was she angry with her husband about any unspoken matters between them—such as whether or not to get pregnant or who should be paying the bills?

Chrissa came back for a checkup three months later. She had had the beginning symptoms of a UTI only once, and they had gone away very quickly with the cranberry juice and vitamin C. She told me, "I realized that the key factor in whether or not my body actually got a UTI was my emotions. As soon as I found myself feeling 'pissy' toward my husband, I forced myself to talk over my concerns with him so that my body wouldn't have to do the talking for me. I also made sure that I never had sex with him when I was feeling angry. I realized that was a setup for an infection. I'm thrilled that I finally know that my body is not betraying me with these infections. There's a lot I can do to prevent them, or at least nip them in the bud."

STRESS URINARY INCONTINENCE

Though many women find it difficult to talk about, even to their doctors, fully 30 to 50 percent of us will experience urinary incontinence (the involuntary loss of urine) from time to time. Ten percent of these women are under the age of forty. In most, it's just an occasional problem that occurs when coughing or sneezing or laughing really hard. But about one in six women between the ages of forty and sixty-five has a significant problem that interferes with her lifestyle. The problem is also common after age sixty-five.

There are a number of types of incontinence. Stress urinary incontinence (SUI) is the most common one, and the one I will be addressing here. SUI occurs whenever you increase your intra-abdominal pressure so much (by coughing, sneezing, or laughing) that your urethral sphincter, the muscle that holds the urethra closed, can't hold back the urine that's in the bladder.

Common Causes

Common reasons for weakness of the urethral sphincter are the following:

- Overall weakness of pelvic floor muscles
- Pregnancy (the SUI usually ends after delivery)
- Damage from childbirth (this is much less likely to happen when a woman is encouraged to birth in a relaxed, conscious, and fully supported manner)
- Genetic factors that result in connective tissue weakness (women with this problem will often have many female relatives with problems related to prolapse of pelvic organs)

~ Persistent, chronic cough, usually from smoking, which results in repeated chronic intra-abdominal pressure that overrides the strength of the urethral sphincter

~ Excessive abdominal fat, which increases intra-abdominal pressure

Treatment

Strengthening your pelvic floor. The first line of treatment for SUI is to strengthen your pelvic floor through Kegel exercises. Pelvic floor strengthening should be part of every woman's health care routine, not only for optimal sexual functioning but also if you have a tendency toward SUI. When your pelvic muscles are strong, they can better support the urethra so that it doesn't give out when you do anything that increases intra-abdominal pressure.

Unfortunately, the vast majority of women who are told to do Kegel exercises are not instructed in how to do them properly, and that's why so many women (and their doctors) don't think they work. When properly and consistently done, these exercises have been found to help up to 75 percent of women overcome their SUI problems.[77] Kegel exercises involve squeezing the pubococcygeous (PC) muscle (the same muscle you use to stop the stream of urine). I recommend the following set of Kegel exercises:

SLOW CLENCHES: Squeeze your PC muscle and hold it for a slow count of three. Relax for a count of five, then repeat. Over a few weeks, gradually work up to holding for a count of ten.

QUICK CONTRACTIONS/FLUTTERS: Squeeze your PC muscle quickly and release—one contraction per second. Work up to ten flutters.

Do five of these sets three to five times per day, with ten repetitions per set. After a week, add five reps to each exercise, for a total of fifteen reps per set. Add five the following week until you are doing twenty reps per set, all the time continuing sets of three to five per day. Results are noticeable in six to eight weeks—and those results include better sex. The exercises need to be performed regularly to keep up the beneficial effect. (See chapter 8.)

Kegel exercises will not work if you contract your abdominal, thigh, or buttocks muscles at the same time that you are squeezing the vaginal area. In fact, this only increases intra-abdominal pressure and aggravates the problem. To make sure you're doing the exercises correctly, put two fingers in your vagina, spread them apart slightly, and squeeze the vaginal muscles—you should feel the muscles tightening around your fingers. These are the only muscles that should be contracted. To make sure that you don't contract your abdominal muscles, put your other hand on your lower abdomen as a reminder to keep your belly soft and relaxed. Video- and audiotapes are available to help you learn Kegel exercises properly.

There are other ways to strengthen the pelvic floor muscles besides Kegels. One method, which is based on ancient Chinese techniques, involves inserting a weighted cone into your vagina and simply holding the cone in place for a few minutes twice a day. (See Resources.) You start with the heaviest cone that you can easily hold in for one minute, work up to five minutes, then gradually move on to the heavier cones, and finally shift to a maintenance program. Holding the cone in the vagina automatically uses and thus strengthens just the right muscles, so you don't have to think about whether or not you're doing your Kegel exercises properly. I have been recommending these cones for several years and have had excellent results with them. They work well if you have a stress urinary incontinence problem with no other factors present (such as infection, the effects of drugs such as diuretics, or caffeine consumption).

You can also purchase an effective Kegel exerciser called the Kegel-Master 2000 on the internet. (See www. www.kegeltoner.com.) This device provides fifteen adjustable resistance levels, so you can increase resistance as your muscles strengthen. I also recommend the Feminine Personal Trainer (FPT), which is a stainless steel vaginal weight that allows women to greatly strengthen their pelvic floor through resistance training in about 10 minutes. It comes with an excellent video and guide. (Available from As We Change; 800-203-5584 or 619-213-2200; www.aswechange.com.) To achieve optimal results in strengthening and healing your pelvic floor I strongly recommend working with a physical therapist fully trained in pelvic floor rehabilitation.

Though strengthening the pelvic floor won't cure every type of urinary incontinence, it is always worth a try before resorting to surgery or drugs. Developing a strong pelvic floor not only helps prevent or cure urinary stress incontinence, it also increases the blood supply to your pelvis, making you more resistant to diseases such as urinary tract infections. It also enhances the ability to reach orgasm and improves vaginal lubrication during sex. You can do these exercises anytime and anyplace if you're doing them properly, and not a soul will know. You have nothing to lose, and a lot to gain.

Nutritional aspects. Many women have stress incontinence only when their urine output is increased, especially from drinking coffee or tea. Even decaf coffee is a diuretic—and so is cold weather (I never drink a cup of coffee in the morning if I'm going skiing, otherwise I'll have to go back to the lodge after every other run). Many women also have increased urinary output on the first day of their period, because they're getting rid of all that premenstrual fluid. Under those conditions, urinary stress incontinence will always be worse because your bladder is always fuller. And coffee is also a bladder irritant. I've "cured" several cases of SUI just by telling the patient to stop drinking coffee! It is also helpful to lose excess body fat. (See chapter 17.)

Hormones. Some women begin to experience urinary stress incontinence after menopause for hormonal reasons and for the same reason that they sometimes experience UTIs—thinning of the estrogen-sensitive outer third of the urethra. (See section on hormones and UTIs.) If this describes your situation, all you need to do to restore the urethral tissue and regain urinary control is to use a small dab of estrogen cream daily for a week and then once or twice per week thereafter. I prescribe estriol 0.5 mg cream, as opposed to other types of estrogen cream such as Premarin, for this purpose because this type of estrogen works very well locally and has a very weak systemic effect. This means that you can safely use estriol vaginal cream to help restore your vaginal and urethral tissues even if you've had breast cancer or another estrogen-sensitive cancer. Estriol vaginal cream is available by prescription from any formulary pharmacy that carries natural hormones. (See Resources for how to locate a formulary pharmacy.) The usual dose is one gram (one-quarter teaspoon) once daily for one week, then two or three times a week as needed thereafter.

Pessaries and urinary control inserts. For mild stress incontinence, simply wearing a menstrual tampon is often helpful because they push on the vaginal wall, compressing the urethra. In one study, 86 percent of women with mild SUI stayed dry during exercise when using tampons, although only 29 percent of women with severe incontinence were helped. If you use tampons for this purpose, remember that they must be changed regularly to avoid toxic shock; don't leave the same tampon in all day long.

Pessaries, plastic or rubber devices that are inserted into the vagina to help women with uterine prolapse, can also be used successfully for those with SUI. Unfortunately, many doctors have never been trained in their use and therefore patients may not be offered this option.

Specially designed "incontinence pessaries" lift the bladder neck and restore the proper bladder angle so continence is restored while it is in place. They work very well for women who aren't candidates for surgery, who have an incontinence problem only intermittently, or who have failed to get help from surgery.[78] (See Resources for more information.)

A new prescription product called FemSoft Insert (by Rochester Medical Products) is a silicone tube inserted into the urethra and surrounded by a liquid-filled sleeve. The sleeve creates a seal at the neck of the bladder, preventing leakage. It must be replaced after urination. (For more information, contact Rochester Medical at 800-243–3315 or visit www.1800femsoft.com.)

Surgery. Surgical approaches to SUI are often very successful. Seek out a surgeon specially trained in urogynecology. Another excellent option for some women involves injections of Teflon or collagen into the urethra.

(For more information on incontinence, contact the National Association for Continence at 800-BLADDER or visit www.nafc.org.)

Regardless of where you currently stand in relationship to this area of your body, know that each of us has inherited the effects of generations of silence or misinformation surrounding the genital and urinary regions. The only way out of this legacy of shame is to talk about our needs, educate ourselves, and reclaim a healthy attitude toward our genitals. As we each begin to listen to and reclaim the wisdom of these areas, we will discover that, like all the other parts of our bodies, this part of our body will respond beautifully to our care, compassion, and respect.

10
Breasts

I am... struck with how often women *sense* in their bodies, especially in the breast and heart area, when they are giving, loving and responding to the needs of others.
— Jean Shinoda Bolen, *Crossing to Avalon*

The mammary fixation is the most infantile—and most American—of the sex fetishes.
— Molly Haskell, American film critic and writer, in *The Quotable Woman*

OUR CULTURAL INHERITANCE

In a culture in which women and men alike are brought up on Barbie dolls, Miss America pageants, and Playboy images, breasts are a very charged part of our anatomy, both physically and metaphorically. Dr. Norm Shealy once remarked, "Freud had it all wrong. I've never seen a woman with penis envy, but I sure have seen a lot of men with breast envy." On some level, many people when they were children didn't get nearly the ideal amount of contact with their mothers' breasts; too many of us have been nurtured not by maternal breasts but by cold, plastic nipples and chemical formula made by multinational corporations. No wonder our society is so hung up on the female breast! No wonder the stage gets set so early for distress in this area of the female body.

Our cultural ideal is of a woman with a matched set of erect eighteen-year-old breasts (that are at least a C cup, judging from media images of the last twenty years). Women who don't match this ideal—the vast majority—tend to feel that something is wrong with them. This perception, if accompanied by enough distress, might even contribute to breast symptoms...and certainly contributes to the desire for implants.

I wish that every woman could have an opportunity to know how truly diverse breast sizes and shapes are, could see how much they vary among women. They would then realize how skewed our perceptions normally are about our breasts. We'd have a chance to begin loving the breasts we have, instead of comparing them with an impossible ideal. (I was reviewing some teaching DVDs recently from the Sinclair Institute [see www.bettersex.com], which specializes in optimizing sexual function. What a pleasure to see so many attractive women with normal breasts!)

Undeniably, an occasional woman has a size discrepancy or other abnormality related to her breasts that is striking and a source of great psychological pain to her. Others have breasts that are so large, they cause back pain. Plastic surgery can correct such problems and can be a blessing. But most cosmetic breast surgery is undertaken because women feel they don't look as good as models in magazines or as good as their lovers want them to look, or because our breast-obsessed culture so favors large breasts. This size concern is medicalized in plastic surgery jargon, which writes the indication for breast augmentation as *chronic bilateral micromastia*. That simply means "two small breasts that have been there for a while."

Women often feel that their breasts exist for the pleasure and benefit of someone other than themselves. I've heard former colleagues of mine discourage women from breast-feeding because it would "ruin their breasts." Some husbands forbid their wives to breast-feed because of their jealousy of the baby! Clearly, the current trend toward breast implants is a symptom of a much deeper, culturally supported discontent. (I discuss implants later in this chapter.)

Breasts are the physical metaphor for giving and receiving. In ancient times they symbolized nature's abundance and nurturing qualities. That the breasts are symbols of nurturing was demonstrated well by the case of a woman whom I saw in the early 1980s. Jennifer, four years past menopause, had been referred to me with two very large cysts in her right breast that had manifested almost overnight. (They were five and seven centimeters in diameter.) When I asked her if anything was going on in her life in the area of nurturing others, she told me that her last child was leaving home for college and that a beloved cat, a pet for fifteen years, had recently died. Jennifer was grieving the loss both of her daughter and of her pet. The night before the cysts appeared, she dreamed that she was nursing her baby daughter—the same child who was now about to leave home. When I aspirated the fluid from the cysts, I found that they were filled with milk! Jennifer's body had manifested the fluid of maternal nurturing in response to the change in her own nurturing *role*. (Dixie Mills, M.D., a breast surgeon colleague, saw an increase in nipple discharge and bloody discharge after September 11, 2001, when the country was grieving.)

Our culture has skewed the nurturing metaphor in such a way that women too often will give themselves away to others, without nurturing themselves. Women give and give and give without regular replenishment until the well runs dry. If men and women generally went around without shirts, people would see that the major wound for women is the mastectomy scar. In contrast, the major scar for men would be the coronary artery bypass scar down the center of their chests—because many men need to learn how to reopen hearts that were shut down in childhood.

Mona Lisa Schulz, M.D., Ph.D., a medical intuitive and scientist, says that in women who have an "overdeveloped nurturance gland" she can often "see" in their left breast, near their heart, the energy of significant people they've taken care of in their lives. She says the reason for this is that these women have learned nurturance as the primary expression of love. Though there is nothing wrong with nurturance, nurturance at the expense of oneself can set the pattern for ill health. Dr. Schulz doesn't see this pattern in healthy women or men.

Much breast cancer is related to our need to appear to be self-contained and self-nurturing, which is impossible. Everyone needs the support of others to be fully healthy. Caroline Myss notes, "The major emotion behind breast lumps and breast cancer is hurt, sorrow, and unfinished emotional business generally related to nurturance." Breasts are located in the fourth-chakra energetic center, near the heart. Emotions such as regret and the classic "broken heart" are energetically stored in this center of the body. Guilt over not being able to forgive oneself or forgive others blocks the breasts' energy. (The other organs in the fourth chakra, e.g., lungs, are also susceptible to this energy pattern.)

An important 1995 study found that the risk of developing breast cancer increased by almost twelve times if a woman had suffered from bereavement, job loss, or divorce in the previous five years.[1] It is important to note that long-term emotional difficulties were not associated with breast cancer. Another researcher also showed that severe life stress (determined before the diagnosis of breast cancer was made) was associated with increased risk for the disease.[2] Similarly, severe losses occurring after the diagnosis of breast cancer have been shown to be associated with increased risk of later recurrence of the cancer.[3]

As far back as the 1800s, the medical literature has noted associations between breast cancer and loneliness, sorrow, and even rage and anger.[4] Women with breast cancer frequently have a tendency toward self-sacrifice, inhibited sexuality, an inability to discharge anger or hostility, a tendency to hide anger and hostility behind a facade of pleasantness, and an unresolved hostile conflict with their mothers. There is evidence that women with breast cancer who perceive themselves as having high-quality emotional support from a husband or other source have an enhanced immune response.[5] In one study, breast cancer patients were more likely than women without breast cancer to be committed to maintaining an external appearance of a nice or good person. They were also more likely to suppress or internalize their feelings, particularly anger.[6] In fact, one study found that the suppression of anger over many years is correlated with adverse changes in the immune system.[7] Given our society's tendency to suppress, ignore, or denigrate women and their anger, it is easy to see why so many women have breast problems. A nurse-practitioner once told me that several months before one of her friends died of breast cancer, her friend had the following insight: "I finally realized that I didn't have to die of cancer in order to rest." Studies have demonstrated that severe emotional losses such as divorce, death of a loved one, or loss of a job may set the stage for cancer, depending upon how a woman deals with the loss.

It is not the loss itself that causes the problem—it is the inability to express one's grief fully, release it, and respond to the situation in a healthy, adaptive fashion. In the 1995 study noted above, the researchers demonstrated that the coping styles of women influenced whether or not they got breast cancer. Compared to the control group, those with cancer were more apt to have a type of coping strategy characterized by engaging with the problem, confronting it, focusing on it, working on a plan for action, and lobbying for emotional support in this process. What the researchers noted is this: In most severely stressful life events (loss of a loved one, loss of a job, or serious family illness), the person has no control. Therefore, engaging in efforts to change or control the situation and recruiting others to support one in this strategy, as opposed to letting go, ultimately doesn't work and actually increases stress (and risk of cancer). Examples of this would be working tirelessly with organizations that seek to eradicate breast cancer rather than spending time and energy investigating what you need to do in your own life to grieve, let go, and heal. Severe loss is inescapable and part of the process of life for most of us. What helps is grieving fully, making meaning of the situation, and surrendering to something bigger than we are. This is a painful and difficult process that I call radical surrender.

Ryke Geerd Hamer, M.D., an internist and oncologist, has done extensive research on more than twenty thousand cancer patients and has demonstrated that in every case the development of cancer followed a severe emotional shock or loss within a year or two of the diagnosis. (Dr. Hamer understands the mind/body connection in cancer on a personal level as well. He was diagnosed with cancer following his son's death from a random act of violence.) Most important, his research shows that "the tissue starts to augment from the time of the onset of the actual conflict and will stop growing as soon as the conflict has been resolved." To read more about Dr. Hamer's research go to www.newmedicine.ca or read *The Cancer Report: The Latest Research in Psychoneuroimmunology (How Thousands Are Achieving Permanent Recoveries)* by John Voell and Cynthia Chatfield (Change Your World Press, 2005). (For more information, visit www.cancer-report.com.) This book is a compendium of the work of many experts in the holistic treatment of cancer. It is the most practical, helpful, and uplifting manual on the subject I've ever seen.

ANATOMY

The female breast is designed to provide optimal nourishment for babies and to provide sexual pleasure for the woman herself. The breasts are glandular organs that are very sensitive to hormonal changes in the body; they undergo cyclic changes in synchrony with the menstrual cycle. They are very intimately connected with the female genital system: nipple stimulation also stimulates the clitoris and increases prolactin and oxytocin secretion from the pituitary gland. These affect the uterus and can cause contractions. Breast tissue extends up into the armpit (axilla), in what is known as the tail of Spence. Lymph nodes that drain the breast tissue are also located in the armpits. After a woman has had a baby and her milk comes in, she may develop striking swellings under her arms from engorgement of the breast tissue in that area. Breasts come in all sizes and shapes, as do nipples. Most women have one breast that is slightly smaller than the other. Some women (and men) have a third nipple.

BREAST SELF-EXAMS

One of the sacred cows of women's health is the monthly breast self-examination (BSE). Women are told to do it as a way to "save their lives." The truth is that very few women actually perform monthly breast self-exams in the way they're taught. Nevertheless, it is women, not their doctors, who find the vast majority of breast abnormalities (not including those picked up on mammograms).

Women's reluctance (even female nurses and doctors who are supposed to know better) to do breast self-exams is rooted in two things:

1) Fear about what you're going to find

2) Innate inner guidance that knows that making a breast exam into a "search and destroy" mission is not only counterproductive, it may even be harmful

By the law of attraction, that which we focus on tends to expand. So who in their right mind would consciously approach their breasts every month thinking, "cancer"? In fact, studies have shown that that's exactly what happens! (See below.)

Transforming the Breast Self-Exam

The first thing I want all women to know about the breast self-exam (as currently taught) is that it doesn't change breast cancer mortality! But it does increase the likelihood of having a biopsy for benign disease. A 2002 study published in the *Journal of the National Cancer Institute* followed 260,000 women in Shanghai for five years. Half of the group was trained in BSE and had that training reinforced at work, while the other half had no BSE training and was not encouraged to practice BSE at all. At the end of the study, the women in the BSE group had found more benign breast lumps than the other group, although the breast cancer mortality rate was the same in both groups. The researchers concluded that "women who choose to practice BSE should be informed that its efficacy is unproven and that it may increase their chances of having a benign breast biopsy."[8]

There is a healthy alternative, however. You can get to know your breasts in a healthy, loving way that enhances your health on all levels. A good time to change how you think about and do your breast

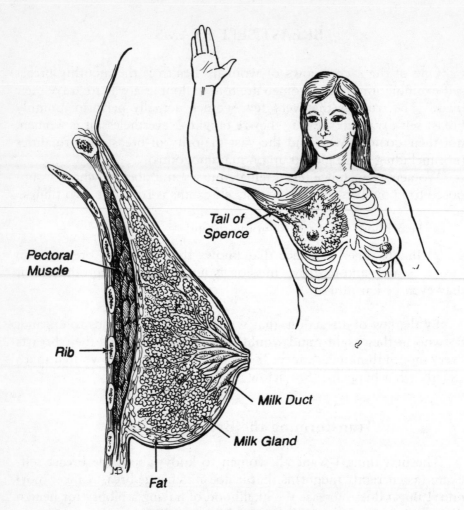

Tail of Spence

Pectoral Muscle

Rib

Milk Duct

Milk Gland

Fat

FIGURE 9: BREAST ANATOMY

exams is right after you've had a normal exam with your health care practitioner and you know that everything is currently normal. If you don't know what "normal" feels like, here's what to do. When having your breasts examined by your doctor, ask her (or him) to tell you exactly what she is feeling. Then repeat the exam yourself so you know what "normal" feels like in your breasts. From then on, whenever you touch your breasts, do so with loving kindness. Rub your hands together until they are warm. Then cover your breasts with them, visualizing your hands transferring love and care to your breasts. You may well feel a tingling in your breasts from increased circulation when you do this.

Approach your breasts with respect. If you are currently afraid of

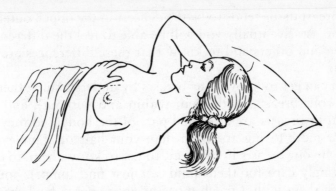

FIGURE 10: BREAST SELF-EXAM

your breasts and find them "too lumpy," start changing your attitude toward them by paying special attention to them during your daily bath or shower. When you wash this area of your body, pay attention to how the skin feels under your fingers. Imagine that you have healing power in your hands (which you actually do). As you wash your breasts and under your arms, do so in the spirit of blessing this area of your body. As you do so, you will be learning the basic contours and feel of your own breasts. Do this daily as part of your bathing until you have reclaimed some respect for your breasts as an important part of your anatomy. Your breast tissue will respond positively to your intent!

Once you are completely comfortable with this exercise, proceed with learning how your breast tissue feels when you use deeper pressure. You might approach this step in a spirit of curiosity, the same way you might examine your own hand or the sole of your foot. Your breasts are a vital part of your woman's wisdom, and you want to learn to listen to them. Lie on your back with one hand behind your head. This will flatten your breast tissue against your chest wall and make it easier for you to feel and appreciate your breast tissue as it lies on top of the underlying muscles and ribs. With your right hand, using the flat part of your fingers, not your fingertips, explore your left breast. Fingertips are so sensitive that they pick up the little ductules. You may find this frightening until you know what is normal for you, so use your fingertips to explore your breast tissue only after you have become completely comfortable with your breast anatomy and trust yourself. Repeat the exercise, using your left hand to explore your right breast. It is initially helpful to divide your breast into four quadrants and examine each one separately. Then move up to your armpit and back to your nipple so that you can feel the differences in the different breast areas. Breast tissue tends to be the densest in the upper, outer quadrants of the breast. Eventually you will be able to feel the difference between this area and others and to know that these differences are all normal for you.

You can get to know your breasts by understanding their anatomy, feeling your breasts (both from within and without), and looking at them. Your breasts are a normal part of the body and they deserve as much or more loving attention than your hair or complexion. If you approach your breasts in this way, to get to know them, to consciously and lovingly care for them (and *not* just find lumps), you'll be surrounding them with a much more positive energy field than the usual energy engendered by the breast self-exam, in which you examine to find what you don't want to find. Examining your breasts in a spirit of fear simply increases the fear and is the opposite of what you need to create healthy breast tissue. One of my former patients who had had a lumpectomy for breast cancer embodied this healthy way of examining her breasts. She felt her breasts regularly and knew their anatomy well. And every morning, before she got up, she said to them, "Girls, you're safe with me!"

I have another patient who said she liked to visualize the Divine Mother blessing her and her breasts when she touched them. She told me, "It always helps me feel better and dispels my fear."

MONTHLY SELF-NURTURING BREAST MASSAGE RITUAL

Here's a monthly self-care breast massage ritual in which you consciously create breast health. This massage assists the lymph system in removing toxins and impurities from your body tissue because the stroking accelerates the transportation of those impurities to the lymph nodes for processing. (Note: do not do this ritual if you have been recently diagnosed with breast cancer that hasn't been treated yet, because it may increase tumor spread.)

Before you begin, put on your favorite music (I like anything by Jim Brickman or Enya) and scent the bath with rose or lavender aromatherapy oil (rose helps dissipate anger, and lavender is very calming). If you don't like baths, use your favorite scented massage oil. Use a light touch, moving the skin instead of massaging the muscles. Enjoy the sensual nature of touch as you do this. The more pleasure you feel, the more healthful the exercise.

1. With the first three fingers of your right hand, find the hollow spot above your left collarbone. Lightly stretch this skin, stroking from your shoulders toward your neck. Repeat five to ten times.

2. With the fingers of your right hand held very flat, cover the hairy part of your left armpit and stretch the skin upward five to ten times.

3. Keeping the fingers of your right hand flat, lightly stroke or pet the skin from the breastbone to the armpit. Do this above the breast, over the breast, and below the breast, repeating each path five to ten times.

4. Finally, with the fingers of your right hand still held flat, lightly stroke your left side from your waist up to your armpit, repeating five to ten times.

Now change hands and massage the right side of your chest.

(A visualization and breast exam to music on CD and tape entitled *Honoring Our Breasts,* recorded by Dr. Dixie Mills, is available to help guide you through this process with attention to your own inner wisdom. To order, visit www.drdixiemills.com.)

BENIGN BREAST SYMPTOMS: BREAST PAIN, LUMPS, CYSTS, AND NIPPLE DISCHARGE

The most common reason women seek medical consultation for breast symptoms is breast lumps or cysts. Though most of them are benign, these must be closely monitored to make sure that they are not cancerous. (Nipple discharge is a less common symptom but can still be cause for concern.)

Approximately half of all women who go to doctors go because they have some kind of pain in their breasts. Cyclic mastalgia, or breast pain that comes and goes depending on the menstrual cycle, is usually caused by excess hormonal stimulation of the breast from hyperestrogenism, excessive caffeine intake, or even chronic stress. It is *not* a risk factor for breast cancer.

My colleague Dr. Mary Ellen Fenn once remarked, "Have you

noticed that men *never* complain about pain in their testicles, but that women are always complaining about pain in their breasts and even their ovaries? Do you suppose it's because men know that if they complain, someone would want to cut into them? Or is it because in our culture, these organs in men are not as much at risk?" If women learn how their inner guidance is advising them through breast symptoms to give more time and energy to themselves, they can appreciate their breasts in a different way.

"Fibrocystic Breast Disease"

Currently about 70 percent of women have been told by a health care provider that they have "fibrocystic breast disease." In the 1970s and early 1980s a few studies seemed to indicate that women with so-called fibrocystic breast disease had a two to three times higher incidence of breast cancer. A panic ensued, and women were told conflicting stories by different doctors. When the National Cancer Association Consensus Committee investigated the issue in 1985, it discovered that 70 to 80 percent of what is called fibrocystic breast disease is actually normal changes in breast anatomy and is *not* associated with an increase in breast cancer. Yet many women still believe it is.

Breasts are composed of fat and connective tissue. Over time, the ratio of connective tissue to fat changes. It is therefore normal for some areas of the breast to be denser on examination than others—breast tissue is not homogeneous. One area may be denser than another simply because there's more connective tissue in that area than another. Most women normally undergo what pathologists call fibrocystic changes in their breasts, so the chance of finding them on a biopsy is very high. Unfortunately, because the term has been used to describe just about any breast thickening, tenderness, or other symptoms, women whose breast tissue is merely dense with connective tissue are sometimes given the diagnosis of fibrocystic breast disease, as are those who simply have variations in tissue density throughout their breasts, all of which are variations of normal.

Like the term *cervical erosion,* which simply pathologizes a normal change in the cervix, *fibrocystic breast disease* is basically not a disease. I think the term should be discarded.[9] Misinformation about fibrocystic disease, the constant media exploitation of women's breasts, and our culture's ambivalence toward breasts set up a psychological dynamic that is loaded with potential harm for many women. Not only are they made to feel that their breasts are too small, too large, or the wrong shape, but now they are told by someone whom they trust that their breasts have a disease!

Nipple Discharge

Nipple discharge most often happens after nipple stimulation, usually from lovemaking. It is not dangerous. After a woman nurses a baby, it may take a year or more for milk discharge to disappear completely. In cases of persistent nipple discharge that are not associated with nipple stimulation—the discharge can be anything from milky to greenish clear fluid—a blood test to measure the hormone prolactin should be done to be certain that the woman doesn't have a rare pituitary tumor known as a pituitary microadenoma. A bloody discharge should always be investigated to be certain there's no cancer. Sometimes, however, this very rare condition is caused by benign growths in the ductal tissue of the nipple.

Breast Cysts

Breasts are very sensitive to hormonal changes, and nonmalignant lumps or thickenings often go away over time. But it is a standard medical recommendation that you tell your health care practitioner immediately about any lump you find. You want to know if the lump is a cyst! Breast cysts are very common in women in their forties when their hormone levels are changing. Breast cysts, which are fluid-filled, are diagnosed by placing a needle in them under local anesthetic and aspirating the contents. Sometimes a physician cannot tell a solid lump from a cyst on examination, so ultrasound is needed to make the distinction. If the lump is a cyst, its contents, usually yellow or greenish brown fluid, can be aspirated. Most experts feel that cyst fluid can be discarded because it is rarely helpful to analyze. The cyst will disappear following aspiration in most cases and no further treatment is required. If there's any suspicion, however, the aspirated cells should be tested for cancer. If the ultrasound clearly shows a simple cyst, and the woman does not want a needle stuck into her breast, the cyst can be watched. Many women track their cycles and stress levels by their cysts. When a cyst gets too painful or too large or sticks out, then she can go in and get it aspirated. Most cysts disappear with menopause.

If a lump is *not* clearly a cyst, the patient should be referred to a general surgeon with an interest in breast problems or to a comprehensive breast care center. I feel strongly that women should get the best medical opinions possible about their situation before they embark on any treatment for a breast problem. In women younger than thirty-five (with some exceptions), a breast mass can be watched for several menstrual cycles to see if it goes away.

TREATMENT FOR BENIGN BREAST SYMPTOMS

The vast majority of women have breast pain from time to time. Breast pain (also known as mastalgia or mastodynia) is the number one reason why women visit clinics specializing in breast care and is present in 45 percent of the women who visit these clinics. But it's so common that almost all general physicians see women with this problem. Unfortunately, like so many other women's health issues, breast pain has been too often viewed by the medical profession as a neurotic all-in-her-head kind of disease, and so it hasn't received the attention and care that it deserves. Breast expert Dixie Mills, M.D., says she is waiting for someone to be awarded the Nobel Prize for discovering the cause and cure for breast pain. But every one of us knows that pain is a sign of imbalance somewhere in our lives. And breast pain is no exception.

The burning question that most women with breast pain want answered right away is this: "Is my pain a sign of cancer?" The answer to this is almost always no. But there are a few cases in which the answer is yes. One study showed that breast pain alone is a symptom in only 7 percent of women who had early-stage breast cancer, and another 8 percent presented with both pain and a lump. Another retrospective study suggested an increased risk for breast cancer in women who have had a history of chronic cyclic breast pain compared to those who did not.[10] Since we don't know what causes breast cancer and can identify only 20 to 30 percent of the known risk factors for this disease, it is clear that more and different kinds of studies are needed to fully address this issue. I'm going to assume that if you have significant breast pain, you have been to a physician, received a thorough breast exam, and have had a normal mammogram or sonogram if indicated. My own experience with seeing hundreds of women with breast pain over the years is that the link between breast pain and breast cancer is very low. In fact, in one study of women with breast pain in whom no breast cancer was found on routine screening exams, less than 1 percent

(0.5 percent, to be exact) actually went on to develop subsequent breast cancer at some point in the future.[11]

What Causes Breast Pain?

To get relief from your breast pain, you first have to understand why it may be there. There is no doubt that the most common type of breast pain occurs premenstrually and is related to the hormonal changes in your body that are part of your menstrual cycle. In the luteal phase of your cycle (the two weeks before your period begins), all women have an increased tendency to retain fluid and to gain a pound or two. But in susceptible women, this slight fluid increase, as well as other hormonal changes associated with the menstrual cycle, can cause pressure or inflammation in the breast tissue, resulting in breast tenderness. The same inflammatory chemicals such as prostaglandins and cytokines that cause menstrual cramps can also cause breast tenderness! Your breast tissue actually goes through cyclic changes each month that mirror those that are happening in your uterus. The difference is that the buildup of fluids and tissue in your uterus passes out of your body in the form of your menstrual flow. But the buildup of fluid and cellular tissue in your breasts simply gets reabsorbed back into your body. So it's not difficult to see how pain might result in many women. These cyclic hormonal changes also explain why women are so often offered a variety of hormonal therapies for their breast complaints—which I'll address in a minute.

Some women experience breast pain that is not related to the menstrual cycle at all. No one knows what causes this. Some sources think it is related to inflammation in the body, whereas others think it is related to neuroendocrine changes resulting from subtle interactions between our environment, our perceptions, and our hormonal and immune systems (breast pain has been linked to alterations in steroid and protein hormones, including estrogen, progesterone, LHRF [luteinizing hormone releasing factor, made by the hypothalamus], and prolactin). It is not surprising that one scientific study showed that many women with severe breast pain also suffered from anxiety, panic disorder, and a number of other chronic pain syndromes. Many of these women are not helped by the numerous medical treatments that their health care practitioners suggest. The key to pain relief here is following an inflammation-reducing diet and supplementation program (see chapter on nutrition)—and at the same time acknowledging and then releasing the various emotional states, including trauma, depression, anxiety, and learned helplessness, that have been shown to alter the body's immune and hormonal systems.[12]

A Program for Breast Symptom Relief

Choose from the options in this section on the basis of what appeals to you and what you can easily do without stressing yourself out unduly. You don't have to do everything I've listed here all at once, unless it feels right to you.

First, consult your physician. This is to make certain that you have no signs of breast cancer. It is ideal when your physician can also offer you the emotional support you need for dealing with breast pain, a breast lump, or both.

Minimize estrogen and inflammation. Follow a diet that minimizes excess estrogen and also decreases cellular inflammation (see chapter on nutrition) in your system. Breast tissue is exquisitely sensitive to high-fat, high-refined-carbohydrate diets, which raise estrogen levels. Excessive estrogen production stimulates breast tissue, resulting in breast pain and cyst formation in many women.[13] Many cancerous breast tumors are stimulated by hormones such as estrogen. Tamoxifen, a drug used to treat breast cancer, works by lowering estrogen's effect on breast tissue. The higher the body fat, dietary fat (especially saturated fat and trans-fatty acids), and insulin levels from too many refined carbohydrates, the higher the estrogen levels and the greater the risk for breast and other gynecological cancer.[14] Body fat itself manufactures estrone, a type of estrogen, through the conversion of cholesterol to androsterone, so it's helpful to decrease your total body percentage of fat, if possible.

Plenty of soluble fiber in your diet from vegetable sources helps increase the excretion of excess estrogen. The cruciferous vegetables (cabbage, broccoli, kale, Brussels sprouts, and turnips) all contain indole-3- carbinol, which has been shown to decrease estrogen's ability to bind to breast tissue. This substance is also available as a supplement. The same is true for soy foods such as tofu, miso, and tempeh. Include these foods in your diet regularly. About 80 percent of women with cyclic breast pain get a good response to dietary change alone because a whole-food, inflammation-reducing diet changes hormonal levels and has been shown to significantly reduce the severity of breast tenderness and swelling.[15]

Eliminate dairy products. Stop eating all dairy foods for at least one month as a trial run. Over the years I've seen this relieve the breast pain of many women. If it hasn't helped after one month, then you can add dairy foods again. Though I know of no studies that document this specifically, I have found that dairy foods are associated with breast tenderness and lumps in some women. I believe that the reason for this is that when cows are fed large amounts of antibiotics and hormones to increase their milk supply, these pass into their milk and when consumed by humans can potentially affect human breast tissue. Women who use organically produced dairy foods seem to experience fewer problems.

Eliminate caffeine. Stop all caffeinated beverages, colas, and chocolate—even decaf coffee and decaf Pepsi or Coke. The methylxanthines in cola, root beer, coffee, and chocolate can cause overstimulation of breast tissue in some women, though not all. Scientific studies show conflicting evidence about this issue, but I've seen women who were so sensitive to these substances that eating one piece of chocolate a month resulted in breast pain. So, as with dairy food, a trial run of elimination (usually for one full menstrual cycle) is worth it.

Progesterone. Make sure you have enough progesterone in your system. Because breast pain is often related to estrogen overstimulation, it can be alleviated by increasing your levels of progesterone. Progesterone down-regulates estrogen receptors in your breast after you've been on it about a week or so, which means that your breasts will be protected from the effects of too much estrogen. In fact, studies have shown that when a 2-percent progesterone cream is applied directly to the breasts, it decreases the cellular proliferation of breast tissue, whereas applying estradiol (a form of estrogen) to the breast increases cellular proliferation. Uncontrolled proliferation of breast tissue is associated with an increased risk for breast cancer.[16] Apply one-quarter teaspoon (about 20 mg) once or twice a day for up to three weeks before menstruation. Give progesterone about one month to work; 2-percent progesterone cream may increase breast tenderness initially because it increases estrogen receptors initially, but then they decrease.

Don't overdose with estrogen. If your breast pain started when you started taking estrogen replacement therapy (or birth control pills), chances are your dose is too high. Have your dose adjusted accordingly. You can also add progesterone as above. (See chapter 14.)

Try supplements. There is an ever-increasing body of literature on the anti-inflammatory properties of omega-3 fats, such as those found in flax oil, hemp oil, and cold-water fish.

I also recommend omega-3 fatty acids such as fish oil, walnut oil, macadamia nuts, flaxseed oil, and sesame oil. These oils help with breast pain for the same reason that they help decrease dysmenorrhea. They help decrease inflammation, which stops breast pain. (See section on dysmenorrhea and chapter 17.) There is evidence suggesting that fish oil may also be protective against breast cancer. One recent study of women with breast cancer showed that the composition of breast tissue was altered in a positive direction following the addition of fish oil supplement for three months.[17] I recommend adding omega-3 fats plus supplements (1,000–5,000 mg/day) for optimal breast health.

This includes a good multivitamin-mineral supplement containing high levels of vitamin E in the form of d-alpha tocopherol, or you can add vitamin E (400 to 600 IU per day) to your regimen. Studies have shown that many women with breast pain are helped by the antioxidant vitamins E and A and selenium and that vitamin E actually decreased serum pituitary hormone levels (LH and FSH) in women treated with it for breast pain.[18]

Take vitamin D, as well. It is well documented that many women are deficient in vitamin D. Those with the lowest levels (less than 25 mg/dl in blood) have a higher risk for breast, ovarian, and colon cancer. In addition to moderate sunlight exposure (about ten to twenty minutes or so per day), I also recommend taking at least 1,000 IU of vitamin D-3 per day.

Note: All the studies done on the various supplements that help breast pain studied a particular supplement individually. Since all of these factors work together, it's best to take them along with or as part of a balanced multivitamin formula.

Apply castor oil packs. Castor oil packs applied to the breasts three times per week for one hour, over two or three months often eliminates breast pain, particularly if there is inflammation of breast tissue. A maintenance program of once per week thereafter is recommended.

Increase your intake of iodine. I have prescribed iodine supplements for women with breast pain for years with excellent results, usually within only two weeks. The iodine decreases the ability of estrogen to adhere to estrogen receptors in the breast.[19] An easy way to add iodine to your diet is to eat sea vegetables regularly. Try a small amount of wakame or kombu: soak it until it's soft, then cut it up and add it to soups. You'll never taste it and you will get a lot of good minerals and iodine from it.

Another option is to have your doctor prescribe potassium iodide, 70 percent solution (30 mg iodine per drop). Any formulary pharmacy can make this up for you. Start with two drops per day in water or juice, and increase up to eight drops per day as needed. You probably won't need more. I haven't found that this dose causes thyroid problems in anyone, but if you have a thyroid condition in addition to your breast pain, you'll want to check this out with your doctor.

A third way to get iodine safely into your system (which also helps your thyroid gland function) is to apply tincture of iodine to your skin. Dr. Mills recommends painting a quarter-size dot right over the painful spot on the breast or on the nipple once a night for two weeks.

Change bras. Stop wearing an underwire bra (at least most of the time). Too often this kind of bra cuts off the circulation of both blood and lymph fluid around the breast, chest wall, and surrounding tissue. Tight bras can also cause chest pain.

Learn about your breasts. Understand your breasts' anatomy and keep a calendar, noticing how your breasts change with your menstrual cycle, so that occasional cyclic breast pain doesn't scare you. Talk to your breasts. Ask them, "What are you trying to tell me?" And watch what you say. "My breasts are killing me" is not a useful slogan. Do the breast massage ritual on page 342.

Avoid certain drugs. Don't take the following drugs for treatment of breast pain unless you feel you have no other choice. All of these have very significant side effects.

- Danazol (Danocrine): This drug causes a decrease in levels of estrogen and is also used for the treatment of endometriosis. It often has the following side effects: changes in menstrual cycle regularity, weight gain, acne, flushing, breast reduction, hirsutism, voice change, and depression.

~ Bromocriptine: Bromocriptine is also used to suppress lactation after childbirth. It can cause nausea, vomiting, low blood pressure, dizziness, and depression.

~ Birth control pills: These are made from synthetic hormones. Though I have often prescribed them for birth control, there are better options for the treatment of breast pain.

~ All drugs can have side effects for different women. Some statin drugs (cholesterol-lowering medications), SSRIs (antidepressants), and cardiac pills can cause breast pain, so women should look at what new drugs they have been taking.

Accept support. Be open to accepting support from others in your life. Breast symptoms are often the body's way of getting us to nurture ourselves more fully and allow others to help.

Dixie Mills, M.D., has noted that women with a history of emotional and psychological trauma often have breast pain. These women often have difficulty creating nurturing relationships and have issues with never wanting to feel dependent on others in their lives. They greet the world with a brave and stoic face—the classic stiff upper lip. (Boy, can I relate!) Dr. Mills notes that women with particularly severe mastalgia frequently come to the clinic alone, without a support person. I agree with her observations completely.

Discovering the Messages Behind the Symptoms

Sometimes a woman's breast pain persists until she addresses a deeper cultural wounding. One of my patients got over her breast pain only after she remembered that at the age of five she had been playing in a barn and some boys forced her to pose nude for them. She remembered that her chest was a major focus of this activity. After her breasts grew at puberty, her emotional and psychological discomfort at this kind of attention became chronic and eventually manifested as physical pain.

A forty-seven-year-old woman told me that when her daughter turned thirteen and became quite independent from her, she became acutely conscious of her breasts for a while. She said that they ached at times, as though they were longing to nourish or cradle a baby. She hadn't given birth to her daughter but had adopted her. She said, "Heading into menopause, I remembered that I never beheld her infant face, nor did she drink from my breast. I experienced an intense desire to hold a baby for as long as I needed to. Several months later, a thickening in my left breast was found during my routine annual exam. It was near my heart. I knew what it was about. I needed to deal with renewed feelings about my infertility and its losses. I felt intense sadness over not giving birth to this wonderful child of mine. Now for the first time, my body was letting me know that it too was sorry." Two months after she had this realization, her breast thickening was gone at her follow-up exam. Sometimes the body heals simply when you give yourself permission to listen to its messages.

Breast Biopsy

Any persistent mass requires further testing for definitive diagnosis, most often (but not always) in the form of a biopsy of some kind. High-resolution ultrasound has decreased the number of biopsies required. Most breast biopsies are done on an outpatient basis under local anesthesia by a general surgeon with a special interest in breast care. Increasingly, a needle biopsy can be done in an office setting under ultrasound or mammographic guidance, thus saving the patient from disfiguring lumpectomy for benign lumps and giving her a diagnosis quickly. In fact, in some breast care centers, diagnosis can be made virtually the same day as the needle biopsy. Sometimes, however, the diagnosis must wait for several days until the pathologist can perform further diagnostic tests on the breast tissue. Many women worry that the needle will spread the cancer. Yet years of experience haven't borne this out. Dr. Mills has only seen two cases of this in twenty years, and those were of a rare variant of breast cancer.

One of the most unpleasant experiences a woman can have is living with the uncertainty about whether a breast lump is cancerous. Therefore, if there are any doubts about a breast mass, or if a woman herself is inclined toward further testing, she should seek out a surgeon who has a special interest in breast care. In the past decade, many breast care centers devoted to a multidisciplinary approach to breast care have opened around the country. In these centers, surgeons, pathologists, radiologists, and support staff all work together to give women the care and answers they need in a timely fashion. This is a very significant step forward.

A note on progesterone. Several studies have strongly suggested that premenopausal women who have breast surgery for suspected or already diagnosed breast cancer during the luteal phase of their menstrual cycle (after ovulation and before the onset of menses) have a better prognosis than those who have surgery during another stage of their cycle. In a study of 289 premenopausal women with operable breast cancer who were followed from 1975 to 1992, women with node positive breast cancer who had serum progesterone levels greater than 4 nanograms per milliliter at the time of surgery had a survival rate that was 70 percent higher than those with lower progesterone levels at the time of the surgery. This may be because progesterone decreases blood-clotting effects and also increases the natural killer cells in the immune system. It also decreases breast cell proliferation. Given these three factors, it is possible that progesterone works by decreasing the chances of tumor cells seeding themselves in remote places when breast surgery is done for cancer.[20] I would recommend that any premenopausal women facing breast cancer surgery make sure that her progesterone levels are optimal before proceeding. This can be done by using 2-percent progesterone cream at the dose recommended on page 349. There is also a substantial body of evidence that women who have adequate progesterone levels during their menstrual and perimenopausal years may be at decreased risk for breast cancer development. (Note: I'm talking about physiologic levels of progesterone, not megadoses. Theoretically, the body can convert high levels of progesterone into estrogen. It's a question of balance.)

MAMMOGRAPHY

A mammogram is an X-ray study of the breasts used to diagnose breast cancer in its earliest stages, before it can be felt on clinical exam. Though authorities agree that annual mammograms are helpful for early diagnosis of cancer in women over the age of fifty, there is disagreement over how often women in their late thirties and forties should have them. In 1996, the National Institutes of Health appointed a panel of prestigious experts who spent over six weeks reviewing more than a hundred scientific reports on mammograms and hearing thirty-two oral presentations. The conclusion of this group was that there was not enough evidence to support a recommendation that women in their forties should get routine annual mammograms. Though there was a great hue and cry about this conclusion, I certainly agree with it. A report in the July 2005 edition of the *Journal of the National Cancer Institute* found no benefit in terms of lives saved from mammography screening performed in the community setting.[21] Later in 2005, another study showed that half the decrease in mortality from breast cancer could be attributed to mammography.[22] The controversy continues, and women deserve to be informed about the risks and true benefits. Mammography has its limitations. Many women in their late thirties and forties have breast tissue that is too dense to make mammography readings helpful. The key here, as elsewhere, is individualization of care. Some women might do well with yearly mammograms in their forties if they have a strong family history of breast cancer and have breast tissue that can be easily read on a mammogram. Others will want to wait until they are fifty. And some will choose to avoid mammography altogether. You and your health care provider need to discuss how often you should have a mammogram.

Mammograms aren't foolproof for diagnosing all breast cancers—they miss 10 to 15 percent of them overall, and in young women, they miss up to 40 percent. If something is called "probably benign" on a mammogram, the odds of it being cancer are less than 2 percent, according to most radiologists at academic medical centers. The rate of false positive mammograms (saying that there's something abnormal when there isn't) is about 10 percent and it increases with time. One study estimated that after ten mammograms, about half of women (49 percent) will have had a false positive result, which will have led to a needle biopsy or an open biopsy in 19 percent.[23]

Mammogram reports sometimes can seem punitive and confusing to women. Here are a few examples. A routine mammogram in a thirty-eight-year-old woman who had completely normal breasts was reported this way: "The breasts are extremely dense and poorly suited to mammography." For reading this, one would think that breasts were created *for* mammography and that this woman's breasts were to blame! Having breasts that are dense to an X-ray beam is *not* an abnormality—it is perfectly normal for a woman in her thirties, and even for a woman in her fifties who is on estrogen replacement therapy. It is not your fault if your breasts are dense, it is the medical field's fault for not being able to think out of the box and find a new screening tool. (See "The Picture Problem: Mammography, Air Power, and the Limits of Looking," by Malcolm Gladwell in the December 13, 2004, issue of *The New Yorker*.)

One of my patients, a forty-five-year-old woman who had completely normal breasts, went in for a routine screening mammogram. She had benign calcifications in a small amount of her breast tissue, which is quite common and no cause for alarm. Her mammogram report, though normal, was written in extremely convoluted and frightening language: "Trabecular derangement and mazoplasia cystic with adenosis bilaterally. Some prominence of the suspensor ligaments. No evidence for superdensities, skin thickening, or unifocal hypervascularity. Scattered acinar, punctate, singular calcifications in both breasts, the largest 1.5 mm. They are quite discrete and do not have the same appearance as microcalcifications associated with malignancy." Talk about confusing!

Every radiologist reads a mammogram a bit differently. Reading them is an art, practiced by imperfect human beings—it's not an exact science. Women are led to believe, however, that a normal mammogram reading is a kind of guarantee that everything is all right. They don't understand the limitations of the test. (One of my good friends just had a normal mammogram reading but a biopsy she insisted upon having showed cancer!) On the other hand, thousands of women with benign breast findings are put through an incredible amount of anxiety each year due to mammogram reading. Some, of course, do get diagnosed with early stages of breast cancer as a result of the test. Many physicians believe that diagnosis in the early stages is the best strategy for saving lives, but this is controversial. Many women undergo a breast biopsy because of abnormal findings on a mammogram. Even though most biopsies are benign, a lot of women go through hell thinking they have cancer, and the experience understandably makes them fearful. Almost everyone has had a friend die of breast cancer. No wonder we cling to mammograms in hopes they'll provide a lifeline!

Some women don't want mammograms and won't get them. One of my patients once said to me, "I've seen far too many women have a mammogram that was positive who then became frozen with fear. I can't help but think that's a threat to their health. I've watched them go downhill very rapidly." This is the same reaction that some people have to getting a diagnosis of AIDS. Fear and the feeling of helplessness are indeed very detrimental to health. This same woman said, "I'll have a mammogram as soon as I'm ready to deal with the consequences, no matter what they are. For now, I believe that I may be creating cancer daily—but I also believe that my body probably handles it." Interestingly, my friend Deena Spear, a vibrational healer, says that cancer goes in and out of physical form constantly. But once the diagnosis is made, it tends to begin growing in earnest, probably in part because of the law of attraction.

Another of my patients, a vibrant and healthy woman in her fifties, said that she didn't want a yearly mammogram, even though that's the current recommendation for a woman of her age. She felt that yearly radiation exposure to a radiation-sensitive organ is probably not benign. As she put it, "I intend to live into my nineties. I'll be damned if

I'm going to zap my breasts once every year. That adds up to over forty X-rays!" She's on to something—research shows that mammograms may actually raise the risk of breast cancer.

Most mammogram reports also contain a statement that reads: "A negative mammogram should not preclude biopsy of a clinically palpable lesion." This is dictated into the report for legal reasons, to put the doctor and patient on notice that there are limitations to the diagnostic capabilities of mammograms (as there are with all diagnostic tests).

Digital mammography (taking pictures of the breast on a computer rather than film) got a lot of press recently when it was found to be better for younger women with dense breasts. This method usually involves just one or two compressions; technicians can tweak additional views with the computer. But it still involves radiation exposure, and it is a one-dimensional, black and white photo. Digital mammograms are extremely expensive and only available in about 10 percent of centers. Their usefulness and cost effectiveness is still under study.

Breast problems should be diagnosed via a multimodal approach that combines physical examination, mammogram where applicable, sonogram (see page 361), aspiration of lumps, and surgical or needle biopsy if necessary. When a woman knows her own breasts well, this entire process is enhanced because she trusts herself to know what is normal and what is not. I don't doubt a woman's ability to find an abnormality, and it's important that health care practitioners pay attention when a woman who is tuned in to her body tells them that something is wrong. If a woman or her doctor feels a lump that hasn't been there before, a biopsy is necessary to rule out cancer, even if the mammogram is normal.

Over the years, I saw some women with stable lumps in a breast for many years who decided not to have biopsies of these areas. The lumps didn't change, the women themselves knew these areas of their breasts intimately, and they took full responsibility for avoiding a biopsy. On the other hand, I've seen women with recent-onset breast lumps who have delayed seeing a doctor for months even when they knew the lump was there. One of my patients who was eventually diagnosed with breast cancer delayed diagnosis and treatment for two years because she was immobilized by her grief about the loss of her father several years before. She was a working woman and told me that she simply "didn't have the time or energy to seek help." This is a dangerous attitude to have toward your health, and it's also part of the breast cancer "archetype." Well-informed and well-supported women often come in to be examined for reassurance and diagnosis very shortly after noticing a change in their breasts that is unusual.

When this happens, it's important to ask yourself, "What is going on in my life around self-nurturance and partnership? Am I striking the right balance between nurturing myself and nurturing others?" I always ask women with breast problems what is going on in their lives, especially how they are nurturing themselves or others. This is the heart of the matter, along with an exam and further diagnostic testing if it is warranted. Regardless of the diagnosis, a woman needs to know that she is being asked by her breast to look within and to tune in to her inner guidance system. Dr. Mills always asks her patients what their relationship is with their breasts.

Mammograms: The Limitations of a Gold Standard

Fear of breast cancer is a very real issue for many women. A 1995 Gallup poll found that 40 percent of women believe they will die of breast cancer, even though the actual risk of death from the disease is less than 4 percent! Though mammograms have been the gold standard for early diagnosis (and the perception of a greater chance of cure), mammograms are associated with some very real risks. For example, Danish researchers Ole Olsen and Peter Gotzsche published two studies in *The Lancet* of their reviews of seven randomized controlled studies on the benefits of mammography in reducing mortality from breast cancer. They found that five of the seven studies were so flawed they couldn't even be reviewed. In the remaining two, they also found major design flaws and limitations. They concluded that mammograms had no effect on deaths attributed to breast cancer. The studies also showed that, in many cases, mammograms led to needless treatments and were linked to a 20 percent increase in mastectomies, many of which were unnecessary.[24]

As I've already pointed out, most cancer screening modalities identify the slow-growing lesions that women would die "with," not "from." In other words, they would never become life-threatening if left alone. In 2002, a National Cancer Institute advisory panel concluded that the benefits of mammography are uncertain and the chance of receiving a false positive result is substantial. Despite these substantial limitations, all traditional medical groups continue to support the regular and continued use of mammography. In fact, nineteen medical organizations, including the American College of Obstetricians and Gynecologists, urge women to continue receiving annual mammograms. The National Cancer Institute even extended its recommendations to include annual screenings for women age forty and older, despite contrary advice from its own panel. This isn't difficult to understand. Both inside and outside of medicine, we as a culture have come to rely on screening to save us. And even though the evidence doesn't support it, individual women and their doctors often feel safer if they perceive that they've "covered all the bases."

There have been a number of other negative studies on mammography in the medical literature—though they usually don't get much press. In 2000, the *Journal of the National Cancer Institute* pointed out that the cumulative risk of having false positive mammograms is quite significant in many women. While this is possible in any age group, it is most common in women in their forties because they tend to have denser and more fibrous breasts that get read as false positive mammogram readings that then require biopsy. Andrew Wolf, M.D., an associate professor at the University of Virginia School of Medicine, supports these findings. In an August 2003 review article on breast cancer screening in *Consultant,* Dr. Wolf states, "If a woman begins getting regular mammograms at age 40, there is virtually a 100 percent chance that some kind of abnormality will show up that will warrant at least a follow-up mammogram, an ultrasound scan, or a call from the physician recommending a six-month follow-up examination. It is also likely that over the course of a lifetime, she will undergo an unnecessary breast biopsy."[25]

For me, the biggest concern about mammography is that it doesn't appear to reduce mortality from breast cancer any better than simple breast exam (which also doesn't decrease mortality!). According to a 2000 study from the *Journal of the National Cancer Institute,* after following nearly forty thousand women between the ages of fifty and fifty-nine, researchers found that annual mammograms were no more effective than standard breast exams in reducing breast cancer mortality. Mammography didn't increase the survival rate of those who were diagnosed with breast cancer.[26] Another study published in the *Journal of the American Medical Association* found that women age seventy and older benefited very little from mammography.[27] The cancers detected at this age would never have killed them. Then there are those researchers who doubt the safety of mammography because of radiation exposure. A 1994 study published in *The Lancet* addressed another concern that many women have brought up with me—that the breast compression that occurs during a mammogram may cause small, in-situ tumors to rupture, thereby spreading cancer cells into surrounding tissues and potentially leading to more invasive cancers and metastases.[28]

Cornelia Baines, professor emerita at the University of Toronto and former deputy director of the Canadian National Breast Screening Study, recently said, "I remain convinced that the current enthusiasm for screening is based more on fear, false hope and greed than on evidence."[29] I agree with Dr. Baines completely.

The bottom line is this: when it comes to mammograms, things are not as cut and dried as they seem. There's a lot we simply don't know. After discussing all their options with a knowledgeable health care practitioner, all women will need to follow their own inner guidance when it comes to mammograms, taking full responsibility for their choices. Intelligent, informed women can be trusted to do what's right for them, including forgoing mammograms—and I support them wholeheartedly.

The Limits of Early Detection

Doing breast self-exams and getting mammograms (or sonograms) regularly is not the same as *prevention*. In other words, it is not the same as brushing and flossing the teeth, which actually prevents cavities and periodontal disease. As one of my colleagues said of breast cancer, "We identify the risks, but we don't know what to do until they manifest as disease." Our culture uses mammograms as a fix but doesn't encourage women to change their diets, stop smoking, and learn how to be in relationships that nurture them. These are preventive changes that I believe would result in healthy breasts. But as one researcher has said, it's difficult to put together a constituency for prevention. It is treatment that gets our attention. If your sister or mother dies of breast cancer, you usually give money to programs that do research to produce better treatments; you don't start a whole-food restaurant in your neighborhood or advocate teaching eighth-grade girls how to appreciate their breasts. This culture likes to act only after the horse is already out of the barn.

There is a third option, however. You can use mammography and other disease screening as an external guidance system. And if any abnormality appears, you then have the opportunity to ask the abnormal cells what they need that they're not getting. The earlier in the disease process you make adjustments to your diet, beliefs, and lifestyle, the easier it is to transform your cells.

Breast Ultrasound: An Adjunct
(and Sometimes Alternative) to Mammography

In many women, ultrasound screening of breast tissue (reading breast tissue by sending sound waves through it and reading the echoes on a screen) is more appropriate and helpful than mammography. With the advent of high-resolution ultrasound, some authorities feel that this modality may become the method of choice for detecting an invasive breast carcinoma, with mammography reserved for localizing intraductal carcinoma marked by calcifications.

In the diagnosis of a nonpalpable mass (one that you can't feel but that is discovered on mammography), ultrasound can be invaluable for guiding fine-needle or core-needle aspiration. High-resolution breast ultrasound has also made it much easier to delineate palpable breast lumps. An ultrasound can easily tell the difference between a cyst and a lump. And if a breast mass is solid, the ultrasound has a 98 percent specificity in terms of being able to distinguish a benign lesion from a malignant one. In fact, some studies have shown that ultrasound is the single most accurate diagnostic test for those women with palpable breast masses, yielding a 99.7 percent positive predictive value if it's used by those who are skilled in this technique.[30] If there's any question about the findings, a needle biopsy can now be done in the office setting to determine whether or not a breast mass is malignant. This has spared many women from disfiguring breast biopsies and the anxiety that comes from not knowing what she's dealing with.

There is another reason why ultrasound is important. Mammography is often not helpful in women who are younger, have dense breasts, have postoperative scarring, suffer from acute or chronic radiation effects, are on hormone replacement, or are less than forty-five to fifty years of age. Sonograms are also more accurate than mammograms for diagnosing breast problems accurately in women who've had breast implants. The highest-risk women are those who've already had radiation to their breasts. Sonography is often a good alternative for these women. It is also painless and without risk of radiation. Mammography is still the screening modality of choice for most asymptomatic women, but ultrasound definitely has its place. Many centers will not do screening ultrasounds because it is very time-consuming and it is difficult to compare pictures from year to year. However many centers do offer screening ultrasounds for high-risk women.

MRIs (magnetic resonance imaging) are the latest tools in the breast cancer detection department. But they will most likely never be used as a screening test—they are too expensive (at least $2000), too hard to do (women have to lie still for up to an hour, often medicated), and there are too many false positives. MRIs do have a role in high-risk women with dense breasts or suspicious mammograms, though. I would recommend having them done only at a breast center whose personnel are highly experienced in their use.

Thermography is an old test that is regaining popularity because new technology has improved the capabilities of the infrared cameras to measure heat variances in the breast. Thermogram usage is still investigational. Many technicians recommend repeating the thermogram in three months to check stability. At this point, thermography is not recommended in place of mammography and is not covered by insurance.

The DCIS Dilemma

Mammograms can pick up very early breast abnormalities that may not go on to become actual invasive cancer. These early changes are known as ductal carcinoma-in-situ (DCIS), or mammary dysplasia or atypia. DCIS refers to cancer cells that are still contained within the microscopic breast ducts and have not broken out or invaded the fatty or fibrous tissue of the breast and formed a lump. DCIS is considered Stage 0 breast cancer and many people consider DCIS a pre-cancer.

However, this may be an oversimplification. The multistep progression to breast cancer is not at all clear, and in my experience DCIS may be arrestable or even reversible. Nevertheless, because the natural history of DCIS has not been studied over a long period of time, some doctors automatically assume that all such abnormalities are fast-growing and potentially lethal. Since these lesions usually occur in many areas of the breast, mastectomy is often recommended.

Dr. H. Gilbert Welch, a general internist and senior researcher at the Department of Veterans' Affairs in White River Junction, Vermont, has researched the problems associated with the ability of technology to overdiagnose diseases such as breast cancer. He cites a study that showed that in the breasts of women who died of other causes, 40 percent had microscopic precancerous changes in their breasts. These same types of lesions commonly show up on mammograms, and no one knows which ones will remain dormant and which ones will actually become invasive cancer.[31] In fact, it is now well documented that the majority of women diagnosed with ductal carcinoma-in-situ of the breast do not go on to develop invasive breast cancer.

A 1996 article in the *Journal of the American Medical Association*[32] and a 2005 article in the *Annals of Internal Medicine*[33] summarized the current dilemma well. Both studies show that the incidence of DCIS has increased dramatically since 1983 because of mammography screening. At least 20 percent of breast malignancies detected by mammogram are DCIS. A 2005 study from the Fred Hutchinson Cancer Research Center published in the April 2005 issue of *Cancer Epidemiology, Biomarkers, and Prevention* found that the diagnosis of DCIS has increased sixfold since 1980 while the incidence of true invasive breast cancer has remained flat. The researchers also found a fourfold increase of a less common condition called lobular carcinoma in situ (LCIS) which is also noninvasive.[34] While early detection of invasive breast cancer is beneficial, the value of DCIS detection is currently unknown: I am very concerned about the large number of DCIS cases that are being diagnosed as a consequence of screening mammography, most of which are treated by some form of surgery. In addition, the proportion of cases treated by mastectomy is inappropriately high, particularly in some areas of the United States.

Current treatment options include lumpectomy (although there is no lump per se), lumpectomy with radiation, adding tamoxifen, or mastectomies. While having a mastectomy for such an early stage cancer seems paradoxical, Dr. Mills is seeing more women opting for this surgery. While it is very sad for them to lose a body part, when it is clearly their decision made after weighing all the information, medical and personal, she can understand their choice. And so can I. There is no one right way to treat DCIS once a woman knows she has it, and the whole issue is very controversial at this time. Surgeons tend to recommend surgery for it. Radiation oncologists recommend radiation. Medical oncologists recommend tamoxifen or other antiestrogen pills. Chemotherapy is only recommended when there is evidence of invasion. Women should clearly recognize that they have plenty of time to consider all their options. DCIS is not growing out of control. We know that some untreated DCIS can go on to invasive cancer, but we do not know which types, when, or why. Researchers are looking for markers but unfortunately have not found the perfect one. Others are looking at the "cross talk" between cancer cells and normal cells around them and how they keep a balance. The good news is that the chance of dying from DCIS is very, very low, about 1 to 2 percent. Treatment efforts go into minimizing the risk of the DCIS recurring in the breast. Dr.

Mills and I both feel that many times the angst, fear, and confusion women go through when diagnosed with DCIS create more havoc with their health than the actual disease. Regardless of your treatment choice, however, I would recommend a program to improve your breast health and your ability to heal DCIS from the inside out.

BREAST CANCER

Currently, one in eight women in the United States between the ages of one and ninety gets breast cancer. This does not mean that one in nine forty-five-year-old women will get it. To put this into perspective, you need to know that only women age ninety and over have a one-in-eight risk of getting breast cancer. According to the National Cancer Institute, at age twenty, the risk is 1 in 2,500; at forty, 1 in 63; and at sixty, 1 in 28. Though breast cancer is the leading cause of cancer death among American women who are forty to fifty-five years of age, lung cancer is by far the leading cause of cancer death in women of all ages. Cardiovascular disease trumps them both—killing six times more women than breast cancer.[35]

When I was in medical school, I was taught that one in twenty-five women would get breast cancer. No one is sure whether the incidence of breast cancer is actually on the increase or whether we are simply diagnosing it earlier these days, with the increase in mammography and public awareness. Regardless of statistics, however, most of us know at least one person who has had or currently has breast cancer.

For this to be the case, clearly something is out of balance. Evidence is accumulating that certain environmental pollutants contribute to estrogenic activity and may contribute to the incidence of breast problems in the industrialized world.[36] But whether or not breast cancer is on the increase statistically, and whether or not industrial toxins and pesticides are a contributing factor, every woman has to be proactive about her breast health now. Why wait until further studies on environmental toxins come in or the definitive treatment for breast cancer is figured out when you can start, through your thoughts, emotions, and daily choices, to create breast health now—even if you've already got cancer!

The breast is an estrogen-sensitive organ. Many women who have been on birth control pills or estrogen replacement have found that the medication resulted in enlarged and often tender breasts. The effect of these medications, plus the inflammation-causing standard American high-fat, high-carbohydrate, low-fiber diet, which overstimulates breast tissue, is a setup for breast cancer. I'm also concerned about the possible effects of bovine growth hormone (BGH), which is given to cows to increase milk production, on breast tissue.[37]

With the current rates of breast cancer and DCIS, how would we even know if we had an epidemic of the disease? It's already far too common to wait for the medical profession or the government to do something. Fortunately, it's possible to decrease your risks now!

The Breast Cancer/Diet-Hormone Link

Breast cancer has been associated with high levels of dietary fat and low levels of certain nutrients for many years. As far back as 1977, a study at the National Cancer Institute showed that countries with the highest intake of animal fat had the highest mortality rates from breast cancer.[38] But it's not so simple. In 1996 an analysis of 337,000 women in seven prospective studies suggested that there is no association between women's intake of dietary fat and their risk for developing subsequent breast cancer. The researchers found no difference in breast cancer rates between those whose intake of dietary fat ranged from more than 45 percent of their calories to less than 20 percent. It didn't seem to matter whether the fats were from saturated, monounsaturated, or polyunsaturated sources.[39] Somewhat confusingly, an Italian study showed a decreased risk of breast cancer with increased fat intake but an increased risk of breast cancer when the intake of available carbohydrates in the form of starch (breads, pasta, etc.) was increased.[40] Scientific data are rapidly accumulating on the link between sugar, insulin levels, and breast cancer.[41]

Here's my current thinking. High-fat diets in industrialized societies almost always include large amounts of partially hydrogenated fats and are usually associated simultaneously with high consumption of refined carbohydrates and sugar along with a low intake of fresh fruits and vegetables and antioxidants. This combination is a setup for chronic inflammation at the level of the cell—especially when you add in the biochemical effect of certain emotional states, which I've already mentioned. In addition, environmental contaminants such as PCBs, PBBs, and mercury are probably significant. Excessive estrogen (relative to progesterone) over the life cycle that is related to diet and obesity also appears to be associated with increased risk of breast cancer, at least in some individuals. Emotional stress, a nutrient-poor diet full of refined carbohydrates, low in vitamin D and omega-3 fats, plus environmental toxins—any and all of these lead to change in cellular inflammation. And inflammation precedes cancer!

Program to Promote Healthy Breast Tissue

~ Maintain optimum progesterone levels. I recommend that all women with concerns about breast cancer, or who have a history of breast pain, PMS, fibroids, or other evidence of estrogen dominance, make sure that they have enough progesterone in their system. Your health care provider can arrange for hormone testing to determine your hormone levels.

~ Limit consumption of animal fats. Animal fats may stimulate colonic bacteria to synthesize estrogen from dietary cholesterol, thus possibly contributing to hyperestrogenism in the body.

~ Maintain a healthy body composition. Your percentage of body fat should be 26 percent or less. More than that creates an estrogen factory in your body that can lead to overproduction of estrogen, which stimulates breast tissue growth because body fat makes estrone.

~ Get enough dietary fiber. Hyperestrogenism can be modulated by a high-fiber, low-fat diet, because dietary fiber increases fecal excretion of estrogen.[42]

~ Get enough phytoestrogens (e.g., soy, flax) in your diet. Asian women who consume a traditional diet—including the soy-based products tempeh, tofu, miso, and natto—excrete estrogen at a much higher rate than those who don't. They also have a much lower risk of breast cancer. These soy products, rich in what are known as phytoestrogens, which are plant substances that have biochemical properties similar to weak estrogens, appear to be protective against breast cancer, in part because their weak estrogenic activity tends to block estrogen receptors on the cells from excessive estrogen stimulation from other sources.[43] A Singaporean study showed that diets high in soy products conferred a low risk of breast cancer in premenopausal woman.[44] Studies also show that soy exerts a protective effect on breast tissue.[45] Laboratory studies have also shown that phytoestrogens inhibit the cell growth of human breast cancer cells.[46]

~ Get enough lignans. Another study found that vegetarians and women in areas with low breast cancer risk have high urinary lignan levels, whereas those women in areas of high risk have low levels.[47] (Lignans are building blocks for plant cell walls that, when eaten, break down into enterolactones and enterodiol, which have potent anticancer and estrogenic effects.) Flax seed has one of the highest lignan concentrations of any food. It can be eaten as ground-up seeds (I recommend one-quarter cup three to seven days per week, mixed with soup, yogurt, or other foods) or in capsule form as Brevail, a natural plant extract available at health food stores.

~ Eat your vegetables. A compound called indole-3-carbinol (I3C), which is a plant chemical obtained from cruciferous vegetables (such as cabbage, broccoli, Brussels sprouts, kale, and collard greens), changes the way estrogen is metabolized. It has the ability to make the body's own estrogen less apt to promote cancer.[48]

~ Take supplements:

~ Selenium: Women with breast cancer have been shown to have selenium levels that are lower than those of women without cancer.[49] Selenium is a trace mineral that is often lacking in refined-food diets. In fact, a double-blind, randomized cancer prevention trial that supplemented selenium at levels of 200 mcg per day for more than six years showed a 50 percent reduction in total cancer mortality.[50]

~ Bioflavonoids: The use of bioflavonoids (found in the vitamin C complex) may inhibit estrogen syntheses.[51]

~ *Lactobacillus acidophilus*: Hyperestrogenism and possibly breast cancer itself may be decreased by including *Lactobacillus acidophilus* in the diet. This beneficial bacterium helps metabolize estrogen properly in the bowel.[52] It is available in capsules from health food stores. Health practitioners can usually suggest a reliable brand; I recommend PB8, which doesn't require refrigeration. Most commercially available yogurt does not contain enough of the live bacteria to make a difference, but organic brands do.

~ Vitamin A: In one study of women with breast cancer, low serum retinol (a vitamin A by-product) was associated with a decreased response to chemotherapy.[53]

~ Vitamin D: Take at least 1000 IU of vitamin D-3 per day.

~ Coenzyme Q10: Studies have found that about 20 percent of breast cancer patients have levels of coenzyme Q10 that are below the normal range. Coenzyme Q10 (also known as ubiquinone) is a natural substance necessary for the production of ATP—the main molecule that powers our cells. It has also been shown to enhance immune functioning. In one recent study from Denmark, thirty-two breast cancer patients were given up to 390 mg per day of CoQ10, together with antioxidants and essential fatty acids. Seven showed partial or complete regression of their tumors.[54] Although these results are preliminary, I recommend CoQ10 as part of a supplement program for every woman who has concerns about breast cancer. The usual dose is 30 mg to 90 mg per day. For those women with already diagnosed breast cancer, 300 mg per day is definitely worth a try. Several of my colleagues who treat breast cancer have reported results similar to those found in the Danish study. CoQ10 is available in health food stores. Note: Statin drugs greatly reduce CoQ10 in the body. Women on these drugs should take supplemental CoQ10.

~ Decrease alcohol consumption: Alcohol consumption is associated with breast cancer risk.[55] In one excellent study, this link was felt to be due to the fact that alcohol consumption increases hormone levels in the blood. In women age fifty and over, the type of alcohol associated with the highest risk was beer.[56] Given the fact that many women drink to medicate their emotions, women's unexpressed emotions may enhance the alcohol–breast cancer link.

~ Exercise regularly: An exciting study from Norway found that women who exercise regularly (four hours per week) had a 37 percent reduction in risk for breast cancer compared to sedentary women.[57] Data from the Nurses' Health Study (covering more than eighty-five thousand women) showed that those who did daily moderate to vigorous exercise were 20 percent less likely to get breast cancer than those who exercised less than one hour a week.[58] The most likely reason for this is that regular exercise is associated with lower levels of body fat and less total circulating estrogen.

~ Get plenty of sleep: Some of the newest research shows that getting adequate sleep (in a dark room) is more important to breast health than most of us realize. A 2005 Finnish study of more than twelve thousand women found that those who consistently sleep nine hours or more a night have less than one-third the risk of breast tumors compared with those who get seven or eight hours of sleep nightly.[59] Several other recent studies have shown that exposure to bright light late at night may increase the risk of breast cancer (and indeed, female night-shift workers have about a 50 percent greater risk of developing breast cancer than other working women).[60] Researchers discovered that nighttime light (if it's bright) interrupts the production of the hormone melatonin. Inadequate melatonin levels can promote breast tumor growth.[61] Women with above-average melatonin concentrations are less likely to develop breast cancer.[62]

~ Get it off your chest: Acknowledge any grief, sadness, fatigue, or loss that you are feeling. Get help and support. Remember, all human beings deserve and need social support. There's nothing to be gained by suffering in silence! Have compassion for yourself.

~ Intend to get more pleasure and nurturance: Remember that your breasts are designed for nurturance and pleasure. And that's what keeps them healthy. Make sure that you use your own power to get more of these in your life.

Family History of Breast Cancer and the Breast Cancer Gene

Certain families have been identified as having genetically higher chances of early-onset breast cancer and sometimes ovarian cancer.[63] The men in these families have increased rates of colon and prostate cancer. Though genetic testing is now commercially available to screen for the BrCa1 and BrCa2 genes, most experts agree that this test should be limited to people participating in research studies because we really don't know what the results mean or what should be done about them. Here's why: In some families studied, those members who carry the gene have an estimated lifelong risk of developing breast cancer of 85 percent and a 50 percent risk of ovarian cancer. But other families who have the gene *don't* have a high incidence of breast or ovarian cancer. This raises serious questions about whether or not the 85 percent figure is an overestimate.

It's clear that the genes we are born with are only one part of the story. How they get expressed to breast disease is another story entirely. Diet, environment, specific emotions, and behavior influence whether or not a gene actually gets expressed and causes disease. It is clear that in certain settings the BrCa1 gene is less lethal than in others.[64] The majority of women diagnosed with breast cancer *don't* have a positive family history of the disease; nor do they have the BrCa1 gene. In one major study, only 10 percent of young women with breast cancer had the gene. But a woman who doesn't have the gene still faces a lifetime risk of breast cancer of 12 percent. The first thing I tell my patients who have a positive family history—usually a mother with breast cancer—is that they are *not* their mothers and that genetics is only *one* part of whether somebody gets a disease.

A Word About Genetic Profiles

With the completion of the Human Genome Project in 2000, an ever-increasing body of research is showing that certain gene mutations run in families that may predispose them to an increased risk of breast cancer, heart disease, etc. These "genomic profiles" typically consist of tests for combinations of gene variants; the specific combinations are considered proprietary and are usually not disclosed in online or printed product information.

A critical evaluation of genomic profiling for guiding individualized health promotion and disease prevention concluded that this approach is "not ready for prime time" yet because there are still so many variables involved and questions that haven't been answered. In other words, it's still a research tool.[65]

Still, I believe that this type of testing will become a very valuable tool in the future. For example, one of my medical colleagues has a mother who has had two different types of breast cancer. A practitioner of functional medicine who understands the link between our genes and our environment, she had her mother and herself tested for the type of gene mutations that are associated with some types of breast cancer. Sure enough, she and her mother had exactly the same genomic profile in the area of estrogen metabolism. But rather than feel as though she is a "sitting duck" for developing cancer, she used the data to spur her on to do what she already knew she should do! Exercise more, increase her intake of indole-3-carbinol, decrease sugar, etc. Increasingly, genomic profile blood tests—and the ability to change how our DNA gets expressed—will be the medicine of the future. If you work with a skilled health care practitioner who knows how to interpret a genomic profile and help you improve your lifestyle, then getting one might be worth it. For the vast majority of people, family history is all the genomic profiling they need. The key is to make the changes they already know they should make! (To find a practitioner who is combining genomic profiles with specific lifestyle suggestions, check out the website of the Institute for Functional Medicine at www.functionalmedicine.org.)

Changing Your Legacy: Prevention from the Inside Out

Here's the story of one woman, a social worker, who has resolved her family history eloquently. "Life had been hectic for some time. Working as a social worker in a large Boston teaching hospital, I covered the oncology unit and the two ICUs [intensive care units] and had a beeper that went off nonstop. At home, I felt continuously assaulted by the noise from the street and from the huge radios that every kid on the block played. I vowed that by the age of fifty I would retire from the rat race and find someplace quiet where I could do some teaching and consulting and have a small private practice and a big garden.

"I had been working in oncology for a few years. Initially, I felt somewhat compelled to do so, knowing that it had to do with my own mother's death, at the age of forty, from breast cancer. It was something of a death-defying act. If I could learn as much as possible about cancer, it would never 'get' me. All I had to do was get past the age of forty. In my own therapy, as I approached forty, I faced the issue of 'having' to do oncology work. After some struggle, I finally decided that I did what I did because I was very good at it, and that when the time came to work in some other sphere, I could do it.

"The age of forty came and went. And the angst remained.

"In September 1990, I came to Maine for a vacation. I was having dinner with an acquaintance and we were talking about our dreams for the future. When I said that my dream was to retire to a place like this when I turned fifty, she challenged me with the question 'Why not now?'

"My answer was that I made good money for a social worker, I had a manageable mortgage, and I was vested in the hospital pension plan. Her observation that I was being held by the 'golden handcuffs' irked me, because I like to think my values are elsewhere. 'Besides,' she said, 'what makes you think you'll get to fifty?' Not only did my mother die young, but every day I was working with people younger than I who were dying.

"At that moment I know that my life changed. I felt it in every cell of my body. And I *knew* there was no reason not to come to Maine. The next day I told a Realtor what I wanted, and on the following morning at nine A.M. I walked into the house that I now own. The first house that I looked at was just what I had dreamed about.

"In January I moved to Maine and continued to work in Boston, never minding the commute, which was made easier by a flexible schedule. In March, Claudia, a young leukemic of whom I had become very fond, died. I had worked with Claudia and her family for four years. I dreaded her death. The morning she died, I experienced chest pains. Knowing that there was no physical problem with me, I paid attention and tried to figure out what my body was saying to me. By the end of the day, I had named the pain 'collective heartbreak.' I realized that I knew more dead people than live people and decided that I needed a weekend away to think about things. A few Sundays later, I was sitting out on the rocks in front of a big resort, looking at the ocean. My thoughts were of Claudia, of many of the others I had worked with who had died, and eventually of my mother.

"For some reason I was curious about exactly how old my mother had been when she died. Surprisingly, I had never done the arithmetic that would give me that information. Simple calculations told me that she had been forty-one and nine months old when she died. On that very day, I was exactly forty-one years and nine months old! And I had been working on the oncology unit for five and one-half years—the same length of time she had been sick with her breast cancer. I had done it! I had survived!

"The next day I handed in my resignation. I took the summer off to think about what to do with my life. Those few months turned into a few more, and before I worked again, nine months had passed—an appropriate amount of time to be reborn.

"During that time, I had the birthday my mother never had and began to rethink my identity and priorities. Eventually, I began what has turned into a very successful psychotherapy practice. I get to teach now and then, do a bit of consulting, and have that big garden. And I know for sure that although I'm my mother's daughter, I never have to *be* her.

"As part of my journey, I have come to believe in the strength of the body and spirit—a helper even in the most impossible situations. In the 1950s, when my mother had breast cancer, I know that there were few options for a Roman Catholic woman stuck in a bad marriage, even fewer if she had been physically disabled in childhood, as was my mother. I now believe that my mother's breast cancer was her only way out of an impossible situation, a bad marriage, a stultifying existence of guilt and self-sacrifice. I regret that her escape cost her her life."

Breast Cancer Treatment

Treatment modalities for breast cancer are beyond the scope of this book and are not my specialty. I'm not particularly happy with the cure rate from the current approaches. Though the experts may disagree somewhat on the statistics, the data suggests that the overall mortality rate from breast cancer is going down. Though it is reported that the age-adjusted mortality rate for U.S. Caucasian females with breast cancer dropped 10 percent from 1975 to 2000, I'm not sure how meaning-ful this figure really is, given the large number of noninvasive ductal carcinomas-in-situ that have no doubt been included as part of these statistics. In some areas of the country, mastectomies are still being done, even though lumpectomy to preserve the breast has, in most cases, been proved equally effective. I urge every woman faced with breast cancer treatment decisions to seek a second opinion if mastec-tomy is the only option she is given or if she has the feeling that her sur-geon isn't comfortable with lumpectomy and therefore doesn't offer it.

One major advance in the surgical treatment of breast cancer is the sentinel node biopsy, whereby a surgeon is able to remove a single ax-illary lymph node, the sentinel node, which is the first to process can-cer cells. When this node is negative, no further nodes are removed. This prevents women from getting so much pain and swelling from re-moval of large numbers of lymph nodes. Studies are looking at leaving the rest of the lymph nodes even when the sentinel node shows some cancer cells. The lymph nodes are after all part of the body's immune system and exist to help the body fight the cancer, so removing large numbers of them doesn't seem logical. However, I do not treat breast cancer, and so I must defer treatment decisions to those who do. Women who are planning lymph node dissection should begin a phys-ical therapy program as soon as possible after surgery to decrease the risk of developing lymphedema, swelling of the arm and hand that re-sults from lymph node removal. (See Resources.)

Women now have access to information from other people, books, and the internet as much as they could want. Some feel overwhelmed by it, while others make a thesis project out of it. Every woman has her own unique decision-making process and should feel validated in using it. Everyone can read the same statistics and feel differently about them. Some want everything done even if the benefit is statistically very small (less than 5 percent). Others perceive treatment risks as higher and are willing to trust their own intuition. Different doctors can present sta-tistics to patients in different terms. While doctors are rarely malicious, some oncologists (because they deal with so much death) can be quite frightening and full of doom and gloom. A woman should feel she has a support system of health care providers whom she can trust and who trust her.

One new online innovation is AdjuvantOnline.com. (Currently, you can only use the site with a password from a health care provider, so you might have to ask yours for one.) Women can plug in information such as tumor size and characteristics, and the site—using data from clinical trials and published studies along with the National Cancer Institute's

SEER (Surveillance Epidemiology and End Results) database—calculates a statistical estimate of their ten-year survival rates and ten-year relapse rates with different treatments or no options. The presentation includes easy-to-read colored graphs.

Another online resource I recommend is *The Moss Reports* by Ralph W. Moss, Ph.D., an expert on alternative cancer therapies. His reports, a periodically updated electronic library of more than 200 documents on various cancer diagnoses, contain information on the most successful treatments and most promising innovative therapies for various types of cancer, including breast cancer. (For more information, call Dr. Moss's office at 800-980-1234 or 814-238-3367 or see Dr. Moss's website, www.cancerdecisions.com.)

Whatever the form of treatment, women all over the world today are transforming their experience of breast cancer and healing at the deepest levels to go on and live full, dynamic, and creative lives.

Inner reflective work to change emotional patterns associated with breast cancer, certain types of support groups, and dietary improvement are important parts of treatment, regardless of whether one has a lumpectomy or undergoes mastectomy, radiation, or chemotherapy. Though the vast majority of women with breast cancer choose surgery, chemotherapy, or both for treatment, I've worked with several women whose choice has involved dietary change and inner healing work only—without any aid from conventional medicine besides the initial biopsy to make the diagnosis. After several years, some of these women now have clear mammograms and no evidence of cancer anywhere. One was called at home by her surgeon at the time that she first refused treatment and was told that if she didn't have the recommended surgery she would die. She refused, and now ten years later she's cancer-free.

Many women choose some, but not all, of the treatment options offered to them. Mildred was forty-three years old when her diagnosis of breast cancer was made. She was married to a university professor and lived in a midwestern college town. She had never worked outside of her home, having chosen instead to marry in her early twenties and raise three children. Shortly after she turned thirty-five, she realized that her husband had been having a series of affairs with students. For financial reasons, she chose to stay with him until their children were older. When her diagnosis of breast cancer was made, however, she left her marriage, went back to school, and got a job. She is now living happily and independently. She had a lumpectomy only. When her daughter asked her why she didn't get a mammogram and exam every six months, Mildred replied, "I know why I got breast cancer. I know I will not get it back again." She knew that she could not maintain her health and stay in a marriage with a man who was sexually unfaithful to her. After more than ten years, she hasn't had a breast cancer recurrence.

Brenda Michaels was first diagnosed with cancer at the age of twenty-six. She battled her disease for seventeen years and had three major surgeries. Finally, after her third diagnosis, and a prognosis that gave her less than a year to live, she took charge of her life and committed to listening to her inner wisdom. She wrote me the following: "Indeed, the emotional issues I had with martyrdom were enormous. I chose to view my cancer as a teacher and a wake-up call in my life and then take responsibility for my health. This decision led me to exploring not only alternatives with respect to my physical body, but also to begin to heal my deep, repressed emotions and the spiritual roots that were associated with my disease. I feel this is where most of my healing occurred, which ultimately led me to the health and vitality I experience today." Brenda is now a nationally recognized speaker with the American Cancer Society and is the first person to work extensively with this group who has used alternatives outside of conventional treatments to heal her cancer. She now hosts a show on internet talk radio (www.conscioustalk.net).

Another of my patients, Julia, was thirty-eight when she had a lumpectomy. The biopsy showed that not all the tumor had been removed during this procedure. A mastectomy and lymph node dissection were recommended because of the nature of her cancer. Instead, she chose to return to her childhood home in the South and confront her demons— a lifetime of codependence and a marriage she had outgrown. This process was accompanied by a deep emotional cleansing and a letting-go of her past ways, unhealthy behaviors, and habits. Julia also changed her diet to a healthy vegetarian one. Though she is cancer-free at this time, she knows that she must stay in touch with her innermost needs and her bodily wisdom. She recently felt called to move to the Southwest. Though unsure of how she would make a living, she decided to go anyway. Almost immediately she found a job at a bed-and-breakfast. Her circumstances there were very healing and afforded her not only room and board but a great deal of time and space alone and close to nature. Julia is extraordinarily courageous and continues to do well.

Another of my patients, Gretchen, was diagnosed with a type of breast cancer that is known to be very aggressive and fast-growing. She refused conventional treatment and instead changed her diet and left an abusive marriage. She eventually found a job in a publishing house doing work that she loves. Three years later, she had no obvious cancer. But she lives from day to day and doesn't think in terms of "being cured." She says, "The essence for me is living my life one day at a time." Gretchen believes that the lifestyle changes she made have been the major factors in her healing.

Women's Stories

Caroline Myss and other healers teach that cancer is the disease of timing. It can result when most of a person's energy is tied up dealing with old hurts and resentments from the past that they can't seem to release. These old hurts need a witness—someone who validates the wounds—before healing can begin.

Our relationship to time can and does make us sick. Sonia Johnson says, "Time is not a river, we all have all the time there ever was or ever will be right now. Linear time, itself, is a workaholic construct."[66] In a materialistic, addictive culture, we learn that time is money and that we should spend each minute of our lives accomplishing or producing more and more. Instead of enjoying each moment we have and living our lives fully, we are instead taught at an early age that there is never enough time. We are always running out of time. Far too many of us suffer from "hurry sickness." We rush around, our hearts beating faster, feeling that there is too much to do and not enough time to do it. The state of our bodies and the cells that constitute them reflect this.

Monica: a summer of healing. Monica was forty-eight when she first came to see me. She had recently had a positive biopsy for breast cancer. Her general surgeon wanted to do a mastectomy as well as remove the lymph nodes from underneath her right arm. Monica and her partner owned a used-book store and ran a service for procuring hard-to-find books. Both of them had read extensively on the topic of breast cancer. She objected to the mastectomy and, after full discussion, the surgeon stated that he felt comfortable doing a lumpectomy. However, he found that her tumor margins were not clear on the specimen, leading to a concern that cancer cells still remained. Monica and her partner had been to see an oncologist and knew that chemotherapy was a standard recommendation for her type of cancer. But they wanted to find out about other things that she could do in addition to conventional treatment.

I suggested to Monica that she could switch to a diet that would lower her circulating estrogen levels, apply castor oil packs to the affected breast to enhance her immune system functioning, and begin a good supplementation program. I stressed that these measures were not considered "cures" in a conventional sense and that they hadn't been studied nearly as well as surgery and chemotherapy. She understood that. I told her that it was imperative that she spend the next few months learning how to take care of herself and do things that brought her pleasure. She and her family left to consider all her options, and I planned to see them three months later, in September.

When Monica returned three months later, she looked fifteen years younger and was radiant with health. I asked her what she had done. She told me, "When I left here, I knew that I had to change my life. This summer I decided to do whatever felt wonderful and healing. So I rode my bike every day and spent long hours lying in the fields looking up at the sky and the clouds. I took summer into every cell of my body. I haven't had a summer like this one since I was a kid. It seemed to go on forever."

Monica had changed her relationship to time, stopping the clock and bringing her cells into the present. Many of us need to take the time to "take summer into every cell of our bodies." It has been more than ten years since Monica has had any evidence of cancer. Though she eventually decided *not* to have chemotherapy or further surgery to try to eliminate tumor cells, she has remained cancer free.[67]

Serena: releasing the past. Serena was forty-eight when she first came to see me following a mastectomy for a fairly large breast mass that was a poorly differentiated breast cancer—a tissue type associated with faster growth and a poor prognosis. She had just moved to the East Coast from California. Two years earlier she had broken up with a man with whom she had lived for ten years when he fell in love with and married another woman. This man was the creator and founder of a very popular self-help group, and the group activities, workshops, and trips had not only provided Serena's income, but also functioned as a family and support system for her. In addition, Serena had contributed substantial money toward a center where this group met regularly. When her significant other left her for another woman in the group, Serena found herself on the outside, and was no longer welcome at group activities in the same way as in the past. When Serena moved back to the East Coast following the breakup of her "family," she immediately went into therapy (both individual and group) to help her deal with the rage, grief, and abandonment she felt. As a result of this experience, she found herself meeting many other women who also found themselves in the position of being taken advantage of financially, sexually, and in other ways. She had always eaten a whole-food diet and simply continued this. In the breast cancer support group she attended, she found women who had followed a whole-food diet for years, others who had exercised all their lives, and others who were on all kinds of supplements. She told me that it certainly was not clear, at least from the group members' experiences, that diet or supplements were the answer.

When I first met with Serena, I told her that she needed to make sure that every relationship she was in was a true partnership, in which she gave and received in equal measure. Though she had been involved in alternatives to conventional medicine for years, her inner guidance led her to chemotherapy, which she went through without any problems by using meditation and relaxation. (See "How to Prepare for Surgery (or Chemotherapy)," page 677.)

Soon after her relationship breakup, she consulted a lawyer to help her get her money and personal belongings back from the group. This lawyer told her that, given the legalities of her situation, it was highly unlikely that she could get her money back. After talking with members of her support group, she decided to get another lawyer and "take it to the Supreme Court if necessary."

Though she continued to eat well, take supplements, and exercise, Serena found herself feeling fatigued and listless. She wondered why this was so, given that she had finished her chemotherapy and radiation almost a year before. I suggested to her that she take a retreat and make a list of all aspects of her life that were working and another of all aspects that needed to change. Then, having meditated on the lists, she could come up with a plan for changing those things she was willing to change right now. She went off by herself to a meditation center. While there, she had the following dream: She was on a raft and saw a house burning in the distance. Her former friends from her self-help community were in the house. At that point in the dream, she realized that she had a choice: to go to the burning house and rescue them, or to stay on the raft and allow the river to take her where she was supposed to be going. In the dream, she noticed that making the choice to leave the river and go to the house was associated with feeling tired and struggling. Even though her mind was pulling her toward the house, her heart (and body) were drawn to going where the river was taking her. She woke up abruptly and knew what she had to do. She had to allow herself to float on the river of a new life.

Even though all her thoughts told her that the community owed her financially, she realized at a very deep level that continuing to hang on to that old community was draining her life's energy away from her—and keeping whatever energy she still had stuck in the past, so nothing new or better could come to her. One week after she returned from her retreat and had her dream, she stopped her legal proceedings against the old group and created a ceremony to release her past and let her move on to a new life. In time, she also stopped going to her support group, since she realized that this experience simply re-created her past. She also noticed that when she went to the meetings, she always felt more tired when she left than when she went in. She knew that, though the group had originally been very helpful, it was now time to leave.

Two months after this healing phase, Serena was offered a job in publishing—something she had always dreamed of doing. She took it, and while there met a new man to whom she is now married. This marriage, unlike her former relationship, is a true partnership of the heart for Serena, and she is able to look back on her breast cancer as her inner guidance coming to her at a critical time. She feels that it gave her the gift of a new, better life. She continues to do well. Most of the time she does not worry about breast cancer. And when she does, she "turns it over to her higher power."

Though Monica and Serena chose different healing approaches, both have changed their relationship to time, and both know that they've chosen the right path for themselves. Most important, they are no longer afraid of breast cancer.

COSMETIC BREAST SURGERY

Implants: Are They Safe? Should You Get Them?

Breast augmentation is extremely popular right now, fueled in part by the constant bombardment (and perhaps alteration) of our senses by media images of enhanced breasts. In fact, it's rare to see a non-augmented breast on a popular television show, in music videos, or in movies. The new "ideal" models of feminine beauty are seen in the hugely popular Victoria's Secret catalog. So the "bar" has been raised artificially high on what we culturally consider an ideal breast size and shape. The "average" implant is a C cup—many are even bigger. To put the entire area into perspective—and to make sure that women are really informed about it, let's first start with a little history.

The first silicone injections were done into the breasts of Japanese prostitutes in order to satisfy the desire of their American G.I. clients for larger breasts in the 1940s and '50s. Problems were reported with silicone leaking into other areas of the body because it was never confined to an implant. Little wonder why these women reported health problems! Later, given the "bigger is better" American desire for larger breasts, the first silicone breast implants were developed by two plastic surgeons from Texas: Frank Gerow and Thomas Cronin in the 1960s. And in 1962, a woman named Timmie Jean Lindsey became the first woman to receive silicone breast implants.[68]

At the time of the first implants, these devices were not regulated by the FDA or any other agency. In the ensuing three decades, it is estimated that anywhere from eight hundred thousand to one million women received the devices.[69]

No one questioned the safety of implants until the 1980s when some of the women with implants began to attribute their symptoms to having breast implants. Chronic fatigue, arthritis, immune system disorders, and connective tissue syndromes such as lupus were said to be associated with silicone implants. This resulted in a decade of controversy in which emotion took precedence over science. Though there was never any convincing evidence that implants were, in fact, associated with connective tissue disorders, that didn't stop a series of huge class action lawsuits against Dow Corning and an enormous amount of fear in women who had had implants. It also resulted in difficulty in obtaining raw material and fear of litigation in manufacturers of other silicone medical devices including vital shunts, catheters, artificial heart valves, and Dacron grafts.[70]

In the end, researchers could find no solid data linking implants, per se, with an increased risk of death. In fact in June 1999, a panel of experts appointed by Congress to study the issue under the auspices of the Institute of Medicine (part of the National Academy of Sciences) failed to find any scientific evidence connecting silicone breast implants with an increased risk of death. This group released a 400-page report prepared by an independent committee of thirteen scientists that concluded that although silicone breast implants may be responsible for localized problems such as hardening or scarring of breast tissue, implants do not cause any major diseases such as lupus or rheumatoid arthritis. The committee did not conduct any original research; instead they examined past research and other materials and conducted public hearings to hear all sides of the issue. Despite this lack of data on their harm, silicone breast implants were taken off the market in the U.S. and replaced by saline implants.

Since then, only two studies have been done on the long-term mortality among women with silicone implants. A 2001 study by the National Cancer Institute found that women with breast augmentation were more likely to die of brain cancer or lung cancer compared to other plastic surgery patients. In fact, the results showed a doubling of brain cancer and a tripling of lung cancer, emphysema, and pneumonia in women with implants. There was also a fourfold increase in risk of suicide among implant patients.[71]

A second study done in Sweden confirmed some of the results of the American study. Researchers studied about 7,500 Swedish women with implants from 1963 to 1993 and found that there was a 50 percent increased likelihood of suicide among women who had breast augmentation, and also more deaths from cancer than expected.[72] The cancer deaths were explained by the number of women with implants who smoked. And the increased risk of suicide was felt to be related not to any effect of implants but more likely because the link between desire for plastic surgery and psychiatric disorders is well documented.[73]

Having seen dozens of women over the years who have done very well with their breast implants (and some who haven't), I'm convinced that the women who are most likely to do well are the ones who generally already feel good about themselves and their worth but are getting the implants to enhance how they look in clothes or because of their professions, e.g., models, actresses, etc. (See stories, below.) They are not getting implants to get or keep a man or because they don't feel feminine enough.

It's intriguing that both brain cancer and suicide risk appear to be higher in women with breast implants. Those are both sixth emotional center issues—perception, thought, and morality. In other words, it is not the implants themselves that are causing the problem. It is how each woman is thinking about and perceiving herself and her worth that either sets the stage for health or illness concerning implants.

The uproar over silicone implants masks a deeper cultural problem: on some level women know that our concern with breast size is not healthy, but we haven't yet found out what healthy is. It doesn't take a sociologist to figure out why women would want to look like the images that have been burned into our brains since childhood by everything from *Playboy* to MTV. (By the time my daughters were eleven and thirteen, they had been concerned with their body shape and weight for several years.) Women's bodies are cultural battlegrounds, and we have taken on the impossible task of trying to look perfect according to standards that are not based on reality.

I disagree with those who feel that women who have had plastic surgery have "sold out." If there were an easy way to move fat from the buttocks to the breasts, I might consider having an augmentation myself! But when I first watched a breast augmentation and saw the amount of tissue damage done by lifting the chest wall off the underlying tissue, I instinctively held my own breasts protectively. I realized that I could never elect to have this procedure, as it is currently performed, done to me for cosmetic reasons. For one thing, implants (now filled with saline instead of silicone) can decrease or eliminate nipple sensation, which is part of a woman's sexual pleasure. The implants can become very hard, and they can cause the breast tissue to develop fibrous capsules around them. (To prevent this, take omega-3 fats as supplements, 1,000–5,000 mg/day; see chapter on nutrition.) In some cases they make it difficult (though not impossible) to nurse a child.

There are other risks associated with implants that all women who plan to get them should keep in mind. The FDA has approved saline breast implants made by two manufacturers, Inamed and Mentor. The FDA came to the conclusion that saline implants were "reasonably safe" for most women for the three years that were studied. They have not been studied for long-term safety yet. Saline implants by companies other than Inamed and Mentor are not considered to be "reasonably safe" by the FDA. "Reasonably safe" is not a guarantee. Data show that about 40 percent of augmentation patients and 70 percent of mastectomy reconstruction patients have at least one serious complication within three years after getting their saline implants.

Within the first three to five years after surgery, 12.5 to 25 percent of breast augmentation patients can expect to have additional surgery, and within ten to twelve years, most women will need at least one additional surgery. The reason is that by then, at least one implant is likely to have ruptured. Like most new products, the majority of implants are often fine for the first few years. Then like anything (e.g., a car), problems can happen over time. The older they get, the more likely they are to rupture. The ruptures are not always obvious.

All breast implants have the same basic design. They are made up of a silicone envelope with a filling of some kind—usually saline unless you have silicone gel. Silicone implants have a more normal feel than saline and a big advantage of the newer ones is that it's impossible for them to leak. The silicone is in a matrix, sort of like a gummy bear candy, so it adheres to the shell that encases it. Even if the implant develops a hole or a tear, called a rupture, the silicone stays put and can't migrate into the body and cause tissue reaction. This is thought to be why the newer silicone imlants are less likely to develop hard encapsulations around them.[74]

Unfortunately, silicone implants are currently available only to women having breast reconstruction. According to Dr. David Fitz, a plastic surgeon to whom I've referred patients for years, reconstruction includes women who are getting implants following breast cancer surgery and also women who are having a breast lift with augmentation. It's currently illegal to use a silicone implant in a woman who simply wants breast augmentation alone—which obviously makes no scientific sense. This will undoubtedly change given the proven safety of the newer silicone implants.

Saline implants have a valve. If you have saline implants, the surgeon will place the empty silicone envelope in your chest and then use the valve to fill the envelope with saline. If the valve is defective or breaks, it will leak.

Mammograms can potentially cause an implant to break, especially with older implants or with a technician who is not trained to work with breast implants. (Make sure the mammogram technician knows you have implants and is qualified to do the procedure.)[75] Women who have had implants after a mastectomy do not need mammograms of the reconstructed breast. MRIs are useful for imaging both the breast and the implant when mammograms are not helpful or intolerable.

Women are also given the choice between a round or a teardrop-shaped implant. Though the teardrop seems like the best-looking choice, round implants are more resilient and have less chance of rupturing. The shape of the implant doesn't determine the shape of the breast. Rather, the pocket that the surgeon creates to put the implant into determines the shape of the breast because the implant will take the shape of the pocket.[76] (Before getting breast implants, check out the information at www.breastimplantinfo.org.)

At the end of the day, I would never judge women who have had implants or who want them, any more than I would judge women who have had their nose size and shape cosmetically altered.

Breast implants and the newer breast reconstruction methods can give women who have lost a breast to cancer a body image that approaches wholeness. This surgery can be key to a woman's healing. Dr. Sharon Webb, a plastic surgeon who specializes in breast reconstruction following breast cancer surgery, says that she often receives letters from her patients and their family members telling her how grateful they are for her work and how much the surgical breast reconstruction has contributed to their overall sense of well-being.

None of us is immune to our cultural inheritance and its impact on how we approach our breasts, and we need to exercise compassion for our own and other women's choices. Each woman has to decide for herself what feels best for her body and why. Here are a few stories concerning cosmetic breast surgery and its consequences.

Women's Stories

Janice: family pressure. Janice came to see me ostensibly for a routine annual physical exam. She had been there on two previous occasions for diaphragm fittings. A working woman, she was slim and attractive.

When I entered the exam room, she said that she had some other issues she wanted to discuss after her exam, so afterward she came into my office.

Janice told me that she had had a breast-enlargement procedure a few years before and that everything seemed fine. (My exam had confirmed that.) In my office, however, her eyes filled with tears, and she said she was afraid she would cry because she had something to ask me that she had never before asked a doctor. I suggested that she stay with her emotions because whenever we're moved in this way, we are on to something very important. She continued, "I first went to see a gynecologist when I was sixteen. I was having terrible menstrual cramps, and I wanted to see if anything was wrong with me. He wouldn't let my mother remain in the room with me when he examined me. His exam was very painful and I asked him to stop, but he wouldn't. Then when he saw my breasts, he laughed and said, 'Maybe if you marry and your husband fondles you enough, they'll grow.'" He prescribed birth control pills for her cramps, and she left the office feeling humiliated.

Janice went on to describe her early breast development. She said that at first her nipples had grown and started to stand out. It felt, she said, as if she had a walnut-size mass under each nipple. The tissue grew to about the size of an avocado pit and stopped. What she was describing was normal breast budding, with normal glandular tissue underneath the nipple. This had happened around the time she got her first period. I told her that it all sounded very normal to me. She cried again. Her breasts were naturally small, but her mother, her brother, and a sister had always referred to her as "deformed."

One day while clothes shopping with her mother, her mother commented on Janice's "deformity" and told her that if she ever wanted anything done about it, she'd be willing to pay for it. (I frequently hear stories of mothers telling their daughters that their breasts are not big enough. Sometimes they suggest that their daughters wear padded bras or stuff their bras with tissue.) Janice surprised her mother and said that she did in fact want something done. Soon after, she had an augmentation mammoplasty, or breast-enlargement procedure, with silicone implants.

I asked Janice how she felt about her breasts now. She replied that she had mixed feelings because of the circumstances under which she had had the surgery. Since she was also having acupuncture treatments and was more interested in natural healing than she had been in the past, she was afraid that she'd messed herself up by doing something so "unnatural."

My reply was to share with Janice that many women have elected to have their breasts enlarged and have been very happy with the procedure. The women who are happiest with it are those who have given it a lot of thought beforehand and are doing it to please themselves and not anyone else. These women usually have good results and no complications. When someone feels positive about a decision such as this, I believe that her immune system function is enhanced and that the complication rate is apt to be lower. I wanted Janice to know that I didn't think that having the breast surgery had damaged her health in any unalterable way.

Most important, I affirmed that she was normal, not "deformed," and that she had always been normal. She simply had small breasts, like all the women on her father's side of the family. Unfortunately, she had grown up in a family that was emotionally abusive about her body at a time when she was very vulnerable. Her visit to the gynecologist had reinforced that pathology.

Now, at the age of thirty-three, Janice was finally ready to bring up this history about her body. Before she left, she said to me, "You have no idea how important it is for me to hear this stuff from a doctor." I suggested that she spend the rest of the day staying with her tears and any other emotions that came up. I asked her to express them through sound. All of the tears and all of the emotions that we stifle stay in our physical bodies as unfinished business and are waiting for us to attend to them. Janice now had the opportunity to finish a significant amount of healing. She was ready to heal on all levels her relationship with her breasts.

Sarah: implants to please her husband. Sarah was about fifty-five when I first saw her. She had raised several children and had been married for twenty-five years to an alcoholic but was now divorced. As is so often the case with people like Sarah, her father had also been an alcoholic. Fifteen years before, Sarah's husband had become impotent. He had blamed her for his condition, telling her that her body just wasn't the way it needed to be for him to be able to get an erection.

Like so many women who are in dominator relationships, Sarah believed him and took on his problem as her own. Her husband said that maybe he wouldn't be impotent if her breasts were bigger. She dutifully went to New York and had breast implants placed. She hated them from the first, and her husband's impotence remained—except that now he told her something must be wrong with her vagina. Their relationship continued to deteriorate, and his drinking worsened.

Several years later Sarah's husband left her. (He is now with a younger woman, for whom we can all feel sorry.) Sarah went into code-pendence recovery and realized that she was *not* the cause of her hus-band's impotence and never had been. But now she is stuck with silicone implants that she hates. She said that when it's cold outside, her breasts don't get warm because it takes so long for the implants to warm up. She had apparently looked into having them removed but was told that it would cost her thousands of dollars, which her insurance wouldn't cover. Every day she is reminded of the price she's paid with her body. (Sometimes insurance will cover implant removal. And many plastic surgeons will remove them for a minor fee.)

Kim: implants to please herself. Kim is a vivacious woman in her late thirties. She works in the fashion industry now, but she was a teacher for years. When she was a teenager, she had large hips and very small breasts. She was never able to buy a suit because she could never find a top and a bottom that both fit. For years she was unhappy with her figure, even though she was a multitalented woman. She exercised and followed diets to correct as much of the imbalance as she could, and she elected to have her breasts enlarged after giving it years of thought. The procedure went beautifully and was healing for her because she chose this procedure under optimal circumstances: She did it for herself. She already had high self-esteem, and her expectations for the procedure were appropriate. She has never had a problem.

Beth: caught in the middle. Beth was a patient of mine for years. She had two pregnancies and nursed both children. Her husband left her after her second child was born, and she was raising her children by herself. She was independent and strong. Several years ago, she had a breast augmentation. After childbirth and nursing, her breasts seemed to be flaccid. She couldn't find a bra to fit, and she was uncomfortable with her appearance. She had always had a very at-tractive body. (I realize that this concept is loaded: Attractive to whom? Why? For what purpose?) In any case, though she had a very low income, she managed to get the money together to have her breasts enlarged. The outcome was excellent, and she was very pleased with the results. An anthropologist might say that her "so-cial" body was improved by this surgery. (She's currently at work on overcoming her uncanny ability to attract men who aren't support-ive of her.)

*   *   *

I believe that the circumstances surrounding a woman's breast implantation—why the surgery was done—are as crucial to her freedom from side effects as any potential problems from the silicone. Kim had implants so that she would be happier with her own appearance. Now everything matches, and she's content. I spoke with her recently, and she said she loves her implants and is certain she'll have no trouble with them. She was not concerned about the media hype that broke out shortly after her surgery. Now, nearly ten years later, she continues to be healthy. I believe that the same holds true, in general, for postmastectomy reconstruction patients and for those who have had implants to equalize the size of their breasts.

A HEALING PROGRAM FOR IMPLANTS

- You should understand that thousands of women have *no problems* with implants.

- If you're angry about any aspect of your implant procedure or care, give yourself a defined amount of time in which to express it and work it through, and then move on to forgiveness. Forgive yourself for everything you didn't know. Don't waste any of your precious energy beating up yourself—or anyone else.

- If you want to breast-feed, know that recent studies have failed to show any increased incidence of immune problems in babies whose mothers had silicone implants. (One study showed that women with implants were three times more likely to experience breast-feeding difficulty than women who haven't had breast surgery, but over 40 percent had no problem at all. Implants placed through an incision in the nipple were associated with the least success.)[77]

- Make sure that your diet supports your immune system. Include vegetables rich in beta-carotene, phytoestrogens, and plant lignans. (See chapter 17.) I also recommend a multivitamin-mineral supplement. Consider consulting a nutritionist.

- Castor oil packs applied to the breasts once per week are an excellent immune system enhancer and are also relaxing and soothing. I believe that taking the time to use packs lets your breasts know that you care for them. This could decrease any adverse effects from the implants. Regular breast massage also helps prevent hardened capsules from forming around the implants.

~ Understand that only you can decide what is best for you concerning implants or any other cosmetic surgery.

~ Take lots of omega-3 fats. I've been very pleased by how well the encapsulation on implants softens when women follow an inflammation-reducing diet that includes enough omega-3 fats.

Breast Surgery to Decrease Breast Size

Sharon's breasts started to develop when she was only eleven years old. By the time she was fifteen, she wore a size 38D bra. She felt embarrassed at school and was self-conscious about sports. Running was uncomfortable for her, and in the summer she developed painful rashes under her breasts from sweating. Buying clothing was difficult because her hips were slim relative to her chest. At about thirty she had a reduction mammoplasty—a breast-reduction procedure. Even though she now has visible scars across each breast, she is thrilled that she had the procedure done.

Erin, a strikingly beautiful woman in her thirties, came to see me for a tubal ligation. During her physical, I noticed that she had the characteristic scars of a breast-reduction procedure and asked her when she had had the surgery. She told me that she'd had it in her mid-twenties, because she had simply been tired of all the attention that she got from being both beautiful and having an ample breast size. Though her size had only been about 38C—not unusually large—she still had elected to have the procedure.

One of my friends has a jogging partner who is about a 38C as well. Men slow down their cars and make comments as she jogs by. Even twelve-year-old boys feel that they have the right to follow her on their bicycles and make comments!

These experiences are typical of women who have chosen to have their breast size reduced. Though this procedure often decreases or eliminates nipple sensation, leaves scars, and may make it difficult for a woman to nurse her baby, most of the women who've had this surgery are very happy with the results. Dr. Janet Hurley, a family physician and breast-feeding advocate in Calgary, Alberta, told me that in her practice, women can often nurse successfully following reduction mammoplasty, as long as they feel good about their choice to breast-feed and have no difficulty appreciating their breasts' normal function.

Women have had a range of experiences with cosmetic breast surgery. Plastic surgery of the breast or any other area of the body is neither right nor wrong—the demand for it merely reflects the values of our culture. The changes it effects can be very rewarding, but as Naomi Wolf so aptly points out in *The Beauty Myth*, they are not a panacea. Surgery will not heal a woman's life or her relationship with her body. The most important factor in a successful outcome, aside from a skilled surgeon, is the context in which the procedure is done and the expectations that the woman has of it.

The Power of the Mind to Affect Your Breasts

Research has shown that it is possible to increase breast size and firmness through hypnosis and creative visualization. In four separate studies, hypnosis not only increased breast size and firmness in those who completed twelve weeks of treatments, but it also resulted in decreased waist size and even weight loss in some. In one study, volunteers were asked to feel the warmth of a towel on their chests, or to otherwise feel a sensation of warmth in their breasts. Then they were asked to feel a pulsation in their breasts, and to merge that with their heartbeat, allowing heart energy to flow into their breasts. They were instructed to practice this same imagery in their home once per day for twelve weeks. At the end of this time period, 85 percent experienced measurable breast enlargement (the average was 1.37 inches). In this study, those who were good at visual imagery got better results, but even those who weren't good at it also got results. It did not matter how small a woman's breasts were to begin with; the technique also worked for women over age fifty.

In another study, the subjects were asked to go back in time, while in a mild trance, to an age between ten and twelve, when breasts normally start to grow. The suggestions for this group included feeling swelling sensations, tightness of the skin over the breast, and slight tenderness. The subjects were asked to put their hands on their breasts during the sessions, and the suggestion was made that the subject could feel her hands being gently pushed upward as her breasts grew larger. Usually, the subjects' hands could be observed to rise a few inches off the chest during the course of the suggestions. The third component of the treatment consisted of telling the subject that she was at a point in time two to three years later. It was suggested that she imagine herself after a shower, standing nude in front of the bathroom mirror. She was asked to inspect her appearance, noting the larger and more attractive breasts that resulted from the posthypnotic suggestions. The authors of this and other studies suggest that the reason breasts may not have achieved their full growth potential in adolescence is because there was some adverse message the girl was receiving about her femininity or her breasts. In one study, the researchers worked with the study participants to clear this material, but not always successfully. In the first study, more than half of the subjects dropped out "for personal reasons"; obviously, using hypnosis to regress to this vulnerable time may be fraught with emotional peril for some women, though if a woman can work through this safely, the potential for emotional healing (and getting full breast development) exists.

In a third study of eight women, ages twenty-one to thirty-five, who underwent hypnosis, all gained from one to two inches in breast size except one woman who didn't want to be a female at all and instead wished she were a man. The greatest breast-size gain in this study was made by the older women in the group who were married.[78] (Hypnosis CDs for increasing breast size are available on the internet; check out the products by certified hypnotherapist Wendi Friesen at www.wendi.com.)

Clearly, if women can use the power of focused intent and visualization to change their breast size and consistency, we also have the power to maintain and create healthy breasts by imagining our breasts as healthy and beautiful. If our bodies are nothing but a field of ideas, let's make sure that those ideas represent our best interests.

CARING FOR YOUR BREASTS

Our task as women is to learn, minute by minute, to respect ourselves and our bodies—whether we have small breasts or large breasts, implants or mastectomies. When we can appreciate our breasts as potential or actual sources of nourishment and pleasure for both ourselves and others, our breast health begins to improve immediately.

When you touch your breasts each month, do so with respect and caring. Thank your breasts, chest, and heart area for being a part of your body. Forgive yourself if you've continually showered messages on them that they're too large, too small, too droopy, or too lumpy. Commit to respecting your breasts and accepting them as worthy parts of your body. If you still think they're ugly after a week or so, respect them anyway—as an act of courage. Eventually, your attitude will soften. Remember, thoughts and feelings have *physical* effects. Open yourself to receiving help, nourishment, and compassion from yourself and others. When you experience events that cause you sorrow, resentment, or pain, allow yourself to quite literally get these feelings off your chest by experiencing your emotions fully, grieving fully, and then letting go so that you can "make a clean breast of it."

Dr. Barbara Joseph, an OB/GYN who was diagnosed with breast cancer while nursing her third child, wrote the following to-do list during her healing process. It works equally well for prevention.

- ~ Be gentle with myself
- ~ Love myself
- ~ Be kind to myself
- ~ Take care of myself
- ~ Ask for what I need
- ~ Say no to what I don't want

I would add to this list: Nourish yourself well. Enjoy eating delicious whole, high-quality food daily.

If You've Had Breast Cancer

If you've had a mastectomy, touching your scar with respect and reverence is a help—an acknowledgment of your sacrifice. A thirty-eight-year-old midwife whom I met at a conference had had a breast removed at the age of twenty-one. She said that in looking back, she realized that she had profoundly rejected her breasts early on in life because she'd been given the message since birth that she should have been a boy. She attributed her breast cancer to her chronic negativity about being female. Now, more than twenty years after her mastectomy, she has decided to discard her prosthesis. She told me that the "fake" breast created a block between her chest, her heart, and the loving energy that this part of her body needed to feel. She said that now when she gets a hug from someone, all of her chest gets in on that loving energy, too.

Breast reconstruction following mastectomy can be a blessing. If this is your truth, spend some moments regularly appreciating the work of the surgeon, combined with the healing power of your body.

Acknowledge that your body knows how to heal and be healthy, regardless of where you are now. Get support from those who've been there and transformed the experience. A good starting place is Dr. Barbara Joseph's book *My Healing from Breast Cancer* (Keats, 1996).

Brenda Michaels, whom I mentioned earlier, told me that when she was diagnosed with her third recurrence of cancer, she didn't think in terms of "fighting" her cancer. Instead, she figured that her body had created it for a reason and that her body could heal it. So she asked her cancer what it needed from her. The answer was love. At first she was afraid that if she gave it love, it would grow. But then as she thought about it more, she realized that love won't make a cancer grow; rather, it will help the body transform any abnormality. As she allowed more and more love and appreciation for herself and others to work their magic in her life, her cancer (and her life) were transformed. Brenda's is not an isolated case. Research on women who had recurrence of their breast cancers showed that those who expressed more joy tended to live longer than those who didn't. This finding was highly statistically significant.[79]

Ask yourself the following: Which aspects of my life could use more appreciation? Which aspect of myself could use more appreciation? Which relationships am I in that fully nurture me? Which ones do not? Spend five minutes each day appreciating some aspect of your life, no matter how small. What we pay attention to expands.

Take fifteen seconds five times per day and think about someone or something (like a pet or a young child) you love unconditionally. Put your hand over your heart area when you do this. With practice, you'll be able to feel a warm, tingling sensation in your chest area. This is energy that heals your heart—and your breasts.

11
Our Fertility

A fertile, sexually active woman using no contraception would face an average of fourteen births or thirty-one abortions during her reproductive lifetime: altogether, a mind-boggling disruption in this period of hoped-for independence and equality for women.
— Dr. Luella Klein, former president of the
American College of Obstetrics and Gynecology, 1984

A broader vision of fertility is one that is not solely determined by whether or not one has a biological child. Fertility is a lifelong relationship with oneself—not a medical condition.
— Joan Borysenko, Ph.D.

Ideally, prenatal life, close to the mother's heart, is bliss for the unborn. Women need to choose to live out their pregnancies wisely, because the way they do so affects both themselves and their offspring. Though Sigmund Freud coined the term "infant amnesia" to explain the fact that most people don't recall much that happened to them before the age of three, several decades of research reported in peer-review literature (plus the experience of many clinicians and their patients) has established beyond a shadow of a doubt that parents have a huge influence on the mental and physical attributes of their children—and this influence starts long before birth.[1]

All of us retain the imprint of our entire lives within our cells, starting before birth. Our lives begin in the water of amniotic fluid, our first environment. If, during those vulnerable first nine months, a mother is emotionally unavailable to her baby—for whatever reason—her baby will pick up on this. Prenatal and birth memories, and their potential impact on the unborn, are one of many reasons why women must learn to manage their fertility well and learn how to conceive consciously. We must become conscious vessels.

When a child perceives that she is loved and wanted from the very beginning, her sense of safety, security, and belonging creates an enormously resilient immune system as well as bone and blood health that set the stage for a lifetime of health. On the other hand, many women have told me that they knew their mother didn't want them, and that they had felt it their entire lives. "I know I was conceived during my mother's grief for a son who died nine months before," one woman said. "I remember taking this on in utero. I vowed to try to make it better for her. I've spent sixty-four years trying to do that for her. It has never worked." One menopausal woman, Beverly, said that her mother visited her on her fiftieth birthday with balloons and a rose, then proceeded to tell her, "You are fifty. Your life is downhill from now on. You're not a kid anymore." She told her daughter how much she had suffered in giving birth to her, and she went on to say that when Beverly was born, she had been ugly. She sang the praises of her son, however—Beverly's brother—saying that that labor had been virtually painless and that her son had been beautiful ever since birth. Listening to her mother, Beverly felt that in a perverse way she had been given a true gift on her fiftieth birthday. Her mother had confirmed what she had always thought—that she had been rejected since birth.

An existential depression can be felt by people who have been gestated and born under circumstances in which they are not wanted. One woman described feeling ashamed for breathing the air and for taking up space—she had a sense of never belonging, that she was causing someone else pain simply by being here. She told me that she had felt this as far back as she could remember. She knew that she hadn't been wanted.

Another woman, a physician in her fifties, said that she recently had gone through an emotional healing session in which she realized that she had never felt safe in her mother's womb—that she knew she hadn't been wanted. She had been trying to compensate for this her whole life by studying, becoming a doctor, and having a series of relationships. But none of this ever fulfilled a need that had been within her since before she was born—the need to be well loved and desired as a child. As she recalled, "My mother's heartbeat, so close to my own, was *not* a comfort and reassurance to me." Though her mother is now dead, she had gone through the process of forgiving her. In tears she said to me, "Now I finally miss the mother I never had. I realize that she was doing the best she could. She never had a chance for herself."

ABORTION

For many women, abortion is an area of "unfinished business," and as such it deserves a thorough discussion. If we lived in a culture that valued women's autonomy and in which men and women practiced cooperative birth control, the abortion issue would be moot. If abortion were forced on women in the United States as it is in China today, it would hold a different meaning here than it does now.[2]

Abortion deliberately ends one potential life. But *not* allowing an abortion potentially murders two lives. The bond between mother and child is the most intimate bond in human experience. In this most primary of human relationships, love, welcome, and receptivity should be present in abundance. Forcing a woman to bear and raise a child against her will is therefore an act of violence. It constricts and degrades the mother-child bond and sows the seeds of hatred rather than love. Can there be any worse entry into the universe than forcing a child to inhabit a body that is hostile to it? Life is too valuable to inhibit its full blossoming and potential by forcing a woman to bear it against her will. Since we know that the early lives of criminals and societal offenders are often filled with poverty and despair, it may even be dangerous to bring a being into the world who isn't wanted. (In their best-selling book *Freakonomics* [William Morrow, 2005], authors Steven Levitt and Stephen Dubner hypothesize that the reduction in crime over the past few decades can be traced to the legalization of abortion!) The specter of more and more women trapped in unwanted pregnancies looms on the horizon as women's reproductive capacity is treated as political barter.

On some level, everyone knows this—even those who publicly would deny women the right to control their own fertility. During my residency in Boston, it was not uncommon for pregnant young Catholic women to be brought to me by their parents, who would say, "We don't believe in abortion, but if our daughter has this child, it could ruin her life. Can you arrange something?"

One thing I've learned over the years is that there is no such thing as sexual freedom. I think that's why I've always been uncomfortable with the phrase "abortion on demand." Having worked in the area of women's reproduction for years, I realize that the current abortion debate is a symptom of the much deeper problem I described in earlier chapters: As long as women continue to misunderstand how to meet their erotic needs, as long as they continue to sacrifice their bodies for the sexual pleasure of men, we will get nowhere. And as long as abortion is seen solely as a "women's issue," we'll get nowhere.

I performed abortions for years, and I will always be a proponent of reproductive choice for women. But along the way I've come to see how complex the issue of abortion is, and I've learned that there are no easy answers.

Abortion is always a loaded topic because it forces each woman to face her deepest feelings about men's ability to impregnate women and women's power to either retain or reject the result of this impregnation. Abortion hits at the heart of our society's beliefs about the role of women. Is society committed to women's full participation in the economy? What is our appropriate role in the home and in society? "Abortion exemplifies political control of the personal and the physiological," writes historian Carroll Smith-Rosenberg. "It thus bridges the intensely individual and the broadly political. On every level, to talk of abortion is to speak of power."[3]

I always felt as though I were sitting in the middle of a minefield when I performed abortions. Sometimes I got angry when I performed a fourth abortion on a woman who simply didn't use contraception. At other times I'd perform abortions on women who really didn't want them but felt they had no alternative. Of course many unintended pregnancies happen in women who use contraception religiously and their method failed.

The call for "abortion on demand" implies that women need take no responsibility for their sexual behavior or its consequences. It implies that it's fine to have intercourse with whomever we wish, whenever we wish, and without having to deal with the consequences—just as men have done for centuries. Many women who have had repeated abortions have told me that they later came to realize that their sexual acting-out with men was a form of self-abuse, stemming from their self-loathing and lack of self-esteem. "Abortion on demand" implies that having sex somehow can and should be divorced from the other aspects of our lives, such as the need to be nurtured, held, or respected. It implies that the same behavior that we find abhorrent in men—having sex with no heed for its consequences—is okay for women. Why would women want to imitate (some) men in the sexual arena? We should be resisting *any* sexual contact with men who don't also respect our souls and our innermost selves.[4] As we begin the twenty-first century, many women are rethinking their sexual programming. The first step in this process is to get clear on what that programming is.

When a woman chooses to have an abortion on behalf of herself and her own life, she is swimming against a five-thousand-year-old tide of conditioning, of social agendas propounded by churches and other male-dominated institutions, that say that women's primary purpose is to have children and to serve her children and her husband. Allowing women to choose the course of their own lives goes very deeply against a very old grain.

Over the past twenty years, as the number of women going against this grain has vastly increased, the political and societal forces that want to "keep us in our place" are becoming more vocal—and more destructive. A century and a half of rhetoric designed to make women feel guilt and shame surrounding abortion and choosing self-development over motherhood (at least for a time) leaves little wonder that abortion is not an easy issue for women to talk about freely. Yet if every woman who ever had an abortion, or even one-third of them, were willing to speak out about her experience—not in shame, but with honesty about where she was then, what she learned, and where she is now—this whole issue would heal a great deal faster.

Since the first edition of this book, many women have written to me expressing their gratitude that I have addressed this issue. And they have written about how their willingness to tell the truth about their abortion experience has healed them. Kris Bercov, a therapist who offers abortion resolution counseling, has written a poignant booklet entitled "The Good Mother: An Abortion Parable."[5] When she sent me a copy, Kris wrote, "The abortion experience has tremendous potential to either wound or to heal—depending on how it is handled and interpreted. As you well know, so many women go through the experience unconsciously—leaving their bodies the challenging (and sometimes dangerous) task of communicating the women's unresolved feelings." Kris's book is revolutionary specifically because it helps women feel their way through the experience—and thus heal it. It has been used effectively in several abortion clinics. (See note 5 for ordering information.)

The cultural climate of any historical era can have profound effects on the overall emotional and physical well-being of that era's people. It is estimated that in the 1840s half of all pregnancies ended in abortion.[6] Currently, as women's power is rising, so is the antiabortion rhetoric. Though no culture at any time in history has been a stranger to abortion, Carroll Smith-Rosenberg's research documents that abortion becomes a political issue only when there are "significant alternations in the balance of power between women and men, and of male heads of household over their traditional dependents."[7] At just such a time, these changes are reflected in laws concerning women's right to manage their own fertility.

Healing Postabortion Traumas

The technical aspects of the various abortion procedures are very simple and don't usually cause women any physical problems, though it is always somewhat of a shock to the body when the process of gestation is abruptly halted via outside intervention. All the studies done so far on the long-term health consequences of abortion, whether done by D&C or suction, have failed to show an increase in infertility or other problems. The antiprogesterone drug mifepristone (formerly known as RU486) is even safer than D&C or suction abortions. When it is used with misoprostol, a prostaglandin, its efficacy rate is 95.5 percent, and it can be administered confidentially in a health care practitioner's office. This drug works to block the action of progesterone and is usually used within fifty days of a woman's last menstrual period. Medication abortions are very effective and safe—and a big step forward in women's health. (See www.plannedparenthood.org.)

With decades of guilt and shame as an emotional backdrop, however, many women never adequately process the emotional aspects of abortion. Many have never even told another person that they had one. Not infrequently, a woman will tell me not to tell her husband about the abortion she had prior to their relationship because she doesn't want him to know about her sexual history. Through the years, I've heard many women's stories about illegal abortions—some of them painful, and some quite healing. Several women in their sixties, for example, have told me that they were raped by the abortionist before he performed the procedure—"just to relax you," he would tell them. Because they were so scared and so dependent upon his services, they simply went through the humiliation and said nothing about it for decades. Another woman who had gone through an illegal abortion said that she would be forever grateful to the wonderful man who did her procedure. She felt that his gentle touch and medical skill were a godsend to the many unfortunate women such as herself, in a time when choice wasn't available. May we never see that time again.

The physical results of a woman's shame and regret about abortion can live on in her cell tissue for years. This is one of the reasons why, when the supposed link between abortion and breast cancer was first reported, it seemed plausible; however, a 1996 study failed to substantiate this link.[8] Unresolved emotional pain becomes physical and can set the stage for later gynecological problems such as fibroids and pelvic pain. Remember, it is the *meaning* surrounding an event or procedure that gives it its charge and potential to harm or heal—not necessarily the procedure itself. Despite the safety of abortion, I believe that repeated abortions weaken the *hara,* or body energy center, of the female.

The most difficult abortions I ever did were in those women who had already had one or two children and had homes and resources, but who found themselves pregnant at inconvenient times. I told one of these women, whose husband didn't want the pregnancy, that she might well find herself grieving after this abortion, since she herself clearly wanted the child and was having the procedure mainly to keep peace with her husband. She assured me that she had made a firm decision—that she was finished with car seats for infants and diapers and that she wanted to get on with her life. So I went ahead. Exactly one week later, this woman was back in the office crying, "Why didn't you tell me how bad I'd feel? Why didn't you talk me out of this procedure?" She decided that she wanted to get pregnant again as soon as possible, to "relieve her sense of loss."

Time and time again, women have abortions that they don't want because the men they are with insist upon it. Under these circumstances abortion is a self-betrayal, even a kind of self-rape. It can poison the relationship unless the issues are dealt with openly and honestly. The first step is for a woman to be totally honest with herself about how she really feels.

A patient of mine in her fifties developed continual spotting and an abnormal condition in her uterus called cystic and adenomatous hyperplasia of the endometrium, accompanied by pelvic pain. (See chapter 5.) This problem, she feels, was triggered by watching her daughter give birth to a girl and experiencing her husband's unconditional support for this birth. This birth experience caused her to feel a great deal of anger at her husband and a sense of deep sorrow—emotions that she couldn't understand intellectually. Later, after letting herself sit with these feelings, she realized that she still had unfinished business about an abortion she'd had years before that she hadn't wanted. Her husband hadn't been supportive of the pregnancy, so she had gone ahead with the abortion. She is now in the process of doing some belated healing.

In the mid-1980s, I stopped doing abortion. I was tired of mucking around in women's ambivalence about their fertility, and I was tired of performing repeated abortions on women who came back every year for the procedure. I needed to take a break from this arena for a while and preferred to work on other aspects of the problem—like helping women understand their sexuality and their need for self-respect and self-esteem, regardless of whether they had a male relationship.

At this time, many women are simply neither ready nor able to assume dominion over their own fertility and sexuality. We are still evolving on this point. Abortion as a means of contraception will be necessary in this country for a long while to come, and I will support its availability. Still, I look forward to the day when abortion is rare, when women and men in cooperation will conceive carefully, thoughtfully, and purposefully, and every child will be wanted and cared for.

HEALING PAST ABORTION: THOUGHTS TO CONSIDER

~ Were you well supported, counseled, and well informed?

~ Did you take time off from your daily routine for a day or two?

~ Did you grieve at all? Did you feel the need to?

~ Did you feel guilty about it? If so, do you still feel that way?

~ Did your early religious upbringing reinforce the idea that having an abortion and choosing your own life were wrong?

~ Can you forgive yourself now for what you didn't know then?

~ Were you able to share the experience with your family or a trusted friend? Did they support you? If you had it to do over again, would you?

~ Can you reframe the abortion in your mind as an act of courage—an act of reclaiming your power?

~ For some women, the choice of an abortion is a celebration on behalf of self. If that is the case for you, congratulations. If not, what did you learn?

Another View of Abortion

I first heard about communication with the unborn from Gladys McGarey, M.D., M.D.(H.), in her book *Born to Live* (Inkwell Productions, 2001). Dr. McGarey writes of her many years of delivering babies both at home and in the hospital. Her deeply spiritual approach to medicine and women's health care has been a great comfort and guide to me over the years, particularly as it relates to the abortion issue. She tells the following story: "I can see that abortion is frequently reasonable, understandable, and the 'right' thing to do. The new light dawned with a story one of my patients told me some time ago. This mother had a four-year-old daughter, named Dorothy, whom she would take out to lunch occasionally. They were talking about this and that, and the child would shift from one subject to another, when Dorothy suddenly said, 'The last time I was a little girl, I had a different mommy!' Then she started talking in a different language, which her mother tried to record.

"The magic moment seemed over, but then Dorothy continued, 'But that wasn't the last time. Last time when I was four inches long and in your tummy, Daddy wasn't ready to marry you yet, so I went away. But then, I came back." Then, the mother reported, the child went back to chatting about four-year-old matters.

"The mother was silent. No one but her husband, the doctor, and she had known this, but she had become pregnant about two years before she and her husband were ready to get married. She decided to have an abortion. She was ready to have the child, but her husband-to-be was not.

"When the two of them did get married and were ready to have their first child, the same entity made its appearance. And the little child was saying, in effect, 'I don't hold any resentments toward you for having the abortion. I understood. I knew why it was done, and that's okay. So here I am again. It was an experience. I learned from it and you learned from it, so now, let's get on with the business of life.' "[9]

My own sister, the mother of three strong-willed and active sons, became pregnant inadvertently when she ovulated during her menstrual cycle—a rare event. She knew that the pregnancy was not right for her—in fact, she felt that it was actively *wrong* on all levels. So she began to work on communicating with the unborn baby, asking its soul to leave. She continued this inner work daily for two weeks. Still she remained pregnant. Finally, she called an abortion clinic to make an appointment, a step she had never dreamed that she would make. No sooner had she hung up the phone than the bleeding started. She miscarried later that day.

Stories such as this one shed a whole new light on abortion. Caroline Myss is very clear that the energy of spirits remains behind after abortion and needs to be fully released. Many ancient traditional cultures acknowledge this as well. (See the story of a patient who went to a Native American shaman for healing around three past abortions that were still emotionally unresolved, in chapter 6.)

In 1985, while I was attending an international meeting of the Pre- and Perinatal Psychology Association, I participated in a healing abortion ritual performed by Jeannine Parvati Baker, author of *Conscious Conception* (North Atlantic Books, 1986). Baker had learned the ritual from a Native American medicine woman. All the women at the meeting who had had abortions and those who had been deeply affected by them sat in an inner circle. Included in this group were a man whose mother had unsuccessfully tried to abort him, and a man whose wife had aborted a child he had wanted. In an outer circle surrounding this one sat all of us who had ever seen or done an abortion. We were considered the "eyes" that had witnessed abortion. The outermost circle also included people whose friends and loved ones had had abortions. They were the "ears" that had witnessed abortion. Throughout an entire afternoon and into the evening, both men and women spoke of—and let go of—years of previously unvoiced personal pain surrounding abortion. Baker, representing a conduit between the worlds, helped release the energy of the aborted spirit. For many, it was a powerful healing.

Each woman's situation is unique regarding whether to have or keep a pregnancy, and no one but that individual woman can or should decide. Whatever her choice is, however, there will be consequences. What is important is that each woman be clear that she had a choice.

EMERGENCY CONTRACEPTION: ABORTION PREVENTION

Emergency contraception has been available in the United States and Europe for more than twenty years as an off-label use of birth control pills. An example would be to take two tablets of Ovral brand at once, followed by another two white tablets twenty-four hours later. In 1997, the FDA declared this regimen both safe and effective in preventing pregnancy. In September of 1998, the first dedicated emergency contraceptive product (known as Preven Emergency Contraceptive Kit) was approved for sale in the United States.[10] The most recent brand of emergency contraception is known as Plan B and consists of the progestin levonorgestril. Studies have shown that having emergency contraception available to sexually active young adults does not result in an overuse of the emergency contraception. In fact it is estimated that regular use of emergency contraception could cut the number of unintended pregnancies and abortions in half.[11]

Emergency contraception prevents pregnancy by inhibiting or delaying ovulation or altering the lining of the uterus, making it inhospitable to implantation of an egg. It also alters sperm and egg transport. (It does NOT cause abortion of an established pregnancy.)

If a woman needs emergency contraception, she needs to take a pregnancy test first. If she is not pregnant, she should take her first dose within seventy-two hours of a previous act of intercourse. The next dose should be taken twelve hours later. Side effects include nausea in some patients. To counteract this, a doctor can prescribe an antinausea drug, which should be taken one hour before each dose of pills. The vast majority of women will menstruate within twenty-one days after treatment. Having an IUD inserted will also prevent pregnancy; I recommend this only for those who are at a very low risk for sexually transmitted disease, are in a monogamous relationship, and will want to continue this birth control method.

The emergency contraceptive Plan B is so effective and safe that in 2004 the FDA's Center for Drug Evaluation and Research strongly recommended that it be granted over-the-counter status. Unfortunately, on August 26, 2005, the FDA decided to disregard the findings of its own scientific panel and delay its approval. In an editorial in the *New England Journal of Medicine*, Susan Wood, assistant commissioner for Women's Health and director of the Office of Women's Health at the Food and Drug Administration, explained why she resigned from her position. She wrote, "The agency leadership had chosen to delay indefinitely a decision about switching emergency contraception to nonprescription status. I believed that in doing so, they were disregarding the scientific and clinical evidence and the established review process and were taking an action that harms women's health by denying them appropriate access to a product that can reduce the rate of unplanned pregnancies and the need for abortion."[12]

In a dominator society, many ideologic battles are, unfortunately, fought on the soil of women's bodies and choices. (See Resources for more information, including a toll-free hotline and website that can help you locate a provider in your area.)

Taking Matters into Our Own Hands

I've always felt that ancient women must have known how to control their own fertility through methods that have been lost in the mists of time. In Chinese medicine, there are twenty-four acupuncture/acupressure points that are known as the Forbidden Points. When Jeanne Blum, acupressurist and holistic healer, began to research these points, she found that they have been called "forbidden" for centuries precisely because of their power to terminate a pregnancy. What Blum also found, however, was that by learning these points and manually stimulating them at the right time, women could learn how to control their cycles at will. Thus, the Forbidden Points system can, with practice, be used as a form of birth control or to terminate an early pregnancy.

Though I could find no research documenting use of the points in this way, Blum's ongoing work with many clients and the feedback she has received from women using her book attest to the effectiveness of this system if used properly. The points and complete instructions for their use can be found in her book *Woman Heal Thyself: An Ancient Healing System for Contemporary Women* (Charles E. Tuttle, 1996). These same points can be used to relieve and heal PMS, endometriosis, dysmenorrhea, and other menstrual problems.

CONSCIOUS CONCEPTION AND CONTRACEPTION

If women expect to improve our personal and professional status in the world, we have no choice but to assume responsibility for our creations and to reclaim our power. This is especially true when it comes to having babies. Women have now reached a time in our planetary history when we must learn to procreate from our conscious choice, not just to fill up an empty space inside ourselves or to try to keep a man. These latter reasons for getting pregnant are remnants of an unconscious tribal programming that no longer serves us. Jeannine Parvati Baker describes herself as both prochoice *and* prolife: When she was seventeen, she made a decision that she was ready to become sexually active. She also vowed that she would never make love with a man whose child she wouldn't willingly bear, should she become pregnant inadvertently. She says that it took her three years to find such a man. Now that is a powerful example of taking responsibility for what we create! Baker's story, like the stories of birthing women in chapter 12, are beacons for how women might be if they loved and appreciated their bodies and their creative capacities.

To women who are contemplating pregnancy, I suggest that they spend some time meditating and praying alone or together with their partner for guidance around the prospect of having a child. Traditional Tibetan women have always spent time in prayer and meditation before conceiving. I believe that there are thousands of souls waiting to incarnate. Not all of them are highly evolved. When you raise your vibration through conscious prayer and meditation, you make it more likely that you'll conceive a like-minded soul! You can do this even if you're considering single-parenthood through donor insemination! The important point is to see your body as a channel for a new spirit and to surrender yourself to the experience—to be open to all that it has to teach you. (For those women who are considering single motherhood, I recommend the book *Single Mothers by Choice* [Times Books, 1994]) by Jane Mattes, C.S.W; for more information on single motherhood and support for single mothers, visit www.singlemothers.org.)

All the currently available methods of birth control—pills, IUDs, diaphragms, condoms, and the rest—have their place. (See table 6, page 412.) Unfortunately, many health care practitioners do not present birth control methods objectively. When I was in medical school and residency, there was a tendency to push oral contraceptives as the optimal method of birth control and to downplay the reliability of the diaphragm and condoms. This hasn't changed in over thirty years. Given our cultural approach to control of the female body, this is not surprising. The pill (and now the patch) is easy to prescribe, easy to take, very reliable, and very convenient. We can use it to manipulate our menstrual cycles, avoiding periods altogether or on weekends. In short, it fits our cultural ideal. The pill is the most-studied medication in history. Unfortunately, because it's made from synthetic non-bioidentical hormones, it has more side effects than it should!

Most other birth control methods require more education about the body and more active participation than the pill. They are not geared to the average busy doctor's schedule. Many physicians feel that women will not use barrier methods of contraception, such as diaphragms, condoms, or contraceptive foam, because they have seen too many "failures." This is true of some women but not all women. The data show that in the women who are ideal users—who use the method correctly every time—barrier methods and even "fertility awareness" (natural family planning) can be 95 to 98 percent effective.[13]

It is important to distinguish between the failure of a birth control method itself and the failure of a woman to use it properly. Many women are socialized to be available for sexual intercourse without involving their partners in contraceptive responsibility. Many women are involved with men who will not cooperate with contraception and feel that it is the woman's job. Though I'd like to suggest that it is not worth having sex with such men, I know that this is not always an option—especially in the all-too-common situation when domestic violence is an issue. Obviously, it is best for women in this situation to use a contraceptive method that requires no male cooperation. Such methods include birth control pills, the birth control patch, NuvaRing, the IUD, Depo-Provera, tubal ligation, and the Reality female condom. Methods that require conscious partner participation, such as condoms, simply are not appropriate for these women. In fact, in one study, when the Philadelphia Department of Public Health offered a choice of birth control to a group of low-income women, the majority chose the Reality female condom because this method gives more control over their risk of pregnancy and infection than they otherwise would have experienced.

In order to choose the right birth control method for you, you need to decide *honestly* where you are in your own life—and how much responsibility you are willing to assume over your fertility. Some women don't even want to think about getting to know their times of ovulation and checking their cervical mucus, let alone inserting a diaphragm before each intercourse. That's fine—they often do well on the pill or another "automatic" method. Other women prefer barrier methods, such as diaphragms, and I encourage these methods, too—but only in those women who are committed to using them consciously. I've worked repeatedly with women who've had three or four abortions from failure to use so-called unnatural contraceptives; the pill would have been a better choice for these women, given their sexual behavior. But they refuse to put anything "unnatural" in their bodies. I counsel that there is nothing *natural* about abortion when a woman fails to use her "natural" method of birth control conscientiously. These women, though conscious about food and the environment, often suffer from the mind/body split we've all inherited—that it is part of being a desirable woman to be available sexually, without asking our partners to share in the responsibility. This is a shame, particularly given that there are so many ways to express oneself sexually without the risk of unintended pregnancy. (See chapter 8, "Reclaiming the Erotic.") I recommend that all women make every effort to put their own sexual and fertility needs first in every relationship. Doing so takes courage and support.

Intrauterine Device

The intrauterine device (IUD) is a good choice for some women, though it may carry an increased risk of pelvic infection. I've worked with women who've done beautifully with the IUD for up to twenty years. IUDs are associated with an increased risk of tubal pregnancy. They are also associated with increased cramping and bleeding in some women. They work best for women who've had a child.

When I was a medical student, I noticed that women with IUDs seemed to get more infections. The manufacturers of these devices and many doctors denied the problem for a while. At that time, Dalkon shields were being touted as *the* contraceptive of choice for young women who'd had no children. The results were devastating for the many women who tried the product and became victims of its side ef-

●

fects. The Dalkon shield has since been taken off the market. Other far safer IUDs are now available and are, in my opinion, underutilized given their safety and effectiveness.

Combined Hormone Methods

Oral Contraceptives (The Pill)

Oral contraceptives have been a boon for many women, though they may contribute to suboptimal nutrition and an increased incidence of yeast infection in many (the pill has been associated with lowered serum levels of B vitamins and other metabolic changes).[14] It is also associated with a slightly increased risk for cervical adenocarcinoma[15] and elevated triglyceride levels.[16] Although the announcement didn't get much press in the U.S., the World Health Organization has classified birth control pills with combined estrogen and progestin (as well as combined-hormone HRT) as carcinogenic. (The latest such designation came after the cancer research agency of the World Health Organization convened a group of twenty-one scientists from eight countries in France in June 2005. Reviewing the scientific literature on the pill and cancer, the group pointed to evidence for an increase in cervical cancer, breast cancer, and liver cancer in making its decision, while also stressing that convincing evidence existed for a protective effect against endometrial and ovarian cancers.)[17] Yet other authorities don't think the slightly increased relative risk for breast cancer is significant.[18] In my experience, the pill is also associated with mood swings, weight gain, and decreased sex drive in many women.

Going off the pill makes many women feel much better, although not all symptoms always subside. Ironically, new research is showing that oral contraceptives might actually contribute to long-term sexual dysfunction in some women. The January 2006 issue of *The Journal of Sexual Medicine* reports that the pill lowers levels of testosterone, even after the women have stopped taking oral contraceptives. Such problems occur because pill users have elevated levels of a protein called sex hormone binding globulin (SHBG) that binds testosterone, rendering it unavailable for use by the body. Such low values of "unbound" testosterone potentially lead to side effects such as decreased desire, arousal, and lubrication and increased sexual pain. Although the research showed that such problems persisted even after the pill was discontinued, long-term studies are still needed to determine if the problems are permanent.[19]

Health benefits of the pill also include lowered risk of ovarian cancer, endometrial cancer, acne, and pelvic inflammatory disease. In general, the pill's benefits outweigh its risks for the vast majority of women because the health risks from unintended pregnancies far outweigh any risk from the pill. Women who are on the pill should take a good multivitamin-mineral supplement containing B complex. The majority of women who have serious health problems with the pill are smokers. Smokers should not use the pill after the age of thirty-five. Oral contraceptives are now being used for women right up until menopause, at which time these same women may start on estrogen replacement therapy. Such women are on chemical birth control or hormone replacement for most of their adult lives. When a woman uses hormones in this way, she misses out on the messages she'd normally get from her uterus and ovaries (as discussed in chapters 6 and 7).

The Ring (NuvaRing)

The contraceptive ring, approved by the FDA in 2001, is a flexible ring about two inches in diameter that is inserted into the vagina and held in place by the muscles in the vaginal wall. The ring is worn continually for three weeks (including during sex) and then it's removed for seven days to allow a menstrual period. After seven days, a new ring is inserted.

Like the pill, the ring contains low doses of estrogen and progestin, which are absorbed by the walls of the vagina and distributed throughout the bloodstream in a steady supply to suppress ovulation. Because users don't have to remember to take a pill at the same time each day, women who use the ring have fewer hormonal ups and downs. As with the pill, users also experience more regular, lighter, and shorter menstrual periods, and fertility returns quickly after use of the product is stopped. When used as directed, the effectiveness rate is 99 percent.

Initial side effects are similar to those of the birth control pill and include weight gain or loss, nausea, moodiness, and breast tenderness. However, some users have also reported increased vaginal discharge, vaginitis, and irritation. The risk of getting blood clots may also be greater with the type of progestin in this product than with some of the low-dose pills on the market. As with the pill, women over the age of thirty-five who smoke should not use this form of birth control.

In addition, certain medicines—including the antibiotic rifampin, certain drugs used to treat mental illness or to control seizures, certain oral anti-fungals prescribed for yeast infections, or certain HIV protease inhibitors—may make the ring less effective. (For more information, see www.nuvaring.com.)

The Patch (Ortho Evra)

The birth control patch, also approved by the FDA in 2001, is applied to the upper arm, upper torso, abdomen, or buttocks, and replaced once a week for three consecutive weeks. It's then removed for one week to allow a menstrual period. Like the ring, the patch delivers a steady flow of estrogen and progestin absorbed into the bloodstream to prevent ovulation. It's also 99 percent effective when used correctly.

Most side effects are similar to those of the pill, although trials showed that breast discomfort and dysmenorrhea are significantly more common in women using the patch than in those using the pill. Also, the estrogen levels in women who use the Ortho Evra patch are 60 percent higher than estrogen levels in women taking standard birth control pills. The increased estrogen may raise the risk of blood clots (some of which are fatal) and may also, after several years of use, cause other side effects, as well. Studies are currently looking into the risks of this higher estrogen level.[20] Some women also report an increase in depression, changes in sexual desire, and a skin reaction at the site where the patch is applied.

The patch may also be less effective for women weighing over 198 pounds, those taking St. John's wort, or those using the same medications listed above that make the contraceptive ring less effective. And as with the ring and birth control pills, women on the patch who smoke are at greater chance for cardiovascular problems. (For more information, see www.orthoevra.com.)

Progestin-Only Contraceptives

Norplant (which is no longer available) and Depo-Provera are both made from synthetic progestins. Norplant is a set of capsules that were inserted under the skin of the upper arm under local anesthesia. Women who've had them inserted can still continue to use them until their effectiveness expires. Depo-Provera is given as a shot at twelve-week intervals. Synthetic progestin of all kinds can result in headache, bloating, and irritability in some women. This last effect is so common that a professor of OB/GYN with an interest in natural hormones once remarked, "It's no wonder Depo-Provera works for birth control. It makes women so ornery, they don't want anyone near them." Irregular spotting and acne are other problems with these methods. On the other hand, they are highly effective and "automatic" compared with other methods, and they work well for some women.

Barrier Methods

A wide range of barrier contraceptive methods are available. Condoms have the distinct advantage of protecting individuals from STDs. Many couples alternate between condoms and diaphragm use, thus sharing responsibility for contraceptives. See table 6 (page 412) for a list of barrier contraceptive options, all of which have their place.

Outercourse

Outercourse is just about any form of sex play that does not involve intercourse, making pregnancy impossible (as long as care is taken that no semen gets onto the vulva or in the vagina). Some of the most common forms include oral sex and manual stimulation, but activities such as erotic massage, fantasy, and role-playing and the use of vibrators or other sex toys also fall into this category. As long as it also eliminates exchange of bodily fluids, outercourse also reduces the risk of sexually transmitted diseases. Another big benefit of outercourse is that it can enhance orgasm because like foreplay, it helps build excitement. (See Steve Bodansky and Vera Bodansky's book *Extended Massive Orgasm* [Hunter House, 2000] for great instructions.)

Fertility Awareness: Natural Birth Control

My colleague Joan Morais teaches natural birth control at UC Davis. She wrote, "The most common response I have gotten when I tell people I am a fertility awareness instructor is 'Is this the method that Catholics have used that doesn't work?' They presume it is the old and unreliable rhythm method that Catholics used many years ago. They have already made up their minds that it sets women back a hundred years and takes away our reproductive freedom. I can relate as I also used to think this. I opposed Natural Family Planning and I thought the birth control pill was the best thing ever. I took the birth control pill on and off until my late twenties. I didn't do well on it. I couldn't feel my cycles. I couldn't feel my body! I became depressed and I lost my libido. Somewhere inside me I had an innate wisdom that was telling me that the birth control pill wasn't right for me.

"There is another way besides chemical contraceptives, devices, and sterilization. Fertility awareness is a beautiful way that allows a woman to feel her cycles as she wanes or waxes while also preventing pregnancy. This fundamental knowledge of a woman's fertility and infertility should be taught to every menstruating girl and woman. It is our birthright. These are the operating instructions of our female body that somehow got thrown out along the way. Fertility awareness includes natural birth control, knowing your cyclical body, your menstrual cycle, your reproductive health, and your fertility and infertility. To know how to prevent pregnancy naturally or to consciously know when you can become pregnant is the most profound and empowering knowledge a woman can learn. There are only five days a month a woman may become pregnant, yet we medicate our bodies twenty-four hours a day, three hundred and sixty-five days a year. This is like medicating our body every day to prevent a monthly headache."[21] I completely agree with Joan and wish I had known about fertility awareness years ago. Though it's not well known, fertility awareness and natural family planning are well studied and very effective.[22] Fertility awareness is not the outdated rhythm method.[23]

Dr. Joseph Stanford, a family physician and expert in natural family planning, defines fertility awareness or fertility appreciation as "the use of physiologic signs and symptoms of the menstrual cycle to define the fertile and infertile phases of the menstrual cycle. This information can be used for natural family planning or the diagnosis and treatment of infertility." Fertility awareness involves learning how to determine your time of ovulation. This can be done in a number of different ways: cervical mucus checks, observation of vaginal discharge of cervical mucus, or measurement of basal body temperature (BBT).[24] Observation of cervical mucus, combined with monitoring BBT and other symptoms that occur around ovulation, is called the symptothermal method of natural family planning. Commercially available ovulation indicators that test urine pre- and postovulation are also available in most pharmacies, but it is much easier, and cheaper, to learn how to determine your own ovulatory time from changes in cervical mucus. Salivary testing can be very helpful, too (see page 418). I also recommend a highly detailed and feature-rich software program called Ovusoft that's made to correspond with the highly successful methods developed by Toni Weschler, M.P.H., author of *Taking Charge of Your Fertility* (HarperCollins, 2002). Ovusoft Fertility Software not only automates Toni's methodologies but also allows for individual preferences and personally tailored formatting, forecasting, charting, and reporting. (For more information, visit www.ovusoft.com.)

Studies have shown that symptoms sometimes associated with ovulation in some women, such as breast tenderness, *mittelschmerz* (midcycle pain associated with ovulation), and change in the position of the cervix are not always accurate indicators of ovulation. In a comparative study of fifteen different methodologies, including variations of the most common methods used to determine ovulation, it was found that the observation of vaginal discharge alone, known as the Ovulation Method, was the most precise and practical way to determine time of fertility.[25] The addition of basal body temperature graphs did not improve accuracy over the mucus discharge alone.

TABLE 6

COMPARING CONTRACEPTIVE METHODS

˙ Assumes perfect use every time. Effectiveness rates of actual use may vary significantly from those shown. Effectiveness statistics from Planned Parenthood (see www.plannedparenthood.org), except for Essure, which was provided by Conceptus, Inc.

Method	Effectiveness	Requirements	Advantages	Disadvantages
FERTILITY AWARENESS	91%–98%	Conscious understanding of fertility cycle Continual conscious commitment Willingness to use barrier methods of birth control or abstinence during fertile periods	Maintains natural hormonal/ fertility cycle	Requires cooperation and high awareness Medication that affects cervical mucus, body temperature, or menstrual regularity may compromise effectiveness
DIAPHRAGM, WITH CONTRACEPTIVE CREAM OR GEL	94%	Fitting by health professional Faithful use at each intercourse	May protect against pelvic infection and cervical abnormalities Maintains normal hormonal/ fertility cycle Can be inserted hours before sex It holds blood in nicely during menstruation, making sex less messy.	Unacceptable to some people May cause genital irritation Failure rate is higher if intercourse frequency is greater than 3X/week Must be resized after pregnancy, some miscarriages, or abortions, weight change of 20 percent May cause frequent urinary tract infections in some women
CONDOM	98%	Conscientious use for maximal effectiveness	Protects against STDs Decreases risk of cervical dysplasia Does not require a prescription	Requires male partner to be cooperative Unacceptable to some people Some people are allergic to latex condoms (other kinds are available)

Method	Effectiveness	Requirements	Advantages	Disadvantages
CONDOM (cont.)			Can help premature ejaculation	Erection must be maintained Loss of sensation
REALITY FEMALE CONDOM	95%	Conscientious use for maximal effectiveness Faithful use required at each intercourse	Protects against STDs Protects labia and base of penis during intercourse Can be inserted up to eight hours before intercourse Decreased risk of cervical dysplasia Can be used without partner participation Stronger than latex and less likely to break External ring on condom may stimulate clitoris	One-time use only Unacceptable to some May be noisy May be difficult to insert May cause genital irritation May slip into vagina during sex
BIRTH CONTROL PILL	99%	Prescription from a health care professional Taking a daily pill	Decreases risk of ovarian and uterine cancer Decrease in monthly bleeding and chance for iron deficiency Decrease in menstrual cramps and PMS Decreased risk for benign breast tumors Acne improvement Requires no planning	Blocks natural hormonal/fertility cycle May lower sex drive May increase risk of cervical adenocarcinoma Increased incidence of depression Increased risk of chlamydia infection Increased risk of thrombophlebitis, pulmonary emboli, stroke—especially in smokers Nausea and vomiting Headaches

Method	Effectiveness	Requirements	Advantages	Disadvantages
BIRTH CONTROL PILL (cont.)				Certain medications compromise effectiveness May cause spotting, breast tenderness, moodiness, headache, nausea, and weight gain
IUD (Progestasert, Copper T)	99%	Insertion by health professional	Requires no planning	May increase risk of pelvic infection following insertion or in women exposed to STDs May cause spotting Periods may be longer and heavier May cause cramping after insertion
SPERMICIDAL FOAM, CREAM, JELLY, FILM, OR SUPPOSITORIES	85%	Conscientious use for maximal effectiveness	Provides partial protection against STDs Free from systemic effects No advance planning required Available with no prescription	Unacceptable to some people May cause genital irritation Must reinsert with each act of intercourse May be messy
LEA'S SHIELD	85% (Note: figure is for typical use; stats for perfect use not available)	Prescription from a health care professional Conscientious use for maximal effectiveness	Can be inserted hours before sex and worn for forty-eight hours	Can be difficult to insert Can't be used during any vaginal bleeding including menstruation May cause frequent urinary tract infections in some women

Method	Effectiveness	Requirements	Advantages	Disadvantages
SPONGE	80%–91%	Conscientious use for maximal effectiveness	No prescription necessary Can be inserted hours before sex Can be worn for thirty hours after insertion, and intercourse can be repeated without additional preparation during the first twenty-four hours	Use during vaginal bleeding, including menstruation, may decrease effectiveness Slight increase for toxic shock syndrome Spermicide used with it may cause genital irritation
CERVICAL CAP	71% (Note: figure is for typical use; stats for perfect use not available)	Prescription from health care professional required Conscientious use for maximal effectiveness	Requires no planning Provides continuous protection for up to forty-eight hours, no matter how many times intercourse occurs	Current caps come in only three sizes—therefore accurate fit is not always assured Some risk of toxic shock if cap is left in longer than forty-eight hours May cause odor problems with some women if left in too long Not as effective in women who've had children Not as effective after a recent abortion Can be difficult to insert Use during vaginal bleeding, including menstruation, may render less effective
THE RING	99%	Conscientious use for maximal effectiveness	Decreases risk of ovarian and uterine cancer	May be less effective in women weighing more than 198 lbs. May decrease libido

Method	Effectiveness	Requirements	Advantages	Disadvantages
THE RING (cont.)			Decrease in monthly bleeding and chance for iron deficiency Decrease in menstrual cramps and PMS Decreased risk for benign breast tumors Acne improvement Requires no planning	Increased risk of thrombophlebitis, pulmonary emboli, stroke—especially in smokers Nausea and vomiting Headaches Certain medications compromise effectiveness May cause spotting, breast tenderness, moodiness, headache, nausea, and weight gain as well as skin irritation at site of application May cause increased vaginal discharge or vaginal infection or irritation
THE PATCH	99%	Conscientious use for maximal effectiveness	Decreases risk of ovarian and uterine cancer Decrease in monthly bleeding and chance for iron deficiency Decrease in menstrual cramps and PMS Decreased risk for benign breast tumors Acne improvement Requires no planning	May be less effective in women weighing more than 198 lbs. May decrease sex drive Increased risk of thrombophlebitis, pulmonary emboli, stroke—especially in smokers Nausea and vomiting Headaches Certain medications compromise effectiveness

Method	Effectiveness	Requirements	Advantages	Disadvantages
THE PATCH (cont.)				May cause spotting, breast tenderness, moodiness, irritability, headache, nausea, and weight gain as well as skin irritation at site of application
WITHDRAWAL	96%	Conscientious use at each intercourse Great self-control, experience and trust of partner	Requires no planning	May decrease sexual pleasure The male pre-ejaculate (fluid at the end of the penis after erection) may contain sperm Less effective in men who ejaculate prematurely
INJECTABLE PROGESTIN (Depo-Provera)	Almost 100%	A shot every three months	Requires no planning Can be used by women who can't take estrogen May help prevent endometrial cancer Fewer and lighter periods	Spotting and headaches, moodiness, irritability, and decreased sex drive May not be used for more than two years in a row Takes an average of nine to ten months to regain fertility after stopping May cause temporary bone thinning
VASECTOMY	Almost 100%	Surgery	Requires no planning	Irreversible
TUBAL LIGATION	Almost 100%	Surgery	Requires no planning	Irreversible

Method	Effectiveness	Requirements	Advantages	Disadvantages
TUBAL BLOCKING	Almost 100%	Nonsurgical procedure in the doctor's office	Requires no planning Insertion does not require incisions or anesthesia Does not block the blood supply in the fallopian tube or to the ovary	Irreversible

The advantage of becoming familiar with your fertility cycles simply through the changes in vaginal discharge over the month is that you will be able to tell beforehand when you are becoming fertile. This is very empowering and helps women embrace their fertility, not worry about it.

Lovemaking without intercourse is then possible as an alternative at ovulation time—so is using a barrier method at that time, though some experts point out that, depending upon the barrier you use, this may make cervical mucus changes more difficult to interpret. Highly motivated couples work this out together. Dr. Stanford, who has both personal and professional experience with this method, told me, "Fertility is not a disease, even though it is often treated like one. It is a part of who we are. When a couple uses this method, they often develop a deep respect for each other, for their fertility, and for their sexuality. This enhances all aspects of the relationship. It is a spiritual thing." Though I did not know about the accuracy of the Ovulation Method at the time I conceived my children, I did use basal body temperature recordings to help time conception. I found it very empowering.

Fertility awareness techniques (with or without barrier contraceptives during ovulation) can be highly effective birth control techniques. (It would also be worthwhile to add the Forbidden Points system to this approach.) The Creighton Model Ovulation Method has been studied the most rigorously. Three major studies show method effectiveness rates to avoid pregnancy of 99.1 to 99.9 percent, while actual user rates ranged from 94.8 to 97.3 percent. The differences in these figures were attributable to teaching- and using-related errors.[26]

Knowing when you ovulate can enhance chances of conception considerably. It is generally accepted that the probability of conceiving in one cycle for couples with normal fertility is in the range of 22 to 30 percent. But with fertility-focused intercourse, the chances can increase considerably. In one study of couples using fertility-focused intercourse, 71.4 percent of the clients who had a previous pregnancy achieved pregnancy in the first cycle. With those clients who had never had a pregnancy, the rate was 80.9 percent. By the fourth cycle, 100 percent of those who had never been pregnant had conceived.[27]

In couples who are having difficulty conceiving, using the Ovulation Method alone without any other testing can considerably enhance the chances of conception. Dr. Stanford notes that "of couples referred to the NFP [natural family planning] center at Omaha for inability to achieve pregnancy [for an average of three years], 20 to 40 percent have achieved pregnancy within six months of use of the Ovulation Method, before any further medical evaluation and treatment is undertaken."[28] The Ovulation Method also works well for those who have irregular periods, are breast-feeding, or are peri-menopausal.

I would strongly recommend the Ovulation (or Billings) Method to any committed couple. Dr. Stanford, like other experts in fertility awareness, always refers patients to a thoroughly trained natural family planning counselor, because although the method is simple, it requires support and education, especially in the beginning. This is partly because one member of the couple may find himself or herself experiencing resentment and frustration initially. Obviously, introducing fertility consciousness into the whole area of sexuality and working with it daily is a pretty new concept for many. Adequate personalized instruction by qualified teachers is essential for the successful use of natural family planning in general and the Ovulation Method in particular. It is not learned well from a book, most likely because of the emotional and psychological issues it brings up. The quality of a woman's (or couple's) experience with this method often depends upon the quality of instruction given and follow-up care received. (I recommend *Taking Charge of Your Fertility: The Definitive Guide to Natural Birth Control, Pregnancy Achievement, and Reproductive Health* [HarperCollins, 2002] by Toni Weschler.)

Couples who use fertility awareness effectively throughout their reproductive lives experience no side effects and often find an increased intimacy in their relationships, which includes a shared responsibility for their combined fertility. Though we tend to associate interest in natural family planning with certain religions, many women are drawn to this method because it is, inherently, a holistic approach to fertility. In a random telephone survey of 1,267 women in Germany, for instance, 47 percent of the respondents were interested or very interested in learning about NFP, and 20 percent indicated a high probability of future use of NFP. Religious factors were notably absent as a motivating force.[29] I suspect that if this method was more widely known and supported by health care professionals, it would be more widely used. Whether or not you use fertility awareness for contraceptive or conception purposes, it is empowering to know your fertility cycle. Here's a brief overview of the method.

Determining the fertile phase. The egg lives anywhere from six to twenty-four hours after ovulation. Sperm viability depends on the presence of fertile mucus. Sperm can live for up to five days in fertile mucus. Without fertile mucus, they die in a few hours. Therefore, there is about a seven-day time period during every cycle when pregnancy could theoretically occur. One study found that among healthy women trying to conceive, nearly all pregnancies could be attributed to intercourse during a six-day period ending on the day of ovulation. Though no one in the study conceived on the day after ovulation, the authors of the study concluded that there was probably a 12 percent chance of conceiving on the day after ovulation and also on the seventh day before ovulation. The study also concluded that for those couples trying to conceive, having intercourse every other day was just as effective as every day. Practically speaking, if you are trying to get pregnant, have intercourse four times during your most fertile week. This is usually more effective, and less stressful, than trying to stick to an every-other-day schedule.[30] It has been my experience, however, that despite the best information science has to offer, sometimes when a soul is meant to come in, it will—no matter what you do or don't do.

Mucus checks (natural birth control). Studies have shown that almost all women can easily learn to check for the presence or absence of fertile E-type (estrogen-stimulated) mucus by the routine observation of vaginal discharge on the vulva.[31] As menstruation stops, cervical mucus is at a minimum. You feel dry. There is no mucus in the vaginal opening and no discharge on your underwear. This lack of mucus is associated with being infertile. These "dry" days are usually safe for unprotected intercourse. The cervix begins secreting E-type mucus about six days prior to ovulation, so, using this method, you will know when ovulation is apt to occur before it happens. When you see mucus on your underwear or can wipe it off with toilet paper, you know your fertile time is beginning. E-type mucus, when looked at under the microscope, contains channels that help the sperm swim up through the cervix. It also dries into a characteristic ferning pattern. Fertile mucus is similar in feel and quality to uncooked egg white. Some women may even notice that it wets their underwear. You are fertile from the time when fertile mucus first appears until the fourth day after your peak mucus discharge. The last day of any mucus that is clear, stretchy (greater than or equal to one inch of stretch between thumb and index finger), or lubricative is called the "peak" day of mucus discharge. This "peak" mucus day is highly correlated with ovulation, which occurs plus or minus two days from this "peak" day over 95 percent of the time.[32]

G-type mucus (progesterone-stimulated) appears immediately after ovulation. This type of mucus lacks elasticity. It also has an opaque and adhesive quality. G-type mucus, when looked at under the microscope, lacks the channels that facilitate the swimming of sperm. This type of mucus actually blocks the passage of sperm. Following ovulatory mucus discharge, cervical mucus may cease (you become dry) or become thicker and more dense (G-type mucus). Either way, the change is distinct and noticeable. Your period will start about twelve to fifteen days after the peak ovulatory cervical flow.[33]

As already mentioned, saliva also changes cyclically with your hormonal cycle. As your hormones change during your cycle, your saliva, when dry, develops a special microscopic ferning pattern that matches that of the cervical mucus. Special small microscopes are available and widely used in Europe and Japan as yet another way for women to learn about and therefore make the best use of their fertility cycle, whether the goal is to conceive or avoid pregnancy.

Keep a record of your basal body temperatures for three months to see if you are ovulating. Though learning how to assess your cervical mucus is more accurate, taking your basal body temperature and recording it for a few cycles is an interesting way to learn about your body and its internal rhythms. It may also enhance your ability to correlate your cervical mucus and/or salivary changes with ovulation.

The temperature rise that occurs with ovulation is due to the effect of progesterone. If you become pregnant during the period in which you have been taking your basal body temperature, you will notice that it stays up and doesn't drop down again. This temperature elevation on BBT is a very early sign of pregnancy. (When women are pregnant, they have a great deal of progesterone in their

FIGURE 11: FERTILITY AWARENESS:
OVULATION AND BASAL BODY TEMPERATURE

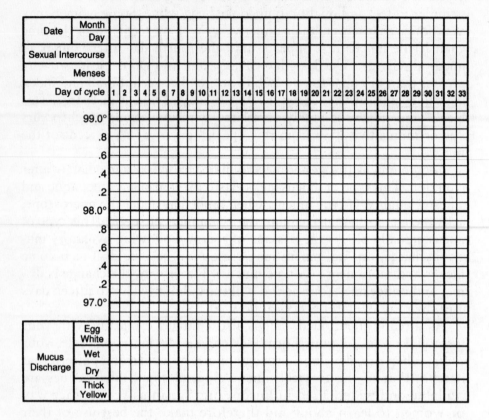

systems and their temperature is higher than in the nonpregnant state. Pregnancy was the only time I could comfortably swim in the ocean in Maine.)

Take your basal body temperature first thing each morning starting on the first day of your menstrual period. (This is considered day one of your cycle.) Do this for three cycles, and chart each cycle separately. You can then use your temperature graph to record cervical mucus and salivary changes. (See figure 11.) Ovulation is accompanied by a rise in basal body temperature of about 0.6 to 0.8 degrees, and it occurs somewhere between the time when the temperature begins to rise and the time when it reaches its highest point. The fertile time generally is over at the end of the third day in a row of elevated temperature. (See figure 11.)

If your cycles are quite regular, you can get a general idea of the length of your fertile and infertile times by charting the following:

FIGURE 11: FERTILITY AWARENESS:
OVULATION AND BASAL BODY TEMPERATURE

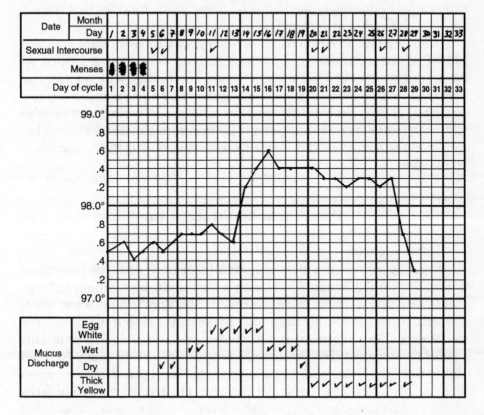

Record cycle length for at least six months to determine the earliest possible day that your ovulation could occur. The follicular phase of the cycle (from day one of your period until ovulation) is variable in length. The luteal phase (the time from ovulation to onset of your period) is generally fixed at fourteen days. To determine the earliest day of the cycle when you could ovulate, subtract fourteen from your shortest cycle length. Therefore, if your cycle ranges in length from twenty-six to thirty-one days, the earliest you could ovulate is day twelve (26-14=12). Depending upon your cervical mucus, you could probably have intercourse until day eight or nine of your cycle and avoid pregnancy. (In doing these calculations, you can easily see why charting mucus flow or salivary ferning patterns is generally more accurate than this "calendar" method.)

The consistency of your cervix also changes over the monthly cycle. During ovulation, it is much softer and the opening becomes wider than at other times of the month. You can easily feel your cervix by squatting and inserting your index or middle finger into you vagina. (You can also do this in the bathtub.) Some women notice that the position of the cervix also changes.

In summary, there is no right or wrong way to work with your fertility. Each of us, however, must look at how deeply programmed we have been to believe that we can't trust our bodies without external hormonal manipulation. When you understand this, you can make a conscious choice. Some of my patients who are in loving relationships with supportive men do not use any contraceptive method at all. They simply enjoy sex when they want to, knowing that if they conceive, it will be fine.

Permanent Contraception

Tubal Ligation

Tubal ligation is the most common form of permanent contraception in the United States. Many women are ambivalent about it, however, even when they know intellectually they don't want more children. Most of us value the *ability* to conceive, even if we choose not to use that ability. Permanent contraception closes a door that usually cannot be reopened. For centuries, women were valued solely for their ability to bear children, and bearing children has been the most important socially acceptable outlet for women's creative power. Voluntarily giving up this capacity stirs primitive fears. Yet many women find that being free of the fear of pregnancy is health-enhancing and rejuvenates their sexuality.

Tubal ligation is an excellent choice for some women—but not all! I chose this procedure after waiting until my younger daughter was four. Somehow, though there is no logic to it, this made me feel that she was "safe" and "permanent." At about the age of thirty-seven, my path was split in front of me in terms of childbearing. I knew that having another child would mean at least another five years of energy diverted to the needs of the child and away from my own pursuits. I still went mush sometimes looking at babies in airports, and I harbored a secret fantasy of having the ideal pregnancy and the ideal labor, in which I would rest and really enjoy the pregnancy *and* the new baby—things I had not done fully with my other two children.

But I had seen far too many women become pregnant "accidentally" in their late thirties and early forties, just as their lives were settling down after a decade or so devoted to the demands of raising children. I was at a point where I had to make a conscious choice one way or the other about having another child. I wouldn't have had an abortion if I became pregnant at this time in my life. (If I had become pregnant during my training years, however, I would have had an abortion without hesitation.) Still, I didn't want a pregnancy just to happen. I wanted to be a conscious decision maker, not have my life decided by "fate."

My husband assured me that he didn't *need* a son to feel complete. Right after I pushed out our second daughter, he had said to me, "You never have to do that again for me." Like many women, I would gladly have had a third child if my husband had wanted to try for a boy. I was and am very pleased to have two daughters. I know I would love them just as much if they were boys, but I didn't feel incomplete without sons. Neither my husband nor I really wanted more. We made our decision together, though the final choice was mine. Making the decision to have a tubal ligation was not difficult. I knew that I personally didn't want to bear any more children—so I felt that I should have the procedure, even though vasectomy is technically easier to perform. In the event that I acquired another sexual partner one day through a change of circumstances, I wanted to be sure I would not get pregnant. Besides, I had performed many tubal ligations and felt comfortable with the procedure. (Other couples feel much more comfortable with vasectomy. It is safer and cheaper than tubal ligation.)

A tubal ligation changes the blood supply to the ovaries somewhat. There may even be a slight risk of an earlier menopause following tubal ligation if the blood supply to the ovary becomes severely compromised, but this is rare. Some women develop "post–tubal ligation syndrome," an ill-defined problem characterized by increased cramping, irregular periods, and heavier bleeding. (Many studies do not show this effect, so its existence is controversial.) This is mostly a problem for women who have been on the pill prior to their tubal surgery and haven't experienced natural periods for years. Indeed, they may have developed bleeding problems anyway when they went off the pill, not necessarily *because* of the tubal ligation. Tubal ligation may even be somewhat protective against ovarian cancer.[34]

Tubal ligation lowers progesterone secretion significantly and even a year after the ligation, these levels may not recover fully to what they were previously. The menstrual pattern isn't affected, however.[35] This data certainly does explain, in part, why some women develop PMS following a tubal ligation.

ESSURE: NEW TUBAL BLOCKAGE PROCEDURE WITHOUT SURGERY

The first permanent method of birth control for women that doesn't involve surgical incisions or general anesthesia, called Essure, was approved by the FDA in 2002. I predict that this will replace conventional tubal ligation procedures pretty quickly if it lives up to its initial promise. Essure is just as effective as tubal ligation and is performed in the doctor's office in about half an hour. The doctor inserts a small scope through the vagina, cervix, and uterus and uses it to place a tightly coiled springlike device one or two millimeters long into each fallopian tube. Most women return to their normal activity the same day or the next day. The body then starts to develop scar tissue around the coil, which becomes thick enough to fully block the fallopian tubes in about three months (so an alternate method of birth control is necessary until the physician confirms that the scarring is sufficient).

In addition to the benefits of not requiring anesthesia and a hospital stay, Essure doesn't block the blood supply in the tube or interfere with the blood supply to the ovary at all. Another plus is that it's available to women who aren't good candidates for tubal ligation, such as those who are obese, those with previous multiple abdominal surgeries, and those with heart disease or other contraindications to general anesthesia. (For more information, call the Essure Information Center at 877-377-8731 or visit www.essure.com.)

Though some ancient Taoist traditions feel that tubal ligation or vasectomy interferes with the energy flow of the body, my medical intuitive consultants say that the life-energy around the body simply reroutes itself—that there is no permanent damage to the body after a so-called sterilization procedure. Caroline Myss says that the only problem with a tubal ligation or vasectomy is when the person is ambivalent about it and really doesn't want it done. As with abortion, it's not the procedure itself that can potentially cause problems—it's the *meaning* of it.

I was very clear that the potential problems associated with tubal ligation were *nothing* compared with the disruption that an unplanned pregnancy would cause in my life. So I made an informed choice. Then I called my sister.

Moving into Greater Creativity

My sister Penny had her miscarriage a year before I decided to have a tubal ligation. (We're eleven months apart in age—the doctor asked my mother if she had poked holes in her diaphragm.) After the miscarriage, I said to her, "Why don't you have a tubal ligation and be done with the worry?" She said, "I'll do it when you do." So when I finally decided to do it, I called her up and asked her if she wanted to join me for the event and schedule them at the same time. She said she did. I made arrangements for both of us to have our procedures done in the office via a technique known as a minilaparotomy (small operation). After I made the appointments, I hung up and experienced about thirty seconds of sorrow about what I had just done. I vowed that if this feeling of loss continued, I'd cancel the procedure. But the feeling passed very quickly.

We decided to make this a meaningful event for both of us. Penny has no daughters; I have no sons. Each of us had to make peace with that. We named our operations and the ceremony we had beforehand "Moving into Greater Creativity" because we saw our lives after childbearing as rich with potential to develop ourselves further. (By the way, that is exactly what has happened for both of us.) I've always hated the word *sterile* because of its negative connotations—"barren" women are sterile; a bare, cold room is sterile; hospitals are sterile. I didn't consider myself sterile before the tubal ligation, and I certainly didn't see how having my fallopian tubes cauterized would change how I felt about myself. I had simply chosen to be proactive about avoiding future pregnancy.

Our operations were scheduled at nine and nine-thirty on a Friday morning in May. Springtime—a perfect time to celebrate newfound fertility and also, according to Caroline Myss, a good time to have surgery, as the energies associated with spring bode well for healing and new growth. The night before, Penny and I participated in a beautiful ceremony—one prepared for us by Judith Burwell, a friend who guides people via ritual through significant life changes. Another friend, Gina Orlando, had made us two exquisite spring flower wreaths to wear on our heads during the ceremony. I felt like a bridesmaid—virginal in the true sense of the word, a woman complete unto herself.

Each of us spoke in turn about how she felt taking this step—and about how, when we make a conscious choice, there's always grieving for the choice not taken. Yet we must fearlessly go forth and consciously work with our circumstances to the best of our ability, working to manifest our dreams. In the ritual Penny and I made space to grieve aloud our unborn children—me for my unborn sons, and

Penny for her unborn daughters—knowing full well that Mother Earth doesn't really require more people right now, that that part of the Earth's history—the order to go forth and multiply—is over. "For now," I said, "may we go forth and multiply many spiritual children and give birth to ourselves."

The next morning we arrived at the doctor's office, three miles from my house. We had brought a special music tape with us to listen to during our surgery, which was to be performed under local anesthesia with a very light intravenous sedative. My sister went first. I held her hand and checked to see that her tubes were cauterized in just the right way—not so much that the blood supply would be compromised.

Penny walked into the recovery area, and then it was my turn. It was all quite painless. The doctor at one point said, "Do you want to see your tubes? They are very long and perfect." I said, "No, I'd just as soon have a mind/body split right now." I didn't like the idea of actually burning nice healthy fallopian tubes, something that so many women would love to have. But I had made my choice. If I had changed my mind even *during* the procedure, though, I would have told the doctor to stop.

Afterward, my husband drove us home and fed us lunch and dinner while we rested on the couch, kept ice packs on our lower abdomens, and watched all the episodes of *Anne of Green Gables* on videotape. We developed shoulder pain, which often results when the abdominal cavity is opened and excess gas from room air or carbon dioxide gets trapped under the diaphragm and then is "referred" to the shoulder because the nerves that supply the diaphragm are connected to the nerves that innervate the shoulder. This gas gets reabsorbed after a day or two, and the pain goes away. The intensity of our shoulder pain was unexpected, but we were very happy with our choice.

The following morning we gathered spring flowers from the yard and floated them in the bathtub while we sat on the side, soaked our feet, and talked about our parents, our childhoods, and how happy we were to be celebrating this momentous event together. While listening to the singing of Susan Osborne, we gave each other a foot massage. Then we rested some more.

Later that afternoon, we drove into Portland to a special store called the Plains Indian Gallery. I bought a piece of art called *Tree Momma,* a magical figure of a woman made out of a weathered wooden branch, fur, and some clay. Penny bought a painting that had deep meaning for her of two Sioux warriors riding away from a burial platform. These purchases were personal symbols of our conscious choice to shape our destiny by clarity and intent—not chance!

Neither my sister nor I had any regrets. One chapter of our lives closed, but we each opened an entirely new one. At a family reunion in which we watched our then teenage children have fun together, we remarked on the wisdom of our decision.

TRANSFORMING INFERTILITY

Almost all women assume that they will be able to have children someday, even if they're not sure they want to; the potential to have them is important even to women who never intend to use that potential. The ability to conceive and bear children can profoundly affect the way a woman feels about herself on a very deep level. So when a woman finds that she is unable to have a child, she's often thrown into great despair and feels a sense of injustice: "Why me?" Seeing teenage mothers having no problems getting pregnant becomes almost impossible to bear, unless the woman can find some meaning in the experience and come to terms with it. The pioneering work of Alice Domar, Ph.D., founder and executive director of the Domar Center for Complementary Healthcare in Waltham, Massachusetts, has clearly documented that women who've been diagnosed as infertile are twice as likely to be depressed as a control group, and that this depression peaks about two years after they start trying to get pregnant. And even though infertility is not life-threatening, infertile women have depression scores that are indistinguishable from those of women with cancer, heart disease, or HIV.[36]

Approximately one in every six to ten couples has a problem with infertility. About 40 percent of the problems are related to a male factor and 60 percent to a female factor. Statistics show that sperm counts have been gradually falling over the past century. Decreased sperm counts are associated with cigarette, marijuana, and alcohol use as well as with environmental factors. Humans cannot pollute this planet and their own bodies without consequences, and infertility is one of them. Conditions on the Earth may not favor fertility the way they used to. It's as though the collective species brain were generating a great deal of energy toward making many women and men infertile, due to the stresses of today's families, social environments, and personal addictions, and to stress on the planet itself. Too many stressful childhoods remain unhealed; too many children grow up too fast. We're not allowing nature's rhythms to click into gear naturally. The preliminary data on reproductive problems associated with toxic chemicals and with electromagnetic field disturbances support the idea that fertility is down.[37] But that doesn't mean that an individual woman's fertility will necessarily be adversely affected.

Fertility is affected by many different factors, such as diet and environment, but in about 20 percent of the cases, the causes are unknown—meaning that medical testing cannot explain the problem. In my experience those couples who are most willing to look at and work with the mind/body connection in addition to the other aspects of fertility are the ones who are most successful either conceiving or healing their relationship with fertility.

The most common (and often interrelated) factors affecting female infertility are the following:

- Smoking
- Following a high-glycemic diet with inadequate micronutrients
- Irregular ovulation
- Endometriosis
- A history of pelvic infection from an IUD or other source, causing scarring of the fallopian tubes
- Unresolved emotional stress that results in subtle hormonal imbalances
- Immune system problems—some women make antibodies against the sperm of some men and not others. Likewise, they can make antibodies against the fertilized egg that is created with some partners but not with others.[38]
- Age

A certain percentage of women who've been told that they are infertile for a "medical" reason get pregnant even without treatment. Infertility is never a completely straightforward affair. Many physical, emotional, and psychological factors are involved in conception, so many that it is ridiculous to try to reduce fertility to a matter of injecting the right hormone at the right time. An infertility specialist I met once said, "I do all the latest high-tech surgery and hormone treatment to try to make someone pregnant. When it is all said and done, I still don't know who will get pregnant and who won't and why. After all my years of training, this area is still a big mystery that I can't control."

The conventional "management" of infertility generally focuses on the body as a hormonal machine and in large part ignores emotional, psychological, and even nutritional factors that have physical and hormonal manifestations.[39] Though the mind/body connection in infertility has been appreciated for decades, only recently has this important link begun to be explored more seriously. As our society has become more technologically focused, the study of the mind/body connection in infertility holds the potential to help many couples, and a thorough psychological interview should be a routine part of every fertility investigation.[40] When we focus only on the extremely expensive and invasive technology currently available for fertility, and forget the hearts and spirits of those going through these procedures, the results are often disappointing and even devastating.

In 2002, more than 45,000 infants were born as a result of ART (assisted reproductive therapy or technology), which represents 1 percent of the births in the U.S. Despite its popularity, ART is not without significant risk. It is well documented that ART increases the risk of multiple gestations, preterm delivery, low birth weight, chromosome abnormalities, adverse neurodevelopmental disorders, birth defects, eclampsia, prenatal mortality, placenta previa, and increased rate of C-section delivery.[41] Over $1 billion is spent annually on overcoming infertility, and this figure is increasing.[42] The bottom line here is that Mother Nature has some checks and balances that technology can't bypass entirely.

Psychological Factors

On a personal level, many women do not get pregnant because in their hearts they really do not want to—they are afraid of the demands a child will make on them. In one study, women who were unsuccessful with fertility treatments were found to be more successful in the outer world than those who conceived. The authors of the study interpreted this result as "an exaggerated positive attitude as an attempt to overcome inner fears, doubts, and ambivalence" about having a child.[43] Caroline Myss explains that women have only so much second-chakra energy. If a woman is using her ambition for career success and is already very busy in this area, she may simply not have enough energy circuits available in her body to conceive a child unless she cuts back on other commitments. Many infertile women are working sixty to eighty hours per week and are exhausted; then they pursue having a child as though they were writing a Ph.D. dissertation. A prospective study done in Italy of women going through IVF (in vitro fertilization) or ET (embryo transfer) found that both vulnerability to stress and working outside the home were associated with a poor outcome of IVF or ET treatment, even though the straightforward medical causes of infertility were distributed equally throughout the study group.[44]

Conceiving a child is a receptive act, not a marathon event that can be programmed into your Day-Timer. Several studies have indicated that excessive focus on the goal of having a child may result in premature maturation of the eggs in the ovary and subsequent release of eggs that are not ready for fertilization![45] I'd like to stress that having a job or career need not affect your fertility; problems can arise as a result of other factors that are often associated with today's careers, such as a perceived inability to get your needs met; a sense of lack of control in your life; and not feeling good about the work you're doing, what that job represents in your life, or a career that is not an extension of your inner wisdom.

One fascinating study of heterosexual women undergoing donor insemination noted that after the first several attempts to produce pregnancy, the women, who were previously ovulatory, actually stopped ovulating. The authors concluded that artificial insemination—and any other mechanized, unnatural technique for "forcing" pregnancy—is on some level a traumatizing procedure that leads to the inhibition of the very process it is trying to accomplish. (This may or may not be true with lesbian couples or single women choosing motherhood because donor insemination is the only method for achieving pregnancy in these situations.) Interestingly, orgasm has been found to enhance a woman's chances of conception. Involuntary vaginal and uterine movements that promote conception accompany orgasm. Failure to achieve orgasm may lead to circulatory changes in the blood flow to the pelvis, which can affect fertility.[46] High-tech conception techniques, by their very design, completely ignore this aspect of fertility.

Whenever a woman feels conflicted over birthing, children, or the restrictions that children may impose once they arrive, infertility may result. Some studies from the 1940s through the 1990s have suggested an association between infertility and ambivalence toward pregnancy and children.

The relationships between husbands and wives who are infertile have also been studied. Many of the women in these studies had an actual aversion to intercourse; they had low levels of orgasm when they did have intercourse, and they felt a marked sexual disharmony in their partnership. When these women found more suitable partners, how-ever, they became fertile.[47] I have seen this phenomenon repeatedly in my practice, just as I have seen countless so-called infertile women con-ceive shortly after adopting a baby! Psychological testing done on 117 husbands in infertile couples in one study indicated that the men had a pronounced lack of self-confidence, were introverted, and had de-creased social assertiveness.[48]

The fertility-stress link remains controversial in conventional science and it's difficult to document a causal link between psychosocial distress and fertility. Though many studies do show that women with infertility are more apt to have depression and anxiety, most doctors believe that the depression and anxiety are the result of infertility, not the other way around. In any case, studies tend to be conflicting, not well-controlled, and there are no prospective studies. In their review of forty years of re-search on psychological distress and infertility, psychologist Dr. W. A. Fisher and his colleague A. M. Brkovich summarized the viewpoint of most conventional doctors when they wrote: "Much research has been done to try to corroborate the proposition that psychological factors may be casually related to the occurrence of infertility, but no study has been able to confirm a causal relationship to date. In fact the very as-sumption of a psychological distress–infertility link has become quite controversial because some feel it blames women for their inability to conceive."[49]

Despite this conventional opinion, failing to explore the psychoso-cial aspects of fertility is a big mistake and robs a woman of all her op-tions. The conflicts that are associated with infertility are not at the conscious level and you can't get at them by simply asking a woman (or a man) if she or he is conflicted about having a child! Doing so makes them feel "to blame," which is the exact opposite of what anyone needs to feel in order to heal. Still, there's no doubt that subconscious fears about having a child can and do exert a powerful influence over the subtle endocrinologic processes that are required for conception. Perceived stress changes the way the hypothalamus of the brain func-tions, which affects ovulation. It also changes the immunologic func-tioning of the cells in the reproductive tract as well as elsewhere. When a woman learns how to modulate her stress effectively, her fertility can change. This was demonstrated by Alice Domar, Ph.D., based on her work with a group of women with unexplained infertility in her mind/body program at Beth Israel Deaconess Hospital in Boston. Thirty-four percent of these women became pregnant within six months— which is much higher than the average pregnancy rate for infertile couples at six months. The mean duration of infertility had been 3.3

years.[50] There is enormous potential for healing infertility when a woman is willing to acknowledge the role of her beliefs and commit to bringing them to consciousness and healing them. The first step—and the hardest step—in healing one's adverse subconscious programming about anything is being willing to accept yourself fully and unconditionally right now. This process involves never beating yourself up for "failing" to conceive because you waited too long, or "failing" at anything else! It's just the opposite of blame.

I've seen many women get pregnant once they committed to healing themselves on the deepest levels. On of the most striking examples of this is the story of my colleague, Julia Indichova, who, at the age of forty-three, was unable to conceive a second child. She was told that her FSH level (the follicle stimulating hormone from the pituitary gland—often used to judge whether a woman is still producing fertile eggs) was too high. But her inner wisdom told her that wasn't true. She changed her diet, began to do some deep soul searching, read everything she could, got her FSH down naturally, and eventually conceived and delivered a healthy daughter. Her book, *Inconceivable: A Woman's Triumph over Despair and Statistics* (Broadway Books, 2001), tells her story. Julia now leads workshops for women diagnosed with infertility and has helped many heal their fertility and their lives. (For more information, see Julia's website, www.fertileheart.com.)

Niravi Payne, author of *The Whole Person Fertility Program* (Three Rivers Press, 1997) is another colleague therapist who has devoted her professional life to helping couples conceive through her Whole Person Fertility Program. (See www.niravi.com.) Her view of current fertility problems is both enlightening and empowering. It's no accident, she says, that so many baby boomers have had problems with fertility. A series of complex psychological, sociological, and political factors has led to unparalled changes in our society in the last twenty-five years and has given rise to the decision of many to delay childbearing, thus altering the reproductive life patterns familiar to their parents and the thirty thousand generations before them. Niravi writes, "In the space of one generation, middle- and upper-class Americans decided to defer childbearing for ten to twenty years. This may be the most radical voluntary alteration of the lifestyle of all of them, and, unquestionably, there have been physiologic consequences."

Millions of boomers rebelled against the circumscribed lives that they saw their mothers living in the 1950s and 1960s. They said no to early marriage and childbearing and yes to defining and developing themselves. And many mothers of baby boomers, recognizing the lack of fulfillment and frustration that characterized their own lives, encouraged their daughters to seek college educations and professional careers. Ironically, many baby boomers had their first abortions around the same time that their mothers had their first children. Acknowledging how factors such as these may be affecting her in the present is often a woman's first step toward healing her relationship with fertility.

Time and again, I have witnessed how unconsciously absorbed beliefs about pregnancy, sexuality, and having children can, in some cases, actually block fertility. For example, some women are actually very unhappy with their current partner but are afraid to say so because they feel they have no alternative but to stay with him. Other women were told by their mothers that having babies could ruin their lives. Many of our mothers had no choice but to stay home and raise children, even when they had lots of talent and ambition in other areas. Their daughters often picked up on this and blame themselves for their mothers' frustrations. They don't want to risk passing this pain on to the next generation. And there's another fear: the fear of "having it all." Our mothers were taught that they could have a family or a career, but not both. The baby boom generation has clearly charted brave new waters for all the generations of women coming after us. In those women who are willing to come to terms with unconscious beliefs such as these, Niravi reports a subsequent pregnancy rate significantly higher than expected.

Mind/Body Program to Enhance Fertility

If fertility is an issue that concerns you, I highly recommend that you explore the mind/body connection thoroughly. The steps below will get you started.[51] I'd recommend that you have your journal ready as you read through this so that you can write down any thoughts, feelings, or beliefs that arise as you go through the steps I've outlined. Your responses will be an invaluable guide on your journey toward healing your fertility.

The mind/body approach to fertility is based on the premise that knowledge is power and that a change in perception based on new information is powerful enough to effect subtle changes in your endocrine, immune, and nervous systems. Regardless of what you've been told about your fertility, you need to know that your ability to conceive is profoundly influenced by the complex interaction among psychosocial, psychological, and emotional factors, and that you can consciously work with this to enhance your ability to have a baby.

The first thing that's needed in the area of fertility is a new language. Few labels are more damaging to women (or to men) than the label "infertile." It strikes at the very heart of one's self-concept and self-esteem and results in a punishing internal dialogue in women who are going through this experience. Many feel inadequate, guilty, and to blame for their condition, which creates a vicious cycle inside them. The word *infertility* conjures up images of barren, dry, sterile earth that can't bear fruit. If you currently carry this label, try replacing it with the following: "I am a sensual, sexual, fertile being with a great deal of love and nurturing to give to others—and to receive for myself." Internalizing the feeling that goes along with these words will help you change your self-concept (and physiology). Remember that changing your self-concept is a process, not an event. Give it time.

~ Step one: Look at the big picture. Know that you're not alone—millions of women are charting new territory when it comes to balancing personal and professional lives. Your fertility situation may, in part, be the result of the sweeping psychosocial forces that have unconsciously influenced an entire generation, with very real physiologic effects.

~ Step two: If you are over thirty-five and trying to get pregnant, examine your programming about your biological clock! The popularity and widespread publicity surrounding assisted reproductive technologies have made it seem as though every woman over the age of thirty-five is apt to have problems conceiving. But this just isn't true. Here are the statistics: about one-third of women who defer childbearing until their mid to late thirties will have a problem with fertility. But fully two-thirds won't have any problem. And 50 percent of women in their early forties won't have a problem either.[52]

Though statistically a woman's fertility decreases with age, it's important to keep in mind that statistics are based on the experience of an entire population. Within a given population there are very big individual differences. For example, the oldest spontaneous pregnancy in modern times recorded in the *Guinness World Records* was in a woman in Portland, Oregon, who delivered at the age of fifty-seven. In earlier times, it is reported that a Scottish woman delivered six children after the age of forty-seven—the last one at age sixty-two.[53] Interestingly, Brant Secunda, an American-born shaman trained by the Huichol Indians, who live in a remote region of Mexico, reports that Huichol women routinely get pregnant in their fifties and even in their sixties.[54] (Perhaps because they haven't been told that their eggs are too old, their fertility doesn't suffer much with age.)

This information is evidence of just how miraculous the human female body is when it comes to fertility! Things are not always what they seem. Indeed, research from Jonathan Tilly, Ph.D., and colleagues at Harvard Medical School found that female mammals are able to create new eggs even into adulthood.[55] This preliminary research has exploded one of the most sacred tenets of reproductive biology! When it comes to fertility, there's a big difference between chronologic age (age in years) and biologic age (age of one's tissues). We all know women in their early thirties who are going on fifty and women in their forties and even fifties who look like they're no older than thirty.

The birth rate for women aged forty to forty-four years has more than doubled since 1981, and in 2003, the Centers for Disease Control reported that the birth rate for women aged forty to forty-four topped 100,000 in a single year—the first time that has ever happened.[56] That number continues to rise. A lot of women over forty may not realize how fertile they are. Fifty-one percent of pregnancies that occur among women in their forties are unintended.[57] This may be one of the reasons why women over forty are second only to women between the ages of eighteen and twenty-five in frequency of abortions. So who says your eggs are too old?

~ Step three: Make the connection between your emotions, your family, and your fertility. The crux of the mind/body approach to fertility is discovering how the messages you internalized from childhood are currently affecting your ability to conceive. It is very clear that your physiology may well be responding automatically and unconsciously to situations directly related to your early childhood and family conditions. Though most people, especially other family members, may believe that it's easier and healthier to forget painful childhood experiences, and may urge you to avoid emotionally volatile subjects, your willingness to remember and release your emotional ties to past experiences will free up energy that will help you heal your fertility. Please remember that recalling painful childhood experiences is not done at the expense of happier memories. Usually, you'll find that this work will be a mixture of profound joy and sadness that ultimately leads you to a place of greater love and forgiveness for both yourself and your parents.

To get started on this, construct an *ephistogram*. An ephistogram is an emotional and physical family health history that diagrams family patterns. It was developed by Niravi Payne as an adaptation of the genogram used by family therapists. It can help you understand what circumstances, over many decades, may have caused you to experience reproductive problems. "Filling it out," writes Niravi, "is a powerful method for creating new pathways for healing, conceiving and carrying a baby to term." To create an ephistogram, you use the same diagram you would use when drawing a genealogy, or family tree, except that in addition to the names of your grandparents, parents, aunts, uncles, and siblings, you also put in any illnesses or physical symptoms they had, any emotional patterns you remember, and any reproductive difficulties they may have had. This is like detective work. Remember, for better or for worse, your family served as the model for your current intimate relationships. Ask yourself the following questions about each member of your family tree: What message did I receive from this person about having children? Was it positive? Was it negative? Did I internalize any of it? What did they lead me to believe about the process of conception, pregnancy, labor, and birth? Were there any family secrets, such as miscarriages or pregnancies that were kept hidden?

Niravi points out something very empowering: "The real freedom from our negative parental conditioning occurs when we stop denying that we are like them. Rather, asking ourselves how we feel, think, act, and react like our parents is the beginning of our separation and healing process. When we look at our lives in this way, it is easier to bring to light multigenerational ambivalence about conception that the ephistogram outlines." And this brings us to the next step.

~ Step four: Name your ambivalence. It is perfectly normal to be somewhat ambivalent about having a baby. It is possible to very much want a baby and to be terrified of the process at the same time. Why wouldn't you be? It changes your life permanently and in ways that you can't really plan for. I certainly was ambivalent... so much so, in fact, that when I was pregnant with my first child, I didn't buy a single baby item until after she was born! And I went about my duties in the hospital as though nothing were happening to my body. Ambivalence is a problem only when it isn't acknowledged and worked through. Many women desire pregnancy but are unsure about raising a baby. Others want children but don't want to go through a pregnancy, believing that it will be too painful, too damaging to their figure, or whatever. Others are afraid that they will treat their children as they were treated by their parents. These feelings of ambivalence need to be brought to consciousness so that they won't interfere with conceiving. Ask yourself the following and write the answer in your journal: why don't I want a baby? Be completely honest when you do this exercise.

Other Factors to Consider

Unabated Stress

Unabated emotional stress results in high adrenaline and cortisol levels. This leads to imbalances in other hormones that are important for optimal fertility including thyroid, progesterone, and estrogen. One of the most tried and true ways to decrease emotional stress and its physiological effects is with guided imagery, meditation, breathing through the nose, and relaxation. A wide number of well-documented modalities are available to help with this.

Mindfulness meditation and techniques such as Herbert Benson's relaxation response[58] (see PMS section) have been successfully used by Alice Domar, Ph.D., to help women heal from the stress of infertility while also increasing conception rates substantially.[59] A practical guide to Dr. Domar's program can be found in her books *Healing Mind, Healthy Woman* (Henry Holt, 1996) and *Self-Nurture* (Viking, 2000).

Mindfulness and relaxation training are especially important if you're going through any high-tech medical fertility treatments, since it is clear that unresolved and unexpressed emotional and psychological stress has physiologic consequences that may hamper the effectiveness of fertility treatments.[60] But when emotional stress is addressed and resolved, pregnancy rates go up. Helpful, guided imagery for enhancing fertility has been created by my colleague Belleruth Naparstek. (See www.healthjourneys.com.)

The Male Factor

When people hear the word *biological clock* we usually think "women." But this simply isn't true. Fully 40 percent of infertility problems lie with the man, not the woman! Because treating female fertility is far more lucrative and well-accepted than thoroughly investigating and treating male fertility problems, however, the male factor often remains hidden. According to urologist and male infertility specialist Harry Fisch, M.D., author of *The Male Biological Clock* (Free Press, 2005), roughly 10 percent of men trying to father a child—about 2.5 million men in the U.S. alone—are either infertile or subfertile. Many don't know they have a problem because they haven't been tested or tested thoroughly enough. As Dr. Fisch notes in his book, "Men's fertility is often checked only by a simple semen analysis. If a man seems to have enough sperm and those sperm seem healthy, he is presumed fertile. This kind of cursory 'exam' fails to detect a host of problems that could contribute to a fertility problem—most of which can be fixed relatively easily and inexpensively."[61] So the problem remains undetected and medical attention shifts to the female. This is a tragedy that is completely preventable.

Many of the factors that affect female fertility also affect male fertility. For example, sperm quality is greatly affected by nutrition. Recently I had the pleasure of having the husband of a former patient come up to me to show me pictures of his children. He said, "I can't thank you enough for recommending vitamin C and zinc to me so many years ago. We got pregnant within three months of my cleaning up my diet and starting those supplements."

An article in the July 2005 issue of *Fertility and Sterility* also showed that acupuncture can significantly improve both total sperm counts and sperm function in men.[62] Unabated stress and the hormonal imbalance that results are also often a problem. "Over the decades that I have been in this line of work," Dr. Fisch writes, "I have seen firsthand that the male biological clock can be slowed down, or even reversed, and problems with sexuality or fertility that arise at any point in a man's life can usually be fixed.[63]

Though male factor infertility is beyond the scope of this book, I urge every couple who is undergoing fertility evaluation to read Dr. Fisch's book, which gives a detailed plan to enhance male fertility and overall health.

Artificial and Natural Light

Living in artificial light without going outside into natural sunlight regularly can have adverse consequences on fertility, because light itself is a nutrient. Far too many people not only are stressed at work, but don't get outside much. When I was trying to conceive my first child, my basal body temperature rose very slowly at ovulation. (As I've already mentioned, ovulation causes a rise in basal body temperature of about 0.8 degrees. The ovary produces progesterone at ovulation, which in turn produces this rise in body temperature.) I decided to walk outside in the sunlight without glasses or contact lenses for twenty minutes each day. (To be effective, natural light has to hit the retina directly; we shouldn't look at the sun directly, but we must be out in the daytime.) Within one menstrual cycle, my basal body temperature began to rise very sharply at ovulation—a big improvement in the pattern. I got pregnant within two cycles of doing this, having tried for five months before. Though this isn't scientific proof of anything, it is an example of a simple change that had immediate measurable effects. The scientific literature on light and human biocycles is extensive.[64]

Nutritional Factors

Nutrients affect every hormonal interaction in the body, and adequate levels of them are clearly important in human reproduction. The standard American diet, high in processed foods and low in nutrients, is a setup for suboptimal nutrition at the time of conception. Studies have shown that taking vitamin C (500 mg every twelve hours in one study) and zinc supplements has helped infertile couples.[65] Other studies have shown beneficial effects from folate and B_{12} supplementation.[66] A double-blind placebo-contolled study on nutritional supplementation done at the Stanford University School of Medicine Department of Obstetrics and Gynecology and published in 2004 documented the benefits of nutritional supplementation in fertility patients. Researchers gave infertile women ages twenty-four to forty-six years a nutritional supplement containing vitamins, minerals, green tea extract, and chaste berry. After five months, fifteen women (33 percent) of the nutritionally supplemented group were pregnant. None of the placebo group had conceived. There were no side effects.[67]

If a woman has been on the pill, especially if she is coming off it to conceive, I recommend that she take a good multivitamin if she isn't doing so already. Given the standard diet today and the stress levels of modern life, I suggest that all couples who are trying to conceive begin taking a multivitamin-multimineral supplement. (Nutritional deficiencies can affect sperm quality in males.) It's also important to follow a diet that decreases cellular inflammation. (See chapter 17, "Nourishing Ourselves with Food.")

Eating disorders have also been associated with infertility because they are associated with endocrinologic disturbances. In one study, the investigators determined that 16.7 percent of their infertile subjects had eating disorders ranging from bulimia to anorexia. They recommended that a nutritional and eating disorder history be taken in infertility patients, particularly those with menstrual abnormalities.[68] (See chapter 17 for more on nutrition.) Once the eating disorder is successfully resolved, endocrine balance is often restored.

Smoking, Drugs, and Alcohol

Smoking, drugs such as marijuana and cocaine, and alcohol intake have been shown in many studies to have adverse effects on all aspects of reproduction, from conception (both women's and men's roles) to labor and delivery. Smoking causes significant increases in miscarriage and prematurity. Women who smoke are less successful with fertility treatments of all kinds than are nonsmokers. If you're serious about becoming pregnant, get help for your addictions. (See How to Quit Smoking in chapter 17, "Nourishing Ourselves with Food.")

Tubal Problems

In order to become pregnant, the fallopian tubes have to be able to pick up an egg and assist its passage to the waiting uterus. This process is dynamic and can be affected by myriad factors, one of the most common being scarring of the tubes from previous pelvic infections that are often the result of sexually transmitted diseases. This can be treated with a variety of techniques including deep tissue massage (see next page). In cases where the tubes are open but not fully functional, emotional work may need to be done. Tubal problems, says Caroline Myss, are centered around a woman's "inner child," while the tubes themselves are representative of unhealed childhood energy.

Helpful New Modalities for Enhancing Fertility

Traditional Chinese Medicine (TCM)

Though our culture is quick to bring in the big-gun technologies when it comes to fertility enhancement, these are often not necessary. One of most helpful modalities for enhancing fertility is Traditional Chinese Medicine (TCM). I've been referring patients to practitioners of acupuncture and herbology for years with great success. It's the first place I go for any health problem myself! My colleague Randine Lewis, Ph.D., has dedicated her life to helping women enhance their fertility through the use of TCM. Dr. Lewis, author of *The Infertility Cure* (Little, Brown, 2004), was in medical school when she began to have fertility problems herself. After exhausting the western medical approach, she discovered the ancient wisdom of Traditional Chinese Medicine. Not only did TCM resolve the imbalances that were leading to her own fertility problems, Dr. Lewis realized that it was the perfect solution for many other women as well. She eventually dropped out of medical school to pursue training in Traditional Chinese Medicine. Following training in China, she returned to the U.S., where she opened a clinic helping women achieve optimal fertility with a 75 percent success rate. Her fertility enhancement work also supports women who are using assisted reproductive technologies, helping them achieve better outcomes. Her fertility enhancement program includes three sections:

1. New Hope: Enhancing Ovarian Response—opening up to source energies to improve the function of the reproductive system.

2. Paradigm Shift: Improving Reproductive Capacity—improving the endocrine system's hormonal status and the energies between all the glands.

3. Nurturing the Mother Within: Opening to Implantation—the coming together of ovarian and hormonal responses, and allowing the body to receive.

Dr. Lewis points out that in Chinese medicine, *it takes a disturbed ovarian cycle a full ninety days to regenerate.* That's why she urges her patients to complete a ninety-day program. TCM, like most holistic methods, is aimed at rebalancing the body from the inside out. It's not a quick fix the way western medicine claims to be. Dr. Lewis offers Fertile Soul Retreats four to six times per year that include personalized evaluation and recommendations. (See www.thefertilesoul.com.)

Deep Tissue Massage

Pelvic adhesions that interfere with fallopian tube function have long been associated with fertility problems as well as chronic pain. It is estimated that approximately 40 percent of female infertility is associated with scarring of the pelvic organs either from prior surgery or infections. A noninvasive, nonsurgical type of deep tissue massage performed by specially trained physical therapists (known as the Wurn Technique after its founders, Larry and Belinda Wurn—both physical therapists) has been shown, in initial studies, to do the following:

- More than 75 percent reversal of fallopian tube occlusion in women with diagnosed tubal occlusion

- More than 70 percent infertility reversal in women who were physician-diagnosed infertile

~ Significant improvement in IVF results when therapy was performed prior to IVF transfer

This technique also helps relieve many other conditions including inability to reach orgasm, severe recurring menstrual pain, irritable bowel, painful intercourse, endometriosis, and pelvic pain. (For more information, contact Clear Passage Therapies at 866-222-9437 or visit www.clearpassage.com.)

Maya abdominal massage, a technique used for centuries by indigenous healers in Central America, is another form of deep tissue massage that has been used to successfully treat infertility as well as other reproductive and pelvic disorders. (See the dysmenorrhea section of chapter 5, "The Menstrual Cycle," for a fuller explanation; for a directory of certified practitioners of Maya abdominal massage, visit www.arvigomassage.com.)

Women's Stories

Grace: childhood fears. Grace was a successful businesswoman from the Midwest at the time when she first came to see me about her infertility. Married for three years, she had been unable to conceive. Like many of my patients, she preferred to avoid extensive and invasive testing to investigate her problem unless it was absolutely necessary. Her reason for this was that she didn't want anyone "mucking around in there."

Grace ovulated regularly, had a normal pelvic exam, and regular pain-free periods. She had no history of infection, IUD use, or prior pelvic surgery. In short, nothing about her history would lead me to think that there was anything wrong with her reproductive system. Her husband's sperm count was normal.

Over the course of her care, she got in touch with a memory from when she was four years old. At that age, she recalled, she had become so ill that she passed out with a high fever and ultimately had to be taken to the hospital. Though she'd felt sick for several days, she had not said anything to her parents until she was quite ill and had developed urinary retention. In the hospital she had to be held down by several nurses and orderlies while they inserted a urinary catheter into her bladder. Her mother felt that this represented very unseemly behavior on her daughter's part.

After Grace's recovery, her mother took her by the hand and made her apologize for being a "bad girl" to each of the nurses and orderlies who had taken care of her. She remembered acutely how ashamed she had felt. She had always felt that she had had a happy childhood, though she admitted that she couldn't remember much about it. But her hospital experience and her mother's abusive behavior had left a very deep wound. I suspect that her childhood was not nearly as happy as she remembered it.

After Grace told me about that childhood hospitalization, her reluctance to undergo invasive testing became understandable. As of this writing, she is working with a therapist and has decided to put her fertility workup on hold so that she can transform her old fears. She recently told me, "I realize I'm not ready to have a child now. I have too much work to do on myself. I don't want to pass my own unfinished business on to a child."

Margaret: the ovarian window. Margaret was twenty-seven when she first came to see me. She was not married at the time, but she told me that she wanted children someday and had always dreamed of becoming a mother. From the time she started her menstrual periods, Margaret had had very bad cramps and excessive bleeding, often resulting in missing days of school. At the age of eighteen she decided that she could no longer live with the problem and went to see her mother's gynecologist. He suggested surgery immediately and admitted her to the hospital. He performed major pelvic surgery, removing an ovarian cyst, and he told her she had endometriosis.

Postoperatively in the hospital, Margaret developed what is called a paralytic ileus—her bowels wouldn't move. She was given a soapsuds enema daily, which she said hurt so much she wanted to die. She also developed a fever that wouldn't go away. She had her mother bring in aspirin to bring her fever down so that she could go home. She said that the hospital treatment was so abusive, she wanted to get out of there at any cost. During this time, her parents were going through a divorce—and although they visited her at the hospital, they used her room as a place to fight. Her postoperative recovery was far from ideal.

After her surgery, Margaret's cramps lessened a bit, but they were still present for most of her menstrual cycle. This went on for several years and she simply put up with it. At about the age of twenty she decided to become sexually active and went to a gynecologist for a diaphragm fitting. He told her, "Your pelvis is destroyed. You are definitely sterile. You'll never have kids." She told me that she took in this message "at a cellular level" and that she didn't see another gynecologist for a long time after that. When she finally did see another doctor, he said to her, "Have your children now, or you may never have any." Since she was just finishing nursing school, was not in a relationship, and was in the process of moving, conceiving a child was not high on her priority list at that time.

Around the age of twenty-five Margaret moved to Maine. At a routine GYN exam she was told by a midwife that she had a huge endometrioma (an ovarian cyst filled with old blood from endometriosis). For a second opinion, she saw a gynecologist who was very reassuring and told her her pelvis was normal, which was very comforting to her. But she had by this time gotten a lot of mixed messages. Was she okay or not?

At the same time she was a visiting nurse, teaching pregnant teenagers parenting skills and working with people who had been reported to the Department of Human Services for child abuse. She told me that during this part of her life she simply ignored the issue of possible infertility. It would have been too hard to face, given the suffering she saw every day.

As I mentioned, Margaret first saw me when she was twenty-seven years old. We went over her notes from her prior surgery. The ovarian cyst that had been removed was probably a functional cyst from ovulation. Very little, if any, endometriosis had been seen. (If she had had that surgery today, it would have been carried out via laparoscopy, without a big incision. The scarring that she had as a result of that surgery would most likely not have happened.)

Because she was still having pelvic pain, I suggested a whole-food diet with no dairy foods. Within one cycle her pain stopped, and it has not returned. She got married several years later and tried to conceive. After a year or so of unsuccessful efforts, she went to a specialist in Boston, who did a laparoscopy. He told her, "I did the best I could but I don't think there's much hope. You have too many adhesions in there." Adhesions are fibrous bands that form from inflammation and can block mobility of the organs. (Do you remember using mucilage in school? If you put some of this glue on your fingers and then try to pull the fingers apart, little stringy threads of glue form between your fingers. These are what adhesions look like. Some are firm, and some are quite flexible.) Margaret eventually had a second laparoscopy from an infertility specialist to whom I referred her, to see if there had been any improvement in her pelvis. (It is not uncommon for a woman with infertility to have a number of laparoscopies.) We scheduled this surgery at a time when I could be present so that I could support her psychologically and see her pelvis as well. She had *no* endometriosis. Instead, her fallopian tubes were encased in scar tissue, most likely from the prior surgery. But around one ovary and tube was a clear window that was free from adhesions. Under the right circumstances, she had a chance of getting pregnant.

In the recovery room, this fertility specialist told Margaret, "It looks like a bomb went off in there." (Doctors' words are powerful at any time. In the recovery room, when someone is coming out of anesthesia, they are doubly powerful. I was not happy about that comment to her.)

I told Margaret about the adhesion-free window. Later that night, she dreamt that a wise old man came to her and said, "There's a window there. I can see it. It's a window of opportunity. It's all you need to become pregnant." After this dream, she stayed home and cried for three days. Then she went into high gear and called every fertility clinic in the United States, as well as many adoption agencies. She organized and collated a resource book for herself.

About six months later, she decided to do in vitro fertilization (IVF), and she and her husband went to New York. "It was awful," she told me. "I was on Pergonal and Clomid [drugs that make the ovaries produce many eggs]. The scene in the waiting room at the IVF place was crazy. There were fifteen women, all talking about where they were in their cycles and how much money they'd spent already. One woman was on a protocol that cost $30,000 per cycle. She had just remortgaged her house. The other women were talking about what they still had to sell, so that they'd have the money to keep trying. It seemed as though their whole lives were focused on this one issue."

Margaret had been in recovery for a long time for bulimia and compulsive overeating. "There's no question but that infertility treatment becomes an addiction," she says. "You don't know when or how to stop. And you keep hoping that maybe, just maybe, the next drug or surgery will help."

Margaret and her husband had agreed to give IVF one try. Her husband was, by now, fairly tired of the whole infertility scene and of having to perform "on command."

"I used to get mad at him," Margaret told me. "Sometimes when I was ovulating, he'd be uninterested in making love. I'd wonder why he couldn't be like all the other men—able to produce an ejaculation at the sight of a *Playboy* pinup. He just didn't like making love on demand. When I asked him what the bathrooms were like at the infertility clinics, he told me about all the pornography at the hospitals and clinics in which he'd given sperm samples by this time."

When Margaret told me this part of the story, I realized once again that with all our high-tech infertility technology, we still need the human mind to produce an ejaculation. Margaret's husband's mind was primed with pornographic images at the time of ejaculation, and Margaret admitted that she played right into this. She wanted a child, and he was her sperm donor. But the energetic quality and even the physiological properties of seminal fluid ejaculated during intercourse with a person a man loves, I am convinced, are entirely different in quality from what he produces via masturbation in a hospital bathroom while reading pornography. How much nicer it would be if ejaculations collected for potential egg fertilization were accompanied by a feeling of deep love in the moment, both for the woman and for potential offspring.

Margaret said that the physician who performed her egg retrieval was "so nasty." She and her husband had been told that there was a 5 percent chance that her eggs wouldn't fertilize. They never expected that they'd have that problem, but nine eggs were collected and none of them fertilized. The technicians said that there might be "antisperm antibodies." So she and her husband went to Boston to have special cultures done to check for this. About this time, she remembered feeling punished. She said, "I felt like kicking and crying. I was mad at God. I kept remembering those teenagers who were pregnant. I was pissed." No antisperm antibodies were found.

During the whole time, Margaret remembered, no one ever talked to her about how she was feeling. From my perspective as a physician, she always appeared to be jovial, in control, and upbeat. But she told me later, "Being in control was my way of avoiding my feelings. I wished so much that someone would sit me down and try to piece the whole puzzle together for me."

Still, Margaret had that "window" around her ovary. She heard of another surgeon in Boston to whom she wanted to talk, and I referred her to him. She found him very respectful and helpful. He performed a meticulous laparoscopy, during which he cleared up many of her adhesions. "There was something very special about this surgery," she told me. "This surgeon was a true healer. He was positive. After this surgery, I knew I had done everything that I could possibly do. Now, I was almost ready to turn the whole issue over to my higher power."

By this time, Margaret and her husband had completed their adoption home studies, and in the spring they were told that a baby was available through an agency in Mexico. They adopted a baby boy and have since adopted two more children.

Margaret is now forty-three. Her husband stayed home with their three adopted children when they were under the age of three. Now they're all in school and child care duties are shared. Though she doesn't want any more children, Margaret once told me, "I missed being pregnant. I grieve the fact that I may never experience pregnancy and that I may never breast-feed. My cousin was recently pregnant. Seeing her, I longed to have that kind of belly. I keep saying to myself, 'What do I need to learn from this?' I still don't know. When I hear about other people getting pregnant, I still feel bad. Sex is tainted for me, in a way. I still can't separate it from the goal of getting pregnant. My husband and I are in a support group with other parents who've adopted children. People think that now that we've adopted, I'll get pregnant.

"I keep thinking, though I know that it isn't helpful, that if I had done my interpersonal work, I'd get pregnant, and that there must be something I still have to learn from this. I keep thinking that if I could just figure it out, I'd get pregnant. It's as if getting pregnant would be *proof* that I was doing everything right!" Margaret's feelings are very common—though not helpful. This thinking comes from the illusion of control so common in our culture.

Eventually, Margaret went to New York and worked with Niravi Payne. Through insightful work on her family history, she discovered that her mother had unconsciously never wanted children, though she had always said she did. Margaret had picked up on her mother's conflict in utero and internalized it. She discovered that her maternal grandmother also had not wanted children. Margaret was now going to break the chain of pain passed down to her. As a result of uncovering and naming the family conflicts about childbearing that she had internalized, she was able to release the whole issue of "longing for pregnancy." She feels free for the first time in years.

I learned a great deal from Margaret. She told me that none of the books on infertility talk about how abusive the infertility rat race is to one's self-esteem and self-worth. Many infertile couples stay on the infertility quest for years. Our current technology is very costly and complex, although it keeps improving. According to the Centers for Disease Control, the number of live births that began with assisted reproductive technology increased 128 percent between 1996 and 2002. In fact, almost 29 percent of all ART cycles now end in a live birth. The most successful transfers are with fresh (as opposed to frozen) embryos from donors. (Usually donor eggs are fertilized with the husband's—or another donor's—sperm.) The success rate for that group is as high as 50 percent! Even the group with the lowest success rate—transfers of frozen embryos with non-donor eggs (meaning a woman's own eggs fertilized in vitro) is now a respectable 24.8 percent.[69]

Now, with the advent of so many pregnancies from ovum donors and fertility-drug-induced multiple pregnancies requiring selective "fetal reduction" to get rid of the excess babies, we've entered completely uncharted territory. How all this will play out in the psyches of the children and parents involved is an unknown. What is known is this: there will be consequences, and how we deal with them will depend upon how conscious we choose to become about what we're doing.

As long as technology keeps holding out yet another chance, infertile couples often don't grieve their loss fully and get on with their lives. They're caught in an emotional holding pattern—hostages to their hope. After a time, it is important for their health to move on. The mind/body approaches that I've outlined here are helping many couples do just that.

Whitney: healing from infertility. One of my patients, after a long bout with endometriosis, surgery, and infertility, healed herself through a process of writing down her feelings and drawing pictures to illustrate them with her left (nondominant) hand. Drawing with the nondominant hand activates the brain's right hemisphere and facilitates getting in touch with imagery and emotions that are important to integrate consciously in the healing process. Memories from childhood often surface as well, because writing and drawing with a hand we don't usually use puts us instantly in a "childlike" state.[70] Whitney's process led to a book that documents and honors her healing.[71]

As a result of her infertility, however, she and her husband became estranged for a while. She wrote, "Over time, a great abyss developed between me and my husband and a gigantic unstable mountain rose between us. I didn't know how to get over, under, or around these obstacles. I had tried everything that I knew how to do. I had gone to couples counseling and to individual counseling as well. I raged. I was loving. I was rejecting. I isolated myself and went on my own way.

"I created a healing ritual for myself. I made a 'child' from pine branches, spruce, pinecones, and berries. All the beauty of the woods went into constructing that child. She had flowers in her pine needle hair. She was angry for not being born. I gave her my name.

"I sat her [the stick child] next to a tree by the pond. She withered and died. I saw her sometimes when I walked by the lake. Now there is nothing left but her stick-bones.

"She didn't 'live' very long but there was energy and beauty in the brief moments of her life. Her coming and going helped me to face the hurt and sadness I felt because I couldn't have another child.

"I read books looking for role models of women who had to deal

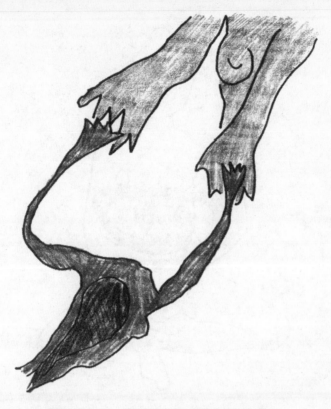

FIGURE 12: SEEKING PARTNERSHIP

with infertility. I didn't find many role models, but in Queen Guinevere I finally found some comfort. She couldn't give King Arthur a child and she suffered greatly. I felt less alone and less ugly when I read that tale. I discovered that not all princesses who get married have children and live happily ever after. There was at least one other woman like me."

Eventually, through her writing and drawing process she began to heal. (See figure 12.) "I have stopped blaming and rejecting my body," she wrote. "I am learning to love my ovaries, fallopian tubes, and uterus. I drew some pictures honoring my reproductive organs. I noticed that at first they were totally separate from my body. In some drawings, they were yearning for a connection. Then I drew them reaching out to me—seeking connection.

"Through this drawing process I began to feel a softening and a tingling in my reproductive organs. Life was returning to my uterus, ovaries and fallopian tubes. They had been feeling dead and hurt for far too long. I named them Queen, Princess, Crowned Jewel, Heart, Warmth, and Love.

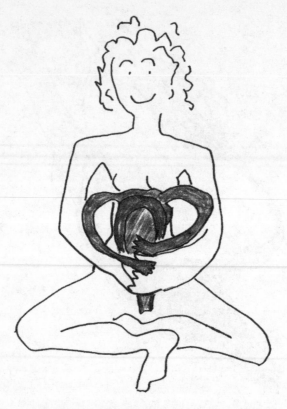

FIGURE 13: REUNITED IN HARMONY

"Finally, through seeing how I had separated my uterus, fallopian tubes, and ovary from my body in my drawings, I was able to create a positive and loving image of myself and return my reproductive organs to their proper place, where I look at them with gratitude for giving me a son [from a previous marriage] and making me a woman." (See figure 13.)

PREGNANCY LOSS

Miscarriage

Approximately one in six pregnancies ends in miscarriage. I tell women that miscarriage is usually nature's way of getting rid of conceptions that will not result in healthy babies. Women who miscarry still must grieve the potential child, though, even if they believe the pregnancy wasn't "meant to be." In some cases, they go through as much grief as women who deliver stillborn babies.

After a woman has a miscarriage, her chances of having another one are not increased, but many women nonetheless lose trust in their bodies after miscarrying. Grieving and learning to trust again are major issues for women following miscarriage. Another major issue is guilt: many women have the mistaken impression that something they did must have caused the miscarriage. But generally speaking healthy babies don't just miscarry. (Women who smoke, unfortunately, do have two times the normal rate of miscarriage. And it appears from studies on the "products of conception" that these are miscarriages of otherwise normal fetuses. Smokers also have decreased success in all aspects of fertility treatments.) There is also some data on the link between mercury exposure (usually from dental fillings) and subsequent miscarriage. Mercury should never be used for filling teeth in any case and it should *never* be used in pregnancy. Far better, less toxic materials are readily available. A study by Claire Infante-Rivard, M.D., Ph.D., of McGill University in Montreal found that drinking an amount of caffeine more than that in three cups of coffee a day during pregnancy nearly tripled the rate of miscarriage.[72] However, a later study of 5,144 pregnant women from the State Department of Health Services in Emeryville, California, Kaiser Permanente Division of Research, and the University of California at San Francisco found no significant increased risk for miscarriage. Among heavy users (300 mg caffeine or three cups of coffee per day) the miscarriage rate increased only slightly. Given that caffeine is a well-documented stimulant and neurotoxin, it's advisable for women to decrease or eliminate caffeine consumption before conception and during pregnancy.[73] If you've had a miscarriage, don't spend a lot of time trying to figure out *why*. Just stay with what you're feeling, and give yourself time to mourn your loss.

Several studies have indicated that in women who have repeated (three or more) miscarriages, there may be an interplay between emotions and the hormonal systems involved in pregnancy. Dr. Robert J. Weil, a researcher on the emotional aspects of infertility, and C. Tupper write, "The pregnant woman functions as a communications system. The fetus is a source of continuous messages to which the mother responds with subtle psychobiological adjustments. Her personality, influenced by her ever-changing life situation, can either (1) act upon the fetus to maintain its constant growth and development or (2) create physiological changes that can result in abortion."[74] The ways in which a woman's body modulates her feelings about her pregnancy are diverse, but all are mediated by the immune and endocrine systems and also by the ways in which our thoughts impact cells directly. Thus, studies have shown that there are endocrinological imbalances resulting from emotional stress in women who habitually miscarry (known as "habitual aborters" in medical circles) and in those who have what is known as an "incompetent cervix," a cervix that dilates too quickly so that the uterus cannot hold on to a baby. Some studies of women who habitually miscarry or who have an incompetent cervix have suggested that some of those women have difficulty accepting motherhood and their feminine role. Femininity, to these women, means being self-sacrificing, passive, and suffering and having to serve and cater to their husbands (yet control them). They became pregnant "because their husbands wanted a child so badly." They also felt that "having a child was a woman's main accomplishment and that not being able to have children meant being inadequate as women."[75] They frequently chose dependent, nonverbal husbands and had restricted social outlets and low adaptability. Due to their aloofness, they were often unable to take part in life around them. The control group of nonmiscarrying women in these studies had much healthier images of womanhood.[76] Another study found that "habitual aborters" basically received their pleasure in life through fulfilling the expectations of others. They appeared to react compliantly to the demands of others, despite tension and hostility building in their bodies. Feeling guilty about directly expressing their anger at other people's demands, their frustration built until their body responded with a physical illness. Miscarrying the child (the "psychosomatic" or "autoimmune" illness in this case) relieved the tension that had built up in their bodies. Interestingly, when many of these same women later underwent psychotherapy and learned how to deal directly with their anger rather than storing it in their bodies, their success rate for subsequent pregnancy was 80 percent, while it was only 6 percent for those who did not go through therapy.[77] Though these studies are fairly dated, they certainly support the role of psychological factors in fertility—factors that are very important to address but not beat yourself up with!

Miscarriage is multifactorial and there's still a great deal we don't know. After his wife had her third miscarriage, science writer Jon Cohen embarked on a thorough investigation of the topic and wrote the most comprehensive book on the subject to date, entitled *Coming to Term: Uncovering the Truth About Miscarriage* (Houghton Mifflin, 2005). Cohen points out the downside of early pregnancy tests—something I've seen repeatedly. Early pregnancy tests have actually increased the rate of so-called miscarriage. By diagnosing pregnancy so early—often before a period is even missed and long before the body has had a chance to say "yea or nay" to the health of a potential embryo—women with a positive early pregnancy test begin to invest emotionally in the pregnancy. And then when the body says "no" to this embryo, which was never meant to reach viability, the woman may experience enormous grief and feel like a failure when in fact her body was acting appropriately. I've seen women repeatedly fall into utter despair over something that is really a gift of wisdom from the body—getting rid of a defective fertilized egg.

Back before early pregnancy tests were available, this so-called miscarriage would have been nothing more than a slightly late or heavier than normal period. And this experience wouldn't be perceived as a sign of failure or inadequacy by the woman herself. (Some experts suggest that up to 90 percent of fertilized eggs never make it to term. And most of these don't even get far enough to make enough hormone for a positive pregnancy test.) I have watched women put themselves in utter despair over this kind of miscarriage, which leads them to believe that their bodies have failed. Nothing could be further from the truth. The good news, as Cohen documents, is that a woman's chance of successfully carrying a baby to term actually increases after each subsequent miscarriage. The books mentioned in the approach to fertility resources for this chapter have helped many women heal miscarriage problems.

Ectopic Pregnancy

A fertilized egg normally implants in the lining of the uterus. Implantation anywhere else is called an ectopic pregnancy. Approximately 1.9 percent of all pregnancies are ectopic, with the risk (higher in nonwhite than in white women) having increased tenfold from 1970 through 2004. These increases have been reported not only for the U.S. but also for Eastern Europe, Scandinavia, and Great Britain. The most likely causes for this increase in ectopic pregnancy are the following: 1. the prevalence of sexually transmitted diseases, which can lead to tubal scarring, 2. the ability of transvaginal ultrasound and early pregnancy tests to pick up the diagnosis in pregnancies that would simply reabsorb on their own, 3. the use of tubal sterilization techniques, 4. the increase in C-sections, which increases the risk of ectopic pregnancies in subsequent pregnancies, and finally, 5. the use of tubal surgery to repair damaged tubes.

The diagnosis of ectopic pregnancy is made in a woman with a positive pregnancy test when an ultrasound fails to find evidence of pregnancy in the uterus (a small sac of fluid surrounding an embryo and known as a gestational sac). When this happens, a series of blood tests several days apart are drawn to determine whether the amount of pregnancy hormone (Beta HCG [human chorionic gonadotropin]) is increasing or decreasing. If it is decreasing, then it is safe to watch and wait and simply follow the patient carefully with blood tests every other day or so. But if the Beta HCG hormone level continues to increase and there is still no evidence of pregnancy in the uterus itself, then the pregnancy is presumed to be in the wrong location. Often it will show up as a mass in one of the tubes on ultrasound. Sometimes you can even feel it on pelvic exam. Since a ruptured ectopic can be life-threatening because of hemorrhaging, ectopics that are growing must be treated. This is usually done with the chemotherapy drug methotrexate, which kills rapidly growing cells. This works in the majority of cases and the tube resorbs the ectopic tissue over time. When medical treatment fails, surgery is necessary. A woman who has had an ectopic pregnancy has a 7 to 15 percent chance of having a recurrence because of scarring in the tube.

Though ectopic pregnancy accounts for 10 percent of all pregnancy-related deaths, the actual death rate from this pregnancy complication has decreased tenfold in the past few decades, most likely due to improved diagnosis and management.[78] Whenever a pregnant woman has pain and bleeding in the first trimester, an ectopic pregnancy needs to be ruled out.

I would strongly recommend deep tissue massage such as the Wurn Technique or Maya abdominal massage for any woman who has had a history of tubal infection, tubal surgery, or ectopic pregnancy. (See chapter 5, "The Menstrual Cycle.") That's because this technique might well be able to help prevent or eliminate the tubal adhesions that favor a future ectopic pregnancy.

Ended Beginnings: The Experience of a Stillbirth

While I was in my residency, a lovely young Catholic woman gave birth to two perfect identical-twin girls. Unfortunately, these twins had gotten their cords wrapped around each other and died just before labor started (a very unusual event). As I was helping the attending physician deliver these two babies, I asked the mother if she'd like to see them and hold them. I had intended to wrap them in baby blankets and spend some time with her after the delivery, sitting with her while she held her babies. But her doctor scolded me, and he said to her, "Regina, it's better if you don't look. We'll just give you something to put you to sleep so you can get on with your life and get this behind you. It will bother you if you see them." An obedient woman, she complied. As a physician in training, I knew that it wasn't a good idea for me to argue with her doctor.

I knew instinctively that this doctor was wrong and that this mother needed to interact with what she had created, lest she go on to dream for years of babies with no faces. Her babies were in fact beautiful. She needed to see their little hands, their perfect bodies and their angelic faces—and to know that her body had created them. It is so much easier to deal with what is than with our fantasies about what is.

Most women need to interact with their "creations"—their stillborn babies. Otherwise, unfinished emotional business may result. When a couple has a deformed baby or a stillborn (or suffers the death of any child or loved one, for that matter), they need to look at and touch this being, take pictures, name the child, and perhaps have a ceremony of some kind that acknowledges that this child existed. Thanks to the vision of Kathy Adzich, many hospitals now provide a room where couples can hold their babies who are sick or who have died, bathe them, and take pictures of them—so that parents have something tangible to hold on to. The process of simply holding the baby and interacting with him or her can be extraordinarily healing.

I met Kathy Adzich, a wonderful, light-filled human being who is obviously doing the work she was born to do, in San Diego in the fall of 2005. Kathy lost her son Jakob to sepsis when he was twenty-six days old (as well as two other infant sons before Jakob). Not ready to have Jakob taken away to the hospital morgue, she asked the nurses if she could have a room where she could hold her baby for a while (and for her, "a while" meant a few days). To their credit, the hospital staff complied. Though some thought Kathy should move on, she felt that staying with her son was perfectly normal. She needed time to sleep with her son nestled in her arms, to keep him close, to stroke him, and bathe him, and sing to him. She made prints of his hands. She invited friends and family to visit, and together they told stories, laughed, and sang. No one thought it was weird or morbid.

And the process helped Kathy transform her grief into a living force to help others. She started a movement to humanize death, committing her life to ensuring that the millions of people who lose loved ones year after year have the resources and space they need to say goodbye. Kaiser Permanente will be opening its first Jakob's Room in 2007, with others to follow. The room will include a rocking chair, hand- and footprint molds, photography access, music, and educational and outreach resources; parents' specific needs will be honored.

Kathy now regularly speaks to hospital staffs, police departments, and parenting organizations to help them create policies that help the bereaved say goodbye instead of whisking the body away and truncating the grief process. (For more information, visit Kathy's website at www.trustingthejourney.com.)

When the work of the late Elisabeth Kübler-Ross, M.D., on grief and dying became better known with the publication of her classic work *On Death and Dying* (Macmillan, 1969), hospitals started to realize that avoiding and denying death didn't help the patients' healing process. Far too many women who have lost babies never grieved properly—in fact, they were often told "You have other children at home" of "You can have more" or "You must be strong." Grief was considered self-indulgent.

But that which isn't fully grieved cannot be released. (This is also a problem with infertility.) Healing from the pain of pregnancy loss or loss of a child is a process. It requires time. It requires that a woman give herself the time and space necessary to grieve and heal.

Barb Frank wrote me the following letter about the unexpected stillbirth of her son, Micah, after a normal and healthy pregnancy. "I was very porous after this experience. It has been a time of intense emotional and spiritual growth for me. Initially it was the opening experience of allowing vulnerability and being willing to openly grieve with my friends...to cry in front of and with other people was really healing and a very new experience. (I am usually 'in control' and a real 'planner.') This also has become an emotionally transforming experience for three women friends who came to the birth center and were able to spend time holding Micah with us and being in the midst of that mysterious energy between birth and death present in that room. Subsequently it has made my compassion and understanding so much deeper; it has affected my work as a pediatric occupational therapist with families dealing with their own fear and loss over their children with disabilities. I am no longer afraid of their tears or even anger, because I've been there. The need to create a space and time for grief and reflection in the midst of busy days has brought me closer to a spiritual discipline of regular prayer/meditation time that I always wanted to make time for, but never did until now, when I've had to for emotional survival. So I guess I'm getting the message."

Barb also created an announcement to be able to share the news of her birth. She used it for everything from shower gift thank-yous to enclosures at the memorial service—and even put it into some Christmas cards. It reads:

Facing the mystery of
life and death
we mourn the loss of our son
—Micah—
who accompanied us through a healthy
and hopeful pregnancy . . . but was stillborn
on September 21, 5 lbs. 6 oz., 19 inches.

At the request of her midwives, she also wrote the following list of the things that helped her in her recovery process. This is a most helpful and universally applicable list of things to help with grieving a loss of any kind. I am honored to share it with you from Barb.

~ Having enough time, initially, with the baby and taking photos to have and share later. Some couples have also dressed and bathed the baby. One couple took the child home with them for several hours.

~ Having friends come and see and hold the baby with us. This validated the whole experience for me, as no one else would get to meet Micah, and in that sense it still isn't "real" for most friends and family.

~ Crying with people, and seeing others cry, made it easier for us. When people tried to hide their emotions in an effort to be "strong" or "professional," it made things feel worse.

~ Notes and phone calls from people who have been there and experienced loss themselves, and could articulate this. Also communication from others who had just spent time thinking about what we have experienced and were able to reflect on it beyond "I don't know what to say."

~ Physical presence of people and physical contact with people, especially in the early days and weeks. I had a need to literally hang on to people to feel grounded and "present" in the world, which is uncharacteristic of me. As time has passed, phone calls still serve that purpose, especially when I need to connect when I'm having a hard time.

~ Creating a "shrine" of important gifts, notes, photos, remembrances of Micah. This has been a tangible way to remember and honor him, and I never understood the importance of shrines/altars in other cultures and churches until this happened. Lighting a candle (and carrying it around the house) still helps a lot when I feel depressed.

~ Getting back in shape physically, getting as much exercise as my body could deal with at each stage.

~ Being involved in purposeful activity. Achieving concrete tasks around the house, in the garden, that gave me a sense of accomplishment but didn't require too much problem-solving (I was easily frustrated, had memory problems, and not much creative energy for a time).

~ Being outside. For me, getting back into work in the garden puts me in touch with the cycle of life and is grounding and gives me a sense of hope and renewal. Going to the beach is good, but the ocean was almost too emotionally powerful at first... so infinite and symbolic as a source of life.

~ Reading the books and handouts on grief and loss of a baby. We read many out loud together, which also let us talk about our feelings. They always made me cry, but it has been important and positive to cry. Afterward I usually feel better. (I highly recommend *Life Touches Life* [NewSage, 2004] by Lorraine Ash.)

Barb went on to give birth to a healthy baby girl. She told me that that pregnancy was difficult because she was always worried about the health of the baby. But with the support of her midwives and the staff of the birth center, she made it through and is now enjoying her new daughter.

ADOPTION

Adoption is receiving more attention than ever these days. In fact, a recent Centers for Disease Control survey published by the Urban Institute reported that between 1995 and 2002, the number of women between the ages of eighteen and forty-four who were interested in adopting increased 38 percent (from 13 to 18 million).[79] Through the years I've worked both with women who have given up babies for adoption and with women who have adopted babies. In the past, adoption agencies operated under the illusions of secrecy and denial. Now, through the efforts of birth mothers and adopted children alike, natural parents and their adopted-out babies are finding one another, sometimes with joyous results but sometimes also with great disappointment. Both giving up a baby for adoption and adopting one have consequences. Giving up or taking in a child is always emotionally stressful for all parties. Adoption is an area in which society is learning that secrets don't work. They especially don't work with matters of lineage. Bloodlines are very powerful—they hold ancient memories.

Even more important, every baby is deeply imprinted in the womb by the prenatal environment created by her mother. There is no way around this except to acknowledge the fact that none of us is a tabula rasa when we are born. On the other hand, any untoward prenatal imprint can be greatly ameliorated by how the adopted child is parented. The birth mother and the mother who adopts both need to know this. All my patients who have adopted children into their homes have put together as much information as they can about the child's circumstances, to share it with the child when the time comes. Most children want to know their heritage. Birth mothers, too, almost always want to know where their children are and if they are all right—even when they know that they themselves are not capable of raising them adequately. In matters of adoption, the only thing that works is honesty.

Currently, a large number of American couples have adopted foreign infants. I can't think of a better way to promote global awareness and intercultural understanding. A patient who adopted two Chinese children told me the following story, which she calls "Listening with the Heart."

In November 1981 Susan and her husband, Bob, went to Taiwan with the intention of adopting a child. One month later, they returned as a family of four with Anio Nicholas, almost six, and Shao-Ma Annie, almost four. "Christmas of 1981 was a wonderful celebration of the birth of our new family," said Susan. The following Thanksgiving Susan invited her extended family of origin to share the holiday with her "new" family. Near the end of that day of celebration, Annie, sitting on the stairs, asked accusingly, "*Why* did you come to get us in that taxicab in Taiwan, anyway?" Susan wondered what had prompted that question. Then it dawned on her that for the first time since the adoption she was sitting in a roomful of people whom she dearly loved, to whom she had been paying a great deal of attention—the kind of attention that up until then Annie had seen her give only to Bob, to Nicholas, and to herself.

Focusing on her daughter's question, Susan told her the truth: that she had had a very happy life, full of friends and family, work and play, but that she had still felt filled with a love that wasn't used up. And so she and her husband had gone looking for someone to love and had found her and her brother. Annie paused, tipped her head pensively to one side, then went off to brush her teeth. Susan joined her for their nightly ritual together. As Annie squirted toothpaste onto both their toothbrushes, she said defiantly, "I want to go back to Taiwan to see my *Chinese* mother"—even though she had been told that there was no record of her mother and that it wasn't known who had brought her to the home. Susan realized that her daughter's desire to go back to Taiwan at that moment was symbolic and important. So Susan asked her, "Would you like me to go with you, or would you like to go by yourself?" Annie answered, "By myself." Susan was struck by a sense of loss, emptiness, and despair. She later told me, "Welling up in me was the question, 'But what about me?' I love you and have loved you with all my heart! Isn't that good enough? What about me?"

Then she looked at her daughter and knew that her longing for her Chinese mother was simply a natural part of her birth history and who she was. "Annie was, in her love for a woman whom neither of us would probably ever meet, sharing with me her deepest self. I could join her now, at the core of her being, in her love, or I could bar myself from it. And so finally, I, the verbalizer, just listened—actively, achingly—with my heart."

Several Christmases later, Susan and Bob were walking together, with Annie swinging between them, holding their hands. She swung high, and as Bob's and Susan's eyes met over her head, she called out to the sky: "Hello, Chinese Mother! How are you? I am happy and I hope you are, too! I love you! Goodbye!"

I once participated in a wonderful adoption ceremony with a couple, long infertile, who had successfully found a child with the help, intent, and prayers of their extended family and community. They brought the baby to a large gathering shortly after the adoption to share their joy with us. I would recommend a similar ceremony to all who are adopting a child. It is a touching and conscious way to bring a child into her or his new community.

In a ceremonial fashion, the woman leading the event had the adoptive parents hold up the baby and carry it around to the members of our community to be welcomed. At the same time, she asked those people who had been adopted to please stand in the center of the circle during this ceremony. As we each welcomed the baby, she addressed the people who had themselves been adopted. "As we welcome this new baby and celebrate his birth and his new parents, may this day symbolize for you that you are deeply wanted, that you were always deeply wanted. And from now on, no matter what has happened to you in the past, may you know how meaningful your birth was and, seeing how deeply wanted and blessed this child is, claim the same thing for yourself." This ceremony was a great healing on many levels for many people and was full of wonder and hope.

FERTILITY AS METAPHOR

We must deal with the economic and social problems that are the root causes of high fertility rates: widespread poverty and the oppression of women... When women everywhere have control over their own reproductive choices, fertility rates drop.
—The Union of Concerned Scientists

Motherhood is not simply the organic process of giving birth... it is understanding the needs of the world.
—Alexis DeVeaux, mother and sponsor of MADRE, a Latin American relief organization

We humans have been clever, producing more and more food from less and less land. The Union of Concerned Scientists writes, "Our species simply cannot survive today's recklessly accelerating population growth, the irresponsible squandering of the Earth's resources, and the continuing destruction of our environment... Every day, there are a quarter of a million more of us than there were the day before. Every week, we must find ways to feed another city the size of Philadelphia. Every month, we must wrest from the Earth additional resources to keep alive another New Jersey. And every year, we are adding another whole Mexico to the burden of this small planet.[80]

The time of endless productivity without replenishing is coming to an end. We as women *must* use our inherent creativity—our womb power—to regenerate our planet as well as to produce the next generation. We can no longer have baby after baby with no thought for the consequences. Many of us already feel bad about disposable diapers because of what we know they're doing to our planet's landfills—but we must also look at the fact that the average child in the United States uses fifty times the resources of a child born in the Third World. Few issues are as controversial as population growth, and I don't intend to go into that controversy here.

In the United States as well as elsewhere, women who have no means of child support bear child after child. These are the mothers who are at risk for developing problems in labor, for having growth-retarded, premature babies. But these women's problems are *symptoms* of the imbalance in our culture—they are *not* the problem. The underlying problem is society's treatment of women and the cycles of poverty, victimization, and abuse in which these young women stay locked.

Sixty percent of teenage mothers are victims of sexual abuse.

Almost instinctively, they mate with men who then abandon them. That is all they know—a premature commitment that keeps them trapped. The only role they perceive as open to them is that of baby carrier. They don't know that they have choices. When they think they can do little else, they have babies. The cycle continues.

But what if we started now to teach our young women that they have inherent worth—and that though they may choose to have a baby, there are many other opportunities open to them as well? What if they knew that their menstrual cycles are part of their sacred connection with the Earth and the moon—and that their sexuality needn't necessarily be shared with a man? That they could have it all to themselves if they chose? What if they didn't measure their worth by whose baby they had or whom they were sleeping with? What if they knew that their wombs, whether or not they had children, are their body's center for creativity and desire—and that the womb is symbolic of our desire and creative power even if we don't use it to have babies?

We need to expand the meanings of *fertility* and *birth*. We must begin to see female birth power for what it is—the basis of all of creation. When enough women sense this creative female power inherent within each of us—not dependent upon what we produce or don't produce with our bodies—the world will change. When women tap in to this power, the children, the ideas, and the new world to which we give birth will be supportive of all beings, including ourselves.

Whether we ever choose pregnancy, every one of us has encoded in our cells the knowledge of what it is to conceive, gestate, and give birth to something that grows out of our own substance. Conception, gestation, labor, and birth are physical metaphors for how all creation manifests on Earth.

On some level we all have miscarriages, abortions, dysfunctional labors, and stillbirths, as well as beautifully formed creations. We don't need to go through these processes physically to understand them and heal from them—they're inherent processes of nature.

Each woman must find her own truth about how to use her fertility or to heal this area of her life. The most important thing to remember is that our creative fertility in the broadest sense is with us for a lifetime—whether or not we have children.

12
Pregnancy and Birthing

For all eternity, God lies on a birthing bed, giving birth. The essence of God is Birthing.

—Meister Eckhard

Pregnancy has great consequences for both mother and child. Though having a baby is rarely a rational or logical decision and cannot be made with the intellect alone, it can still be made consciously and with the heart. My wish for all women is that we gain the courage to choose conception consciously and wisely.

When I recall the reasons that I had children, I see how emotional and instinctual, unconscious and "tribal" my decision was. The biological pull was so strong. Those of us who've had a child or two have often longed to have another baby, even knowing that another child would tax our emotional and physical resources in an unhealthy way. Some women simply love being pregnant. Others adore little babies and want one around all the time. Some women are even addicted to having babies and giving birth—in part because it's the only thing that is totally theirs in their family structure. I've worked with many women who have become obsessed with having another child in their late thirties or early forties, partly so that they could put off deciding what to do with their lives for another five years.

Pregnancy can be used as a way to fill a void in a woman's life that another human being can never fill. We must know ourselves intimately before we can ever be intimate with another human being. When a baby is brought into being to fill the unmet needs of an adult, the child will carry an unfair and often harmful burden of a parent's impossible expectations.

Pregnancy is a miraculous process and should be a time when a woman makes every effort to tune in to her body and baby with the support of her surroundings. The truth is that the vast majority of pregnancies are normal and healthy! For centuries, midwives helped mothers through the pregnancy and birthing processes, standing by them with medical and emotional aid. The very word *obstetrics* is derived from the Latin word *stare,* which means "to stand by." A woman's body knows how to give birth instinctively and will respond in settings in which she is encouraged to move in the ways that feel right and to make the sounds that she needs to make. Modern obstetrics, however, has changed from a natural process of "standing by" and allowing the woman's body to respond naturally into a domineering and often invasive practice. Women's cultural conditioning causes us to turn ourselves over to pregnancy experts, so most of us have lost touch with our innate birthing knowledge and power, as have most of these experts, who rely on tests and machines to tell them how to help. I had the vaguest sense of this during my training, when I wondered why our cesarean section rate was so high. (It's even higher now!) I delivered babies for almost a decade and had two of my own before I really came to appreciate the fact that most women's experience of pregnancy, labor, and delivery is nowhere near as empowering as it could be.

OUR CULTURAL INHERITANCE: PREGNANCY

Pregnancy as Illness

During my mother's era, pregnant women were not expected to go outside their homes much or travel. Maternity clothes, which included that anathema, a maternity girdle, were ugly and did not enhance women's body image. Many women lost their jobs if they became pregnant. And for women who didn't lose their jobs, there was no formal pregnancy leave, even as late as the early 1980s. As the first physician in my former practice to have a pregnancy leave, I experienced some resentment from a few of my colleagues, who felt that pregnancy should not be treated the same as a broken leg because it was, after all, a *chosen disability* over which I had some control. We've certainly come a long way since then, but pretending that a pregnant woman is just like everyone else and has no special needs is shortsighted and puts her and her baby's health at risk. Our culture can't seem to find a happy medium.

An ever-increasing body of research is documenting the fact that prenatal influences set the stage of a child's state of health for her entire life. A baby's gene expression is powerfully shaped and guided starting in utero. In fact, Thomas Verny, M.D., D.Psych., a psychiatrist and psychologist who founded the Association for Pre- & Perinatal Psychology and Health, writes, "In fact, the great weight of the scientific evidence that has emerged over the last decade demands that we re-evaluate the mental and emotional abilities of unborn children. Awake or asleep, the studies show, they are constantly tuned in to their mother's every action, thought, and feeling. From the moment of conception, the experience in the womb shapes the brain and lays the groundwork for personality, emotional temperament, and the power of higher thought."[1] Studies have shown, for example, that suboptimal conditions in utero set the stage for adult diseases such as high blood pressure, heart disease, and diabetes.[2] Therefore, pregnancy needs to be treated as a special (and crucial) time that requires a woman to make some arrangements for increased rest and care. Otherwise, she may experience increased fatigue, premature labor, and toxemia.[3] Studies have shown that women who aren't supported or are highly stressed in their pregnancies have a higher incidence of adverse outcomes. And so do their babies!

PREVENTING PREMATURE BIRTH, PREECLAMPSIA, AND BREECH PRESENTATION

Despite a great deal of research in this area, the rate of premature birth hasn't declined in the past fifty years. It occurs in 12 percent of pregnancies and contributes to more infant deaths than any other factor except severe birth defects. Though many drugs have been used to try to stop labor, these have only limited benefit and haven't significantly affected the prematurity rate. Until the mind/body/lifestyle connection in premature birth is addressed, the rate is unlikely to change. It is well documented that uterine blood vessels are exquisitely sensitive to the effects of sympathetic nervous system stimulation and that the hormones associated with stress of all types can cause changes in blood flow to the fetus.[4] As with cancer and cardiovascular disease, the final common pathway leading to prematurity is cellular inflammation. However, when this aspect of pregnancy is taken into account and addressed, the results are very heartening.

In a study of sixty-four women, for instance, Lewis Mehl, M.D., Ph.D., found that the psychological factors of fear, anxiety, and stress; lack of support from the woman's partner; poor maternal self-identity; negative beliefs about birth; and lack of support from friends and family predicted deliveries that required obstetrical intervention ranging from cesarean section to oxytocin augmentation or induction. In another study, hypnotherapy was found to play a statistically significant role in preventing negative emotional factors from leading to C-section or oxytocin augmentation or induction. Dr. Mehl has also used hypnotherapy to help women avoid giving birth prematurely. Each woman who received hypnotherapy was reassured that she was doing the best she could, asked to state what her stresses were, and then given the suggestion that her body would know what to do to keep her baby safe. As fear and anxiety decreased through supportive hypnotherapy, so did adverse outcomes.[5]

One study followed women with a history of three consecutive miscarriages for which no medical cause could be found. On their subsequent pregnancy, they had a suture placed in their cervix to hold the pregnancy in place. Eighty-nine percent of these women went on to have severe postpartum depression, compared with only 11 percent of the control group who experienced mild to moderate depression. The authors of this study concluded that "these women were forced into motherhood."[6] When women who have severe emotional conflicts about motherhood don't deal with these issues consciously, they can be exacerbated postpartum and result in emotional breakdown. It is clear that adverse pregnancy outcomes could be prevented with approaches that help a woman name and work through the particular stresses that can so profoundly affect her pregnant body and her unborn baby.

In my view, the biggest factor in poor pregnancy outcome is that the pregnancy is unwanted or unplanned or there is some unrecognized ambivalence around it. Current data suggests that at least 50 percent of all pregnancies are unplanned.[7] It's much more difficult to ascertain which ones are unwanted because many women adjust well to unplanned pregnancies and end up desiring them. Maternal ambivalence about pregnancy is a setup for complications unless a woman can resolve her feelings during the pregnancy. (See chapter 11.) A woman who feels (usually unconsciously) that she must end her pregnancy as soon as possible to get on with her life, get the pregnancy over with, or "get her body back" may go into premature labor or develop another condition that ends her pregnancy sooner. Numerous studies have documented the profound effects of psychological variables on birth outcome—in other words, prematurity may correlate with poor maternal emotional and physical investment in the pregnancy.[8] Animal studies have indicated that the death of a baby in utero may also be related to marked maternal anxiety. In pregnant monkeys, guinea pigs, and rabbits subjected to emotional stress, the uterine and placental blood flow were constricted from adrenaline released in response to the stress. As a result, the fetuses did not receive enough oxygen, and many died of asphyxia. Marked maternal anxiety and stress also causes uterine blood vessels to constrict via hormonal and neurotransmitter release into the circulation. This reduces oxygen to the baby and may well be related to pregnancy complications, such as placental abruption, placenta previa (a condition in which the placenta covers the cervical opening, which can lead to bleeding and/or prematurity), a prolapsed umbilical cord, a cord around the neck, or breech presentation.[9]

While mothers automatically communicate stresses they feel through their bodies to their unborn babies, they can also learn to communicate healthful emotions to their babies. After all, the baby is a part of a pregnant woman's own body. My experience has taught me that when women learn how to get in touch with their inner guidance systems, they can learn how to keep their babies safer and even interrupt premature labor and halt the progression of toxemia. Of course, women who develop premature labor and toxemia also have to be willing to stop work, rest more, and change any harmful patterns of behavior and thought. The pioneering work of Dr. Lewis Mehl has shown that prenatal intervention consisting of social support, education, and labor support in a group of minority women reduced alcohol intake, smoking, and stress, and also improved birth outcome significantly.[10]

Preeclampsia

Preeclampsia (or toxemia) is a syndrome in which a pregnant woman develops swelling, high blood pressure, and protein in the urine. It's sometimes referred to as PIH (pregnancy-induced hypertension). Women with kidney disease and preexisting high blood pressure are more susceptible than others. Diabetes also increases susceptibility. Toxemia is a leading cause of prematurity and pregnancy disability. If untreated, it can lead to seizures—the condition is then called eclampsia. No one knows exactly what causes preeclampsia, although there are many theories. In one study, electrodes were placed into the nerves adjacent to the blood vessels of four different types of women: pregnant women with high blood pressure, non-pregnant women with high blood pressure, pregnant women with normal blood pressure, and non-pregnant women with normal blood pressure. The women who had preeclampsia were found to have high sympathetic nervous system activity (more adrenaline in their bloodstream), which resulted in narrowing of their blood vessels with a subsequent increase in pressure and inflammatory chemicals at the cellular level. It is well known that the sympathetic nervous system is involved with the fight-or-flight response and perceived stress. One of the researchers in this study suggested that the reason why the preeclamptic women's blood pressure rises is that they have "a defect in the central conflict processing system," which may increase certain hormone levels that not only contribute to an increase in blood pressure but may be associated with feelings of anxiety and hostility.[11] I don't think there's any such "defect." Quite simply, these women don't have the skills or the resources to get their needs met directly. But they can learn them!

Other studies of pregnant women with preeclampsia suggest that they feel less attractive, less loved, and more helpless than do pregnant women without preeclampsia. They may be excessively sensitive to the opinions of others, and orient themselves to what others expect of them. For these women, pregnancy provides an additional crisis that adds stress to their already overstressed lives. Although they view pregnancy as a crisis, they are ill equipped to deal with their emotions about it. They are unable to cope with what they perceive as others' expectations, taking to heart minor criticisms and injustices done to them. However, they do not show externally that any of this bothers them. Instead, their body reflects this stress as an increase in blood pressure.

This is corroborative with the work of Samuel J. Mann, M.D., a hypertension specialist at the New York Presbyterian Hospital/Weill Medical College of Cornell University and author of *Healing Hypertension: A Revolutionary New Approach* (John Wiley, 1999). Dr. Mann has seen thousands of people with all varieties of high blood pressure. Over time he noticed a pattern that was not in keeping with the common view that stress is linked to this condition. In his book, Dr. Mann writes, "Even patients with severe hypertension did not seem more emotionally distressed than others. If anything, they seemed less distressed. Their high blood pressure appeared to be more related to what they did *not* seem to be feeling than to what they *were* feeling." He began to see that old, unhealed, repressed trauma seemed to be a major culprit in his patients. I certainly agree. Even though pregnancy-induced hypertension is not considered the same as hypertension in the non-pregnant state, I believe that they both have much in common. The bottom line is that it is our hidden emotions, the emotions we do not feel, that lead to hypertension (as well as many other physical conditions).

Not surprisingly, women with preeclampsia frequently have conflicts with their employers, and their blood pressure often rises when they try to negotiate their maternity leaves. They often attempt to get everything settled before the delivery. Compared with women without preeclampsia, these women's emotions manifest physically through the autonomic (subconscious) nervous system: they frequently blush in the face and neck, talk rapidly, and experience rising blood pressure, dizziness, and heart palpitations.[12] One study showed that women with a set of conditions including excessive weight gain, premature rupture of membranes (one of the leading causes of premature birth), and preeclampsia display high anxiety, social seclusion, and hypochondria compared with controls.[13] These symptoms can all be thought of as bodily cries for help and support! If a woman understands what it's like to have a baby in the intensive care nursery, she can begin the process of seeing her own body as the best intensive care space possible for the baby, not to mention the cheapest. And when she begins to name and put her needs first, this is exactly what often happens. A diet that keeps blood sugar stable is also essential. (See chapter 17.)

Breech Presentation

Nowhere is the mind/body connection more interesting than in the case of breech presentation, in which the baby is oriented feet or buttocks first instead of headfirst. By the time a woman has reached the thirty-seventh week of pregnancy, her baby will usually have settled into her pelvis in a headfirst position. But 3 percent of the time, it will be feet first or buttocks first. Though breech babies can turn at any time, the estimated likelihood that a baby will spontaneously convert from a breech to a vertex (headfirst) position after thirty-seven weeks of gestation is only 12 percent. If a woman enters labor with her baby in the breech position, she is almost always delivered by cesarean section. Some babies are breech for structural reasons, such as a septum or wall in the uterus that can interfere with the baby's position. But in the majority of cases, there is no known medical reason for the breech. It's clear that in some cases the baby is breech because of the tension that the mother holds in the lower area of her body. It has been observed that anxious and fearful women have a higher incidence of breech presentation than do others, attributable to the fact that fear, anxiety, and stress can activate sympathetic mechanisms that result in tightening of the lower uterine segment.[14] My obstetrician colleague Bethany Hays feels that a baby may be in the breech position because it is trying to get closer to its mother's heartbeat—to feel more connected to her.

The key to allowing the baby to turn spontaneously is to help the mother release tension in her lower uterine segment. There are a number of ways to do this. Some women have found that acupressure works. (See figure 14.) I have personally had about a 40 percent success rate teaching mothers a type of bioenergetic breathing, which works to relax the lower abdomen and lower uterine segment, thus allowing the baby to turn. Dr. Hays also reports that if she can get women to relax their lower abdominals, she can often turn the breech with ease. (This manual turning is known as external cephalic version, or ECV.) Dr. Lewis Mehl demonstrated that hypnosis can be used to turn breeches, with a success rate of 81 percent—compared to 41 percent for a control group.[15] Dr. Mehl (now known as Dr. Lewis Mehl-Madrona) has also used hypnosis to decrease C-section rates for those at risk and to decrease use of oxytocin augmentation of labor. (For more information, contact the Association for Pre- & Perinatal Psychology and Health at 707-887-2838 or check the resources on their website, www.birthpsychology.com; for information on hypnosis CDs by Dr. Lewis Mehl-Madrona, including *Hypnosis for Breech Presentation, Birth Visualization for Childbirth Preparation* and *Guided Imagery to Facilitate Vaginal Birth After Cesarean (VBAC)*, contact Dr. Mehl-Madrona at coyotehealing@aol.com or visit his website at www.drmadrona.com.)

The Collective Emergency Mindset

Pregnancy is a time when common sense all too often flies out the window, chased by a culture that is out of balance concerning birth. Nowhere is a woman's connection or loss of connection to her inner guidance more evident than during pregnancy. Suddenly, her body is no longer her own. Her entire extended family feels that it is pregnant, and all of them give her advice about what to eat, what to wear, and what to do. I was amazed by how total strangers would approach me when I was pregnant, pat my belly, and offer suggestions. Friends seem to think it their duty to tell pregnant women the worst stories they can think of about cesarean sections, labor pain, and poor outcomes. (This

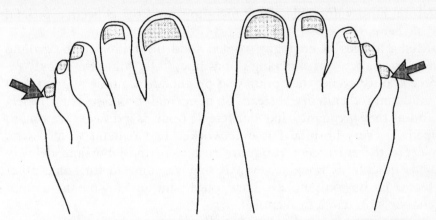

FIGURE 14: ACUPUNCTURE OR ACUPRESSURE POINTS
TO TURN A BREECH

A number of different techniques can be used to stimulate these points, including acupuncture needles or a heat treatment known as moxibustion. If you don't have access to an acupuncturist who is familiar with these techniques, you can try acupressure if your physician approves. Press the point on either toe with your fingernail. Use enough pressure so that the area feels sensitive, but not enough to cause pain. Hold the pressure for one to two minutes once or twice a day. Immediately afterward, get into the knee-chest position for about fifteen minutes. (This position will also help turn the baby.) You can use this technique starting in the seventh month of pregnancy. (Earlier in the pregnancy, the fetus is likely to turn on its own.) Do not attempt this if you have any uterine or pelvic abnormality, a history of habitual miscarriage, or if there have been other problems in the pregnancy. Be sure to consult your doctor before beginning.

is another example of our dominator culture—glorifying pain and destruction over the life-enhancing qualities potentially available through pregnancy and birth.) I felt blessed to be an obstetrician because I was spared hearing all these horror stories. (Perhaps people figured that I had been "socialized" by having already learned these horrible stories firsthand!) War stories about the rigors of birth are often passed down from generation to generation. Mothers not uncommonly tell their daughters that "now you'll see how I suffered with you."

At some very deep level, we are all awed by pregnant women and their power. But instead of emphasizing a woman's awe-inspiring birth power, in classic patriarchal reversal our culture attends to the fear that that power brings up. Pregnant women are emotionally more porous and more in touch with their intuition than usual, and they are therefore more vulnerable. They pick up on all the collective societal fear of them.

Media images of pregnant women suddenly falling to the ground during pregnancy and shrieking things like, "Oh, John, the baby!" reinforce in our psyches the notion that pregnancy is a time of great danger and unpredictability instead of a normal process. They falsely remind us that pregnancy, like our female body, is a disaster waiting to happen. In every hospital I've ever worked in, pregnant women who come into the emergency room are rushed to the labor and delivery floor as quickly as possible, even if they've come in for some other problem. In Boston, the ER crew once sent up a woman in mid-pregnancy who had a broken leg!

This emergency mindset is especially damaging to women who are having babies in their thirties or forties. Most, if not all, pregnant women over the age of thirty are taught by our culture that they are much more at risk for complications than if they were in their twenties. This perception of increased risk is not necessarily true and depends on the individual woman's health. I remember the first pregnant woman I ever met who was over thirty. It was in the prenatal clinic at the Mary Hitchcock Hospital during my second year of medical school, and I thought that she was very unusual and very brave to be having her first baby at age thirty-two. I remember thinking that she was old for attempting this, although I myself was twenty-three at the time and pregnancy and having children were very far from my personal plans. Looking back, I realize that this woman was at the very beginning of a trend that began in the 1970s and has continued unabated through the present—delaying childbearing until later. (As an evolutionary side note, my now twenty-something daughters both feel that marrying much before the age of thirty is awfully young.)

Women having their first babies after the age of thirty-five were once referred to as "elderly primigravidas." Happily, that term has been dropped. Though the term "geriatric" obstetrics is still used occasionally, it should be eliminated, as it sets up all kinds of negativity. Whether or not a woman is more at risk in her thirties must be completely individualized. A forty-year-old in excellent health who has a planned pregnancy is apt to do much better than a twenty-five-year-old who smokes two packs and quaffs a gallon of Diet Coke per day. Too often the medical profession "hexes" women who become pregnant in their thirties and forties by lumping them into statistically high-risk categories that are not necessarily applicable. Older women who are pregnant, as well as infertility patients who become pregnant, have a much higher risk of a C-section. In some places, a woman older than forty will be told that she is very apt to have a cesarean because hers is a "premium pregnancy" (as opposed to a pregnancy in the mother's twenties, whose success doesn't "matter" as much because "you can always have another—you have time"). *Premium pregnancy* means that because the mother is presumed to be or is more anxious (or is *made* to be anxious by her culture and her doctor), we should treat her differently. This is a reflection of the health care team's own unfinished emotional work. And this is the thinking that has led to our current all-time high rate of cesarean birth—which is now 29 percent. (And according to the Centers for Disease Control and Prevention, the cesarean rate has risen 40 percent since 1996!) C-sections are far from benign procedures and our collective trust in them is mind-boggling!

In fact, age doesn't predict anything when it comes to labor and birth. Chronological age (age in years) and biological age (age of one's tissues) aren't necessarily related. One of my friends had her first baby at forty-one. The first stage of her labor lasted only three hours—very short by any standard. And if her hips hadn't been so narrow, she'd have delivered in a total of four hours. Healthy women who are well supported in labor usually do beautifully, regardless of age.

One of the nicest things about women having their first babies in their late thirties and early forties is that by then, these women have established themselves in the outside world of work and career. When they do have babies, they take the time to enjoy them. They already know what it's like "out there." They realize the limitations of the corporate world and are willing to put aside its "benefits" to reassess their lives through the lens of parenting. Many have had time to get in touch with their bodies over the years and are more comfortable with themselves than they were in their twenties. In my mind, such women are actually low risk.

THE TRANSFORMING POWER OF PREGNANCY

Women should savor and celebrate pregnancy, the gestating of the next generation, as the miracle that it is—a crucial time in their own and their child's development. It's a time when we can be in touch with our *hara*—our body center of creation—in the most direct and powerful way possible. Pregnancy is not an illness or a time for us to be treated with kid gloves. Still, it is a period when we need quiet reflective time to tune in to the baby and to rest. The hormone progesterone, released naturally during pregnancy, has calming and soothing effects. (It also relaxes and slows the bowel, which can lead to constipation in some women.) The body is doing a lot of inner work growing a baby. The tenor of the pregnancy itself contributes to the strength of a child's constitution throughout the rest of his or her life. I'm amazed that this culture has been so unable to appreciate the fact that forty weeks of gestation is a *very short* amount of time in a woman's life, relatively speaking. Yet it is a time that is crucial for the health of the next generation.

Because our culture values women more highly during their child-bearing years, and because women tend to take better care of themselves during pregnancy than at any other time, pregnancy is a fantastic opportunity for women to learn more about themselves and their own power. Since the baby is part of their own bodies, positive inner communication between the two translates into a deeper trust of themselves that continues even after birth.

Quality care and education during pregnancy would prevent an untold number of costly problems later, including many cases of prematurity, growth retardation, mental retardation, physical disability, and learning disabilities—all of which make the process of parenting much more difficult. Lewis Mehl's work has also shown that the ill effects of cigarettes, alcohol, and drugs could be vastly decreased, given that most women use these substances to medicate their feelings of fear, anxiety, and vulnerability. The care of pregnant women, who are very powerful and vulnerable at the same time, should be the highest priority in this country.

An Obstetrician Gets Pregnant

When I became pregnant with my first child, I had recently completed my four-year residency training and by then had worked with hundreds of pregnant women, providing them with prenatal care, labor support, and assistance with delivery of their babies. I had been a proponent of natural, drug-free childbirth throughout my residency, and I was very optimistic about my own. After all, the vast majority of pregnancies end with a normal baby—I had seen the truth of this firsthand.

My attitude toward the pregnancy was one of watching an experiment with the uterus. Wasn't this interesting—to see the changes my body was going through! I realize now that I didn't allow myself what I then considered the *luxury* of excitement and anticipation, though mine was very much a planned and wanted pregnancy.

I had learned very well how to separate my mind from my body, so I decided that I didn't want to "bond" much with my baby until after the pregnancy was well along and I knew that the baby was normal—something I would be assured of only *after* he or she was born. Notice the paradox in my thinking here. I felt strongly that everything would be normal, yet I didn't want to make such an investment "just in case." I had watched some women furnish entire nurseries as early as their third month of pregnancy, when the risk of miscarriage is still one in six. I didn't want to go through that kind of grief. I thought that their emotional investment was premature. Years later, I learned that babies know what's going on in utero and hear, feel, and experience emotions long before they're born. When their mothers are detached and not invested emotionally, babies sense this.

Back then I didn't realize for myself, though I taught it to my patients, that a woman's process of bonding with her baby starts when her pregnancy test is positive. At this point, women usually start fantasizing about the baby, thinking about names, and looking at baby clothes and other items. (With the advent of early ultrasound, the bonding process is now earlier and more intense than ever before.) I had never been very interested in babies and could not understand the behavior of women at baby showers—events that I could barely stand. Oohing and ahhing over baby clothes had never appealed to me.

When the nurses asked me, toward the end of the pregnancy, if I had the baby's room ready, I said, "No, I don't even have a T-shirt." I had no baby stuff at all, not even a diaper. My husband was completing a fellowship in orthopedics and was, as usual, busier than I was. He certainly wasn't up for baby shopping. Although I was clear that I didn't want a baby shower, luckily some nurse friends ignored my adamancy. Though I was mortified at the time, I was grateful later. I didn't have a clue as to how to go about buying baby things.

Rather than read parenting guides, I trusted my ability to mother without question. Sentimentality about babies was not, in my opinion, a prerequisite for good mothering. My own mother had been a "lioness" type, with excellent instincts most of the time. She didn't give in much to "experts"—a trait for which I'll always be grateful.

As my baby grew, I watched my body change with interest. I learned a great deal about morning sickness, pain under the rib cage, constipation, excess gas, and heartburn. I'd heard women complain about these things for years, and now I could see why. Although my husband thought my changing body was beautiful, I wasn't convinced. I was concerned about gaining too much weight. How was I supposed to *enjoy* a disappearing waist, puffy cheeks, and increased fat on my hips in a culture that worships quasi-anorexia?

I now regret that I have no pictures of myself while I was pregnant.

I was amazed at my patients who showed me entire photo albums of themselves during pregnancy and delivery—they were proud and unashamed of their bodies. At the time, these women seemed like specimens from a different planet—didn't they "get it" that the culture (and I) didn't think they looked all that great? Two decades have brought about fabulous changes in this area. Now women are justifiably proud of their "bumps."

During my second pregnancy, I lost my waist almost as soon as I conceived and looked pregnant almost immediately, a common event. This time, I was busier than I had been with the first, but I remember taking more time to talk to my baby (except that I thought she was a boy and called her William for nine months—she was much more active than my first, so I made a sexist assumption). Toward the end of this pregnancy, I had difficulty walking because of separation of my pubic bone, which happens so that the baby can fit through the pelvis, but by and large, it was a completely normal pregnancy. Though my belly got a lot bigger, I gained the same amount of weight—twenty-five pounds—in both pregnancies.

I once met a sophisticated professional woman in her late thirties who was in the middle of her first pregnancy. She had finally conceded that she needed to purchase some "ugly clothes" because it had become too hard to "hide" her pregnancy and she had to modify her polished executive look of slim skirts and high heels. Her attitude that pregnancy was something to be endured, ignored, or tolerated used to be all too common—and I was guilty of it myself to a degree. The less pregnant you look, the better everyone tells you you're doing—"Oh, you're so little, you look great—I can hardly tell!" A prenatal-vitamin advertisement in one of the medical journals from the mid-1980s shows a very thin, tall woman who doesn't look at all pregnant, running around taking pictures, working out at the gym, and staying late at the office. The caption reads, "Pregnant, but she won't slow down." The ad reminds me of my own attitude during my pregnancies, when I ran up the hospital stairs to do C-sections or surgery. I didn't want the pregnancies to interfere with my life in any way. Unfortunately, studies have shown that not slowing down is sometimes associated with increased health risks. A pilot study of stress and pregnancy in pregnant physicians and nurses showed that certain hormones (urinary catecholamines) produced by the adrenals and other tissue under physical or mental stress increased by 58 percent during work periods, compared with nonwork periods. The pregnant physicians' catecholamine levels were also increased by 64 percent over those working nonphysicians' control groups of similar gestational age.[16] (And this increases cellular inflammation, which is a setup for all birth complications.)

When I was pregnant with my second child and had to get up at night to go deliver babies, I was so tired that I occasionally walked into walls while I was getting dressed. (My first child, once born, didn't sleep through the night until she was five, so I was up at night for years, whether I was on call or not!) But no one suggested that I slow down. Besides, I was *still* trying to prove myself a worthy professional—especially now that I'd had children!

Woman literally illustrates the on-going life pattern of how energy becomes matter through pregnancy, labor, and delivery.
—Caroline Myss

Program for Creating Optimal Pregnancy and Decreased Risk of Complications

The final common pathway that leads to nearly all pregnancy complications, including preeclampsia, low birth weight, and prematurity is cellular inflammation. Happily, cellular inflammation can be curtailed in many different ways, all of which complement one another. The following program will increase your chances of a healthy pregnancy.

Eat a low-glycemic diet that keeps blood sugar stable and contains adequate protein, essential fats, and micronutrients. (See chapter 17.)

Stop smoking and avoid cigarette smoke. Smoking deprives the fetus of oxygen, resulting in slower growth and therefore low infant birth weight. According to the 2001 Report of the Surgeon General, smoking accounts for 20 to 30 percent of low-birth-weight infants, up to 14 percent of preterm deliveries, and about 10 percent of all infant deaths. The report also states that even healthy, full-term babies born to women who smoke may have narrowed airways and curtailed lung function. Other studies have shown that smoking during pregnancy is associated with learning disabilities and behavioral problems for the child later in life. Many of the same risks apply when partners of pregnant women smoke around them during their pregnancy.

If you think the risks are overstated because you've seen healthy children born to mothers who smoke, consider this story from a non-smoking colleague: "My mother smoked all during her pregnancy and while I was growing up. I weighed 7 lbs. at birth so I was not small, and I was born after forty weeks so I was not early, and I had no learning disabilities (I graduated from college Phi Beta Kappa with high honors). But when I took up scuba diving, the instructors were amazed at how much oxygen I needed. My tank always ran low well before the others'. They said I must be running underwater to use up that much air, and the joke was that I wore Nike fins!" (For support to quit smoking, inquire if your local hospital has a smoking cessation program; see also chapter 17.)

Don't douche. Using vaginal douches is not only unnecessary, it has also been associated with low infant birth weight and bacterial vaginosis.

Take supplements. And start before conception, if possible. For the best results, be sure the potency of the supplements you take is guaranteed and that the supplements are manufactured according to GMP (Good Manufacturing Processes) standards. I recommend a daily supplement with the following vitamins and minerals at the following levels:

Vitamins: folic acid (800 to 1,000 mcg), beta-carotene (15,000 to 25,000 IU), vitamin D (400 to 1,200 IU), vitamin E (200 to 400 IU), vitamin C (500 to 2,000 mg), glutathione (2 to 10 mg), vitamin K (60 mcg), thiamine or vitamin B_1 (9 to 100 mg), riboflavin or vitamin B_2 (9 to 50 mg), pyridoxine or vitamin B_6 (10 to 100 mg), niacin or vitamin B_3 (20 to 100 mg), biotin (100 to 500 mcg), vitamin B_{12} (30 to 250 mcg), pantothenic acid or vitamin B_5 (30 to 400 mcg), inositol (30 to 500 mg), and choline (45 to 100 mg).

Minerals: calcium (500 to 1,500 mg), magnesium (400 to 1,000 mg), boron (1 to 3 mg), chromium (100 to 400 mcg), copper (1 to 2 mg), iron (30 mg), manganese (1 to 15 mg), zinc (12 to 50 mcg), selenium (80 to 120 mcg), potassium (200 to 500 mcg), molybdenum (20 to 60 mcg), vanadium (50 to 100 mcg), iodine (150 mcg), and trace minerals (from a marine mineral complex or from eating sea vegetables such as hiziki, dulse, wakame, or nori).

Eat enough omega-3 fats, especially DHA. Essential fatty acids (also called polyunsaturated long-chain fatty acids or PUFA's) help the body fight and ultimately stop cellular inflammation. Eating enough may help prevent prematurity and low birth weights.[17] The main source of omega-3s are fatty fish, eggs, nuts, seeds, sea vegetables, and green leafy vegetables like spinach, broccoli, cabbage, collards, and kale. Unprocessed vegetable oils (most notably flaxseed, macadamia nut, and hempseed oils) are also good sources.

Talk to your doctor about progesterone. If you are at risk for premature labor, talk to your doctor about progesterone. Studies show that this hormone (available in a weekly shot given from week sixteen through week thirty-six of gestation or as a vaginal suppository) decreases the risk of prematurity.[18]

Get psychological support. Studies have shown that psychological support can decrease the rate of premature birth in those who are at increased risk.[19]

Use guided imagery. Psychotherapist, author, and guided imagery innovator Belleruth Naparstek, creator of the popular fifty-two-title Time Warner Health Journeys guided imagery audio series and author of *Staying Well with Guided Imagery* (Warner Books, 1994), explains that guided imagery is "a gentle but powerful technique that focuses and directs the imagination." Although it has been called "visualization" and "mental imagery," she explains, guided imagery involves not only the visual sense but all of the senses, all of our emotions, and the whole physical body. "It is precisely this body-based focus that makes for its powerful impact," she notes, referring to studies showing that guided imagery has a positive impact on health, creativity, and performance. "We now know that in many instances even ten minutes of imagery can reduce blood pressure, lower cholesterol and glucose levels in the blood, and heighten short-term immune cell activity," she says. "And because it results in a kind of natural trance state, it can be considered a form of hypnosis as well." Belleruth makes hands-down the best imagery CDs on the market. Everything is scientifically chosen and recorded, including the fabulous music. Her CD entitled *The Healthy Pregnancy & Successful Childbirth* is specifically designed to encourage feelings of confidence, support, relaxation, safety, gratitude, and healthy anticipation during pregnancy, as well as labor imagery to ease discomfort, focus breathing, and underline your trust in the divine wisdom of your body. (For more information, see www.healthjourneys.com.)

Start a meditation program. Calm Birth is a form of childbirth preparation that uses proven mind/body and breathing techniques to help create an atmosphere of calmness that decreases fear, pain, and complications for both pregnancy and childbirth. Many medical centers now use this program with good results. The three main methods Calm Birth teaches are the Practice of Opening (allowing the parents-to-be to experience a remarkable access to the development of their unborn child), Womb Breathing (where women learn to breathe into their energy bodies to reach full potential in childbirth and also to enrich the child), and the Giving and Receiving Meditation (which teaches how to transform the energy of fear, anxiety, and tension into light in your own body—and breathe it out). The preface to the program states, "When pregnant women practice meditation, an empowering sense of safety and wholeness is generated from the inside. The Calm Birth Methods were developed to give women direct ways to raise the quality of health in childbirth whether or not medical interventions are applied. These methods have been shown to lower the impact of interventions and also lower medical costs and risks." This is a very powerful program, and I highly recommend it. For those who can't find a Calm Birth practitioner in their area (currently, most are on the West Coast), the organization also offers a CD called *Calm Birth*, as well as a postnatal program called *Calm Healing*. (For more information, contact Calm Birth at 541-488-2563 or visit their website at www.calmbirth.org.)

Get massaged. Massage has wonderful benefits, including boosting endorphins and decreasing stress hormones. Research by Tiffany Field, Ph.D., founder and director of the Touch Research Institute at the University of Miami School of Medicine, has done extensive research showing that pregnant women who receive massage experience reduced anxiety, improved mood, reduced back pain, and increased sleep. They also have fewer complications in labor, less labor pain, and fewer premature babies.[20] (For more information, see the Touch Research Institute's website at www.miami.edu/touch-research.)

Expose yourself to natural light. Morning bright light significantly helps depression in pregnant women, according to a 2002 Yale study. Researchers found that after three weeks of morning bright light therapy, depression ratings improved by 49 percent, and benefits were seen through five weeks of treatment. They also found no evidence of adverse effects of light therapy on pregnancy. Because drugs for depression are best avoided, if possible, during pregnancy, and because depression in pregnancy may be a risk factor for preeclampsia, this is significant news.[21]

The Magic of Labor and Birth

Having a baby is the true "change of life." Women who go through labor and birth fully supported often emerge from the experience changed forever. One of my patients who had her two children at home told me: "My births were absolute peak experiences of ecstasy and spiritual fulfillment. Nothing I've ever experienced before or since has come anywhere close. As a result of my experiences, I now trust my body implicitly." In order to experience the transformational power of birth, women need to know the following:

1. Labor proceeds on its own schedule. The delicate timing that is a result of the delicate interaction between a baby and her mother needs to be respected. (Risky labor inductions for "convenience" and all the complications associated with them [e.g., increased risk of pre-

maturity, C-section, and maternal death] are now on the rise all over the country.)

2. Childbirth is designed by nature to be a peak experience that is joyous, ecstatic, and loving. The body of the laboring woman is flooded with natural morphinelike substances called endorphins as well as oxytocin, the bonding hormone. This kind of ecstasy is seen in centers such as The Farm Midwifery Center in Summertown, Tennessee, where the legendary midwife Ina May Gaskin practices. Her book *Ina May's Guide to Childbirth* (Bantam Books, 2003) is a must-read for all pregnant women. At a recent meeting of the Association for Pre- & Perinatal Psychology and Health, Ina May showed a picture of her niece giving birth naturally with a big smile on her face, something one never sees on television—or in most hospitals!

3. Birth is sexual. This makes sense—after all, the baby is moving down the vaginal canal and stimulating the G-spot and all the nerves connected with sexual feeling. As Ina May says, "The energy that got the baby in is what gets the baby out. Many women experience the most intense orgasm of their lives when they birth in environments in which they are loved, adored, and fully supported."

4. How you do it is what you get. Because of the heightened emotional and neurological receptivity of both mother and baby, the birth experience deeply imprints both mother and baby and impacts their relationship for a lifetime.

5. Natural birth is safe. Studies have repeatedly shown that in healthy mothers with no risk factors, home birth is as safe as hospital birth. Perhaps safer. Ina May Gaskin reports that at The Farm Midwifery Center, the C-section rate is only 1.4 percent—a safety rate unparalleled by hospitals. And her experience is clearly not solitary. A landmark study published in the *British Medical Journal* in 2005 found that natural birth at home, under the care of certified practicing midwives, is safe for low-risk mothers and their babies. This study, which tracked more than five thousand mothers in the U.S. and Canada, also reported that home births with low-risk mothers resulted in much lower rates of medical interventions when compared to the intervention rates for low-risk mothers giving birth in hospitals. For example, the episiotomy rate was 2.1 percent for the home-birth group, compared with 33 percent for hospital births, and labor was induced in only 9.6 percent of home births, compared to 21 percent of hospital births. The rate of electronic fetal monitoring, C-sections, forceps or vacuum delivery, and epidurals were also much lower with home births.[22]

Unfortunately, the American public in general (physicians included) may have a false sense of security about the safety of giving birth today because the statistics on maternal death in the U.S. are misleading. Unlike most other developed countries, the U.S. counts in its pregnancy-related death statistics only women who die within a six-week period after a pregnancy ends. Other developed countries include deaths that occur up to one year afterward. According to a CDC report from 1998, as many as three times more U.S. women may have died as the number reported in our national statistics indicate because not all maternal deaths are classified as pregnancy-related on the death certificate.[23] And when it comes to infant mortality, the figures are even more shocking. According to the National Center for Health Statistics, a division of the Centers for Disease Control and Prevention, in 2002, the U.S. infant mortality rate—already ranking well below most European countries and even Cuba—rose for the first time in forty years to 7.0 deaths per thousand live births. Infant mortality is a very important measure of public health because it reflects factors such as the quality of prenatal care, maternal health, socioeconomic status, and health insurance coverage. So much for the benefits of high-tech birth! Singapore has the lowest infant mortality rate—2.28 deaths per thousand live births. The U.S. comes in thirty-sixth place in the world overall.

6. There are many choices for how to have your baby. In fact, there are more childbirth choices now than ever before—everything from high-tech hospital birth to water birth at home. To choose the care that is the safest and most mother-friendly option, I recommend that you visit the website of the Coalition for Improving Maternity Services (CIMS), a group of individuals and more than fifty organizations whose mission is to promote a wellness model of childbirth. (For more information, read "Having a Baby? Ten Questions to Ask," on CIMS's website, www.motherfriendly.org.)

OUR CULTURAL INHERITANCE: LABOR AND DELIVERY

Labor and delivery very often go well. Yet as a society we continue to treat the normal process of birth with hysteria. The high anxiety about pregnancy and birth in this country is partially the result of our

collective unresolved birth trauma—nearly every one of us has unfinished business about her or his own birth that we keep projecting onto
pregnant women. Most baby boomers, after all, were born drugged
and were then whisked away from their mothers to the glaring lights
and sterility of the hospital nursery. The World War II generation was
born at home. Then birth became medicalized and moved into the hospital. Though the maternal mortality rate fell, we lost a great deal of
birthing wisdom with this shift.

I have seen cemeteries in New England strewn with the headstones
of women who died young, surrounded by the graves of their dead children. Most of these deaths and traumas resulted from poor nutrition,
overwork, and lack of maternal support, *not* necessarily from lack of
sophisticated medical intervention.[24] Data show, for instance, that
women who are unsupported in labor are at greater risk for prolonged
labor and poor outcome. Several excellent studies have also shown that
the presence of a supportive woman called a *doula* who "mothers the
mother" during her labor decreased the average length of labor from
admission to delivery from 19.3 hours to 8.8 hours! The presence of a
doula also resulted in the mother being more awake after delivery so
that she was more likely to stroke her baby, smile, and talk to her or
him.[25]

In so-called primitive hunter-gatherer societies, pregnancies are
often spaced two to four years apart by unrestricted breast-feeding,
which keeps prolactin levels high and acts as a natural contraceptive. In the course of her lifetime, a woman from one of these societies might have twenty periods, as compared to five hundred for
Western women.[26] In these societies, provisions are also made to
support a pregnant woman and her labor. The birth is celebrated
as a community event. Though I don't mean to imply that childbirth
is always a completely risk-free, glorious process, even in societies
in which women have been well nourished and well supported,
we could learn a lot from combining the collective women's wisdom of native, nature-centered people with our current medical
technology.

Women Labor as They Live

Having participated in hundreds of cesarean-section deliveries
and other forms of medicalized birth over the years, I've learned that
our current dilemmas over birthing start *long before* a woman ends
up on the labor and delivery floor. It starts years before she even gets

pregnant! Each of us carries the seeds within ourselves, and we must look at the ways in which we daily participate in less-than-optimal treatment.

A woman's attitudes about pregnancy arrive with her on the labor and delivery floor. One professional woman I know wanted to labor without feeling a thing. She said, "Knock me out—I'm not an Indian." This is the statement of a woman who doesn't understand the power of labor and delivery. It implies that only "primitives" go through labor and that sophisticated intellectuals get babies via technology, keeping their hands clean, their brows uncreased, and their makeup intact.

Studies have shown that women with prolonged labor have certain personality characteristics. They have inner conflicts about reproduction and motherhood and are unable at the time of the labor to communicate and admit their anxiety. (In our culture, where mothers typically receive so little support, who wouldn't have conflicts!) These psychological factors may result in inefficient uterine action and subsequent prolonged labor.[27] It is also a fact of our culture that violence is common in many women's lives, especially during pregnancy, when the woman's pregnant belly is often the target of abuse. This can certainly increase your chances for pregnancy complications of all kinds. Ask yourself the following questions: Within the last year, or since you have been pregnant, have you been hit, slapped, kicked, or otherwise physically hurt by someone? Are you in a relationship with a person who threatens or physically hurts you? Has anyone forced you to have sexual activities that made you uncomfortable? If you answered yes to any of these questions, you're being abused. To get help, call the national toll-free hotline 800-799-SAFE (7233) or 800-787-3224 or your local women's shelter or domestic violence hotline.[28]

Too many women approach labor with the wish, stated or unstated, "Take care of this inconvenience, please. I don't want to feel a thing—just hand me the baby when it's over!" Though what women need most in labor is encouragement and loving support for their abilities to birth normally, too often they don't get this because doctors and nurses hold the same attitudes about labor as they do about a crisis or inconvenience—cure it as soon as possible.

I've learned that a women's entire life leads up to what will happen in labor. Her deepest fears can play out then, not necessarily consciously. Women who have experienced incest or other abuse are prime candidates for dysfunctional labors and subsequent cesarean sections unless they work through this—which is certainly possible! Many of these women have learned at a deep level how to be victims. This plays out in childbirth—a time when, instead of being a victim of their bodies, they need to be at one with the process. One of my patients realized that she had gotten stuck in labor because at some unconscious level she was afraid of giving birth to her father's child. Another sexual abuse victim came to realize that she had learned the victim role so well that she could not *push* her baby out. Like most people living out of a feeling of powerlessness, she simply turned the experience over to the hospital and the staff. On some level she expected them to birth the baby for her. I've worked with countless women who have learned this attitude.

THE Cervix Is a Sphincter

Midwife Ina May Gaskin coined the term "Sphincter Law" to explain why so many women's labors stop progressing the minute they get to the hospital and why so many experience "failure to progress" and end up with interventions. The reason is that the cervix is a sphincter—just like the ones that control urination and elimination. It's impossible to let go and relax a sphincter unless you are totally relaxed and feel safe. That's why so many people get constipated when they travel.

Other survivors of abuse, however, use control as a survival mechanism. During pregnancy these women often come into a doctor's office with a long list of demands: no IVs, no monitor, no medical students, a limit to exams, and no shaving or enemas (despite the fact that shaving and enemas haven't been done for years). Many obstetricians sense that those women who need to control the birth process the most are often the ones who end up with the most interventions. Any birth attendant will tell you that the longer the "laundry list," the greater the chance of an unplanned intervention, such as a C-section. The reason is that the "laundry list" is often a symptom of the woman's illusion of intellectual control, her attempt to control a situation about which she feels completely terrorized and out of control. By trying to control all the variables associated with the birthing process, she thinks she can somehow avoid the terror that she associates with her body, with feeling her body in general, and with the birth process. The more a woman operates from intellectual control, the less likely she will be to surrender to her body's process and the more likely that an intervention will be necessary. And the medical system plays into this seamlessly.

Labor also reveals the bare bones of a woman's relationship with her husband or other labor support people. Sometimes women suddenly, when nine centimeters dilated, lash out at their husbands viciously, simply because they are in transition. I was taught that this just "happens," but it never made sense to me. I've since learned that it doesn't just "happen." Any hostility that emerges between people during labor was already there long before labor began. But because of the essential primitive nature of the process, all pretense at socially acceptable politeness gets dropped, and reality shines through. My father once told me that if I wanted to learn who someone really was, I should go on a camping trip with them. You could say the same thing for the labor and delivery process.

Gayle Peterson, in her book *Birthing Normally,* points out that women labor in the same way they live. Labor is a crisis situation for most women. They approach it the way they approach any crisis: some believe they are powerless, while others try to assume control. A study of the differences between women who had chosen to induce labor and those who had chosen to let labor come spontaneously showed that those who chose induction lacked trust in their own reproductive systems. They were more likely to complain during their menstrual periods, had more complications in their obstetrical history, and had more anxiety about going into labor.[29] Gayle Peterson and Lewis Mehl did a study of pregnant women in which they were able to predict with 95 percent accuracy which of them would get into trouble during labor based on the criteria in table 7, which is supported by the many studies on individual complications.[30]

"Rescuing" Women from Labor

Not uncommonly, a woman in labor will demand that her partner do something to "rescue" her from the situation she's in. How well I remember husbands whose wives sought out their support during their contractions by crying something like "Jer-ry—do *something*!" These men then yelled at me and said, "How much longer is this going to go on? You'd better take care of this soon, or you're going to hear from me." I've been threatened repeatedly by husbands who wanted me to "fix" their wives' labor as soon as possible—or else!

TABLE 7
POTENTIAL RISK FACTORS IN CHILDBIRTH

High-Risk Childbirth	Low-Risk Childbirth
Passivity	Activity
Dependence	Independence
Reliance on others	Self-reliance
Inability to accept support from others	Ability to accept support from others
Rejection of womanhood	Acceptance of womanhood
Repressed sexuality	Healthy sexuality
Self-view as sexual object	Self-view as sexual being
Childlike	Adultlike
Limiting beliefs about birth	Facilitative beliefs about birth
Nonconducive prior acculturation	Conducive prior acculturation
Dishonest, manipulative communication	Clear and honest communication
Spiritual beliefs that interfere with birth	Spiritual beliefs conducive to birth
Self-image of weakness	Self-image of strength
Split of mind and body	Integration of mind and body
Conflictual relationships	Loving relationships
Complete discrepancies in birth plan	Agreement with birth plan
Fear not being worked through	Fear being worked through
Sedentary	Physically active
Frail body appearance	Robust body appearance
Rigid in resisting change and new ideas	Yielding in accommodating to change
Chaotic home	Comfortable home
Does not want child	Wants child
External control of own life	Internal control of own life
Denial of the reality of birth pain	Acceptance of the reality of birth pain

Unable to control their wives' discomfort, and angry at their own feelings of helplessness in a process about which they can do nothing, these men become abusive to the obstetrician—"End this misery!" Their wives, helpless to continue their usual role as "male emotional shock absorber," watch helplessly or expect their husbands to do their "Mr. Fix-It" role. These women become even further out of touch with themselves. Labor is *not* an ideal time to educate a couple about transformative experiences. However, if a couple can be encouraged between contractions simply to stay with the process, understanding that it is normal and natural and not life-threatening, then sometimes they can be helped to work *with* the contractions and the process of labor, and not against them. My associate Bethany Hays, an obstetrician/gynecologist and medical director of the True North Health Center in Falmouth, Maine, reminds husbands or partners that they can't have the baby for their mates; nor can they take away the pain. But what they can do is love their partners. This is a very big gift for most women in labor—simply to be loved through the entire process. Women who are totally supported in labor emotionally and physically have the opportunity to be transformed forever by the knowledge that they *were* able to go through with it, that they have the inner resources after all. Every woman deserves this loving support—and studies show that such women are more loving with their children as a result. Labor lasts a relatively short time. Yet it's powerful enough to transform a woman's entire relationship with her body and its processes. After having her baby normally, one woman told me, "I have never felt so powerful in my whole life. I was so energized by the process. I was flying. I wanted to call everyone I knew and share my joy with them."

Reversing a lifelong pattern of coping behavior during labor, however, is not always possible. When I was still delivering babies, I found that no amount of cajoling, education, or pleading on my part could reverse many women's inherited belief that they *cannot* give birth normally, that they must have drugs and anesthesia to do it.

The medical system participates fully in treating childbirth as an emergency needing a cure. Because of its patriarchal nature, the medical system too often becomes the symbolic "husband" for all the women crying "Jer-ry, do *something*!" And believe me, doctors are trained in many ways to "do something." Each of our doings has a price. Some studies show, for instance, that epidural anesthesia increases the rate of cesarean section because this anesthetic relaxes the pelvic floor muscles, causing the baby to engage with the head in what's called the occiput posterior position—facing up. It's much harder to push a baby out when he or she is in this position; it also slows down the process and may add to the baby's distress. Epidurals are also a metaphor for our current mind/body split approach to childbirth: "I want to be awake and intellectually aware, but I don't want to feel my body." This was illustrated recently when a family practitioner friend of mine was attending the delivery of a woman with an epidural who was almost ready to give birth. She was watching a soap opera on TV and completely unaware of anything going on below her waist. At the point when the baby was crowning and actually being born, she asked my friend, the delivering physician, to please move out of the way so that she could see the TV screen. Though the epidural is not the villain here, it clearly made it much easier for this new mother to stay out of touch with her baby and her birth process—and also made the new mother much less aware of her newborn baby than she otherwise would have been. Pain medications also cross the placenta and may affect the baby. Forceps, episiotomies, vacuum extractors, oxytocin augmentation of labor, and unnecessary cesarean sections are other interventions that are not without risk.

A woman has the power within to birth normally and needs to know that drugs and anesthetics have potential adverse side effects. When I was delivering babies, I was frustrated by women who had no intention of delivering normally, and I tried to change them through education. But this was *my* problem, not necessarily theirs. They wanted all the technology that the hospital could offer. I now realize that it was not my job to change them or anyone. Each woman must look inside and see where she is—and be as honest with herself as possible. My job is to present alternatives in every situation and let each woman choose.

BIRTH TECHNOLOGIES

During the great blizzard of 1978 in Boston, when all the roads were closed and driving was impossible, I skied to a nearby hospital that did not do obstetrics, to deliver a few babies in the emergency room. Laboring women during that storm were being brought into the nearest hospitals by the National Guard. The emergency room (ER) staff, used to dealing with everything from gunshot wounds to heart attacks, were nearly undone by these births. ERs by their very nature are set up to *do something fast*. Births, by their very nature, require just the opposite. They require the qualities of a midwife—standing by expectantly, supportively, lovingly, while *doing* very little in the conventional sense. In most cases, it is the laboring woman herself who delivers the baby, *not* the doctor or staff, who merely catch it.

Hospitals, however, are set up to accommodate and medicate the deepest fears of laboring women. Hospital procedures usually do not address and work through these very real fears, but instead medicalize childbirth. They are designed to "save us" from the discomfort and inconvenience of childbirth, a view of childbirth to which society collectively contributes. Hospital birth practices flow seamlessly out of our adoration for technology and our fear of the process of birth. Doctors have been very willing to use technology to "improve" outcome in obstetrics because our culture believes in technology's superiority to the body's natural wisdom. We trust technology more than a woman's experience of herself and more than the documented benefits of loving human support in labor. And this is at heart of the current cesarean rate of nearly 30 percent!

Unfortunately, the beliefs that support hospital procedures are often so pervasive that even those women who enter the hospital wanting to birth normally often end up with some kind of intervention. This is because a woman in labor is highly vulnerable. If she is not supported in her labor process by people who truly trust labor and see it as normal, she can be talked into almost anything. Peggy O'Mara, editor and publisher of *Mothering Magazine,* summarizes it like this: "A birth plan gives a woman a false sense of security and misleads her to think that she can get the birth she wants if she only plans well enough. It makes her think that she is the one in charge, when, in fact, the philosophy and common practices of her practitioner and birthplace will influence her birth more than any plan. A woman doesn't need a plan when she's compatible with her practitioner. If a woman feels the need for a birth plan, she's with the wrong person or birthing at the wrong place."[31] I agree!

Fetal Monitors and Cesarean Sections

There is no more striking example of the overuse of technology in childbirth than the high cesarean section rates at many U.S. hospitals, as a result of the medicalization of childbirth, fueled by fear of lawsuits if a baby is not perfect. Although the cesarean section rate in most teaching hospitals is now 30 percent, in some cities a white woman with insurance has a 50 percent chance of having a cesarean![32]

During my residency training, when fetal monitoring hit the scene and the cesarean section rate began to soar, I remember thinking, "How can it be that 25 percent of women aren't able to go through a normal physiological event without the aid of anesthesia and major surgery? How could the human race have possibly survived if this many women really need major surgery to give birth? What is going wrong here?"

I was taught that I must treat everyone as though she were going to have a potential complication, as if a normal labor could turn into a crisis at a moment's notice. Whenever a woman arrived in labor, we immediately put in an intravenous line, drew blood, ruptured her membranes—broke the amniotic sac ("bag of waters") surrounding the baby—screwed a fetal scalp electrode into the baby's head, and threaded a catheter into her uterus to measure intrauterine pressure on the fetal monitor. Then, she and her family, the doctors, and the nurses all fixed their gazes on the monitor and pretty much relied on *it* to tell us what to do next. The woman was asked to labor in the position that gave the best monitor tracing—not the one that felt best to her. I recall trying to get these monitoring devices even into women whose babies were about to be delivered when they came through the door. If I didn't have a monitor strip for documentation and there was a bad outcome, I knew that I would be in trouble with my attending physician. Later, studies would show that fetal monitoring did not actually improve perinatal outcome when compared with a nurse listening to the heart rate periodically.[33] What it did do was increase cesarean section rates—a great example of technology "catching on" before all the data were in. (Monitoring has its place—I'm not against it. It simply is *not* a substitute for caring human interaction, though it is often used as one.)

During my second year of residency, I went to a meeting of the International Childbirth Education Association (ICEA) and learned that membranes don't normally rupture until a woman starts to push, and that babies in whom the membranes have been artificially ruptured have evidence of more stress in utero—the pH of their scalp blood samples is lower. I also learned at this meeting that the amniotic fluid is the best "packing material" available. It cushions the baby's body during contractions. Why were we so eager to mess with nature's protection? So that we could put in our technological monitors!

Is it any wonder that when you hook up a vulnerable laboring woman to three or four different tubes and wires, and then rupture her membranes, she, and subsequently her baby, might get a little scared—resulting in some fetal distress? A survey of sixteen hundred women conducted by Harris Interactive for the nonprofit Maternity Center Association showed that 61 percent experienced between six and ten medical interventions during their labor and deliveries, including being hooked up to an IV and being given Pitocin to speed labor—which makes contractions more painful and increases the risk of fetal distress and neonatal jaundice. (In addition, 43 percent had between three and five major interventions—including induction, episiotomy, C-sections, and forceps delivery—and eight out of ten women [and 91 percent of first-time mothers] had pain-relief medication during labor.)

Many cases of fetal distress could potentially have been reversed by soothing the mother and asking her to focus inside on how her baby is—and send it messages of reassurance. Biofeedback has documented the profound effects of thoughts on body systems such as blood pressure, pulse, and skin resistance. The baby is *part* of a woman's body. Her thoughts and emotions can and do have large effects on her baby.

Many obstetricians feel inherently that vaginal delivery is just plain dangerous, leading to increased fetal trauma. I've been in discussions with male and female colleagues who believe on some very deep, probably unexamined level that abdominal delivery is the superior mode of arrival. Recently some are strongly advocating elective cesarean or "vaginal bypass" surgery as a matter of preference!

Approximately 50 to 85 percent of women who've had a cesarean delivery can go on and deliver subsequent babies normally. Though obstetricians used to be taught the dictum "Once a cesarean, always a cesarean," this is no longer the case. The scientific literature documenting the safety of subsequent vaginal deliveries was available by the late 1970s. We routinely offered vaginal birth after cesarean section (VBAC) as an option during my training. Yet this option is *still* not offered to all women who are candidates for it. And for those women who are candidates, it is often not an option they choose because both doctors and patients are afraid of the rare possibility of a uterine rupture. In an article entitled "When Your Patient Demands a C-section," in one of the OB/GYN magazines, Bruce Flamm, M.D., was right on target when he said, "When someone is scared, it is not an indication for surgery. It is an indication for education."[34] Clearly the practice of medicine is a two-way street. Bethany Hays, M.D., commented on reading Dr. Flamm's article, "This is great. We create the fear of vaginal birth, and then we blame it on the patient!"

C-section rates vary tremendously among individual doctors. Some physicians have personal C-section rates of only 6 percent. These tend to be the same doctors who are highly supportive of midwifery.

RISKS OF C-SECTIONS

Although some women elect to have C-sections for convenience or because they fear the birthing process, having a cesarean when there is no medical indication is a controversial practice. And for good reason. A C-section is major surgery that entails some serious risks. The following risks, compiled by the Coalition for Improving Maternity Services (CIMS), are greater in women with C-sections when compared with vaginal birth:

~ Maternal death (five to seven times greater)[35]

~ Injury to the bladder, uterus, and blood vessels; hemorrhage; anesthesia accidents, blood clots in the legs, pulmonary embolism, paralyzed bowel; and infection (up to fifty times more common)[36]

~ Difficulties with normal activities two months after birth (one in ten).[37] (One in four women who have had C-sections report that pain at the incision site is a major problem, and one in fourteen still report pain six months after delivery.)[38]

~ Rehospitalization (twice as likely)[39]

~ Internal scar tissue resulting in pelvic pain, pain during sex, and bowel problems

~ Reproductive consequences, such as subsequent infertility,[40] miscarriage, and premature birth[41]

Risks to a baby born via C-section include:

~ Breathing and breast-feeding problems due to even slight prematurity[42]

~ Being cut accidentally by the surgeon (one to two per one hundred)[43]

~ Lower Apgar scores (50 percent more likely) and admission to intermediate or intensive care (five times more likely)[44]

~ Developing persistent pulmonary hypertension, a life-threatening condition (more than four times as likely)[45]

(For more information, see the CIMS website at www.motherfriendly.org.)

Episiotomy

Another procedure that should be abandoned is episiotomy. It is estimated that one-third of all women who deliver vaginally in the United States (more than one million women per year) undergo episiotomy, the surgical cutting of the tissue between the vagina and rectum. Nationally, 70 to 80 percent of first-time mothers delivering vaginally in the United States undergo this procedure.[46]

Women who have an episiotomy are fifty times *more* likely to suffer from severe lacerations than those who don't.[47] The reason for this is that episiotomy cuts frequently extend further into the vaginal tissues during the delivery. This surgical cut of the perineum can result in excessive blood loss, painful scarring, and unnecessary postpartum pain.[48] The woman's discomfort may affect her bonding with and nursing of the infant.

Studies have shown that whether a woman giving birth has an episiotomy is most dependent upon whether she is attended by a doctor or by a midwife. Midwives are taught how to do normal, noninterventional deliveries. Doctors naturally *do* more—that's what they've been trained to do. Letting a woman push her baby out slowly, gently, and without interference is a rare experience in some hospitals. A retrospective analysis of 2,041 operative vaginal births (meaning that forceps or vacuum extractors were used) in San Francisco showed that the rate of fourth-degree tears (tears extending into the rectum) declined from 12.2 percent to 5.4 percent during a ten-year period as the rate of episiotomy at the hospital fell from 93.4 percent to 35.7 percent.[49] While the rate of vaginal lacerations increased, these are trivial and very easy to repair in comparison to the damage done by episiotomies. They are also far less painful.

A recent highly publicized review has finally laid this matter to rest. (I hope!) In an exhaustive review of every article published in the medical literature from 1950 to 2004, the authors found that none of the benefits previously ascribed to routine episiotomy did in fact exist. "In fact," the study reported, "outcomes with episiotomy can be considered worse since some proportion of women who would have had lesser injury instead had a surgical incision."[50]

A Word About Pelvic Floor Dysfunction

Every since the late 1990s, the potential for pelvic floor dysfunction from natural birth has been used to justify cesarean delivery, especially when there is no other indication. In fact, the American College of Obstetricians and Gynecologists released a statement in October 2003, indicating that although physicians are under no obligation to initiate discussions about elective C-section, a physician is justified in performing the surgery if he or she believes that C-section delivery promotes the overall health and well-being of the mother and baby better than vaginal birth. And the potential protection of the pelvic floor through C-section (which I call vaginal bypass surgery) is one of the justifications.

This statement received wide criticism from many organizations, including the International Cesarean Awareness Network, the College of Midwives, Doulas of North America, Attachment Parenting International, and the American College of Nurse–Midwives. The Society of Obstetricans and Gynaecologists of Canada stated in two press releases, in March 2004, that vaginal birth remains the preferred approach and the safest option for most women because it carries less of the complications in pregnancy and subsequent pregnancies than C-section.

A thorough review of the medical literature on mode of delivery and pelvic floor dysfunction published in 2006 pointed out the difficulties of comparing modes of delivery because of the varying skill levels of practitioners and also the varying conditions under which birth takes place. For example, vaginal births involving forceps deliveries by unskilled practitioners or vacuum extraction, or the use of episiotomy, are far more apt to be associated with pelvic floor problems than births that don't involve these modalities. The authors state, for example, that "gentle birth in nonlithotomy position, without urgent directed pushing and without the routine use of episiotomy, will tend to protect the pelvic floor and the perineum and reduce strain on the very structures that we are reviewing, thereby improving outcomes and reducing difference between vaginal birth and C-section where they exist."[51]

Regardless of the statistics, it is clear that the female pelvic floor is designed to give birth without complications in most women and is perfectly capable of doing so in a supportive environment. I was on a panel with the famous midwife Ina May Gaskin at the Annual Meeting of the Association for Pre- and Perinatal Psychology and Health in 2005. Ina May suggested that it's nearly impossible to birth normally if one is out of touch with her pelvic floor, including her bowel function—a common situation in many women who are terrified of losing control during birth. She jokingly suggested that women might want to follow a horse around so they could see how well the anal sphincter of a horse expands to allow discharge of waste matter and then instantly returns to normal size. The female cervix is also a sphincter that is capable of dilating very nicely under optimal conditions but that is also heavily influenced by how safe and supported a woman feels in birth. The same thing is true of the pelvic floor. A comprehensive website designed to help women prevent pelvic floor problems at birth is available at www.childbirthconnection.org/article.asp?ck=10206.

Anesthesia

Modern anesthesia is a godsend in many instances, but in labor it is used far too often. This culture believes that if a little is good, more must be better. So there are now obstetrical services in which almost every pregnant woman, long before she goes into labor, is sold on the virtues of epidurals—the "Cadillac" of obstetrical anesthesia. The seed is often planted during hospital-sponsored childbirth classes; "You don't need to feel a thing." Anesthesia is offered as a panacea to many. I've heard women say, "I want that epidural catheter put in during my last two weeks of pregnancy!" One remarked, "I'm making sure I get that happy dural!" But the risks include arrest of the first and second stages of labor, fever, increased forceps use, pelvic floor damage, and fetal distress, with a subsequent increase in cesarean section rates.[52]

In a 1996 study of 1,733 women having their first babies, the cesarean rate for those who received epidural analgesia was 17 percent, compared to 4 percent in those who did not receive this type of anesthesia—a fourfold increase.[53] In a study published in 2005, researchers found epidurals were strongly associated with the more problematic fetal occiput-posterior position (the baby's head facing up at delivery, instead of the more ideal position of head down, facing the mother's back), which the researchers suggested might explain the higher rate of C-sections in women who have epidurals.[54] Despite these studies, there continues to be debate on the pros and cons of epidurals. (How the anesthesia is given, by whom, and when during the course of labor are among the factors that can affect outcome.) But the association of epidurals with C-section accords with my own experience working in a large hospital delivery unit.

In another study of 1,657 women having their first babies, 14.5 percent of those who received epidural anesthesia experienced fever, compared to only 1 percent of the women who did not receive an epidural. Because of these fevers, the infants born to the women in the epidural groups were over four times more likely to be evaluated for infection and about four times more likely to be treated with antibiotics than babies born to women who didn't receive an epidural.[55] Yet of the 356 newborns in the epidural group who were evaluated for sepsis, only 3 actually had it. Epidurals put women at higher risk for fever regardless of the infant's size or the length of labor, two factors also felt to be associated with increased risk of infection. The cascade of adverse consequences of having your baby worked up for an infection include having your baby taken away from you and taken to the neonatal intensive care unit; more pain for the baby, because blood needs to be drawn and IVs started; the risks of antibiotics, which kill all the friendly, normal bacteria in the baby's body, thus increasing the risk of infection from antibiotic-resistant strains of bacteria found in hospitals; increased anxiety for both mother and baby; and possible adverse effects on the establishment of successful breast-feeding. Since this sepsis workup takes place right after you've had your baby, it can significantly affect the important bonding period that nature intended following birth.

Supine Position

Women who deliver in a physiologically normal position, such as standing or squatting, are much less apt to have perineal tears and are more apt to have normal, nonsurgical second stages of labor. Many women also feel most comfortable laboring on their hands and knees. In fact, lying supine while pushing out the baby is a position that is actually unfavorable for birth because this position favors excessive pressure of the delivering baby into the posterior vagina, and it *decreases* the diameter of the pelvic outlet—a setup for vaginal tears. (Ever try to move your bowels while lying flat on your back?) This position, known as the lithotomy position, was apparently popularized by Louis XIV in France, who was a voyeur and wanted to watch the births of women in his court without their knowledge of his presence. In the lithotomy position, with her skirts hiked up, the laboring woman couldn't see who was watching. This position caught on because it was associated with the upper classes and therefore was imitated. It also made things easier for the birth attendant.

Probably another reason it caught on was the popularization of obstetrical forceps. Forceps were originally developed in 1560 by Peter Chamberlain, a male midwife who came from a family of male midwives. These tools remained a Chamberlain "family secret" until they were released to the medical profession in 1728.[56] Training in the use of this instrument was given only to men (usually physicians and surgeons), and they were originally used when all else failed and the woman had been trying to push the baby out for hours. The lithotomy position was the one in which the exhausted woman could rest while forceps were applied. It also allowed the obstetrician maximal control over the process of forceps delivery.

During the second stage of labor, women who squat instead of lie supine increase the size of the vaginal outlet naturally, because this position distributes pressure equally throughout the entire vaginal circumference and helps bring the baby's head down. In the squatting position the anterior/posterior diameter of the bony pelvis (front to back) is increased by a half-centimeter or more.[57] The squatting position also keeps the pregnant uterus *off* the major pelvic blood vessels leading to the heart. The blood supply from the mother to the baby is therefore improved, resulting in increased safety for both. (I've seen countless babies go into fetal distress in the delivery room simply because of the mother's position, flat on her back.) Women who are encouraged to touch their perineum and the baby's head get connected up very quickly with their birthing babies and deliver much more easily. In general, it's not advisable for a mother to overexert herself during the second stage of labor. Pushing the baby out slowly and gently is associated with far less pelvic trauma!

Bottom line: when birth technology is truly needed, it is life-saving and miraculous. When a physician is in the operating room transfusing a woman whose placenta simply won't separate from the uterus and who is losing blood quickly, she knows that one hundred years ago, her patient would have died. In the vast majority of cases, however, more "high-touch" and less "high-tech" would do the job.

MOTHERING THE MOTHER: A SOLUTION WHOSE TIME HAS COME

Labor support is centuries old, and it is intuitively obvious that those women who feel most supported in labor are apt to do the best. Marshall Klaus, M.D., and John Kennell, M.D., have proved in six controlled clinical trials that the presence of a female labor support person, known as a doula, shortens first-time labor by an average of two hours, decreases the chance of a cesarean section by 50 percent, decreases the need for pain medication and epidural anesthesia, helps the father or co-parent participate with confidence, and increases the success of breast-feeding. Dr. Kennell has proved that if doula labor support were routinely used, this simple step would save the health care system at least $2 billion a year in the costs of unnecessary C-sections, epidurals, and sepsis workups for newborns. He once quipped, "If a drug were to have this same effect, it would be unethical not to use it."

Too often, when we think of labor support, we think of a labor "coach"—someone who specializes in knowing the right breathing techniques and so on. But a doula embodies women's wisdom. She is a compassionate woman especially trained to give emotional support in labor by tuning in to the needs of the mother and mothering *her*. Doulas create an "emotional holding environment for the mother, encouraging her to allow her own body to tell her what may be best at various times during labor.... A successful doula," write the authors of *Mothering the Mother*, "is giving of herself and is not afraid of love."[58] A doula enters the space of a laboring woman and is highly responsive and aware of her needs, moods, changes, and unspoken feelings. She has no need to control or smother. Every pregnant woman should have the benefits of a doula. This person does not detract from the role of the baby's father or co-parent, by the way. A doula enhances it and leaves him (or her) free to do the very important job of loving the mother.

HOW TO DECREASE YOUR RISK
FOR A CESAREAN SECTION

Though cesarean sections are sometimes necessary, many experts in the field feel that a rate of 15 percent plus or minus 5 percent is far more reasonable than the current overall rate of 30 percent.[59] This means, of course, that many women are having cesareans that aren't truly necessary. Because this surgery is so common, however, many women do not realize that cesarean section is major abdominal surgery fraught with potential complications, such as bleeding and infection. This surgery should be avoided unless absolutely necessary. Here's how to decrease your chances of having a C-section.

1. Check out your beliefs and your doctor's. Do you believe vaginal birth is inherently distasteful and too dangerous or frightening for you to get through? Many women and their doctors actually operate under this belief, and it gets played out seamlessly in what happens in labor and delivery. A 1996 study published in *The Lancet* found that of 282 obstetricians surveyed, 31 percent of the women and 8 percent of the men (17 percent overall) said they would want a cesarean section if they or their wives were pregnant. Many said that they would choose the operation even in uncomplicated, low-risk pregnancies![60] Though I don't know of a similar study from the United States, I've met many physicians who honestly believe that cesarean sections are the superior mode of delivery. And this belief is reflected in their personal C-section rates. Hospitals keep statistics on the C-section rates for individual doctors, so a physician should be able to tell you his or her rate. (Of course, in a practice limited to high-risk obstetrics in a large medical center, the rate will be higher.)

2. If you've had a prior C-section, plan on having a normal vaginal delivery for your next birth. Currently, about 36 percent of all C-sections in the United States are scheduled repeat C-sections, with the only indication for this major surgery being that a woman had a

C-section previously. Though many women don't know it, both the medical literature and the personal experience of countless obstetricians (including me) who have performed VBACs (vaginal birth after cesarean) for years show that the vast majority of women who've had a previous C-section can safely go through a normal labor and delivery. A recent study found that roughly 73 percent of women attempting VBAC were successful. The same study also reported that only one woman out of every two thousand who undergo VBAC will have a significant complication from uterine rupture.[61] This makes VBAC far safer than a routine C-section! If your doctor is not comfortable with this option, find someone who is.

3. Choose your birth place carefully. Plan to have your baby in a place in which you know you're most apt to feel safe and secure. More and more, studies are documenting that home births are safe for carefully selected and well-supported women. Family-centered maternity care centers offer many of the comforts of home with the safety net of a hospital.

A growing number of hospitals and some freestanding birth centers now offer this kind of care, which is characterized by the following: the laboring woman, with her support person(s), labors and delivers in the same room; the labor and delivery nurse is the same throughout her stay; and the mother's nurse is also the primary nurse for the baby, who rooms in with the mother. In short, in family-centered maternity care, the focus is on keeping mothers, babies, and families together in supportive and healthy ways. This is a vast improvement over the childbirth-as-major-operation approach that has been common since the 1950s; this approach requires a labor room, delivery room, and recovery room—all staffed by different nurses. In this model, the baby is sent to the nursery, where yet another group of nurses takes over. This fragmented care, which was experienced by nearly all of our mothers, can be devastating to a laboring mother and her new baby, and it increases the risk of intervention starting from the time a woman enters the hospital.

4. Hire a doula to "mother you" during your labor and delivery. (See page 500.) Better yet, work with a doctor or midwife who automatically suggests professional labor support and is comfortable working closely with these individuals. Such doctors and midwives almost always have a lower C-section rate than their colleagues.

5. Don't go to the hospital too early. It's very common for a woman to go through many hours of "prodromal" mild labor before going into

true labor, which is defined as the active dilation and effacement of the cervix. If you're really in labor, you won't want to talk through a contraction, your attention will be focused inward, and you won't want to move around much during the contraction. Consider hiring a midwife who can meet you at your home or at another convenient location to check your progress before you get admitted to the hospital, where the atmosphere may actually slow your labor or cause it to be dysfunctional. (This is not always the case in a good birth center that offers family-centered maternity care.) Remember, your uterus is very sensitive to your environment. It works best whenever and wherever you feel the most relaxed and safe. This will vary from woman to woman.

Recent studies have suggested that labor may take longer than doctors have been led to believe it should and still be completely safe and normal. Many doctors have been trained to follow now-outmoded charts for determining progress of labor known as Friedman curves, named after a well-known Boston obstetrician whose advice influenced several generations of obstetricians. If your labor doesn't follow these graphs, it may increase your chances for having a C-section even when everything is normal.

A significant number of C-sections are done for "failure to progress," a condition often attributed to the fact that the baby is "too big." This is usually not the case, since many women who have had C-sections for this indication go on to have even bigger babies in subsequent pregnancies following normal labors and deliveries. Failure to progress, in my experience, simply means that the uterus stops contracting efficiently and the mother becomes exhausted. When this goes on for a number of hours, a C-section is often done to get the whole thing over with.

What you want to do is avoid the chain of events that leads up to this in the first place. Tune in to your body's wisdom. Most women will be able to know when they're really in labor. Don't let the collective emergency mindset of the culture invade your physiology here, because once you go on and get all hooked up to the monitor, you may find that your labor slows—or stops altogether if you are really anxious. And try to avoid letting anyone rupture your membranes to "get things moving."

Unfortunately, all too many women and their mates have been indoctrinated by TV shows and movies showing couples rushing to the hospital at the first sign of a contraction, fearful that the baby will simply drop out if they don't arrive in time! Once they are there, the hospital staff will often be subtly (or not so subtly) pushed to do something because the woman is tired of being pregnant and wants it over with. If, in this state, you get into bed, allow your membranes to be ruptured, and then stay immobile waiting for something to happen, you won't be allowing your body and your baby to find their own timing.

6. Plan to labor without an epidural. When you enter labor with the idea that your body will know how to deal with the sensations, you're more likely to be in the receptive mode necessary for optimal uterine functioning. If, on the other hand, you believe you will need an epidural the minute you enter the hospital, you won't be present with your own labor. The contractions will simply be something to be endured until the anesthesiologist gets there. Although epidurals can be very useful under certain circumstances, they are associated with prolonged labor and with relaxing the lower part of the uterus and pelvis so much that the baby's head engages in the wrong position. And, as I mentioned above, even if an epidural does not increase your cesarean risk, it is still associated with maternal fever and the risk of your baby needing a sepsis workup. It also inhibits the release of the neurotransmitter beta-endorphin, which normally increases during labor and is responsible for the euphoria some women feel. Nature designed that euphoria as the best possible state in which to meet and fall in love with your new baby.

If you do find you need an epidural, for whatever reason, wait until your labor is well established and ask for the lowest dose that gives you adequate pain relief.

7. Above all, trust that your body knows how to give birth. During labor more than at any other time, women have the opportunity to experience their body's wisdom in a dramatic way. Move into the positions that feel best. Don't get into bed unless that's the position that feels most comfortable. Don't resist labor—dive in deeply and go with it. I've attended enough labors to know that when women feel comfortable, relaxed, and well supported, their bodies automatically know what to do to keep both themselves and their babies safe.

MY PERSONAL STORY

As a mother and a women's doctor, I have experienced childbirth from both sides of the bed. Every mother has moments that she cherishes from the birth experience and insights and feelings she'd like to share with other women. I'd like to tell you my story and also some remarkable stories of other women.

The due date for my first child was December 7, 1980. I continued my work supervising the residency clinic at a Boston hospital, and flew or drove to Maine every other week to keep my practice going there. I had watched far too many pregnant women stop work early and then mope around the house eating, waiting for the baby to come, sometimes begging their obstetrician to induce labor. I didn't want to fall into that category. I had also seen dozens of women go overdue. I certainly wasn't going to get excited about labor—at least, not until my due date.

On Thanksgiving we went to dinner at a friend's house. Later that evening, back home in bed, I started to experience very mild but regular contractions that didn't hurt. Like the good controlled doctor that I was, I went into the bathroom and decided to examine my cervix to see if I was dilating. When I did this, my water broke. I thought, "Damn, now I know this really *is* it."[62] Shortly thereafter, without the natural "padding" that the amniotic fluid provides, my contractions began coming every two minutes and were much more uncomfortable than initially.

I called my mother, who was planning to help me after the birth, and said, "I'm not going to like this." She said that she understood (after six children, she knew) but that it wouldn't last forever. In the 1940s, Mom had always had to labor alone, strapped down in bed with no pain relief or personal support. For each delivery, she had been knocked unconscious by drugs and was handed the baby later by the obstetrician, as though it were a gift from him and not the fruit of her own labor. Thousands of women like her were never given a choice and didn't even know there were other ways to deliver.

The pain of labor was far greater than I thought it would be. (It's always worse after the membranes are ruptured, a point that doesn't seem to stop some obstetricians from doing it prematurely even when there's no need to.) I had seen hundreds of women in labor after five years of OB training. I had always focused on the women who didn't appear to have any discomfort, and I was so sure I would be one of them. But here I was—stuck. I felt as though I were in a box, and there was no way out except through. My intellect could not get me out of this—and I was determined to go through the process naturally. I already trusted the natural world more than the artificial man-made one. What I didn't appreciate then was the depth of my own programming into and cooperation with that same man-made world.

We called my obstetrician, a sensitive man with whom I had worked in the hospital for several years. He suggested that my husband and I go into the hospital. The only problem was that all I wanted to do was stay on the floor on my hands and knees. Moving *anywhere* seemed to me the most unnatural thing I could think of. It went against every instinct in my body.

I didn't have a bag packed for the hospital, so my husband ran around and put some underwear, a nightgown, and a toothbrush in a bag. Then he tried to get me dressed, out the door, and into the car. He nearly had to carry me. Left to my own instincts, I would never have left my position on my hands and knees on the floor.

When we got to the hospital, a place where I had worked for half a decade, I had to go through the admitting office as a patient. Admissions had lost the correct papers and would not let me go upstairs to the labor and delivery floor, where my nurse friends and my doctor were waiting. This was my introduction to the bureaucracy of hospitals, something I'd been shielded from for years. (Laboring in a hospital hallway alone is inhumane; but for thousands of women, it is their experience.) I simply walked out of the room, went to the back hall elevator, got in, and went up to labor and delivery by myself.

When my doctor examined me, I was four centimeters dilated. (You have to get to ten to be ready to push.) For the next three hours my contractions came frequently. But I failed to dilate beyond six centimeters, where I remained "stuck" for those three hours. The contraction pattern on the monitor was "dysfunctional." Though the contractions hurt a lot, and I never got much of a break between them, they simply were not getting the job done. I had what is known as hypertonic uterine inertia, which means that the contractions, though present, are not efficient—they are erratic, originating all over the uterus at the same time, like the heart when it goes into atrial fibrillation. (The high heart—in the chest—does the same sort of thing as the low heart—the uterus in the pelvis—sometimes.) Instead of beginning at the top and moving in a wave to the bottom of the uterus, the contractions originated in many places at the same time. Labor didn't progress well. It was like trying to get toothpaste out of a tube by squeezing it in fifteen places at the same time with a little bit of pressure, instead of squeezing firmly only at the back end of the tube so that the paste comes out uniformly.

When my doctor told me that I had made no progress in three hours, I knew what was next. (Remember, my intellect thought it was in control of my labor.) "Okay," I said, "start the IV, plug in the fetal electrode, and hang the Pit." Pitocin (oxytocin) is a drug that artificially contracts the uterus. After the Pitocin was started, the contractions became almost unbearable, going to full intensity almost as soon as they began.

No amount of Lamaze breathing distracted me from the intensity of the feeling that the lower part of my body was in the grip of a vise.[63] At one point, I looked at the clock and saw that it was 11:15 A.M. What I recall thinking was, "If this goes on for another fifteen minutes, I'm going to need an epidural anesthetic." I didn't know that I was in transition—the part of labor that is most intense, just before the cervix becomes fully dilated. Within the next twelve minutes I suddenly felt the urge to push. It was the most powerful bodily sensation I've ever felt, and I was powerless to resist it. The thought flashed through my mind, "If I ever tell another woman not to push when every fiber in her body tells her to push, may God strike me with lightning!"

In two pushes, Ann almost flew out of my body. My obstetrician quite literally caught her. Though I was laboring in the "birthing room," I wasn't laboring in the "correct" delivery bed, and I barely made it to the delivery bed in time. (Birthing rooms now are equipped with beds that adjust for delivery of the baby, so that moving from one bed to another isn't necessary.)

Ann cried and cried, and though I put her to my breast almost immediately, it still took quite a while to calm her down. I believe this was because the Pitocin made for a far too rapid second stage of labor. It was too intense both for Ann and for me. Neither she nor I had much chance to recover between contractions.

A primiparous patient—one having her first baby—usually takes an hour or more to push the baby out. From the time the cervix is fully dilated to delivery—the second stage of labor—I went from six centimeters to delivery in less than one hour; my uterus was being pushed by a powerful drug, a very intense and distinctly unnatural experience.

During her childhood, my daughter was not particularly "at home" in her body and was afraid to take physical risks, for instance in skiing or hiking. Though there are various reasons for this, I know deep within me that being propelled into the world with so little time to accommodate herself to the process of labor was a terrifying experience for her. She had difficulty nursing, and she was never a good sleeper. Part of the reason is that she was small (five pounds, eight ounces) and early (38.5 weeks), and part is her personality—but another part is how she was born. I didn't know then what I know now, and I don't for one minute blame myself about how she was born. I allowed myself to feel sadness about the experience, which would be considered a completely normal labor and delivery by most everyone.

After Ann's birth, the cord got pulled off the placenta, so that my placenta had to be manually removed by my doctor. The explosive uncontrolled delivery had left me with some vaginal tears, so removing the placenta was somewhat uncomfortable. But nothing could equal the discomfort of those Pitocin-induced contractions! I was euphoric to have the whole thing over with. I had had a "normal vaginal delivery" and felt lucky to have avoided a cesarean. Most women obstetricians are automatically treated like candidates for high-risk pregnancies and deliveries, because women doctors (and other women who have been highly trained out of their instinctual feminine knowing) often split their intellects from their bodies, mistrust their bodies, and unconsciously set themselves up for the possibility of labor problems. We as a group are also at risk for working too many hours during pregnancy to "prove" that we can "handle it" and compete with the men.

When I look back now, I realize that my being stuck at six centimeters was a perfect metaphor for my ambivalence about having a baby and for how I felt during my labor. I had felt "stuck" and trapped by the pain—something my intellect had not prepared me for. My intellect, you recall, thought I was doing an experiment with my uterus. I wasn't very invested in actually having a *baby*. I had made no room in my life for a baby. I had spent the previous decade proving to myself and to the world that I was as good as any man—and men don't do babies.

Another factor in creating my dysfunctional labor was the process of moving off my hands and knees in my house, getting to the hospital, going through admitting, and then answering insurance and medical questions for forms that I had already filled out several times. All those things are interruptions of the inner focus required for normal labor. I didn't really know that at the time, though I'd seen countless women come to the hospital in active labor, only to have the process become slowed down or dysfunctional when they were "processed by the system."

Now it was me having a baby—something that I was determined would not change my life. I realized that what I needed when I got stuck was a midwife or a doctor with good midwifery skills, preferably some wise woman (or wise man—male midwives and male obstetricians with the souls of midwives do exist) who was a parent and who trusted the process of labor and the messages my body was sending. I needed someone who would have said to me, "Go inside and talk to your baby. Let the baby know that it's okay to come out, that she will be fine." Then the midwife would have taken me for a walk in the hall—a very effective way of getting contractions back on track. She might even have helped me work through my ambivalence about having a baby.

With my second labor, I did go to a midwife. I began labor at home and spent some time in the bathtub. (Studies done in Sweden have shown that women who labor in warm water dilate much faster.) I didn't want to go to the hospital until I had to. My husband was asleep, and I didn't wake him until I knew that the labor was moving right along, several hours later. When he examined me, I was already seven centimeters dilated. We went to the hospital and my colleague Dr. Mary Ellen Fenn met me at the front door and parked my car, a gesture of support that I will always treasure.

When I arrived in the birthing room, I was nine centimeters dilated. I spent the rest of the labor rocking from one foot to the other while standing up. This second baby was a lot bigger than the first—eight pounds, nine ounces. Her head was what is called posterior (she was face up in my body). I never felt the urge to push, but I pushed her out anyway with a great deal of effort. Even after I was fully dilated, the contractions felt the same as they had at nine centimeters. I didn't have any episiotomy—and I didn't tear. My baby, Kate, and I left the hospital an hour after she was born. Kate was calm and collected, and she has been that way ever since. Her personality and body type are entirely different from her sister's. Part of the reason is that I was a different person during my pregnancy with Kate than with Ann.

Having my midwife in the room with me was heaven. I felt so supported. I had much more trust in myself this time—and I had all the baby things ready. I remember thinking during this second labor that every woman deserved this same amount of support. *Every* woman should be able to labor in whatever position her body wants to take. She should be surrounded by beloved friends of her choice. (Not spectators, but supporters—there's a big difference!) Every woman should be massaged and cared for and cherished during her labor.

In this labor I had pain, to be sure, but I went deep down inside myself with it. In my first labor, I had fought the pain and reached out to my husband in desperation—I wouldn't even let him go to the bathroom. But this second labor felt as though it was between me and my baby. I had plenty of time to rest between contractions and to chat with my caregivers. They gave me backrubs that felt fantastic. No drugs interfered with the labor. I learned to trust my body in a letting-go process that feels like a kind of surrendering to a process that *is* you but that is also *greater* than you. I didn't learn any of this stuff in my residency training—I didn't even learn it from watching women in labor, though I believe that it can be learned that way and that I eventually would have. What you have to do is trust nature, expect the best, and get your intellect's death grip off your flesh.

Labor feels very instinctive and primitive, but because our culture teaches us not to trust our instincts, we usually associate the word *primitive* with *ignorant*. The Random House dictionary defines *primitive* as "unaffected or little-affected by civilizing influences." Believe me, that's exactly how labor feels. We cannot labor with our intellect. We women need to reclaim this animal part of us and embrace ancient and necessary wisdom. Preparing for birth with the Bradley Method (see www.bradleybirth.com) or the Calm Birth method (see www.calm-birth.org) surely helps. I now wish I had groaned loudly and let my groans help me expel the baby. But I was far too "professional" (read: out of touch) to do that. I am deeply saddened by all the unnecessarily medicalized births that occur because women in labor don't trust themselves and aren't surrounded by those who could assist them in this process.

TURNING LABOR INTO PERSONAL POWER

Trusting the birth process and knowing how to tune in to the baby are abilities that enhance labor and make it an experience that offers us the opportunity to empower ourselves. Instead of running from these lessons, we as women could learn a great deal if we were willing to embrace them.

Bethany Hays, M.D., mentioned earlier, is the mother of three sons. She once wrote me the following reflections on the pain of labor and how we can work *with* it:

"I used to think that labor was just a matter of dealing with pain and the fear of pain. I knew that with labor the pain was qualitatively different from any other pain experienced in our bodies. I never subscribed to the punishment theory of labor pain. I was looking for a natural and reasonable explanation. I did not believe labor pain was a whim of Mother Nature any more than it was a punishment from God.

"With all other forms of pain, the pain is there to tell us that something is wrong. 'Stop walking on your foot, there's a piece of glass in it.' 'Don't eat any more chili, it's giving you heartburn.' With labor, I knew that the reason for the pain, at least in most cases, is not related to anything being wrong. The physical process of birth is completely normal and exquisitely planned by nature to ensure the safe delivery of an infant with minimal trauma to the mother. Pain was a part of that plan, and I had but to view it in that context to understand its purpose.

"As I observed women through their pregnancies, I began to understand that nature would have to have a signal to get women to stop what they were doing, to find a safe place to give birth, and to gather people around them to help. For some, nothing short of a sledgehammer would do. It needed to be a signal that no one could ignore but that left the mother able to participate in the birth if there were circumstances requiring her to do so."

Certainly, the pain of labor is a strong signal that says, "Stop what you're doing and pay attention." Instead of the "no pain, no gain" cultural mentality that often leads to self-abuse, gaining from the pain of labor is an entirely different way of being with pain. Once a woman has stopped, gathered support people around her, and gotten herself to a safe place to birth, she has reached the point when she must use the pain for something else. Dr. Hays suggests that at this point the pain is something to allow, and she points out that one of the meanings of *to suffer* is "to allow," as when Christ said, "Suffer the little children to come unto me."

Once settled in, women in labor then must *allow* the pain. Thrashing about doesn't help. Going deep within yourself does. Dr. Hays and I were talking recently about the pain of labor and how to help women work with it, and we exchanged a few stories about women who appeared to "go to another place" when they were in labor.

She told me about the wife of a medical student she once worked with who sat quietly in bed with the lights dimmed during her labor and was so focused that her mother and husband figured that she probably wasn't in labor. Not only was she in labor, however, when she finally opened her eyes and spoke, she said, "I think it's time to push."

"After the birth," Dr. Hays told me, "my curiosity prompted me to ask her where she had gone when I instructed her to go 'somewhere else.' [Early in labor, she had seemed to be very disconnected from her body, and Dr. Hays had told her to get comfortable, relax, and just "go somewhere else."] Her answer was totally unexpected. She said, 'Oh, I was concentrating on the pain.' Her answer intrigued me. Could a woman really deal with the pain of labor not, as I had been taught, by distracting herself and concentrating on something else—her 'breathing' or her 'focal point' or her fantasy trip to the Caribbean? Could she, rather, focus on her body—on the work it was doing, on the *pain itself*?"

So Dr. Hays began questioning those women who labored without noise or a lot of activity each time she worked with one. One said, "Well, I was just concentrating on my cervix. You know, letting it open up for my baby's head." The common thread running through all these labors was that the women were *with* the pain. They were going down inside themselves to the place where the pain was and allowing it.

One of Dr. Hays's patients gave her the following beautiful piece of birth imagery in answer to the question "Where do you go during your contractions?" She said, "Well, you know when you are in the ocean, in a heavy surf, if you stay on the surface you will get thrown about against the reefs and the rocks, and you get a lot of water in your nose and mouth and feel like you're drowning. But if you dive down and hold on to something and let the wave pass over you, you can come up in between and feel just fine. Well, that's what I did during labor. When the contractions came, I dived down and let them pass over me." Water imagery is very common when women describe normal birth.

During my own second labor, I realized that I had *allowed* the process quite differently than I had with my first. Labor is a true *process*—with its own rhythm and timing—and it is a process that is bigger than we are. For that reason, learning to go with it—to let it sweep us along—is something that we never forget. And it is great training for the give-and-take of parenting.

Birth and Female Sexuality

Upon leaving the hospital after Ann's birth (I left about six hours after she was born), it was wonderful to get into bed beside my husband, with our new little daughter sleeping in a cradle right beside my head. She was a gift that the two of us had created together. I felt like making love with my husband in that moment, which we did (avoiding actual intercourse, however).

Many women describe birth in natural settings as erotic. Ina May Gaskin, in her classic *Spiritual Midwifery*, writes that women need to be loved in labor, to be treated like Goddesses. Another provocative piece of writing I once read said that the birth of a baby is the completion of the act of intercourse, conception, gestation, and now delivery. With the birth of a baby, the circle is complete. This book suggested the birth take place between the mother and her mate, with her presenting this baby back to him. One woman told me that after her baby was born she said to her doctor, "If I'd known it was going to feel this good, I'd have planned for ten babies!"

Hospital surroundings, in which complete strangers wander in and out, are not very conducive to a woman being in touch with her deepest self. Nor do they support spontaneous acts of affection between the woman and her mate. Such acts make the staff very uncomfortable because they then become potential voyeurs. A husband holding his wife from behind with his hands under her breasts while she is squatting is a problem for some. Also, many hospital staff and patients are taught to be very concerned about keeping a woman's body covered at all times—despite the fact that in the middle of pushing out a baby, most women could not care less!

Bethany Hays writes, "As I began to reexplore my own births, I realized that I too had made an attempt to go inside to deal with the pain. My own births, however, were filled with great violence. I recently found the five-day diary I had written after the birth of my first child, a birth I have always spoken of with great pride in my accomplishment, the delivery of a nine-pound, six-ounce baby using Lamaze.

"The language I used in those days immediately after the birth, however, was that of physical abuse. 'Just get mad and push that baby out.' I remember thinking that the birth was a mixture of loss and accomplishment, of joy and trauma. I remember my mourning over the loss of my normal vagina and perineum after a fourth-degree episiotomy [an episiotomy that goes right into the rectal lining]. I remember being surprised at how little actual physical pain that had caused. I remember that every inch of my body felt like it had been attacked 'by a tire tool.'

"I remember wanting to be alone to find some way to reconcile these powerful, joyful, and at the same time threatening feelings. I remember knowing innately that this was related to my sexuality, to my erotic core. But it was many years before I realized that I had rejected my greatest innate ability to deal with the pain of my births: that very well of elemental energy that kept calling me."

Bethany Hays experienced labor as being split into two people: one who wanted to do Lamaze breathing and carry on a rational conversation with her birth attendants, and another who was drawing her into a "pit down inside" that terrified her. I, too, recall feeling split in two with my first birth. Part of me was fighting the pain, and part was reading the fetal monitor with the practiced eye of a physician who knows that despite wide variable decelerations (dips in the heart rate) on the monitor strip, the beat-to-beat variability (another measure of heart rate) was excellent. (Now I know that that monitor strip indicated that my baby was scared.)

Bethany told me that she realized that the Lamaze method of breathing had worked for her only up to a point. When the cervix was nearly dilated and it was time for the baby to traverse the pelvis, she was suddenly no longer able to do the ordered breathing patterns that, she thought then, had gotten her that far. When it was time to push, she recalls being in a place she could only identify as "somewhere I could not stay." At this point she said she wanted to get rid of the baby at all costs. (Women sometimes yell at this point, "Get it out of there!") For Bethany this included, during her first birth, demanding that forceps be used to accomplish the delivery. (But in her defense, she realized that being strapped to the delivery table flat on her back to deliver a nine-and-a-half-pound baby after one and a half hours of pushing was not ideal.)

In subsequent births she again found herself in that "terrible, unacceptable place" in which she used all her rational powers to "bypass that terrible transit through the pelvis." "Just get tough." "Get mad and get him out!" "Ignore the pain, just push through it." This resulted, she notes, in "considerable pain and trauma to myself." Both of us remember telling similar things to our patients repeatedly: "Just push through the pain—get him out. Get mad!" Labor and delivery staff are trained to do this, too.

Later in her career, Bethany met a woman who taught her—and me—the secret of the second stage of labor, which now seems obvious: Women don't want to push because we feel disconnected from that part of our bodies and because giving birth is a sexual experience, almost taboo with so many people looking on. Instead of pushing through the second stage of labor as though it were an athletic event, women would do well to let their uterus do the work, while allowing their vaginas to relax into the process.

During my residency training, I was accused of being Dr. Pain by the nurses because I didn't insist on a spinal anesthetic for every delivery. Even then, I knew that pushing the baby out took a relatively small amount of time, and I believed that it was far better for a woman to be alert for her new baby than to have the lower half of her body paralyzed from a spinal so that forceps had to be used to pull the baby out. I witnessed many women who had spinal anesthesia for routine deliveries fall asleep on the delivery table. These women were much less "present" to greet their babies than those who had birthed normally.

Back then, I didn't appreciate the fact that birth is part of the continuum of female sexuality and that by numbing the lower half of the body to feeling anything painful, we were also numbing the possibility for feeling anything ecstatic or sexual.

Though most people don't know this, the art of belly dancing originated for the purpose of getting in touch with birthing power. Grandmothers taught it to granddaughters and daughters. There's currently a resurgence of interest in belly dancing. And with it, our reclaiming of our essential female birthing power! There is also ample evidence that the first drummers were women. And the beat of the drum re-created the beat of the heart, which set up an optimal rhythm for women to bring forth life. (For more information, read the book *When the Drummers Were Women: A Spiritual History of Rhythm* by Layne Redmond [Three Rivers Press, 1997].)

Women's Stories

Rebecca's story: reclaiming birth power. The following story is related in the words of Bethany Hays, Rebecca's obstetrician.

"Rebecca was a second-time mother whose first labor had been long, but she did well with the help of her labor support person and a gentle, loving husband. Rebecca arrived at the hospital for her second birth already seven centimeters dilated and feeling great. She walked and talked with her team of supportive people, and she sipped fluids. She tolerated our medical intrusions into her birth with monitor, blood pressure cuff, and thermometer.

"After several hours, Rebecca was still only seven to eight centimeters dilated. She was puzzled and frustrated, wanting to 'get on with it.' We discussed her options, including rupture of the membranes, which might bring the baby's head down against the cervix. The cervix felt ready and soft enough to allow the passage of the head, waiting for some unknown work yet to be done.

"After considering the possible negative effects of it, she chose to rupture the membranes. This was done. Now the contractions got harder, but after some time, the exam showed that she was not quite fully dilated. The head was still high up in the pelvis. She showed some urge to push when squatting, but she was not pushing effectively. Her monitrice [professional labor support person] reminded me that during the first labor, she had also had difficulty pushing—requiring three hours in the second stage and pressure applied to the posterior vaginal wall to encourage her to push.

"Maybe that would help again, someone suggested. So as Rebecca squatted, I knelt on the floor, placed two fingers in her vagina, and pushed firmly on the posterior wall. Her response was an immediate and reflexive withdrawal. I realized that not only was I causing her pain, but I was triggering some much more serious emotional response. My own reaction was equally strong. 'No,' I thought, 'I will not participate in this abuse. This is sexual abuse of another woman's body, and I will not do it.'

" 'Rebecca,' I said, 'let's try something else.' Now, I have always been touched at the faith (often underserved) that patients place in me, and I knew that she trusted me. Whatever the new plan was, she would try it. The joke was that I had no plan. I was flying totally by the seat of my pants. I asked her to get comfortable, and she arranged herself semireclining on the bed, with her husband behind her and wrapped around her. 'Now,' I said, 'I just want you to relax and listen to my voice. First, go down inside yourself and find your baby where he is in your body. When you are with him, tell him he is okay, in case he is scared.'

"As we waited, a slow smile came over her face, and I knew that she was with her baby. The fetal monitor no longer disturbed her. It now showed sudden resolution of the small to moderate variable decelerations she'd been having with contractions. [Variable decelerations are heart rate patterns associated with compression of the umbilical cord, which can sometimes produce stress in the baby.]

" 'Now,' I said, 'I want you just to listen. Many of us women have not owned all the parts of our bodies. We have not allowed ourselves to feel our vaginas and our perineums. They have seemed separate and are not within our control. They have negative connotations: pornographic or dirty. In many ways these parts of our bodies are problematic for us. But the truth is that they are ours. They belong to us like our hands and our lips and our minds. This part of your body is yours, and you can reclaim it. Right now. Take it back as the sensual, enjoyable part of you that it really is. Since it is yours, you are totally in control. You can allow your baby to move through this part of you as fast or as slowly as you like. It does not have to hurt you, but you will feel very strong signals from this part of your body that you are not used to feeling. Allow those feelings and celebrate them as the return of a long-lost friend.'

"Now we were all watching. Rebecca was totally relaxed, lying in her husband's arms. The room was quiet except for the fetal monitor, which was quietly attesting to the continued well-being of the baby. I was wondering if I was deluding myself—pretty sure that everyone in the room must think I was nuts.

"Suddenly I realized that with each contraction, Rebecca's perineum was bulging—the head was coming down. It was working. Occasionally, Rebecca lost contact with her body, became frightened, and clutched her husband. Immediately when this happened, the baby's heart rate pattern showed prolonged variable decelerations with slow recovery. At these points, I would say, 'Talk to your baby again, Rebecca. He's scared. Remember, don't go faster than you want to. This is your body. All of it belongs to you.'

"Once again, Rebecca was quiet, and we saw the baby's head begin to crown [to appear, just before delivery]. Soon, with little or no pushing effort, the baby was born into his mother's loving arms."

After hearing this story, I realized that the second stage of my own second labor might have been different if I'd had a doctor like Bethany Hays. I also realized that I have been involved in the unwitting physical abuse of many laboring women by pushing down on their vagina to try to help them push, and by encouraging them, like a football coach, to "push him out." I wouldn't have done that if I had known what I now know.

Amanda's story: a home birth. Bethany also attended a birth in which one of her patients went further into herself than either of us had known it was possible to go. Amanda's first baby had been delivered by Bethany by cesarean section. "I thought we had done everything right," Bethany says. "She had been healthy, confident, and wanted a normal birth, including labor without anesthesia. She had labor support, family, and friends. Though it seemed perfect, the baby simply wouldn't come. We did everything I knew to do, which at that time was not a lot. I finally did a cesarean."

With her second pregnancy Amanda returned to Bethany's care and said, "I want to have a normal birth this time." Bethany agreed and told her that she thought that was entirely possible. The women who are most motivated to give birth normally are those who did not succeed in doing so with their first child but hadn't lost the desire to try. Amanda also did not want to have her second baby in the hospital, because she felt that the hospital environment had been part of the problem the first time. Instead, she would have it at home.

For years I've had a special place in my heart for those women who choose home birth. The reason for this is that these women trust themselves more than doctors and hospitals. Though they sometimes make mistakes, they have something to teach us. My sister had a home birth, and I wish I had had at least one child at home. Though I left the hospital right after both my children were born and neither one of them went to the nursery, I would still have liked the experience of waking up in labor and not having to get into the car and go someplace. Both times it felt like a very unnatural interruption of my process.

Though Amanda wanted Bethany there, Bethany does not do home births. Finally they reached a compromise. Bethany would be there only as a labor support person, and Amanda herself would hire the best midwife she could find. For an OB/GYN to do a home birth has been politically very unsafe. Many hospitals will not allow physicians who do home births to have hospital privileges, and most malpractice insurance companies won't insure such physicians despite statistics on their safety. But Amanda was determined to have Bethany present, and Bethany was interested in supporting her, as long as she wasn't responsible for being the caregiver.

Long discussions ensued, regarding risks, uterine rupture, fetal compromise, their likelihood, and what Bethany could and could not do if these problems happened at home. Ultimately, Amanda convinced Bethany that she herself was in charge of the safety of her baby and the integrity of her uterus, and that if she felt she could not do this job, she would let Bethany know and they would all go to the hospital.

The day of Amanda's delivery came. Her early labor was long and painful, but she didn't call anyone. When she finally invited her caregivers to join her, they found Amanda in the rocker. "I feel so great," she said in one breath. And with the next she said, "The pain was so bad this afternoon, I thought I would die." Bethany later told me, "I didn't know how to put those two statements together." As the birth neared, Amanda lay in her king-size bed on her side. "As we tried to keep up with her," Bethany told me, "she circled the bed. Her head remained in the center, and her feet made a full circuit around the bed twice, a maneuver that I had not seen before in the hospital. It was very primitive. Though it was not clear to me what it represented, I trusted her need to move in this way as part of her unique birth process.

"There was little talk. Amanda said nothing and made little noise. She pushed her baby out on hands and knees and then kneeled over her. She was somewhere else. We were all commenting on the baby, but she was not looking at her infant. Her body was in a pose of ecstasy. When spoken to, she did not respond. For a moment I was frightened that she might not come back from wherever she was. Then she looked down at her infant and slowly came back into her body—or was it back out of her body?"

Bethany took a picture of Amanda in that ecstatic state, and she showed it at a recent medical meeting in which we both lectured on women's health. From this and reading Vicki Noble's *Shakti Woman* and *Ina May's Guide to Childbirth* (Bantam, 2003), I learned that Amanda's experience of ecstasy is potentially available to all women at birth.[64] Since then, I have talked at length with some of my patients who have had home births. One recently told me that during her home birth she "left her body" and became an eagle flying high overhead. She experienced no pain. She had never told anyone about this. From that moment on, however, she trusted her body completely.

Women have learned collectively, though not necessarily consciously, to fear the birth experience, and every obstacle has been put in our collective paths to keep us from experiencing this power. But as Bethany says, "This kind of birth is possible in many environments. It requires a mother who trusts her body and is connected to all of its parts. She must love and want her baby. She must understand that birth is a sexual event and be comfortable with her sexuality. She must feel safe. She needs to know that the people around her accept her body and the sexual nature of what she is doing and are not embarrassed by it and will not interfere with the process. She needs to know that she can go down inside and come back safely. If she has never been there before, she needs the grounding love of family and friends who will, if needed, call her back."

Those women who have already had babies in standard ways should understand that they are not responsible for what they didn't know at the time. I was born drugged, as were all my brothers and sisters. Though we were breast-fed, we were still left in the hospital's nursery for hours while my mother woke up. This isn't the way she had wanted it, but she didn't know she had a choice.

Remember that *being responsible* simply means "being able to respond." No one is guaranteed a perfect birth. In fact, the concept of "a perfect birth" is part of the perfectionism of the addictive system. Sometimes a baby needs to be observed in the nursery right after birth. Sometimes an emergency cesarean is necessary. When this happens, it is not a failure on the woman's part. She is only one part of a complex and mysterious process. The baby herself (or himself) is also an active participant in the labor process. Each baby makes a unique contribution to her mother's pregnancy, labor, and delivery. We can always learn something from it and use the experience for personal growth. But whatever happens, parents should be involved as much as possible, at all stages of pregnancy, labor, and delivery. They need to understand that their input is very important to their baby's health.

Reclaiming Birth Power Collectively

Imagine what might happen if the majority of women emerged from their labor beds with a renewed sense of the strength and power of their bodies, and of their capacity for ecstasy through giving birth. When enough women realize that birth is a time of great opportunity to get in touch with their true power, and when they are willing to assume responsibility for this, we will reclaim the power of birth and help move technology where it belongs—in the service of birthing women, not as their master.

For many women, having a baby is their first experience of being connected with other women and with their vast creativity. It has the potential to transform the ways in which we think about ourselves. As one patient said to me, "I felt at one with every woman who ever gave birth. I felt powerful and in touch with something within me that I never knew was there. I took my place among the lineage of women as mothers."

13
Motherhood: Bonding with Your Baby

The process of becoming attached to a new baby begins long before the actual birth and continues long afterward. Still, every effort should be made to optimize the labor, birth, and postpartum environment because this is a particularly sensitive period that deeply imprints both mother and baby, setting the stage for their life together. During this time, the bodies of both mother and baby are flooded with prolactin, oxytocin, and beta-endorphin—neurochemicals that have been called "the molecules of belonging" because they help establish a deep sense of trust and belonging in a baby. Like Cupid's arrow, they help a new mother fall blissfully in love with her baby and also with those who have supported her during labor and birth. These neurochemicals also make the mother far more sensitive to her environment. That's why the events associated with birth have a very powerful effect on a mother's feelings about herself, her caregivers, and her new baby.

Our understanding of this biologically programmed sensitive period has come light-years in the last few decades. And voluminous research has been done on the biological effects of prolactin and how it engenders trust. (See chapter 8, "Reclaiming the Erotic.") In a nutshell, labor, birth, and the postpartum period—and all the experiences the mother and baby have during this time—set down the original wiring between the neurological system, the endocrine system, and the immune system—and this sets the stage for one's state of health for the rest of one's life.

When I was a medical student, a newborn baby was quickly wrapped in a sterile drape, shown to the mother only briefly, as though the baby's life depended on being somewhere else, and then whisked off to a "warmer" in the nursery, while the mother looked on with pleading eyes, aching to hold her creation. Early bonding studies reported that new mothers greeted their babies first by touching them gingerly with their fingertips, then finally holding them skin-to-skin, yet this response was nothing more than a cultural artifact, the *result* of immediate separation. During my residency, we began to place babies on their mothers' abdomens instead of putting them immediately into the warmer. If a mother holds her baby skin-to-skin with a blanket over both, the baby doesn't need a warmer; the mother is the warmer—which is as it should be. At a normal birth, the mother swoops her baby into her arms and holds her full frontal against her skin as soon as the child is born. She knows this baby is hers and needs to be welcomed and comforted immediately. It's also very helpful for the new baby to become colonized with her mother's bacteria by being held skin-to-skin. This helps establish healthy immunity.

The birth of a baby also has great significance for the baby's father. The more he is included, the better. Margaret Mead once said that the reason so many cultures banned fathers from births was that if they participated, they would be so hooked by the experience and the new baby that they would never be able to go out, steel themselves, and "do their thing" in quite the same way. I believe that the increased participation of men in childbirth—not as bosses or saviors, but as witnesses to the awe of the moment—holds great potential for balancing our world.

I never wanted my own babies to go to the hospital nursery, because I was aware of how different the atmosphere in the nursery was from what I wanted for them. They had just spent forty weeks listening to my heartbeat, bathed in warm fluid in a darkened space. In the hospital nursery, they would be isolated in small bassinets, alone, under fluorescent lights that were on twenty-four hours per day, cared for by a stranger. I knew that my entire physiology was set up by nature so that my baby and I could become "attached." The breast colostrum (first milk) contains antibodies optimally suited to protect the baby from germs, and the suckling of the child produces hormones that help the uterus contract. Babies are innately most interested in eye contact at a distance of about twelve inches, the distance between a mother's eyes and those of her nursing infant. Looking into my baby's eyes, having her look back at me, having her sleep close to me skin-to-skin—all of these events have been set up by nature as the "glue" that continues the mother-infant bond that begins in utero. I knew that these experiences were important for both of us.

Too many babies are taken to the nursery to "get cleaned up" after birth (to get rid of all that filthy vagina stuff!). The process of bathing can lower a baby's body temperature to the point that the nursery nurses won't let the baby out of the nursery again to be with the mother until the temperature is back up! I figured, why bathe the baby and make her cold? Why not just nurse her, keep her near me, and hang out together?

When I had my first baby, I went to the postpartum floor, but I kept Ann with me. When I got up to go to the bathroom, I took her with me. A nurse came in and yelled through the door, "Where is the baby?" I replied, "In here with me." She said, "You're going to have to learn to leave her sometime." I replied, "Not on the first day of her life!"

I was afraid of my vulnerability postpartum. Too many mothers were undermined by the nursing staff, and I didn't want to risk arguing with the nurses or their rules about when I could and couldn't hold my baby. I wanted my own mother to be able to hold her first female grandchild. In those days, the hospital rule was that only the immediate family could hold the baby, as though the hospital "owned" the child. (Though hospital rules have now changed, I had to fight with the nurse back then to let a baby's grandparents, even those who had driven for hours to see their new grandchild, actually hold her. Sometimes, depending on the nurse involved, I didn't get very far.)

Expecting a hospital stay to be restful was the stuff of mythology, I knew. My home was where I wanted to be, so I left the hospital on the day of delivery both times. The first few weeks of life are a crucial time of adjustment for both the baby and the parents. I wish now that I had spent even more time with my newborns. The first three months after a baby is born are known as the fourth trimester. During this time, the mother's body serves as a kind of "external" placenta for the baby. And the baby herself is considered an "external fetus" who still requires a great deal of contact with her mother's body for optimal regulation of her breathing, temperature, digestion, etc.

Dr. John Kennell is a pioneer in the field of neonatal (newborn) care.[1] *High-risk* refers to any baby who requires intensive surveillance at birth and in the first few days, weeks, or months of life. The majority of high-risk babies are born premature. Many premature babies' bodily systems aren't fully developed at birth and this causes them to have an increased risk of lung problems, developmental and feeding problems, and infection. Dr. Kennell and another colleague, Dr. Marshall Klaus, later turned their attention to preventing the conditions that lead to babies entering the high-risk nursery in the first place. Back in the 1960s and '70s, they found that there was an unusually high percentage of battering by the mothers of babies who were born prematurely or who were otherwise sick and whose care was taken over by the nursery staff with the mothers not included.

Their research, first on mother-infant bonding and then on parent-infant bonding (adding the father), showed that mothers whose babies stay with them from birth onward bond better and are more attentive to their babies' needs than are those whose babies are whisked away to the nursery to be cared for by "experts."[2] (This is especially true in those mothers who have fewer other resources available to them because of poverty, abuse, single parenthood, etc.) These babies are also healthier and more intelligent overall, months and even years later. (The human psyche and soul are very resilient, however. Separation doesn't necessarily cause irreversible damage, but it should be avoided unless absolutely necessary.)

Klaus and Kennell's research has shown what should be common sense to everyone—that human touch and concern have a measurable impact on a baby's health. One study on infant touching—known as "tactile stimulation"—indicated that a group of premature infants who were stroked regularly gained weight much faster than those who weren't touched—even when both groups were fed the same diet! And in a study at the University of Miami the touched babies were discharged from the hospital earlier—a cost savings of thousands of dollars per baby![3] Touch should be thought of as a lifelong nutrient. After all, the skin is derived from the same embryonic layer as the brain and central nervous system. When we stroke a baby's skin (or have our own stroked), it lowers stress hormones, increases the hormones of belonging, lowers blood pressure, and enhances health on all levels. An impressive body of research continues to show these benefits for both mother and baby. (For more information, see the research of Tiffany Field, Ph.D., at the website of the Touch Research Institute at the University of Miami School of Medicine; www.miami.edu/touch-research.)

Touching is so simple, so instinctive. Pregnant mothers automatically stroke their bellies, sending love and energy to the unborn and practicing for when the baby is born. How could we ever have devised a system in which babies were separated from their parents' love and touching in the first minutes of life and sent alone to nurseries run by strangers?[4] No mammal leaves its children unattended and unsuckled the way humans do. A mother bear is at her most dangerous when she's protecting her cubs. She won't let anyone or anything come near them. Many women could use a little more bear energy.

One of the primary ways a baby learns trust and love is through touch. James Prescott, Ph.D., who created and directed the Developmental Behavioral Biology Program at the National Institutes of Health's division of Child Health and Human Development, has done comparative studies of child development in different cultures. His research has found that societies that physically hold and love their children and are not sexually repressive are peaceful. But those societies (like ours) that deprive infants, children, and adolescents of our primal need for touch are far more violent. In fact, children who are touch-deprived often develop a disorder in which they are unable to deal effectively with stress hormone surges, which are a precursor to lashing out in violence. (For more information, visit www.violence.de.) Nature has designed labor, birth, and the postpartum period as a crucial time to maximize touch. This imprints well-being.

Culturally, we've all participated in subtle and not-so-subtle abuse of our vulnerable newborns in the name of science, partly out of fear and doubting of our own natural instincts. Putting burning silver nitrate or erythromycin ointment into infants' eyes to prevent gonococcal infection is one example. Why do this to all babies, even those whose mothers don't have gonorrhea or chlamydia? I signed a waiver to forgo putting anything in my baby's eyes. I knew I didn't have gonorrhea or chlamydia, and I couldn't see why my baby should have to undergo treatment of something I didn't have. The waiver absolved the hospital from all responsibility for my choice, which is as it should be.

Clamping the cord immediately after birth is another example of an overly stressful act against our newborns, which can even be dangerous because it can lead to too little blood volume in the baby—and decreased tissue oxygenation. Nature designed birth so that the baby will receive backup oxygenated blood from her mother via the still-pulsating umbilical cord during the time when her lungs and heart are undergoing the profound changes necessary to switch from a water to an air environment. Once the baby is breathing well on her own and her circulation has been established, the umbilical cord vessels naturally close down on their own. And when the cord is allowed to pulsate until it stops, it also helps normalize blood volume in the baby, making sure that the baby's circulation is adequate. No premature cord clamping is necessary in the vast majority of cases. When babies are sick or premature, the extra-oxygenated blood that they can get from a pulsing umbilical cord helps resuscitate them optimally and can make the difference between life and death. (Far too many premature babies who undergo premature cord clamping end up with hypovolemia, not enough blood volume, and then need transfusions once they get to the intensive care nursery.) Clamping the cord immediately after the baby's birth forces the baby to make the switch over to air more quickly than is necessary. Many mothers and doctors feel that this gives the baby a feeling of panic—that there is not enough air. This practice is like shouting a command, "Okay, breathe now—or else!"

After most normal births, the baby can be placed on the mother's abdomen and the cord can be allowed to gradually stop pulsating on its own. Babies often rest very peacefully while this is going on. They breathe gently and don't cry. In fact, mothers and fathers sometimes worry that something is wrong when their babies are calm at birth. They've learned from the culture that a screaming, terrified newborn is *normal*. (Remember, that which is normal in this culture is not always that which is healthy.) A generation ago, a limp, unresponsive baby was considered "normal." A nurse friend of Bethany Hays, M.D., recalled that at the first Lamaze birth she ever saw, she thought there was something wrong because the baby didn't cry immediately! Unfortunately, the collective emergency mindset that permeates high-tech birth makes premature cord clamping the norm, not the exception. Conventional OB/GYN training argues that delayed cord clamping will increase a baby's risk of hyperbilirubinemia (jaundice). But OB/GYNs have no problem using Pitocin for labor induction or augmentation and/or epidural anesthesia—both of which have been conclusively linked with nonphysiologic neonatal jaundice. In fact, any drug given to a mother or baby is likely to compete with bilirubin sites on blood protein, thus causing more free bilirubin, which contributes to jaundice. Though one could argue about the advantages versus disadvantages of delayed cord clamping in a sick newborn, in a healthy full-term infant, there are untold advantages to delaying cord clamping until after the placenta has been delivered (or the blood vessels have stopped pulsating).[5]

POSTPARTUM: THE FOURTH TRIMESTER

The first three months postpartum are when most women go through enormous physical, emotional, and psychological changes that aren't very well appreciated in this culture. Much of the controversy about sending mother and baby home from the hospital too soon has to do with the fact that for many women, their care and rest end the minute they get home. Though the hospital is often far from an ideal place to rest after your baby is born, it sure beats going home to a sink full of dirty dishes and a load of dirty laundry.

Your body also goes through some unexpected changes. For instance, it is normal to sweat a great deal and have hot flashes during this time—it's part of the readjustment process following the profound adaptations of pregnancy. Also, some women notice that some of their hair falls out from hormonal changes (it grows back). It is also normal to bleed for up to four to six weeks as the placental site heals over in the uterus. The other really common problem many women face is pain during intercourse, especially if they've had an episiotomy. Though many doctors tell women it's okay to have sex after their six-week checkup, this may be far too soon for comfort. Aside from the episiotomy, the hormonal changes necessary for breast-feeding can result in vaginal dryness. This doesn't mean (as some women fear) that you don't love your mate anymore. It just means that you might need vaginal lubricant until postpartum hormonal shifts are completed. You also may find that you're so exhausted from being up at night with the baby that sex is the last thing on your mind.

On the other hand, a fascinating study by Marilyn Moran on do-it-yourself home birthers found that women who gave birth in an environment in which they were totally supported by their husbands and in which they felt safe being sexual, actually experienced a marked increase in their sexual activity postpartum. I find this highly plausible and deeply intriguing. It flies in the face of everything we've been taught about sexuality and birth—probably because what we've been taught (and therefore what we experience) has been deeply tainted by our cultural Madonna/whore split in which motherhood and sexuality are split off from each other. Also, modern high-tech birth environments do not encourage feelings of sexuality during birth! (A full discussion of this topic can be found in *Mother-Daughter Wisdom*, pages 99–100.)

If I were running the country, I'd make sure that every postpartum woman had full-time help for cooking and cleaning for at least two months after the baby was born and that she had time for a nap or two every single day. In some traditional cultures, women with newborn babies are often cared for by their midwives, mothers, or other women for two to three months after the birth of the baby. During this time, their only duties are to nurse, rest, and recover so that they can be fully present for their new babies.

Postpartum Depression

Maternal depression is frequently underdiagnosed. (About 10 to 15 percent of women are clinically depressed during pregnancy itself.)[6] Fully 80 percent of women experience the baby blues for up to two weeks after delivery. Approximately 10 to 15 percent of women will go on to experience some form of mood disorder postpartum, ranging from major depression to anxiety disorders such as panic attack. If a woman has a history of depression, she is at significant risk postpartum. Many women who suffer one postpartum depression will experience the same thing after each birth.[7] True psychosis occurs in only about 1 in 1,000 births, and is characterized as being out of touch with reality, hallucinating, and hearing voices. One of my patients went through this process with minimal medication even though she had to be hospitalized for a time. She said that during that time, she healed a great deal of her past with her mother, father, and, as she put it, "my ancestors before me. It was as though I had to go into this darkness— that was somehow generations deep—so that I could be present with my baby." Her inner knowing told her that her postpartum reaction was important and loaded with information and energy. By staying with the process and not reducing it to a "chemical imbalance," she was able to heal fully—and, ultimately, so was her family.

Women with any history of depression or psychosis should be sure they discuss this with their health care provider before the baby is born, since the right treatment can prevent the problem from becoming severe. Antidepressant medication has been shown to be helpful in some cases. Women with moderate to severe PMS may be at increased risk for postpartum depression, especially those who feel their best during pregnancy and who respond well to natural progesterone. In this group of women, taking progesterone as soon after delivery as possible is often very helpful.[8] Estrogen has also been used successfully.[9]

Women who take adequate amounts of omega-3 fats also decrease the risk of postpartum depression. In fact, omega-3 fats can be used to treat postpartum depression (1,000 to 5,000 mg per day). It's also essential that women keep their blood sugar normal. (Low blood sugar exacerbates depression and it's very common!) The best way to do this is to be sure to start each day with a breakfast that contains healthy protein, and low-glycemic-index carbohydrates. (See chapter 17, "Nourishing Ourselves with Food.") Good choices would be eggs and whole-grain toast or oatmeal with protein powder in it. There are also a wide variety of bars and shakes available for those who don't have the time to cook. A good multivitamin-mineral is also essential to help the body manufacture the neurochemicals involved in mood balance, e.g., serotonin, dopamine, and endorphin. Adequate sleep also goes a very long way toward helping maintain mood. (Please see the Program for Creating Optimal Pregnancy—all of it applies to the postpartum period!)

The bottom line is to reestablish the individual hormonal balance that supports emotional stability. (See Resources.)

Postpartum depression is made worse by any sense of failure or loss of a hoped-for experience. A woman from Europe wrote me the following:

"I'm the mother of a daughter who is now one and a half years old who was born by cesarean section. This cut changed my relationship with my body a lot. Even now, sixteen months later, I still do have the feeling of being wounded, not so much in the physical body, but in the energetic one. So much physical and emotional pain is connected with such an operation. I know quite a few women who've had the same experience, and there's even a support group in town."

Labor that doesn't turn out the way you planned can be very traumatic to the mind and body, and women can be left with a type of post-traumatic stress disorder (PTSD). A great deal of unfinished business may live in our bodies concerning our labors and deliveries if we weren't fully supported. This is because, on some level, we know that many of these surgeries or procedures may not have been necessary if our circumstances, our thoughts and emotions, and our environment in labor had been different. In these cases, I recommend approaches that help clear the energy body and reprogram the subconscious mind. Examples include hypnosis, EMDR (Eye Movement Desensitization and Reprocessing; for more information see the EMDR Institute's website at www.emdr.com), meditation tapes, and CDs using binaural beat technologies (especially Hemi-Sync products from the Monroe Institute; see www.monroeinstitute.org for more information), and Psych-K. Psych-K is a process developed by psychotherapist Robert Williams using whole-brain integration techniques to communicate with your subconscious mind to change those subconscious beliefs that perpetuate sabotaging habits and behaviors. (For more information on Psych-K, visit the Psych-K Centre's website at www.psych-k.com.) This type of therapy or guided imagery is very helpful for those with any aspect of post-traumatic stress disorder. (Visit www.healthjourneys.com for a great CD for PTSD.)

Significant unfinished business with a woman's own mother at the time she gives birth can also increase the risk of postpartum depression.

Sharon had her first baby at the age of twenty-nine. About one week postpartum, she became severely depressed and was considering giving up breast-feeding. I helped her stick with it, which enhanced her self-esteem a great deal. She sought help with a psychiatrist for about six months and eventually pulled out of her depression. She later told me that she felt that the depression was directly related to the fact that her mother, an active alcoholic, simply couldn't be present for her during this critical phase of her life. She said, "She wasn't present for me when I was born because of her drinking, and she wasn't present for the birth of my son for the same reason. Nevertheless, something deep within me really wanted her there, and so I invited her to come and help me out after the baby was born. But she wasn't reliable, never could get it together to help me with anything, and ultimately, I ended up mothering her as well as my new baby. It's so painful to have to give up the fantasy that somehow you will one day find the mother you never had."

A woman can have a similar reaction if her relationship with her father is unsatisfactory. What it boils down to is this: When a woman gives birth, the process releases enormous energy for renewal and healing. Something deep within her longs to connect with and heal her own family. If her relationship with them is lacking in some way, this healing feeling will be heightened. The contrast between what could be and what actually is can add to a sense of loss or grief that contributes to depression.

Regardless of your circumstances, every woman needs to realize that having a baby is the real "change of life" and that she may not be fully prepared for this stressful time, especially if she lacks support. In my experience, most women don't have nearly the support that they need during the postpartum time. Many are sleep-deprived and exhausted. I remember that after my first child was born, I left the house to go get groceries when she was about four days old. I closed the front door and walked out onto the porch. Then I remembered, "Oh, God, I can't just leave. I have a baby." In a moment of panic, I realized that I had altered my life forever and that there was no going back. We were preparing to move at the time, and each day my husband would come home from work and ask me how much I had gotten done. I told him that it was all I could do just to keep the baby fed, get some rest myself, and prepare meals. I was too exhausted and stressed out to do anything else. On top of that, I couldn't seem to get motivated to go into overdrive, as I'd done so effectively for so long in my medical training. But I didn't understand this, and neither did my husband, so my "fourth trimester" was not a healing time, to say the least.

How to Elicit a Child's Natural Calming Reflex

Pediatrician Harvey Karp, M.D., author of *The Happiest Baby on the Block* (Bantam Books, 2002), shares several very helpful suggestions in his book that parents can use to help fussy babies calm themselves and get to sleep. (For more about Dr. Karp's ideas, or to order his videos and DVDs—which brilliantly show how to elicit the calming reflex quickly using actual crying babies—visit his website at www.thehappiestbaby.com.) His advice includes:

~ Using a white-noise machine or a *shhh*-ing sound. Either a white-noise CD or a white-noise machine will work well, as does shushing the baby yourself (as loud as she is crying, and right near her face). This re-creates the noise level in the womb—which is anything but silent!—and makes the baby feel more secure.

~ Rocking your baby or putting her in a wind-up or motorized infant swing.

~ Swaddling, or wrapping your baby tightly in a receiving blanket. The feeling of being tightly held re-creates the security of the womb.

~ Holding your baby on her side or on her stomach. These positions mimic the baby's position in the womb, making her feel more secure. The classic fetal position—tucking the baby's head down a bit, touching her on her stomach, and then laying her on her side—activates position sensors in the baby's head that trigger a natural calming reflex. (But never put a baby to sleep on her side or stomach, which can increase the risk of sudden infant death syndrome, or SIDS.)

~ Allowing your baby to suck (either by nursing her or giving her a pacifier).

CIRCUMCISION

Circumcision of baby boys is another example of a painful procedure that is unnecessary. (See also chapter 8, "Reclaiming the Erotic.") In fact, I've done hundreds of circumcisions—and I am incapable of doing one ever again. Though I often used a local anesthetic, even inserting the needle for this caused the baby unnecessary pain and didn't always work very well. Increasingly, doctors and parents alike are appreciating the fact that babies are born with a nervous system that is fully capable of feeling pain and that circumcision without anesthesia is barbaric.

In the past when I did the procedure, I would ask mothers to come into the nursery to comfort their babies while they were being circumcised, but they wouldn't do it. They couldn't stand the idea. I always made sure I personally took the newly circumcised baby to his mother as soon as I was finished—so that she could comfort her child. I didn't want him wounded and then left alone in the nursery. There is no medical justification for routinely circumcising newborns. Dr. George Denniston sums up the circumcision issue very nicely: "To me the idea of performing 100,000 mutilating procedures on newborns to possibly prevent penile cancer in one elderly man is absurd."[10]

The discussion of circumcision is a perfect example of the strength and influence of first-chakra tribal programming on our thought and emotional responses. This programming is so ingrained that many people cannot even discuss the subject of circumcision without guilt, denial, or other strong emotions. I know that even addressing the subject of the baby boy's bodily integrity, choices, and pain (if the procedure is done without anesthetic) can cause a "kill the messenger" reaction. But first-chakra programming can be successfully questioned and worked through, if desired. Many Jewish couples have rethought the entire circumcision issue and have decided not to have it done to their sons.

Circumcision is known to cause sleep disturbances for at least three days.[11] It also has profound implications for male sexuality. (See chapter 8, "Reclaiming the Erotic.") In fact, it's a form of sexual abuse. We certainly feel that way about female clitoridectomy, circumcision, and infibulation, but we justify male infant circumcision by pretending that the babies don't feel it because they're too young and it will have no consequences when they are older. I was taught that babies couldn't feel when they were born and therefore wouldn't feel their circumcision. Why was it, then, that when I strapped their little arms and legs down on the board (called a "circumstraint"), they were often perfectly calm; then when I started cutting their foreskin, they screamed loudly, with cries that broke my heart? For years, in some hospitals, surgery on infants has been carried out without anesthesia because of this misconception! Women who are going through memories of abuse in childhood know how deeply and painfully early experiences leave their marks in the body.

FORMULA VERSUS BREAST MILK

Artificial infant feeding is another area that requires rethinking. In the 1940s, infant feeding became very "scientific." Mothers sterilized nipples, bottles, and everything else, and the medical profession as a group systematically undermined breast-feeding as inferior. Rubber and glass took the place of a warm human breast. Feedings were timed. Even if a child showed a need for frequent feedings, the mother was warned not to feed her before four hours had passed. This information was based on a very early study of dead babies (who had been sick enough to die!) that found that at one, two, and three hours there was still food in the stomach, but that four hours after a feeding the stomach was empty. Like routine episiotomy, the four-hour feeding schedule was accepted into the culture and after a while simply became standard practice. The needs of the individual child were sacrificed on the altar of efficiency and "science"—with all its measuring and weighing. Can you imagine the pain of an infant who cries out to be held or fed, and yet the mother does not do so because the "experts" have told her to ignore all her instincts so she won't "spoil" the baby? (Babies were often weighed before and after a feeding to make sure they "got enough"—a practice that does *not* yield reliable data.)

Even now, women ask their doctors, "How will I know if I have enough milk?" Here's how you know: if the baby is growing, happy, and healthy, she is getting enough! Since women's trust in themselves has been systematically undermined in every area of their lives for centuries, how could we be expected to trust our bodies' ability to feed our babies? (Thank goodness that over the years a few did!) I don't for a minute expect that every woman will want to nurse her babies. For some, it's too anxiety-provoking, while for others bottle-feeding is the only way they can get child care from their husband, because he will be able to help with the feeding. We all have to start from where we are, but we should start from knowledge—not ignorance. The late James Grant, former executive director of UNICEF, stated the case for breast-feeding very succinctly when he said, "Study after study now shows, for example, that babies who are not breast-fed have higher diabetes, respiratory illnesses, bacterial and viral infections, diarrhoeal diseases, otitis media, allergies, obesity, and developmental delays. Women who do not breast-feed demonstrate a higher risk for breast and ovarian cancers."[12]

Nature set it up so that when a baby is put to the breast right after delivery, the suckling action causes the hormones oxytocin and prolactin to be secreted by the mother's pituitary gland. Prolactin induces mothering behavior as well as milk production. These hormones set the stage for adequate milk supply. Mothers who nurse right after delivery also have fewer problems. These hormones help contract the mother's uterus, for example, which helps the placenta separate naturally and thus decreases blood loss. In addition, breast milk is different from cow's milk or formula, and it is unique in that its composition changes over time *depending on the needs of the baby.*

Children who have been breast-fed have one-third fewer hospitalizations than those who are bottle-fed, and they have many fewer allergies. Babies who are breast-fed have a more normal dental arch and palate than those who are bottle-fed. One meticulous study even showed that premature babies fed breast milk had higher intelligence quotients, which is because of breast milk's beneficial effects on neural development.[13] (This study was unusual in that the babies were fed either formula or breast milk by tube, in order to control for the known beneficial effects associated with actually holding a baby close to the mother's body during breast-feeding.) It is a well-known fact that the composition of human breast milk is superior to that found in any formula, including its balance of the essential fatty acids so necessary for brain development. Thankfully, baby formula is now being manufactured with both DHA (docosahexaenoic acid) and AA (arachidonic acid). (Examples include Enfamil Lipil, Nestlé Good Start Supreme, Similac Advance, Bright Beginnings, and Parent's Choice.) Both of these fats are crucial for optimal brain, heart, and immune system development. Hydrolyzed baby formulas (such as Enfamil Nutramigen Lipil, Enfamil Pregestamil, and Similac Alimentum) are also now available that contain "comfort proteins" that are easier for babies to digest.

Most women have to go back to work when their babies are six weeks old, making it much more difficult to nurse in an unrestricted way. By *unrestricted,* I mean breast-feeding in which the mother doesn't time her feedings but simply responds to the child's needs instinctively. Women who nurse instinctively are usually unable to remember when they last fed the baby. Mothers have often told me that they did not intend to nurse precisely because they had to go back to work in six weeks. But they could nurse for just that first six weeks—or even for the first few days so that the baby could get the colostrum, to give the baby's health a head start that no artificial formula could provide. We only kid ourselves when we think that baby formula can do as good a job as nature. No amount of scientific experimentation can come up with food that is more specifically made for a baby than its mother's milk.

I expressed my breast milk into bottles and froze it so that if I was going to be away, someone else could feed my children with my milk in a bottle. Both children took both the breast and the bottle, so I had a win-win situation. (So-called nipple confusion resulting from both breast- and bottle-feeding is not that common!) Breast-feeding is also more convenient than carrying around a bunch of bottles, particularly while traveling. I nursed discreetly in restaurants, medical meetings, movies, and theaters. Usually no one noticed. Some, like Bernie Siegel, M.D., congratulated me and thought it was wonderful. (Some babies are really loud nursers and sound like little piglets, however, so you have to adapt to their behavior and be considerate.)

Ashley Montagu has said, "We learn to be human at our mother's breast." Breast-feeding is one of the most natural, nurturing things that a woman can do for herself and her baby. Yet we live in a culture in which it's perfectly acceptable to walk down the beach in a string bikini but it is not always acceptable to breast-feed an infant in a public place. That is seen as "obscene." Mothers who nurse toddlers are judged as being somehow "unnatural," fostering unnecessary dependence of the child, though it's been shown that people who feel the most secure in later life are those who had very healthy physical and emotional bonds with their mother in childhood. The newest research on boys shows how important a solid bond with their mothers is—a bond that we shouldn't be overly quick to sever! Children who feel most secure in their childhoods often are willing to take the most risks later in life. Only in a dominator culture would we get the idea that it "spoils" children to pick them up when they cry and to comfort them when they need it. (An aside: why should adults get to sleep with someone, while children have to sleep alone?)

Our culture's priorities are completely reversed from what they should be, especially at a time when it has become so hard for mothers to nurture their children adequately and still make a living. I changed my priorities after my own personal wounding with the breast abscess. On the third day after Kate's birth, I noticed that milk didn't seem to be coming out of my right nipple. Then the full impact of the damage I had done to myself two years earlier hit me fully. I wanted to sob. I remember sitting on my bed, looking down at my beautiful new baby girl, and thinking, "Here you are, and I can't even feed you properly because I screwed up my body two years ago trying to prove I was a man." I *was* able to nurse, but I couldn't maintain an adequate milk supply most of the time and had to supplement with formula, especially whenever I was away from home long enough to miss a feeding.

I came face-to-face with the fact that I had done irrevocable damage to myself. I'd been taught it was normal to feel the "baby blues" on about the third day after a baby was born, but my own depression was exacerbated by the knowledge that I wouldn't be able to nurse Kate completely normally. In fact, on her second day of life I had to supplement her diet with formula. I knew that her stools would immediately start to smell bad. The stools of a breast-fed baby smell like buttermilk because of the bacterial balance. Changing a diaper is a completely different experience with a breast-fed baby. But once you add other food sources, the bacteria change and the smell becomes putrid!

Even though the medical community now strongly endorses breast-feeding, the culture discourages it with the declaration that nursing "ruins" women's breasts. Some women who've nursed a couple of children do notice that their breasts don't look the same. For a while, they can be quite flaccid and can take several years after pregnancy and nursing to regain their shape. This usually reverses over time, but that flat appearance, even when it is only temporary, is not what our culture deems attractive.[14] This was illustrated to me once when a friend who had nursed several children told me the following story. She was undressing one night when her four-year-old son walked in. He looked at her chest, and looked up at her, and said, "Mom, what happened to your breasts? They died!" Rapid weight loss caused by inadequate food intake while nursing or prolonged nursing with adequate food intake can deplete the fat stores in the breasts and exacerbate this effect. Rapid weight loss also decreases milk supply.

The experience of producing milk, nursing a baby, and feeling the milk "let down" in response to the baby's cries, or even in response to a mother's own thoughts about the baby, is an experience that connects women everywhere. The midwife who delivered Kate used to tell me that she felt her own let-down reflex many times when she heard a baby cry or was aware of a child in need—even after her kids were in college. I, too, can still feel that tingling sensation in my breasts occasionally, especially when I'm feeling a great deal of compassion or appreciation for something or someone. It's my body's way of telling me that I have some love to give to a person or situation. Many women experience this. Our breasts, through this feeling, are reflecting the truth of the concept of "the milk of human kindness." (It has also been demonstrated that levels of the hormone prolactin—which is necessary to produce milk—increase when one is feeling this compassion, love, or appreciation.)

When we trust the makers of baby formula more than we do our own ability to nourish our babies, we lose a chance to claim an aspect of our power as women. Thinking that baby formula is as good as breast milk is believing that forty years of technology is superior to three million years of nature's evolution. Countless women have regained trust in their bodies through nursing their children, even if they weren't sure at first that they could do it. It is an act of female power, and I think of it as feminism in its purest form. One of my friends recently said, "Breast-feeding my son gave me more confidence in myself as a woman than anything I'd ever done before. I felt so powerful."

Newborns who are treated gently are very beautiful. I've seen in their eyes very wise old souls in tiny bodies fresh from God. I heard the following true story at my office. After one couple had their second son, their four-year-old kept wanting time alone with the baby. They were a bit reluctant, feeling that sibling rivalry might be a factor. But the four-year-old kept insisting. Finally, they let him have some time alone with the baby. Listening quietly at the door, they heard him ask the baby, "Please tell me what God is like. I'm starting to forget."

MOTHERING IN A DOMINATOR CULTURE: THE HARDEST JOB IN THE WORLD

The only thing that seems eternal and natural in motherhood is ambivalence.

—Jane Lazare

Some women say that the most fulfilling time of their mothering was when their babies were small. Others find it exhausting. For me, having young children was—bar none—the most taxing part of my life, a time that I wouldn't care to repeat again unless I had two beloved nannies, sisters, or friends living with me full-time to help with child care. (I might feel differently about this had my circumstances been different.)

The author Lynn Andrews once wrote that there are two kinds of mothers: Earth Mothers and Creative Rainbow Mothers. Earth Mothers nurture their children and feed them—and they thrive on this. Our society rewards this kind of woman as the "good mother."

Creative Rainbow Mothers, on the other hand, inspire their children without necessarily having meals on the table on time. I know that, beyond a doubt, I'm a Creative Rainbow Mother. I once read the cookbook *Laurel's Kitchen* and fantasized about how wonderful it would be to bake bread daily, relish being what Laurel calls the "Keeper of the

Keys," and create that ever-important nurturing home space. But this is not who I am—and to have tried to be something I wasn't would ultimately have done my children and me a great disservice. I love to be alone. I love to read. I love quiet and music and writing. My soul is fed by long hours of unbroken creative time. Young children require a much different type of energy—a type of energy I don't have in abundance.

When my children were little, I became aware of how difficult it is for women to do *anything* for themselves with little children around. Children get and keep our attention through any means possible. They are phenomenal little energy suckers. (I don't blame them for this—it's normal. They're developing healthy egos when they are young. Our culture, however, expects *mothers* alone to meet all their children's attention needs.) This is a setup.

Roughly one-third of all children in this country—nineteen million—live apart from their fathers. "Among the children of divorce," writes Ellen Goodman, "half have never visited their father's home. In a typical year, 40 percent of them don't see their father. One out of five haven't seen their father in five years...it is no wonder that the search for a man missing in the action of parenthood is such a recurrent theme in our culture and conversation these days."[15]

Sometimes a woman with young children needs free time, space, and sleep. But for many, there's no one to take over the burden of raising a child. I once said to Anne Wilson Schaef that I thought the optimal adult-child ratio was three adults to one child. "I think your workaholism is showing," she replied. Then she went on to tell me about an aboriginal culture of Australia where she had recently visited with the tribal elders. In aboriginal societies, all of the mother's sisters—the child's aunts—are considered the child's mothers. All the father's brothers—the uncles—are considered the fathers. If you ask an aboriginal child who her mother is, she will point not only to her biological mother but to all her aunts as well. Same with the father. If her biological mother feels the need to go "walkabout"—a spiritual initiation—she knows that the child always has a place in the group and is not dependent solely on her, as children so often are in our patriarchal society.

Can you even begin to imagine what life would be like for women if they didn't have the crushing responsibility to provide most of the children's emotional and physical nurturing? What would it be like if we *knew* that our society would care for our child if we had to work late at the office one night? What if our family life were not separate from our work life? What would it be like if a woman could still pursue art, music, computers, or whatever she wished, even if she had just had a baby? What if we lived in a society in which a woman didn't have to choose *between* her needs, those of her job, and those of her family? Dream on that for a while.

No one, male or female, should have to be a prisoner in their own home caring for young children for hours each day without meeting their own adult needs for rest, conversation, time alone, and creative pursuits. I remember that the best time I ever had with my children when they were little (three months and two years) was when I went to visit my mother while my sister and her children were visiting. My sister was also nursing a baby at the time, so when I wanted to go out for a while, she simply nursed Kate for me, as women have been doing for centuries. (Kate looked up at her, wide-eyed, the first time, as if to say, "Who is this?" Then she settled right down to her meal.) Our children played together happily, and I was able to enjoy the company of adults *at the same time* that I was enjoying my children. This was my only experience of what a loving tribe must have felt like. On a recent trip to Italy, it was clear that everyone in the village cared for the children— not just their mothers.

One widely held misperception about raising children has always upset me. That is the myth that prepubescent and pubescent boys are *inherently* easier to raise than girls, and even many feminists subscribe to this belief. I'm told by many people, "You just wait—you'll see how difficult girls are when they get to be eleven or so." Well, I've now had two eleven-year-old girls. I've supported them, in every way that I can, to be strong, even opinionated if necessary, and to be powerful. I didn't want them to "dumbify" themselves when they became teenagers. They were *not* difficult then, and they are not difficult now. (In fact, my thirteen-year-old nephew was much moodier on a regular basis than either of my daughters.) That boys are easier to raise than girls might well be the experience of many. But this difference is cultural, a consequence of the differences between the way boys and girls are treated and reared. In her book *Fire with Fire* (Random House, 1993), Naomi Wolf makes a strong case for the fact that all girls are born with a strong will to power that gets turned inward by what she calls "the dragons of niceness." This innate desire to excel and win, when thwarted, gets turned against a young girl. And girls often turn on each other. But this needn't be the case. (See my book *Mother-Daughter Wisdom* for a full discussion of this.)

It makes sense to me that girls would get moody around the age of twelve or so. They can see what's coming. If girls are socialized to be passive and self-sacrificing, their powerful spirits don't like it! (If someone was actively trying to do that to me, I'd be *very* tough to live with.) Instead of attributing this moodiness to the inherent hormonal inferiority of the female, we should be encouraging girls to speak their minds, not to turn their gifts and talents inward. If a teenage girl is taken seriously and encouraged to follow her dreams, she will be no harder to raise than a boy. Young women need to be cherished, honored, encouraged, and praised for their gifts. Otherwise, the world won't benefit from these gifts, and the cycle of oppression will continue.

Each of us mothers must also learn to mother ourselves, or else we can't possibly be good mothers to our children. Self-sacrifice is not a healthy path to motherhood, even though we've been taught to do this for years and have often witnessed the martyrdom of our own mothers. Mothering ourselves takes a great deal of courage, and I encourage you to try it for your health's sake.

The following meditation on mothering well was sent to me by Nancy McBrine Sheehan.[16]

MOTHERING MYSELF

In a society preoccupied with how best to raise a child
I'm finding a need to mesh what's best for my children with what's
*   necessary for a well balanced mother.*
I'm recognizing that ceaseless giving translates into giving yourself
*   away.*
And, when you give yourself away, you're not a healthy mother and
*   you're not a healthy self.*
So, now I'm learning to be a woman first and a mother second.
I'm learning to just experience my own emotions without robbing my
*   children of their individual dignity by feeling their emotions too.*
I'm learning that a healthy child will have his own set of emotions
*   and characteristics that are his alone.*
And, very different from mine.
I'm learning the importance of honest exchanges of feelings because
*   pretenses don't fool children,*
They know their mother better than she knows herself.
I'm learning that no one overcomes her past unless she confronts it.
Otherwise, her children will absorb exactly what she's attempting to
*   overcome.*
I'm learning that words of wisdom fall on deaf ears if my actions
*   contradict my deeds.*
Children tend to be better impersonators than listeners.
I'm learning that life is meant to be filled with as much sadness and
*   pain as happiness and pleasure.*

*And allowing ourselves to feel everything life has to offer is an
     indicator of fulfillment.
I'm learning that fulfillment can't be attained through giving myself
     away
But, through giving to myself and sharing with others,
I'm learning that the best way to teach my children to live a fulfilling
     life is not by sacrificing my life.
It's through living a fulfilling life myself.
I'm trying to teach my children that I have a lot to learn
Because I'm learning that letting go of them
Is the best way of holding on.*

14
Menopause

Like an electrical charge, menstruation and the ebb and flow of energy
is an "alternating current." During menopause, the flow of energy becomes intensified and steady, like a "direct current." We are charged
with energy to the degree we have opened ourselves to the wisdom of
the Crone.

—Farida Shaw

Menopause refers to the cessation of menses—the term derives
from the Greek *meno* (month, menses) and *pauses* (pause).
This natural process is also known to many women as the
"change of life" or simply "the change." The years surrounding
menopause and encompassing the gradual change in ovarian function
constitute an entire stage of a woman's life, lasting from six to thirteen
years, known as the *climacteric*.

Whatever we call it, no other stage of a woman's life has as much
potential for understanding and tapping in to women's power as this
one—if, that is, a woman is able to negotiate her way through the general cultural negativity that has surrounded menopause for centuries.
This negativity has been challenged and changed significantly in the
past decade as the women of my generation, the baby boomers, enter
menopause by the hundreds of thousands. As a result, this climacteric
experience is now significantly different than it was for our World War
II–generation mothers.

By the year 2000, 45.6 million American women had reached
menopause, according to the North American Menopause Society, with
numbers increasing every year. Worldwide, the number of menopausal
women is expected to reach 1.1 billion by the year 2025. At the same

time, longevity has increased dramatically. American women now enjoy a mean life expectancy of approximately eighty years, up from only forty-eight years for a woman born in 1900. This means that a woman is likely to live thirty to thirty-five years following the menopause, making menopause the "springtime" of the second half of life.

Media attention to the subject of menopause has risen accordingly. Feminist authors as well as many doctors and researchers have produced more books on menopause, including a number of best sellers, than on any other subject in the women's health field.

Though the advice about menopause ranges from exalting hormone replacement therapy to promoting natural menopause without hormones, the important point is that the silence surrounding this process has now been broken by many different voices. The medical profession stands poised to help women through this life stage, and centers specializing in the health needs of midlife women have sprung up all over the United States. Every woman, though barraged with conflicting advice, must listen carefully to her individual inner guidance to hear her personal truth about how best to negotiate this life stage with maximum access to her inner wisdom and power to create health.

In her book *Reclaiming the Menstrual Matrix* (Lantern Books, 2002), Tamara Slayton wrote, "The natural expression of personal power and wisdom available to women during [menopause] is thwarted and frustrated in our culture. This surge of energy is subsequently turned inward on oneself and can result in many unpleasant symptoms such as hot flashes, depression, mood swings, and a general feeling of being lost and unable to find a new and vital identity. Lack of support during this time and a tendency toward nutritional depletion in the American diet generate a negative and self-destructive experience of menopause. When women confront the culture's misinformation and address the nutritional needs unique to females, they have, during menopause, an opportunity to discover a deeper and freer experience of self."[1] That's precisely what is happening to thousands of women.

Joan Borysenko, Ph.D., refers to the years between the ages of forty-two and forty-nine as the "midlife metamorphosis," when a woman begins in earnest to create her life in such a way that her innermost values are lived out in her everyday activities. During this stage, she is more apt to tell the truth than ever before in her life and less apt to make excuses for others. Many women quest for peace of mind against a background of turmoil and change as they end twenty-year marriages, have affairs, get left by their partners, face the empty nest, start new businesses, and explore new facets of their identity.

It is during this stage that a woman is also most likely to begin experiencing skipped periods and the early stages of hormonal changes, making this a perfect time to start improving and building on the health that will sustain her for the rest of her life.

Anywhere from about forty-nine to fifty-five, a woman's hormonal shifts will often be in full swing, and she'll want support for these changes. After that, hormonal balance ensues once again for most women, and they are often freer than ever before to pursue creative interests and social action. These are the years when all of a woman's life experience comes together and can be used for a purpose that suits her.

In Celtic cultures, the young maiden was seen as the flower; the mother, the fruit; the elder woman, the seed. The seed is the part that contains the knowledge and potential of all the other parts within it. The role of the postmenopausal woman is to go forth and reseed the community with her concentrated kernel of truth and wisdom. In some native cultures, menopausal women were felt to retain their "wise blood," rather than shed it cyclically, and were therefore considered more powerful than menstruating women. A woman could not be a shaman until she was past menopause in these cultures. "Menopause," observes Slayton, "when understood and supported, provides the next level of initiation into personal power for women. With our increased life span, our way of thinking about menopause needs updating from these ancient mythologies. I think of perimenopause and the five to ten years following menopause as a time of ripeness. Instead of rose buds, we become rose hips—juicy fruit that contains and nurtures the seeds we will sow later.

"In native cultures postmenopausal women provide a voice of responsibility towards all children, both human and *nonhuman,* to the Earth and The Laws of Good Relationship," Slayton notes. "These older women contained great power and scrutinized all tribal decisions. They were unafraid to say a strong no to anything that did not serve life. They also initiated and educated the younger women into this knowledge and responsibility."[2]

Once a woman understands that the true meaning of menopause has been inverted and degraded, like many of the other processes of a woman's body, she will reverse this programming and make her way through the rest of her life fortified with purpose, insight, and pleasure.

OUR CULTURAL INHERITANCE

Up until very recently, the conventional medical mindset has been that menopause is a deficiency disease, not a natural process. Jerilynn

Prior, M.D., an endocrinologist and researcher, writes, "Our culture finds it easy to blame women's reproductive systems for disease. Linking the menopause change in reproductive capability with aging, making menopause a point in time rather than a process, and labeling it an estrogen deficiency disease are all reflections of nonscientific, prejudicial thinking by the medical profession."[3] Since menopausal women are no longer using their energy in childbearing, their systems are described in terms of functional failure or decline; breasts and genital organs gradually "atrophy," "wither," and become "senile."[4] Menopause, viewed through this lens, is the ultimate in "failed production"—a system that is "shut down."

For years the OB/GYN profession has been steeped in lectures and teaching on "managing the menopause" and the perimenopause. (*Perimenopause* refers to the years leading up to the last menstrual period.) If a woman's health care team approaches this life stage with support and respect for a natural process, she will be helped a great deal. But if the perimenopause (or any other natural process) is approached from the disease model, with the mindset that it requires management (and its subtext, control), then a woman's experience will not be ideal. In our culture, the only ages when female endocrine processes escape potential "management" are the years *before* menarche and *after* the age of seventy.

Fear of Aging: Symptom of an Ageist Culture

We live in an ageist culture, in which most people believe that it's natural for aging people to become depressed, fatigued, incontinent, asexual, forgetful, and senile. Pharmaceutical companies and gynecologists plant in women seeds of fear that as soon as they go through menopause, their bodies will simply fall apart and waste away unless they are on medication.

An example of this was the cover of a magazine called *Menopause Medicine* from the 1990s. A woman stands by an open window with filmy curtains blowing at her side; only her back is visible. She is looking out on the landscape covered by dead trees and parched dry Earth. The caption under this illustration read, "The Fate of the Untreated Menopause."

It doesn't take a degree in psychology to understand how the pharmaceutical companies influence the sensibilities of the average woman or doctor. For most of my career, we OB/GYNs felt enormous pressure to give conventional hormone replacement to everyone, having been led to believe that it was necessary to prevent everything from heart disease to osteoporosis. It's easy to see how the pharmaceutical companies and the media manipulate the stereotypes associated with aging and the deep cultural fears that we women have about them. For decades we've been taught that without hormone replacement, we'd lose our attractiveness to men, we'd dry up, we'd become brittle, like parched, cracked Earth, devoid of moisture and nourishment. Newer research is showing that this doesn't have to be true!

The experience of aging as we know it is largely determined by beliefs that need updating. Though many people *do* decline with age in this culture, this decline is not a natural consequence of aging—it is a consequence of our collective beliefs about aging. My mother, who is now eighty and has never been on hormones, hiked the entire Appalachian Trail in her late sixties, skied around the base of Mount McKinley shortly thereafter, and spent the summer of 1997 going on a three-month extended hiking and kayaking trip to Alaska. She later climbed the two hundred highest peaks in New England with her friend Anne, who is now eighty-five. One of my mother's other good friends turned ninety in 2005. She and my mother climbed Mount Washington together earlier that year and also went snowshoeing in northern Vermont. Yet as soon as my mother turned sixty, her mailbox was suddenly full of ads for hearing aids, incontinence diapers, and various aids for failing vision, none of which she has had any need for! Over time, my mother figured out how to ignore the constant barrage of negative messages about aging. She also told me that though she doesn't feel much different from when she was thirty, she is definitely treated differently. No wonder Bette Davis said, "Old age is not for sissies."

Another reason why so many women are afraid of menopause is a misunderstanding of the Crone or Wise Woman archetype. Medical intuitive Caroline Myss points out that in fairy tales and in our collective unconscious, the Crone is often depicted as an old woman living alone in the woods. She is often associated with witches or eccentric behavior.

Caroline notes that this image of a woman alone in the woods symbolically represents a woman who has freed herself from her original tribal programming. She no longer bases her activities, thoughts, and self-image on the approval of her family (thank goodness!). She is free to come and go as she pleases and on her own terms. She need not be alone, but her relationships are more likely to be partnerships and mutually satisfying. In 1998, I wrote, "What we need is a new Crone archetype—a sort of 'Aquarian Crone'—that reflects these new ways of perceiving this time of life." And that is exactly what is happening. Urban shaman Donna Henes dubs this stage the Queen in her book *The Queen of My Self* (Monarch Press, 2005). (See www.thequeenofmyself.com.)

Deepak Chopra, M.D., an endocrinologist, best-selling author, and internationally recognized authority on how consciousness affects our bodies, has reported on an experiment conducted among the Tarahumara Indians in Mexico, a group known for their running ability. Routinely, certain members of the tribe ran the equivalent of a marathon or more every day, and had regular races between groups. The most intriguing aspect of their culture, however, was that they believed that the best runners were those in their sixties. A team of researchers showed that the best lung capacity, cardiovascular fitness, and endurance were indeed found in the runners in their sixties! Dr. Chopra points out that for this belief to translate into physical reality, the entire tribe has to believe it.

And believe me, our tribe is starting to change our collective beliefs about the aging process. As baby boom women have entered menopause in droves, we are finally seeing many more media images of strong, sexy, vital menopausal women. In fact, today's menopausal women look younger than ever before. We are collectively reversing our cultural negativity about menopause, one woman at a time. We are redefining menopause and aging. And this change in our beliefs and expectations is showing up in our bodies. For instance, my mother had a health reading from Caroline Myss when she was sixty-eight. Her body read energetically as though she were in her thirties. This reading is not surprising since it is well known that chronological age and biological age are two different things.

The more women like my mother ignore what is supposed to happen when we age, the better the chances are that all of us will stay healthy. During and after menopause, I became more flexible and healthier than ever before—and even lost weight! I see this happening everywhere I go as women around the world decide to age with power, strength, and beauty.

CREATING HEALTH DURING MENOPAUSE

To make the most of the menopausal transition, I encourage a woman to think of it as a process during which she'll be creating the healthy body she needs to last her until the end of life. The menopausal transition is an excellent time to focus on the prevention of problems that, while not necessarily directly associated with menopause, statistically appear to intensify at this stage. Menopause is a time when we reach a crossroads in our lives. One road says "Grow"; the other says "Die." We can no longer sit on the fence and expect our bodies to stay vital without some active input and lifestyle changes.

What a woman experiences during this period of her life depends upon a multitude of factors, from her heredity, her expectations, and her cultural background to her self-esteem and her diet. At this time in history, the majority of women in our culture experience some discomfort and some troublesome symptoms at menopause. However, a wide variety of options exists for the treatment of these symptoms, ranging from bioidentical hormones that match those produced in the human female body to homeopathy. The ideal path through the change is one that uses the best of Western medical knowledge concerning hormone metabolism, bone density, and heart health, combined with the complementary modalities of the East, from meditation to acupuncture to herbs, to provide optimal individualized care.

Menopause: A Crossroads

The menopausal years are a time when most women find themselves in a crucible—having all the dross of the first half of their lives burned away so that they emerge reborn and more fully themselves. The midlife transitional years are a time in which we complete some of the tasks that we started in adolescence.

At midlife, a woman looks back at her life and ponders where she has been and how far she has come. Now is the time when she grieves the loss of any unrealized dreams she may have had when she was a young woman, and prepares the soil for the next stage of her life. She grapples with many issues that coincide with but are not directly associated with hormonal function, such as caring for aging parents with health problems. Depending upon her degree of success or perceived success in life, she may find herself in a crisis that is not so much physiological as it is developmental. How she negotiates this crisis will affect her health on all levels as she goes through menopause.

During my lectures, I've shown a slide of Mount Saint Helens erupting to illustrate the stormy emotions that so often characterize these years. This is a time when many women, myself included, begin to manifest some of the fierce need for self-expression that so often goes underground at adolescence. I like to think of midlife women as dangerous—dangerous to any forces existing in our lives that seek to turn us into silent little old ladies, dangerous to the deadening effects of convention and niceness, and dangerous to any accommodations we have made that are stifling who we are now capable of becoming. By the age of forty-five, I found myself deeply engaged in the process of scrutinizing every aspect of my life and my relationships in an effort to eradicate any dead wood that either held me back or no longer served who I had become. My tolerance for dead-end relationships of all kinds began to evaporate. This eventually led to the end of my twenty-four-year marriage and was the impetus for writing *The Wisdom of Menopause* (Bantam Books, 2001). Women in midlife are at a turning point: either we can continue living with relationships, jobs, and situations that we have outgrown—a choice that hastens the aging process and the chance for disease dramatically—or we can do the developmental work that our bodies, and our hormone levels, are calling out for. We must source our lives from our souls now. Nothing less will work. When we dare to do this, we truly prepare for the springtime of the second half of our lives.

Hormone-Producing Body Sites

Though we've been taught to think of menopausal symptoms mostly as an estrogen deficiency state resulting from ovarian failure, this belief is based on incomplete information. First of all, estrogen is not the only hormone made by the ovaries. Androgens, such as DHEA and testosterone, are also made by the ovaries, and so is progesterone. Total well-being at menopause and beyond depends at least as much on having adequate levels of these hormones as it does on estrogen. Androgenic hormones are associated with sexual response and libido, as well as general well-being, and are produced by organs and body sites other than just the ovaries. These include the adrenal glands, the skin, the muscles, the brain, and the pineal gland, as well as hair follicles and body fat. (See figure 15, page 550). Interestingly, as hormone production from the ovaries declines at menopause, a twofold increase in production of androgenic hormones from these other sources takes place. Since androgens can act as weak estrogens and can also be precursors for the production of estrogens, it is clear that the healthy menopausal women is naturally equipped to deal with hormonal changes in her ovaries. Women who are able to produce adequate levels of androgens in their bodies often sail through menopause quite easily.

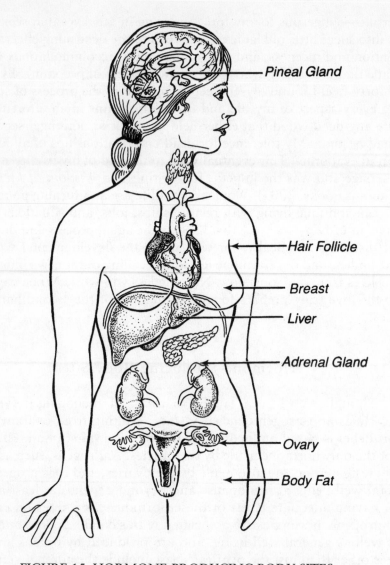

Pineal Gland

Hair Follicle

Breast

Liver

Adrenal Gland

Ovary

Body Fat

FIGURE 15: HORMONE-PRODUCING BODY SITES

Ovarian estrogen and progesterone levels decrease after menopause. Other body sites, however, are capable of making these same hormones, depending upon a woman's lifestyle and diet. The female body, therefore, has the capacity to make healthy adjustments in hormonal balance after menopause.

Nevertheless, some women clearly suffer during menopause. While 15 percent of women are symptom-free, a full 85 percent will experience hot flashes, and approximately one-half of this group does not consider the hot flashes to be tolerable. As time goes on, symptoms of vaginal atrophy (thinning of the vaginal tissue) in postmenopausal women tend to increase; heart disease risk and osteoporosis fracture risk also increase but will not be evident until a woman is in her late sixties or older.

Such menopausal problems are due in part to chronic depletion of women's metabolic resources during the perimenopausal years. The ease of transition into this stage depends upon the strength of a woman's adrenals and the state of her general nutrition. In a healthy woman, the adrenal glands will be able to gradually take over hormonal production from the ovaries. Many women, however, approach menopause in a state of emotional and nutritional depletion that has affected optimal adrenal function. Under these conditions, a woman may require hormonal, nutritional, emotional, and/or other support until her endocrine balance is restored.[5]

ADRENAL FUNCTION:
WHAT EVERY WOMAN SHOULD KNOW

Our adrenal glands provide us with crucial hormonal support that we all need to go through the day with energy, enthusiasm, and efficiency. If your adrenals are depleted from chronic overproduction of the stress hormones norepinephrine (adrenaline) and cortisol, you are much more likely to suffer from fatigue and menopausal symptoms. Here are the signs that your adrenals may need attention: You awaken feeling groggy and have difficulty dragging yourself out of bed. You can't get going without that first cup or two of caffeinated coffee. You rely on sugary snacks and caffeine to get through the day, particularly in the late morning or afternoon. At night, though exhausted, you have difficulty falling asleep as the worries of the day keep replaying in your mind. You wonder what happened to your interest in sex. If this describes you, your adrenals may be running on almost empty, even if all your conventional medical tests are normal.

Functional adrenal testing, which measures the levels of two of the key adrenal hormones over a twenty-four-hour period, has documented that many women who are tired all the time have adrenal glands that simply aren't functioning at their peak efficiency—usually as a result of chronic emotional, nutritional, or other kinds of stress.

Adrenal dysfunction is also associated with symptoms such as foggy thinking, insomnia, hypoglycemia, recurrent infections, depression, poor memory, headaches, and cravings for sweets. But once you know that your adrenals are in need of R&R, there is a great deal you can do to help them recover. Adrenal function can also be measured by doing a simple blood test for DHEA (optimal for women is 550–980 ng/dl).

The adrenal glands are your body's primary "shock absorbers." These two little thumb-size glands that sit on top of your kidneys are designed to produce hormones that allow you to respond to the conditions of your daily life in healthy and flexible ways. But if the intensity and the frequency of the stresses in your life, from inside yourself (such as your perceptions about your life) or outside yourself (such as having surgery or working the night shift), become too great, then over time your adrenal glands will begin to become exhausted—not unlike a horse that continues to be worked or runs too much without adequate rest, food, and water. Eventually your body will produce many different symptoms in an attempt to get you to pay attention and change some aspects of your life—just as a tired horse will sooner or later stop working, no matter how much you whip it.

Here's a list of common stressors that over time can lead to adrenal dysfunction. See how many of these apply to you.

UNRESOLVED EMOTIONAL STRESS

~ Worry
~ Anger
~ Guilt
~ Anxiety
~ Fear
~ Depression
~ Lack of pleasurable experiences

ENVIRONMENTAL AND PHYSICAL STRESS

~ Excessive exercise
~ Exposure to industrial or other environmental toxins
~ Chronic or severe allergies
~ Suboptimal diet

~ Glycemic stress from too many refined carbohydrates

~ Overwork, either physical or mental

~ Surgery

~ Late hours, insufficient sleep

~ Trauma, injury

~ Temperature extremes

~ Chronic illness

~ Light-cycle disruption (shift work)

~ Chronic pain

~ Chronic illness

~ Lack of sunlight

Among the key hormones produced by the adrenals are adrenaline, which fuels the body's "fight-or-flight" response; cortisol, a relative of the drugs prednisone and cortisone; and DHEA. The ongoing balance between cortisol and DHEA is especially important for creating health daily.

Cortisol in the right amounts enhances your body's natural resistance and endurance. It:

~ Stimulates your liver to convert amino acids into glucose, a primary fuel for energy production

~ Counters allergies and inflammation

~ Helps regulate mood and maintain emotional stability

~ Stimulates increased production of glycogen in the liver for storage of glucose

~ Maintains resistance to the stress of infections, physical trauma, emotional trauma, temperature extremes, and so on

~ Mobilizes and increases fatty acids in the blood (from fat cells) to be used as fuel for energy production

But, as in most things, too much cortisol can also cause problems. An excess:

~ Leads to diminished glucose utilization by the cells and increases blood sugar and insulin levels

~ Decreases the body's ability to synthesize protein

~ Increases protein breakdown, which can lead to muscle wasting and osteoporosis

~ Suppresses the sex hormones

~ Increases the risk for hypertension, high cholesterol, and heart disease

~ Causes immune system depression, which may lead to increased susceptibility to allergies, infections, and cancer

Under normal circumstances, DHEA reverses many of the unfavorable effects of excessive cortisol, as well as providing important benefits of its own. It:

~ Functions as an androgen to help the body build tissue

~ Is a precursor for testosterone, the hormone associated with sexual desire

~ Reverses immune suppression caused by excessive cortisol levels and therefore increases resistance to viruses, bacteria, *Candida albicans,* parasites, allergies, and cancer

~ Stimulates bone deposition and remodeling, which prevents osteoporosis

~ Improves cardiovascular status by lowering total LDL (bad) cholesterol

~ Increases muscle mass and decreases percentage of body fat

~ Improves energy and vitality, sleep, mental clarity; reduces PMS symptoms; and helps the body recover more quickly from acute stress such as insufficient sleep, excessive exercise, or emotional trauma

So as you can easily see, an imbalance between your cortisol and DHEA levels can leave you susceptible to fatigue and all manner of illnesses, as well as many menopausal symptoms. Levels of DHEA decline in some women with aging, and replenishing this hormone to normal body levels may have many benefits. However, use of the hormone isn't right for everyone, and once adrenal function is restored, our bodies often have the ability to make enough of this hormone on their own.[6]

To test your current levels of cortisol and DHEA and to see if they are in balance over a twenty-four-hour period, I recommend that you have your health care provider order a test known as the Adrenal Stress Index or the Temporal Adrenal Profile, or get your blood level of DHEA tested. (Laboratories that can do this with a doctor's prescription include Genova Diagnostics, 800-522-4762;

www.gdx.net; and ZRT Laboratory, 503-466-2445; www.salivat-est.com.)[7]

It is not necessary to have your salivary cortisol and DHEA levels measured to benefit from my suggestions for restoring your adrenal glands to full capacity, but I find that most women are more motivated to change when they can see their results on paper, especially if the initial results are not optimal. If you don't want to have the test done at this time, for whatever reason, just follow as many of the following suggestions as you can without stressing yourself further.

Adrenal Restoration Program for a Healthier Menopause

DHEA: The Youth and Health Hormone

Recharge your batteries with the powr of your thoughts and emotions. Studies have shown that your natural ability to produce DHEA can be increased by learning to "think with your heart." This is simple. It means choosing thoughts that feel better, e.g., if you're stressed about something, turn your attention to your heart and think about a puppy, an adorable child, a fabulous meal—anything that feels good and brings you pleasure. Make this a habit. It will change your life! (To get you started, I recommend reading *Ask and It Is Given* or *The Art of Deliberate Creation* [Hay House, 2006] both by Esther and Jerry Hicks.) The Institute of HeartMath in Boulder Creek, California (call HeartMath at 800-450-9111 or visit HeartMath's website at www.heartmath.com), has developed a system of heart-focusing techniques that are taught through training programs and books. One HeartMath technique called Cut-Thru showed that with sincere practice, it could help alter the harmful physiological and emotional responses to emotional stress. The study demonstrated that after one month of using the technique there was a 100 percent increase in the subjects' DHEA levels. Study participants reported significant increases in caring and vigor and significant decreases in burnout and anxiety. The technique helps dissipate emotional static and can help heal emotional patterns of worry, hostility, anxiety, and guilt.[8]

"Thinking with your heart" takes practice, but if you faithfully learn to start thinking with your heart and pay attention to areas of your life that bring you joy and fulfillment, over time you will evoke biochemical changes in your body that will recharge your batteries.

HEART FOCUS EXERCISE TO DECREASE STRESS HORMONES

1. Stop yourself and observe your emotional state.

2. Name what is bothering you—you might even write it down or say it out loud to yourself or a friend.

3. Focus on your heart area (put your hand there if it helps you focus).

4. Shift your attention to a happy, funny, or uplifting event, person, or place in your life that you appreciate, and spend a few moments imagining it.

5. Bring something to mind that allows you to feel unconditional love or appreciation—usually a child or a pet—and hold that feeling for fifteen seconds or more (again, it helps to hold your hand over your heart).

6. Notice how changing your thoughts and your perception has changed how you feel. See that you have the power to shift out of the downward spiral of negativity you may have been caught in.

Make a list of your most important activities and commitments. Let everything else go. Before saying yes to a new task or commitment, ask yourself this question: Will doing this recharge my batteries or deplete them? If the activity will deplete them, then don't do it.

Get enough sleep. Sleep restores adrenal balance more effectively than any other modality. Many women, including me, require eight to ten hours of sleep to function optimally. Get to bed by ten P.M. Getting to sleep on the earlier side of midnight is much more restorative to your adrenals than sleep that begins later in the night, even if you sleep late the next morning to get in your full amount of sleep.

Allow yourself to accept nurturing and affection. If you didn't learn how to do this as a child, you may need to practice it. Every morning before you get up, spend a minute or two reveling in a memory of a time you felt loved. Do the same at night. Imagine your heart being filled with this love. Dwell on the things you really like about yourself.

Concentrate on activities and people that are fun and make you laugh. This stimulates healthy immune function. Make pleasurable activities a priority—every day. Don't wait until later. "Later" rarely comes.

Support yourself nutritionally. Follow the guidelines in chapter 17. Eat a whole-food diet with minimal sugar. Avoid caffeine and junk food as much as possible. Make sure you're getting enough protein— eat some at each meal and snack. Avoid fasting or cleansing programs, which can weaken you further. Check your vitamin-mineral intake, too. Vitamin C is essential for the blood vessels supporting your adrenal glands: take 500 to 2,000 mg in divided doses over the day. Vitamin B_5 (pantothenic acid) is involved in energy production via ATP in the adrenals and elsewhere; take the rest of the B complex along with it (25 to 50 mg of B complex). Also take magnesium 300 to 800 mg a day in divided doses (use fumarate, citrate, glycinate, or malate form); excretion of magnesium in the urine is increased in states where cortisol is too high, so it's easy to see how common magnesium depletion is when you are under chronic stress. (See the supplement recommendations in chapter 17, "Nourishing Ourselves with Food.") My colleague Norm Shealy, M.D., Ph.D., finds that transdermal magnesium is highly effective for raising DHEA naturally. (To order this and other supplements from Dr. Shealy's company, Self-Health Systems, call 888-242-6105 or visit www.normshealy.net.) Zinc is useful as well; take 15 to 30 mg daily. MSM (methylsulfonylmethane) in combination with vitamin C has been shown to raise DHEA. Dr. Shealy has developed a nutritional formula specifically for raising DHEA, known as the Youth Formula.

Your regular multivitamin-mineral supplement may have all of the nutrients I've listed here. Just add more of what is low in your current supplementation regimen.

Try herbal support. Siberian ginseng is often quite helpful for adrenal function because one of its components is related to pregnenolone, a precursor for DHEA and cortisol. Take one 100 mg capsule twice per day. If it tends to be too stimulating, take it before three P.M.

Licorice root contains plant hormones that have effects similar to cortisol. For low-cortisol states, take up to one-quarter teaspoon of 5:1 solid extract three times a day.

Consider hormonal support. If your lab report comes back showing that you have decreased DHEA levels, try the steps listed above first.

It's always ideal to restore adrenal function naturally. If you are not successful, consider supplementing your program with DHEA until your adrenals have recovered. High doses of DHEA over long periods of time can change the normal daily variation in cortisol levels, and I don't recommend them for most healthy women. However, physiologic replacement doses (enough to bring levels up to normal) of DHEA can help your own adrenals get a rest and start to recover faster.

DHEA is available as a skin cream, a pill, or a tincture. The best brands are pharmaceutical grade (look for GMP on the label). (The tincture needs to be made up by a formulary pharmacist.) Each form has a somewhat different effect, but whatever the form, you should start with the lowest dose possible and build up gradually until you notice a difference in your energy. Most women need no more than 5 to 10 mg twice a day; some will need up to 25 mg once or twice a day. Your DHEA levels should be tested again three months later, and if they have been restored to normal, you can begin to taper off the supplementary DHEA.

Progesterone also helps balance the effects of too much cortisol. Use one-quarter to one-half teaspoon of 2-percent progesterone cream once or twice a day on the skin. It also raises DHEA levels.

An occasional individual may also need cortisol supplementation, which can be prescribed for a limited amount of time by your health care provider.

Exercise. Light to moderate exercise is very helpful. But if you feel depleted afterward, you are doing too much. Pushing yourself beyond your limits weakens your adrenals even further, so start slowly—even if it's only walking down your street and back. Then build up slowly. (For more information on DHEA, see *Life Beyond 100: Secrets of the Fountain of Youth* [Jeremy P. Tarcher/Penguin, 2005] by C. Norman Shealy.)

Sunlight. Natural sunlight can be very helpful for restoring adrenal function, as long as you don't overdo it. I recommend working up to ten to fifteen minutes of exposure during early morning or late afternoon (never in midday), three to four times per week. This type of brief exposure, if you are sure not to burn or even redden the skin, will not increase your risk of skin cancer. It's also an excellent way to help boost levels of vitamin D. In the winter, you can use a tanning booth for eight to ten minutes once per week.

KINDS OF MENOPAUSE

Natural Menopause and Perimenopause

The average age of menopause is currently about fifty-two, with a range from forty-five to fifty-five. It is possible for some women to experience menopause as early as age thirty-nine. Most women go through menopause at approximately the same age as their mothers, although this is not always the case.

The climacteric is a biochemical process lasting six to thirteen years. During this process, periods may stop for several months and then return; they may increase or decrease in duration and flow. Some women may experience as much as a year-long interruption in periods only to have them resume once again.

When irregularity in the menstrual cycle begins during perimenopause, a woman's symptoms, such as headaches and irritability, will often be due to increased levels of estrogen relative to progesterone, caused by decreased ovulation. This is known as estrogen dominance. Women who have experienced a difficult puberty, PMS, or postpartum depression are more likely to experience mood swings and other related symptoms during menopause than those who have gone through earlier hormonal changes comfortably. Women in the perimenopause can often be helped dramatically by small amounts of progesterone administered in the luteal phase (second half) of the cycle. The usual dose is 50 to 100 mg of micronized progesterone administered orally one to three times a day from the sixteenth through the twenty-seventh day of the cycle.[9] A 2-percent progesterone cream can also be used. (Some women will fare better if progesterone is administered continuously through the cycle.) Progesterone is particularly beneficial for women with premenstrual migraine headaches.

Many women who begin to skip periods or experience changes in the menstrual flow believe that they are entering menopause. Though the final menstrual period is probably at least five years away, it may be very helpful to order a hormone profile at this time. This establishes your baseline levels of estrogen, progesterone, and testosterone, which may be useful later for prescribing individualized hormone replacement, should you choose that option. (Hormone testing resources include Genova Diagnostics, 800-522-4762, www.gdx.net; and ZRT Laboratory, 503-466-2445; www.salivatest.com.) Hormone testing is still considered controversial at this time. More studies are needed.

While menopause is often heralded by the onset of a change in menstrual flow or skipped menstrual periods, some women simply stop having periods and have no symptoms whatsoever. Others experience hot flashes, vaginal dryness, decreased libido, and "fuzzy thinking." A blood or urine test is often done at this time to "diagnose" menopause. This consists of measuring the levels of the pituitary gonadotropins FSH (follicle-stimulating hormone) and LH (luteinizing hormone), hormones produced by the pituitary gland to stimulate the ovary to produce eggs. During the years of menstruation, FSH and LH peak with ovulation at midcycle each month, producing the emotional and physiological changes discussed in chapter 5. During the climacteric, however, the pituitary gland and the ovaries undergo a gradual change, during which ovulations decrease and FSH and LH levels gradually increase. (The pituitary gland continues to send out LH and FSH because it is not getting the usual hormonal messages from the developing egg to tell it to slow down.) When FSH and LH reach a certain level in the blood, they are said to be in the menopausal range.

I was taught that once a woman's FSH and LH are in the menopausal range, she was indeed menopausal and would stay that way, but this is not always the case. One forty-year-old woman, for example, who had no periods for six months and had menopausal levels of FSH and LH, later went back to having normal periods for years! A recheck of her hormone levels showed that they also had gone back to premenopausal levels. At this point, I don't consider FSH and LH levels very reliable diagnostic indicators of menopause but they can be useful to confirm that a woman is heading in that direction. (It's also fun to watch this trend reverse sometimes when the ovaries and adrenals get the support they need!) It's important for perimenopausal women to know that even though they may be skipping ovulations, they can theoretically still become pregnant up until one year after their last period. For that reason, I recommend that a woman continue to use some form of contraception throughout this time. Though most women will not require hormonal support during perimenopause and menopause, those who've gone through premature menopause or artificial menopause will want to consider it.

Premature Menopause

A small percentage of women experience premature menopause in their thirties or early forties (approximately one in a hundred women goes through the climacteric at age forty or younger). In some cases, this is an autoimmune disorder related to poor diet or chronic stress and resulting in the production of antiovarian antibodies.[10] Women who undergo premature menopause and loss of ovarian estrogen supply have been shown to have increased susceptibility to dementia.[11] It is important for a woman with this history to pay special attention to those things that promote healthy brain function. (See discussion of Alzheimer's later in this chapter.)

Artificial Menopause

Currently, one in every four American women will enter menopause as a result of surgery. Hysterectomy with ovarian removal or bilateral salpingo-oophorectomy (removal of both tubes and ovaries) results in instant menopause in the premenopausal woman, which is very different from natural physiological menopause and should be treated differently. Removal of the ovaries is associated with a dramatic decrease in the production of testosterone and other androgens. Surgical menopause can also result in a major decrease in estrogen production. Symptoms can be severe and debilitating without proper readjustment of hormonal levels.[12] Because normal menopause occurs at around fifty-two years of age, hormone replacement should continue at least until this age but can be continued longer depending on individual circumstances.

Hysterectomy without ovarian removal may still result in accelerated menopause, as mentioned earlier. In some cases, the ovaries temporarily decrease hormone production, causing menopausal symptoms that disappear when normal ovarian function resumes. It has also been shown that progesterone levels decrease significantly for at least six months following tubal ligation.[13] (This is probably not the case with the new Essure method—see chapter 11, "Our Fertility.")

Women who have had chemotherapy for any cancer or who have undergone radiation to the pelvis are also apt to undergo premature menopause. (For women facing chemotherapy or radiation, it has been my experience that undergoing a course of acupuncture and Chinese herbs at the same time as the chemo or radiation can often prevent premature menopause and will also alleviate many side effects of the treatment.) Adding together the women who undergo natural premature menopause and those who undergo artificial menopause means that approximately one in twelve women today faces menopause before the age of forty.

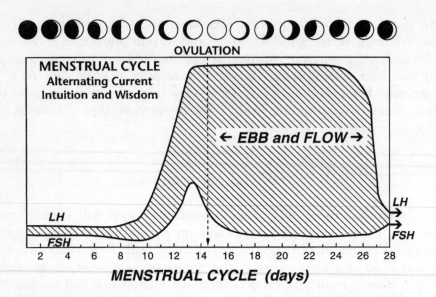

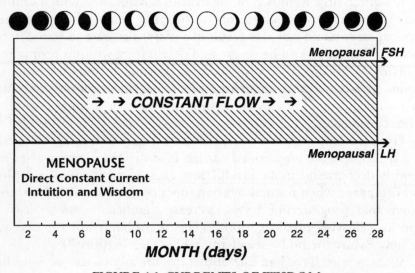

FIGURE 16: CURRENTS OF WISDOM

FSH and LH stimulate ovulation and are realized cyclically each month up until the years surrounding menopause. They then undergo a change during which ovulations gradually cease and FSH and LH levels gradually increase. I believe that these high levels have to do with moving from "AC current" to "DC current." The intuitive wisdom that was once available most clearly during only certain parts of the menstrual cycle is now potentially available all the time.

Note: This figure appears in another form in Mona Lisa Schulz, *Awaking Intuition* (Harmony, 1998).

TABLE 8

Profile of an Optimally Healthy Midlife Woman

~ Normal physiologic menopause at age fifty plus or minus five years

~ No family history of osteoporosis

~ Medium to heavy frame (see chapter 17 for how to determine this)

~ Nonsmoker

~ No long-term use of drugs associated with increased risk for osteoporosis (steroids, high doses of thyroid medication, some diuretics)

~ No history of depression

~ Regular weight-bearing exercise and aerobic exercise (at least three times per week)

~ Nutrient-rich diet that decreases risk of cellular inflammation (see chapter 17)

~ Minimal alcohol consumption (no more than two or three drinks per week)

~ Passion for living

THE HORMONE REPLACEMENT QUESTION

Florence first came into my office at the age of fifty-one for her annual visit. She was having hot flashes, but they weren't really bothering her. She didn't want to take estrogen. But she was concerned about her risk for osteoporosis. She also wanted to prevent heart disease and Alzheimer's. Florence hadn't had a period in three months, exercised regularly, had a healthy percentage of body fat, and had had a hormone profile several months before that showed that her estrogen was on the low side, but her testosterone levels were high normal. Her progesterone was a little low. She had no family history of heart disease, osteoporosis, or Alzheimer's, and her sex life was fine. Her mother was seventy-five and ramrod straight, played tennis every day in the summer, and skied all winter; her maternal grandmother was sharp as a tack mentally, lived alone, and still did all her own gardening at the age of ninety-two. Neither of these women had ever taken hormones.

TABLE 9

PROFILE OF A HIGH-RISK WOMAN: MAY REQUIRE HORMONE REPLACEMENT AND/OR OTHER INTERVENTIONS FOR OPTIMAL HEALTH

~ Premature menopause (age forty or earlier)

~ Artificial menopause before age forty-five, induced by surgery, chemotherapy, drugs, or radiation

~ High umbilical-to-hip ratio (apple-shaped figure)

~ Smoker

~ Strong family history of Alzheimer's dementia

~ Sedentary

~ Nutrient-poor refined-foods diet

~ Perception that there is nothing much to live for

When a woman such as Florence seeks advice on hormone replacement or bone-building drugs, my recommendations are quite simple. She should use the least amount of intervention that will provide symptomatic relief. In this case, I'd recommend taking 400 to 1,200 IU per day of vitamin E, plus some bioflavonoids. And I might have her try a 2-percent progesterone cream daily on her skin three weeks out of every month. Then I'd see how she was doing in three to six months and make adjustments as needed. Because her testosterone level is naturally high, she doesn't need estrogen. She also doesn't need bone density testing because she has no risk factors for osteoporosis.

A Brief History of Conventional Hormone Replacement

Premarin, the first and most well-known form of estrogen replacement, was introduced in 1949. It consists of a collection of more than twenty different conjugated equine estrogens mostly made from the urine of pregnant horses. (Premarin is an acronym derived from the phrase "pregnant mares' urine." If you doubt this, just put a drop of water on a tablet of Premarin and smell it.)

For historical and economic reasons it continues to be the standard against which all other menopausal hormone treatments are measured. It is also the estrogen employed in most major studies. For the past forty years, Premarin (with or without the progestin compound Provera) was considered the gold standard of hormone replacement. In the late 1980s through the 1990s, millions of women were put on this drug because studies strongly suggested that it decreased the risk of heart attack and stroke (the leading cause of premature death in women), increased bone density, and decreased the risk of dementia. Although it was associated with a slightly increased risk of breast and endometrial cancer, these risks paled in comparison to the possibility of saving lives lost to heart disease.

In the early 1990s, the Wyeth-Ayerst company, makers of Premarin, helped fund the huge Women's Health Initiative, which was designed to prove that Prempro would save lives by decreasing heart attacks, etc. The study was stopped in July 2002 when researchers found that Prempro actually increased the risk of heart attack and stroke as well as breast cancer, Alzheimer's, and dementia! Over all, it was felt that the risks outweighed the benefits.

The news about Prempro panicked thousands of women, many of whom stopped taking HRT cold turkey and ended up with insomnia, intolerable hot flashes, and a greatly decreased quality of life.

Then in early 2006, a reanalysis of the data from both the Women's Health Initiative (WHI) study and the Nurses' Health Study found that women who started HRT within ten years after menopause did indeed have an 11 to 30 percent decreased risk of heart disease compared to those who didn't use any hormones. But those who started it ten years or more after menopause were the ones with the increased risk for stroke, heart attack, etc.[14] This adds a new wrinkle to the entire HRT discussion. And makes it more clear than ever that the HRT decision needs to be individualized.

The Need for Bioidentical Hormones

Despite the new reanalysis of the data from the WHI and Nurses' Health Study showing a benefit in decreasing heart disease, I'm still concerned that women aren't getting the right kind of hormones. Back in 1994, concerned about the type of HRT used in the WHI study, I wrote, "In view of the concerns regarding breast cancer associated with estrogen replacement therapy (ERT), the use of synthetic sex compounds with which the human body is not designed to cope would appear to be the equivalent of conducting a vast experiment on the human female population. It is ironic, in this light, that treatment using natural hormones bioidentical to those in a woman's body is designated as 'alternative' medicine."

Premarin doesn't contain hormones that match those in the human body.[15] As Dr. Joel Hargrove, a pioneer in the use of natural hormones and former medical director of the Menopause Center at Vanderbilt University Medical Center, quips, "Premarin is a natural hormone if your native food is hay." In addition, since the women in the Women's Health Initiative were all given essentially the same standard dose, many were undoubtedly being overdosed. A two-hundred-pound woman and a hundred-pound woman on the same dose would likely have *very* different blood levels!

Finding Middle Ground: The Individualized Hormone Solution

Though many of my colleagues and I were disturbed by the way in which the Women's Health Initiative study was stopped and the distress it caused for so many women, the good news is that it changed the HRT paradigm completely. Almost overnight, we went from a "one size fits all," magic-bullet approach to understanding the need to individualize our approach to HRT. And that is likely to remain the standard of care from now on—regardless of what new studies are done in the future.

For those women who require hormone replacement by virtue of their symptoms or other risk factors, there is very good news. The field of individualized natural hormone support has positively blossomed since the first edition of this book was published. And instead of reducing the entire hormone question simply to estrogen, we now know that replacement of hormones may require the two other classes of hormones that the ovaries also produce: progesterone and androgens.

First, a word about that confusing and much-debated word *natural*. The hormone components of Premarin are indeed natural for horses, but the word is more commonly applied to plant hormones (phytohormones) found in foods such as soybeans and wild yams. The human body utilizes plant hormones better than equine hormones, because we have been ingesting them for millions of years, but they are still not the same as those made in the human body.

The "natural" hormones I will be talking about fall into another category. They are derived from the hormones found in soybeans and yams, but their molecular structure is modified in the laboratory to match those found in the human body exactly. That is why they are also referred to as bioidentical hormones. The natural estrogens, progesterone, and testosterone used for hormone replacement are produced in this way and are therefore "bioidentical." The amount of hormone can also be standardized, so that its effects are measurable and pre-dictable. The issue is not whether or not a hormone is produced in a laboratory; if it matches the hormones found in the human body, then it's a bioidentical hormone.

Natural hormone replacement using bioidentical hormones pro-vides no single, uniform program. Prescriptions must be tailored to the individual patient with adjustments made regularly for the first year or so until an optimal dose is reached. This dose may continue to require readjustment as a woman moves through premenopause and meno-pause and her body, lifestyle, and diet undergo changes.

The goal of natural hormone support is to restore hormones (or their precursors) to the normal body levels that were present during a woman's thirties or forties. An integrated approach including all three hormone types (estrogen, progesterone, and androgen) is optimal, even in women whose uteruses have been removed. Currently, most women who have had hysterectomies are offered only estrogen, without any consideration for the role of progesterone or androgen.

Virtually hundreds of combinations of hormones, including estrogen, progesterone, DHEA, and testosterone, are possible and may be adminis-tered by various routes, including orally, transdermally, or vaginally. Because the choices are so numerous and often confusing, I recommend beginning with a hormone profile for every woman who expresses con-cern about menopause or who is exhibiting menopausal symptoms. Such a baseline hormone profile is also ideal when done in the early to mid-forties, when a woman is symptom-free. Then her own ideal levels will be known beforehand, making it much easier to create a replacement regi-men that is tailor-made for her should she require it. That said, there is still a great deal we don't know about how hormones are metabolized in the body and what ideal hormone levels are. Experts in bioidentical hor-mone replacement, such as my colleague Erika Schwartz, M.D., author of *The 30-Day Natural Hormone Plan* (Warner Books, 2004) and *The Hormone Solution* (Warner Books, 2002), ultimately feel that relief of symptoms is the best way to assess the success of HRT, not hormone lev-els. I agree with her! Since the climacteric can last as long as thirteen years, it will be necessary to vary regimens or to reevaluate the need for continued hormone replacement over the course of the menopausal tran-sition. No one knows how long a woman should stay on HRT. Short-term is considered five years or less.

Currently, a growing number of resources exist to help women get the individualized hormone replacement regimens that I consider ideal. Among these are a number of laboratories and independent formulary pharmacies located throughout the United States and Canada that specialize in customized care. (See Resources.) In addition to operating a private practice in New York City, Dr. Schwartz has designed a three-month program combining bioidentical hormones, dietary adjustments, movement techniques, stress management, and lifestyle support. Her results are excellent. The program is tailored to each participant's specific needs and includes telephone consultations and unlimited e-mail support. (For more information, visit www.drerika.com.)

Many clinicians find that blood hormone levels are more accurate than salivary levels, but others disagree. In general, I believe it's prudent to go along with the testing method and protocol used by your health care practitioner. Over time, doctors and other healers get a "feel" for the testing protocols that work best for them. Remember, hormone replacement is as much an art as it is a science. Most formulary pharmacists have a great deal of experience working with health care providers to individualize optimal hormone solutions.

Note: at this time, there are no long-term-outcome studies of large groups of women who have had physiologic replacement doses of balanced hormone replacement. Remember that the WHI—which is considered the final word on HRT—was funded by Wyeth-Ayerst, the makers of Prempro. Given the financial losses that resulted from the outcome of this study, it is highly unlikely that any company would be willing or able to re-create such a significant study of individualized bioidentical hormones at low doses. Without this kind of data, however, we will never really be able to answer the kinds of questions that need to be addressed when it comes to hormone replacement. All hormones, whether bioidentical or not, have physiologic effects, including the possibility of increasing the risk for cancer depending on how they are metabolized and how much is taken. But in my experience, the risk appears to be very low—and the quality of life vastly improved for women who desire or require this type of support.

A HORMONE PRIMER

Estrogen

There are three types of estrogen that occur naturally in the female body: estrone (E1), estradiol (E2), and estriol (E3). Estrone is produced in significant amounts in body fat, which is one reason why anorexic women cease menstruating and get premature osteoporosis. They simply don't have enough body fat to sustain normal hormone function. Estrogen acts as a growth hormone for breast, uterine, and ovarian tissue. Overstimulation of these organs by estrogen is associated with excessive cell growth that may lead to cancer. On the positive side, estrogen elevates HDL (the good cholesterol) and has a beneficial effect on blood vessel walls; these are among the reasons why ERT has been linked with a decreased risk for heart disease. And the newest data shows that when it's given early enough in the menopausal process, it does, in fact, show cardiovascular benefits. Estrogen also helps to prevent osteoporosis by inhibiting bone cells known as osteoclasts, which are involved in the recycling and breakdown of old bone. It also ameliorates hot flashes, prevents vaginal thinning and dryness, and enhances the collagen layer of the skin, which improves elasticity and helps to prevent wrinkles.

The most effective and most commonly used estrogens are estradiol and estrone. These are available in a wide variety of preparations, including transdermal patches and creams, vaginal rings, or oral preparations.

With the exception of estriol, estrogen from any source, natural or otherwise, can be potentially dangerous if the dose used is too high or if it's not balanced by progesterone. The rule for estrogens is this: use the lowest possible dose that gives symptom relief.

The ideal preparations match the hormones found naturally in the female body. These would include any combination of estrone and estradiol from a formulary pharmacy; Estrace and the Estraderm or Climara patch, all types of estradiol; or Ortho-est, a type of estrone.

Note: estrogen given through the skin by patch or cream often results in much higher levels than oral preparations. In some cases, a woman will need only a tenth of the estrogen on her skin that she was taking as a pill. This is one of the reasons why monitoring blood hormone levels can be important.

Estriol

Women who have had breast cancer or an estrogen-associated neoplasia of any kind, as well as any women with concerns about breast cancer, are usually not considered suitable candidates for ERT, although some women will still want to take it. Among them are the famous Suzanne Somers, breast cancer survivor and author of the *The Sexy Years* (Crown Publishers, 2004), which addresses her very positive experience with bioidentical hormones. An alternative bioidentical hormone for these women may be estriol, a somewhat weaker estrogen that seems to have a protective effect against breast cancer.[16] Henry

Lemon, M.D., demonstrated this in a study of women with metastatic breast cancer. In a test group receiving estriol in dosages ranging from 2.5 to 15 mg per day, 37 percent experienced either remission or arrest of the cancer. A later study from Hebrew University of Jerusalem showed that in sufficient dosages, estriol actually has an antiestrogen effect, preventing estradiol from binding to estrogen-sensitive tissue (such as breast and endometrium), which then doesn't form tumors.[17] The most recent study is from Berkeley, where researchers found that rats receiving a three-week treatment of estriol with progesterone had a significantly reduced incidence of breast cancer.[18] Clearly, more research is required in this area.

The bottom line is that estriol seems very promising as an estrogen for those women who are worried about breast cancer. Not only does estriol not cause excessive cell growth in the uterine lining[19] or breast tissue, but it's good at helping hot flashes[20] and preventing vaginal dryness, and it has an equal benefit on the skin collagen layer as the other estrogens.[21] But very high doses (12 mg or more per day) are required to affect bone density. Such doses generally cause nausea and are therefore not clinically appropriate. It is also worth noting that estriol has been linked with otosclerosis in some women, a genetically linked condition in which the three small bones in the middle ear fuse together and thus fail to transmit sound to the brain. The usual oral dose is 2 mg per day.

Progesterone

Bioidentical progesterone is different from the synthetic progestins such as medroxprogesterone acetate (Provera). Unlike Provera, which is known to cause bloating, headaches, depression, and weight gain, and may also increase the risk of fatal coronary artery spasm (see section later in this chapter on heart disease), bioidentical progesterone has no serious side effects at the usual doses and has no adverse effects on blood lipids when compared to Provera.[22] There are occasions when a woman may need the strong pharmacologic effect of Provera, as in cases of heavy bleeding. For purpose of replacement, however, bioidentical progesterone is far superior in regard to both symptom relief and lack of side effects.

For clinical purposes, the usual conversion is 5 mg of Provera equals 100 mg of natural progesterone if a woman is using oral doses. In general, a significant amount of progesterone must be given to down-regulate estrogen receptors in breast tissue and the uterine lining in order to inhibit the growth-hormone effect of estrogen replacement.[23] Transdermal 2-percent progesterone cream at a dose of one-quarter teaspoon (about 20 mg) has also been shown to result in physiologic levels of progesterone, and this is often all that a woman needs to counteract the effects of estrogen, though this must be individualized.

Many doctors believe that 2-percent progesterone creams such as Emerita don't work because they don't result in increased blood levels. Serum levels of progesterone are often low when a woman is on progesterone creams because when progesterone is absorbed into the bloodstream, 80 percent of it will be bound to the plasma membranes of the red blood cells—the part that is thrown out when serum levels are checked. This is also the reason why salivary levels of hormones often measure higher than serum levels. Ideally, hormone levels will be monitored by a physician in a clinical setting. Most clinicians agree that how a patient feels on HRT is, ultimately, a far better measure of effectiveness than a blood or salivary hormone level. This has certainly been my experience.

For effectiveness, transdermal cream should contain a minimum of 375 mg progesterone per ounce. The following creams meet or surpass the standard: Emerita, PhytoGest, Bio Balance, Ostaderm, Progonol, ProBalance, and Serenity. The usual dose of these standardized progesterone creams is one-quarter to one-half teaspoon on the skin one or two times per day. There is virtually no danger of overdose, and many women use 375 to 400 mg, or the equivalent of an entire tube or jar, per week with no ill effects.

Bioidentical progesterone is also available in regular pharmacies in two forms: oral micronized progesterone under the brand name Prometrium and vaginal progesterone under the brand names Crinone 4% and 8% and Prochieve 4% and 8%.

Many preparations sold as wild yam (*Dioscorea*) creams may contain little or no progesterone. Although wild yams are one ingredient used in laboratory manufacture of progesterone and other sex hormones, there are no data to indicate that a yam cream will help a woman in the same manner as standardized formulas. Wild yam may have benefits as a phytohormone (plant hormone); it's just that it doesn't have the same measurable effects.

Although, as I've indicated, there is no standard HRT regimen, Dr. Joel Hargrove, former medical director of the Menopause Center at Vanderbilt University Medical Center, has shown very good clinical results using an average starting dose of 0.5 mg of estradiol and 100 mg of natural progesterone in a single capsule taken orally once per day.[24]

Even better results are obtained with transdermal applications in which the hormone goes right into the bloodstream via the skin without having to be absorbed from the gut and processed by the liver. Dr. Hargrove researched the following formulation: 2.5 mg estradiol and 25 mg progesterone per day, mixed in one teaspoon of fragrance-free body lotion. Dr. Erika Schwartz finds a different ratio has the most reliable and consistent effect: 0.6 mg of estradiol mixed with 200 mg progesterone.

In some cases, a woman will need only natural progesterone to relieve all of her menopausal symptoms. This is possible because progesterone is a precursor molecule that the body can use to produce estrogens and androgens. For example, the body may be able to make adequate DHEA from natural progesterone, which is why a common finding with natural progesterone supplementation is increased sex drive. (Alas, this doesn't work for everyone.)

Androgens

As I pointed out in the section on adrenal function, the androgenic DHEA and testosterone hormones are essential for energy, vitality, and sex drive. Note: female libido also has a great deal to do with thoughts and emotions. Hence some women with low androgen levels have good libido and some with normal androgen levels have low libido. Androgen levels may drop following hysterectomy even when the ovaries are spared; they may also drop following tubal ligation because of the change in blood supply to the ovary. Many women who don't feel their best even on estrogen and progesterone find that taking a small amount of DHEA or testosterone is all they need to feel like their old selves. The usual starting dose of oral DHEA is 5 mg twice per day. It's rare that a woman will need to increase this much beyond 10 mg twice per day. I prefer starting with DHEA supplementation first, since DHEA is a precursor for testosterone. Some women, however, will need testosterone supplementation directly, which can be given in pill form or as a cream. Many women find that natural testosterone at 1 or 2 mg every other day given as a vaginal cream clears up both vaginal dryness and libido problems. A formulary pharmacist can compound this for you with a prescription. More and more research is being done on this and a transdermal patch should be available soon. (Pharmaceutical-grade DHEA is available from formulary pharmacies.)

SYMPTOMS OF MENOPAUSE

What you're likely to experience in menopause has a lot to do with your beliefs, your culture, and your expectations. Given the culture of medicine, it's no surprise that the vast majority of studies through the years have been on women who were experiencing health problems during menopause. The medical system (which is simply a reflection of the larger culture) has only very recently begun to study the menopausal experience of healthy women who exercise regularly, don't smoke, eat a good diet, and lead a healthy lifestyle. And just as one might suspect, these studies are showing that healthy women don't have problems with bone loss, sex drive, cardiovascular disease, or depression!

The research on traditional cultures in which women's experiences are quite different is fascinating. For example, anthropologist Ann Wright studied menopausal symptoms in both traditional and acculturated Navaho women. She found that traditional Navahos exhibited few symptoms, and that economic ranking and social status were clearly related to women's experience of symptoms. Her study suggested that menopausal symptoms are caused by psychological rather than physical stress.[25]

A study of !Kung women in southern Africa showed that their social status increased after menopause. Moreover, there is no word for "hot flash" in the !Kung language. This points to the possibility that !Kung women either do not experience this symptom or experience it in a manner different than Western women and do not view it in a negative light.[26] By contrast, 80 to 90 percent of women in our culture experience hot flashes, and a significant number have vaginal dryness and loss of libido.

HOT FLASHES

Hot flashes, or vasomotor flushes, are characterized by a feeling of heat and sweating, particularly around the head and neck. They affect anywhere from 50 to 85 percent of women at some time during their climacteric years. For most women, hot flashes are simply an occasional sensation of warmth and slight sweating, but about 10 to 15 percent of women experience hourly waves of heat and drenching sweats that disrupt daily activities and can result in sleep disturbance and subsequent depression. Hot flashes usually subside in a year or so, but some women have them for anywhere from ten to forty years.[27] The actual cause of hot flashes is not known, though it is felt to be related to neurotransmitter changes that are poorly understood. Women may experience hot flashes during their adolescence and reproductive years, after having a baby, and premenstrually for reasons other than estrogen deficiency. Hot flashes have also been shown to increase when a woman is anxious or tense.

Treatment

Nutritional treatments. Many, many women notice vast improvements in sleep and hot flashes when they reduce their glycemic stress. (See chapter 17, "Nourishing Ourselves with Food.") Hot flashes almost always improve when you stop wine, sugar, white flour products, and coffee. (Sorry.) The reason for this is that these substances can raise blood sugar and adrenaline levels, thus resulting in imbalances of neurotransmitters. Take vitamin E (d-alpha tocopherol), 100 to 400 IU two times per day,[28] and citrus bioflavonoids with ascorbic acid, 200 mg four to six times daily.[29] Omega-3 fats such as those found in flax seed and fish oil are also very helpful.

Phytoestrogens. Phytoestrogens are naturally occurring estrogens found in more than three hundred plants, including soybeans and flaxseed (two particularly rich sources). Significant amounts of phytoestrogens are also found in cashews, peanuts, oats, corn, wheat, apples, and almonds.[30] Phytoestrogens contain isoflavanoids, which although not identical to, are chemically similar to the estrogens found in the human body. These substances prevent free-radical damage (the number-one cause of premature tissue aging) and appear to block the effects of excess estrogen stimulation of the breast and uterus. (The genistein in soy products also shows promise for decreasing cancer risk.) Phytoestrogens also decrease menopausal symptoms and modulate estrogen levels. It is hypothesized that Japanese women have a lower incidence of hot flashes and other symptoms because of their high intake of soy-based products.[31]

Soy protein, when taken in high enough dosages, has been shown to improve hair, skin, and nails; cool hot flashes; increase vaginal moisture; help with weight loss; and also improve the quality of life of menopausal women. A randomized, double-blind, placebo-controlled three-month clinical trial conducted at Johns Hopkins University in Baltimore showed that women consuming soy protein (in the form of Revival products) reported significant improvement in these areas.[32] Many of my newsletter subscribers and former patients have personally told me how much this high-dose soy product has helped them. One such woman wrote, "Revival has transformed my life! This last summer, my days were plagued by hot sweats, broken nails, and limp hair, plus I was overweight. Now, after four months of using Revival daily, I am twenty-four pounds lighter, my hair and nails are not brittle, and my sweats are completely gone. I am now in a new relationship. I feel like a new woman, young and vital, and I know without the symptoms of menopause I look and feel wonderful. I know I do not look fifty-two years old." (See Resources.)

Botanicals. A wide variety of herbs has been used to alleviate menopausal symptoms since antiquity. One of the most studied at this time is an extract of black cohosh (*Cimicifuga racemosa*), sold under the name Remifemin, and available in pharmacies and natural food stores. A substantial number of controlled clinical trials have shown that black cohosh is equal to conjugated equine estrogens in its ability to improve vaginal lubrication and to reduce depression, headache, and hot flashes. The usual dose is two tablets twice daily.[33] Other herbs that have been shown to be helpful are *Vitex agnus castii,* Siberian ginseng, dong quai, fo-ti, and wild yam.[34] Tinctures and oral combinations of these are widely available in natural food stores. They must be used for four to six weeks before improvement in symptoms is noted. Chinese herbal remedies have also been shown to reduce menopausal symptoms. Several excellent formulations are available, or consult an individual practitioner. (See Resources.) (Please note that botanicals and all natural treatments for hot flashes tend to take longer to work than estrogen. Estrogen is still the gold standard at cooling hot flashes!)

Natural progesterone. Natural progesterone has been shown to help hot flashes in some women.[35] This effect is most likely ascribable to the fact that it is a precursor hormone and also because it down-regulates estrogen receptors.

Estrogen replacement. The standard treatment for hot flashes, estrogen replacement—whether conventional or natural—effects a 100 percent decrease in this symptom when it is due to decreased estrogen levels.

Note that *not* all hot flashes are related to decreases in estrogen. Hyperthyroidism can cause them, as can alcohol intake and out-of-control diabetes. I had hot flashes during my pregnancies and sometimes premenstrually. Many women report similar patterns.

Energy medicine. Meditation and relaxation can help to relieve hot flashes. The relaxation response (see PMS section in chapter 5) has been successfully used by many women to decrease hot flashes by as much as 90 percent.[36] Traditional Chinese medicine and herbs are also very effective. The reason these work is because they all reduce levels of stress hormones that trigger hot flashes. The adrenal restoration program (see page 555) will also reduce hot flashes!

VAGINAL DRYNESS, IRRITATION, AND THINNING

Thinning of vaginal tissue in menopause is associated with decreased estrogen levels. Vaginal tissue is made of many cell layers. When the vaginal mucosa is well estrogenized, it is called "cornified epithelium." *Cornified* refers to cells that are tough and resilient. After menopause, some women lose the outer cornified layers of their vaginal tissue. This can lead to complaints of vaginal dryness and irritation. Such complaints are highly individual and subjective; a woman who has been diagnosed with atrophic vaginitis may not have any symptoms at all. In some women, thinning and irritation are accompanied by an increase of alkalinity of the vagina. At these higher pH levels, bacterial vaginitis sometimes results.

Oral or transdermal estrogen relieves symptoms of vaginal thinning. For some women, an application of estrogen cream directly to the vagina will often be all that's required. Transdermal estrogen or the vaginal ring (Estring) are also very effective.

Urinary frequency and symptoms of urinary tract infection are sometimes also associated with thinning of the vaginal mucosa and urethral tissues. (See section on UTIs and hormones in chapter 9.) This problem is easily alleviated by applying a small amount of estrogen cream directly to the vaginal tissue covering the outer third of the urethra, which you can feel running just beneath the top of the vaginal opening.

Treatment

Botanicals. Remifemin (black cohosh) works similarly to estriol to effect a thickening of the vaginal mucosa. Herbs such as dandelion leaves and oat straw have also been used to restore vaginal lubrication.[37] These herbs should be taken orally.

Lubricants. Crème de la Femme (available from Amazing Solutions; 800-576-7616 or www.amazing-solutions.com) is an oil-based lubricant that is very well tolerated and very effective. Estriol or testosterone can be added by a formulary pharmacist (150 mg of testosterone in oil per ounce of Crème de la Femme). The usual dose is one gram per day. Over-the-counter lubricants such as K-Y Jelly may also be used.[38]

Testosterone. One-half mg to 1 mg transdermally or as vaginal cream, daily or every third day, will restore vaginal mucosa function without the risk of creating excessively high systemic estrogen levels.[39]

Estriol. Estriol vaginal cream is applied in a dosage of 0.5 mg twice a day for one week, then once a day for one week, and two or three times weekly thereafter. Concerns surrounding the effect of estrogens on breast cancer are mitigated by the use of estriol, which exerts a very powerful local action but is weak systemically.[40]

Estradiol vaginal ring. Estring is a vaginal ring made of silicone and impregnated with estradiol. It is placed in the vagina like a diaphragm and continually releases small doses of estradiol for three months. It is a convenient choice for many women. A small percentage of women will experience side effects such as recurrent vaginal infections, headache, and vaginal irritation.

Conventional vaginal creams. Premarin, Ogen (conjugated equine estrogens), and Estrace (estradiol) are estrogen creams for treatment of vaginal dryness, thinning, and other symptoms.

OSTEOPOROSIS

Postmenopausal osteoporosis is one of the most common and disabling diseases affecting women in North America today. Studies have shown a 2- to 5-percent loss in bone mass per year in women over a five-year period during the climacteric. However, as much as 50 percent of a woman's bone loss over a life span is lost before the onset of menopause. Statistics show that 6 to 18 percent of women between the ages of twenty-five and thirty-four exhibit abnormally low bone density. Hip fracture rates for white women in the United States begin to rise abruptly between the ages of forty and forty-four, before the normal advent of menopause.[41] However, two recent studies have shown that a predisposition to falling created by "senile gait"—a shuffling, tentative walking style caused by muscle weakness and general lack of fitness—and poor eyesight is equal to low bone density as a significant factor for hip fracture risk.[42]

Progressive bone loss in women is due to factors far more complex than simply estrogen or calcium deficiency. Women need to realize that taking calcium is only one part of building strong bones. Magnesium, boron, vitamin D, vitamin C, and trace minerals are important. In fact, suboptimal vitamin D levels are increasingly implicated in osteoporosis. So are lack of exercise and depression. And while dairy products are pushed as a panacea to prevent osteoporosis, it's entirely possible to create and maintain healthy bones without eating dairy. (See chapter 17 for alternative calcium sources.) In fact, recent studies in both pre- and postmenopausal women report that consuming soy and soy isoflavones help to support better bone structure.[43] Bone density screening is recommended only for women who smoke, who have a history of excessive alcohol intake, or whose mothers have severe osteoporosis. Other risk factors include lack of exercise; a diet high in refined carbohydrates; deficiencies in calcium, magnesium, boron, trace minerals, and vitamin D; and never having borne a child.

Depression has also been shown to be a significant risk factor for osteoporosis. This is most likely due to the increased levels of cortisol usually associated with this condition.[44]

A history of ovulatory disturbances and subsequent progesterone deficiency can predispose women to osteoporosis. Women with a history of amenorrhea due to a low percentage of body fat, as is often found in athletes and dancers, are at greater risk for osteoporosis than the general population.[45]

The best way to determine your current bone density is through a screening test called dual-energy X-ray absorptiometry (DEXA). It can be used on the hips, spine, forearm, or entire body. It is brief (under ten minutes) and safe, because it uses a very low dose of radiation. A urine test for metabolic breakdown products of bone (Pyrilinks-D) is also helpful in determining a woman's osteoporosis risk.

Bone-Health Program

Although estrogen replacement is very effective for decreasing osteoporosis risk, a program of dietary adjustments, exercise, vitamin D, calcium, and magnesium can also be very effective in preventing, halting, or even reversing bone loss.

One of my patients went in for a bone density test when she went through menopause at the age of fifty-three. It showed that her bone density was low normal. Her mother had died of breast cancer when my patient was thirteen, so she had no intention of going on estrogen. Instead, she was immediately advised to start taking Fosamax, a drug that prevents bone breakdown, and get the scan repeated in six months. She called me, deeply concerned that her bones were melting away. I reassured her that this wasn't the case and suggested a program of weight training, natural progesterone, and supplementation with boron, calcium, magnesium, vitamin D, vitamin C, and trace minerals (see below). Within six months, her bones had shown a significant increase in density. The doctor at the osteoporosis center told her that he was very surprised at her results, and said that she should keep on doing whatever she was doing. She has had a scan every two years since then and her density has remained excellent.

Though the bone-building drugs such as Fosamax, Boniva, and Actonel are probably better than nothing and have been shown to decrease fracture risk, I'd prefer they be used as a last resort. Try the recommendations here first. Fosamax (alendronate) is also associated with severe esophageal ulceration in some cases. Another bone builder, Miacalcin (calcitonin), comes in a nasal spray and can help older women with painful osteoporosis. Boniva can be taken once a month. But once again, I'd prefer more natural approaches as a first line of therapy.

Diet. Switch to a nutrient-rich, whole-food diet. (See chapter 17.)

Exercise. Two forty-minute sessions per week of weight-bearing exercise such as walking, bicycling, or weight training will help increase bone density.

Reduce phosphate consumption. Phosphate consumption directly interferes with calcium absorption. Eliminate cola and root beer drinks, which are too high in phosphate.

Quit smoking and cut back on alcohol. Since smokers, along with women who consume two or more alcoholic drinks daily, are at highest risk for osteoporosis, women should refrain from smoking and limit alcohol intake.[46]

Limit caffeine. Caffeine increases the rate at which calcium is lost in the urine. Daily intake should be limited to no more than the equivalent of the caffeine in one to two cups of coffee.[47]

Vitamin D. We're increasingly finding suboptimal levels of vitamin D in women with osteoporosis. Taking calcium without vitamin D is almost useless. Take at least 1,000 IU of vitamin D per day.[48] (For a more detailed discussion of the importance of vitamin D, see chapter 17.)

Beta-carotene. Take 25,000 units per day (15 mg). Beta-carotene is converted into vitamin A in the body. Vitamin A promotes a healthy intestinal epithelium, which is important for optimal absorption of nutrients, and it also promotes strong joints. It is found in abundance in yellow and orange vegetables such as acorn squash and carrots and also in dark green leafy vegetables.

Natural progesterone. Progesterone's role in bone metabolism is well documented but frequently overlooked.[49] I recommend one-quarter to one-half teaspoon of 2-percent cream daily on the skin.

Vitamin C. This nutrient assists in collagen synthesis and repair. The recommended dose is 2,000 mg per day.[50] The work of Dr. Linus Pauling suggests that optimal vitamin C intake should be much higher than we've been taught. An orange provides only 60 mg per day, but Dr. Pauling's evidence is quite convincing that vitamin C is beneficial and has no side effects at levels around 2,000 mg per day or even more.

Magnesium. Magnesium should be taken at a dose of 400 to 800 mg per day, depending upon the quality of your diet.[51] Magnesium is a constituent of bone and is essential for several biochemical reactions involved in bone building. The standard American diet is low in magnesium. A diet low in magnesium and relatively high in calcium can actually contribute to osteoporosis. Though blood levels of magnesium are often normal, this is misleading. A more accurate test is red blood cell magnesium, which is often low in cases of depression and fatigue. (See the section on magnesium in chapter 17.) Overconsumption of processed food is usually the culprit in magnesium deficiency. This nutrient is found in organically grown vegetables, whole grains, sea vegetables, and meats such as turkey.

Manganese. This nutrient should be supplemented in the form of manganese picolinate. The recommended dose is 15 mg per day.

Calcium. One thousand to 1,500 mg per day should be taken in the form of aspartate, citrate, or lactate. You can take less if you obtain significant amounts from your food. Despite widespread promotion of the antacid Tums as a way to obtain needed calcium, better supplements are available. Although the calcium carbonate found in Tums has been shown to increase bone density, it also exerts an alkalizing effect on stomach acid, thereby inhibiting calcium absorption and increasing the risk of kidney stones.[52]

Boron. Boron is a trace element found in fruits, nuts, and vegetables. It has been found to reduce urinary calcium loss and to increase serum levels of 17-beta estradiol (the most biologically active estrogen); both of these effects help bone health. The minimum daily dose of boron needed (2 mg per day) is easily met with a diet rich in fruits, nuts, and vegetables; supplements can be taken up to 12 mg per day.[53]

SEXUALITY IN MENOPAUSE

What we believe about sexuality and menopause has a lot to do with our sexual expectations and experience. A very common misconception about menopause is that sexual desire and activity significantly decline during this period. The newest research fails to show any significant link between menopause and decreased sexual functioning.[54] Because our society has viewed menopause as "failed productivity" and associates reproductive capacity with sexual capacity, many women have bought the belief that their sex drive is supposed to go away. But in humans, the capacity for sexual pleasure and the capacity for reproduction are two distinct functions. We can always have one without the other.

The most recent research shows that in healthy, happy women, there's no significant decline in libido, let alone in sexual satisfaction, frequency of sexual intercourse, or genital responsiveness, and ease or difficulty reaching orgasm after menopause. In fact, a woman's relationship satisfaction, attitudes towards sex and aging, vaginal dryness, cultural background, and overall mental and physical health have a much greater impact on sexual functioning than does being in menopause. Many of my menopausal patients who left unsatisfying marriages and remarried more compatible mates ended up having better sex lives than ever. Particularly striking was one very proper seventy-five-year-old woman who always came in dressed formally in blouses with high lace collars. She was having a problem with some vaginal dryness and was worried that she'd have to stop her sexual activity. Newly married, she was regularly having seven orgasms per lovemaking session with her husband, after being anorgasmic for her entire forty years of marriage with her first husband. She told me that she had had no idea how wonderful sexual activity could be. All she needed was a bit of estrogen cream and some reassurance that she was normal.

Another woman, age fifty-five, was at her most sexually fulfilled when she began a relationship with a man fifteen years younger than she. There is some evidence that in prepatriarchal times, the older women initiated the younger men in sexual learning that would be especially pleasing to women. The combination of an older woman and younger man in this regard makes perfect sense—though up until very recently, this has gone against everything that our culture has taught us! (No one blinks an eye when a fifty-five-year-old man marries a twenty-five-year-old woman, however.) Sexual preference may also change at midlife. Several of my patients have found themselves sexually attracted to women after menopause, although they had defined themselves as heterosexual beforehand.

Some women truly do notice a decline in libido at menopause. One of them told me that her lack of libido is not a problem for her personally, but she does worry about her husband getting enough sex. I suspect that this concern is shared by many. One of the reasons that libido falls during perimenopause for some women is that their life-force, or *chi,* is simply exhausted from years of stress and they have nothing left over for sexual desire. Many women also find their energy turned inward for a time as they reinvent themselves at midlife. It is also clear that levels of testosterone, which play a role in sexual desire, decrease in many older women for a wide variety of reasons.[55] If the levels are low, these androgenic hormones can be replaced to normal levels.[56] (See section on adrenal restoration in this chapter.)

For other women, however, the climacteric and postmenopausal period is associated with heightened sexual drive and activity. For many, it is the first time that they are truly free from the fear of unwanted pregnancy. Many physicians mistakenly believe older women who are not sexually active lack sexual drive. But studies have shown that the reason they are not sexually active is usually that they have no partner, or their partner is ill, or they have vaginal thinning leading to pain with intercourse (a condition that is easily remedied with one of the remedies on page 576). For some women, the availability of a suitable partner is more important to their sexual interest and desire than any other factor. Of greatest importance to continued sexual desire and interest is marital happiness.[57]

Another problem for many heterosexual women is that their male partner's ability to get and maintain an erection may change as he ages. If the male perceives this as impending impotence, he may avoid sexual activity altogether. Many women have told me that they would like to enjoy regular sexual activity, but their husbands won't participate anymore because of their fear of impotence. Because these women are afraid of offending their husband's ego, however, they keep quiet instead of getting help. Drugs like Viagra, Levitra, and Cialis have helped this situation. However, new risks for these drugs are coming to light. The Health Research Group of consumer advocacy organization Public Citizen has asked the FDA for a black box warning on these drugs because reports of unilateral vision loss (loss of sight in one eye) have been linked to them. Men should also know, however, that the same diet and supplement programs that help support menopausal hormone balance in women also help men maintain optimal sexual function without drugs.[58] Usually all the help most men need is a bit of education. Still, antihypertensive and other medications can interfere with erection and even orgasmic capacity in some men. Lifestyle changes such as weight loss, improved diet, supplementation, and increased physical activity can reverse hypertension in those who are motivated to make them.

Ancient Taoist cultures taught special exercises (like the ovarian breathing exercises described in chapter 7) to the women of royal families, who were reported to retain their youthful appearance and sexual potency long after menopause as a result. These exercises all involved using the mind to flow life-force energy throughout the body. Especially important to these practices was (and still is) the rerouting of potent ovarian energy to other organs of the body. Mantak Chia, a master teacher of these techniques, writes, "With the Ovarian Kung Fu method as it is now taught, a woman can continue sexual activity for as long as she desires because no energy is lost; in fact, energy is gained through the transformation of her sexual energy." He adds that many Taoist women consider the results of these exercises to be the best cosmetic in existence.[59] You don't need to get into ancient Taoist techniques to keep your sex drive strong. What you have to do is actually train your body to be able to receive more pleasure. This takes care of the life-force all by itself. (See chapter 8, "Reclaiming the Erotic.")

Treatment

Treatment for lack of sex drive must be highly individualized, but, as I mentioned, all women with this problem should consider having their testosterone and DHEA levels measured. Some women report feeling more like their former selves on estrogen replacement. Others note an increase in libido following the use of a transdermal 2-percent progesterone cream, which may work, in part, because natural progesterone is a precursor molecule and can be turned into androgens and even estrogen when the body needs more of these hormones. Testosterone is the major androgen associated with libido. In those women who don't seem to be able to produce enough of their own androgens, DHEA or testosterone in the form of a skin cream, a gel, or a capsule can be given. (The first line of treatment is to follow the program for adrenal restoration on pages 555 of this chapter.)

If both DHEA and testosterone levels are low, I prefer replenishing DHEA first, because it is a precursor of testosterone, and when women take it in the usual doses (10 to 25 mg per day), their testosterone levels increase by one and a half to two times.[60] When given with progesterone, DHEA can enhance well-being in those women who don't respond to progesterone alone. Some older women have naturally high levels of DHEA, so not everyone needs it. The side effect of too much testosterone or DHEA is a slight increase in hair growth on arms and legs and sometimes the face.

The dose of testosterone for those who don't respond to DHEA is 1 mg daily or every other day, depending upon the individual.

Other women have done well with homeopathic remedies, acupuncture, or herbs. Whatever therapy you choose, there is likely to be a placebo effect on the libido simply because you are doing something to help yourself. Remember, sometimes it's your *life* that needs "medicine." When you make positive changes (including adding more pleasurable activities), your hormones will balance themselves. Because sexual function and libido are so intimately connected to our thoughts and emotions, it's also important for women who want to enhance libido to actually take the time to think about sex more often. Reading erotic material, watching erotic movies, and spending time self-pleasuring can often jump-start a flagging libido.

Note: Estratest is a combination of equine estrogens and synthetic methyltestosterone. It is often the only solution offered to women with libido problems. However, the dose is too high for many women and it is difficult to make adjustments. The hormones in it are also foreign to the female body. I do not recommend it.

THINNING HAIR

Up to one-third of menopausal and postmenopausal women in this culture have problems with thinning hair. Confusingly, hair loss on the head may be accompanied by excess hair growth on the face. This is because all hair follicles are not created equal in their response to hormones. Much of this problem is related to subtle imbalances of hormones, at the level of the androgen-sensitive hair follicle, that do not show up on standard testing. These imbalances are associated with insulin resistance and overconsumption of refined carbohydrates.

Treatment

- Follow a diet that normalizes blood sugar and insulin and also decreases inflammation. (See chapter 17.)
- Lose excess body fat.
- Take a good multivitamin-mineral supplement.
- Use laser acupuncture or traditional needle acupuncture.
- Use the Chinese herbal nutritional supplement known as Shou Wu Pian. This supplement, if taken regularly for at least two to three months, can restore the natural color of hair if it has gone gray, tends to increase overall energy, and also helps restore hair growth in many individuals. (To order Shou Wu Pian, call Quality Life Herbs at 207-842-4929 or visit www.qualitylife-herbs.com.)

MOOD SWINGS AND DEPRESSION

Research shows that menopause itself does not contribute to poor psychological or physical health. In fact, menopausal women age forty-five to sixty-four actually have a significantly lower incidence of depression than younger women. Moreover, the major stress in the lives of menopausal women is most often caused by family or by factors other than menopause.[61] For example, approximately 25 percent of women in the menopausal years are caring for an elderly relative, according to some studies, which certainly can be stressful.[62] Dr. Sonja McKinlay, an associate professor of community health at Brown University, who researched a group of healthy menopausal women who were not seeking medical advice, says, "For the majority of women, menopause is not the major negative event it has been typified as. That is basic mythology." She noted that only 2 to 3 percent of the women in her study expressed any regret at moving out of their reproductive years. One unique feature of this study is that it was done on healthy women who were not seeking medical advice. Clearly, many physicians have a negative view of menopause in part because they see only women who have menopause-related complaints.

As I pointed out earlier, however, menopause is a time when we may come up against the unfinished business that we have accumulated over the first half of our lives. We may find ourselves grieving for losses never fully grieved, wanting to get a college degree that we never completed, or longing for another child or a first child. It is as if we have gone down into our basement and found boxes and boxes of stuff to be sorted through and weeded out. If a woman is willing to deal with her own unfinished business, she will have fewer menopausal symptoms. She will find that her symptoms are messages from her inner guidance system that parts of her life need attention. And her changing hormones will provide the impetus to make long-needed changes.

Treatment

When a woman is willing to resolve the unfinished emotional business of her life, often no treatment of her mood swings is necessary. The inner work discussed in part 3 of this book is a good place to start. Dietary improvement and exercise can often work wonders. Many women with depression have been following a diet that is so low in fat, they can't make the proper brain chemicals to lift depression. (See chapter 17.)

Other women will need physical support of their endocrine, energy, and emotional systems through ERT, homeopathy, acupuncture, and/or other approaches. Among the botanicals, Remifemin can help to alleviate these symptoms.[63] Saint-John's-wort (*Hypericum perforatum*) has also been shown to be very helpful in mild to moderate depression, allowing many women to get off their other antidepressant medication. Look for a standardized 0.3 percent formulation. The dose of Saint-John's-wort is 300 mg three times per day with meals.[64]

Hormone replacement lifts depression in some women but has no effect on others. Each case has to be examined holistically to determine optimal treatment.

FUZZY THINKING

Many women talk about a perimenopausal change in their thought process. This "fuzzy thinking" is most commonly described as an inability to think straight, and is a normal development that is self-limiting. Marian Van Eyk McCain, in her book *Transformation Through Menopause* (Bergin & Garvey, 1991), calls this "cottonhead," or feeling unable to use the left brain or intellect for such tasks as balancing the checkbook or getting organized.[65] I have asked many women about this and have found it to be common. Many are very relieved to find that it is normal, because they are afraid they are getting Alzheimer's disease. There is no evidence to support the commonly held myth that women (or men) normally lose their memory or get "senile" as they age.[66]

After I read about "cottonhead," I realized that I felt this same way after having my children. I seemed virtually unable to concentrate on linear tasks. My brain felt fuzzy. I wanted to watch movies, be with my baby, and not have to think, at least in the limited way that our culture defines thinking. The way I understand this "cottonhead" state is that it may disconnect us temporarily from our frontal lobes, the part of the brain that is involved with rational, linear, planning-for-the-future thought. We now have a chance to think with our hearts. If we allow this process to unfold, if we don't fight it or see it as a dysfunction, it can be an initiation into a whole new way of experiencing the world, a far more intuitive way. For many women the ability to express themselves in art, writing, or sculpting comes from allowing their "cotton-headedness" to center them and help them withdraw from the world ruled by the steely organized intellect. Neuropsychiatrist Mona Lisa Schulz, M.D., Ph.D., author of *The New Feminine Brain* (Free Press, 2005), points out that temporarily forgetting names or where you put the phone are not caused by memory loss, per se. These lapses are related, instead, to attention. Many perimenopausal women turn their attention deeply inward—a natural way to do healing work.

If you want to be proactive, however, several clinical trials have shown that eating soy helps prevent memory loss.[67] Researchers believe this may be due to the ability of soy isoflavones to protect nerve cells from oxidative stress. In one study, postmenopausal women ages fifty-one to sixty-six years consuming 60 milligrams of isoflavones per day for six weeks showed an improvement in nonverbal short-term memory, mental flexibility, and planning ability. Other studies have shown that soy supports memory in premenopausal women, as well (and men, too).

When Peggy, a fifty-eight-year-old kindergarten teacher, went through menopause, she began to experience an inability to concentrate in her classroom. "After thirty years as a teacher," she said, "I couldn't remember the names of the kids in my classes, and sometimes I couldn't even remember how to spell words." Every fiber of her being told her to take a sabbatical from teaching to give her inner life some attention. Her "thinking" problem became so bad that she eventually started crying in front of her classes. She realized that she needed a change. She left school, traveled to California, and lived in a small cottage near the beach for a year. During that time, she began to knit. She found that the knitting was exactly what her brain needed for meditative activity.

On a hunch, Peggy began to teach senior citizens the knitting techniques she was learning. She mailed a beach chair to me. She had hand-knitted the seat and the back in beautiful and unusual designs. She found that her skills were in great demand. In addition to her knitting, she allowed herself to grieve fully for the end of her marriage ten years before. She forgave herself for the impact that it had had on her son. By the time I saw her a year later, she was a healed women with a great deal of trust in life. She had accepted the challenge of menopause, moved into her intuitive side, and begun a whole new life. She now spends half the year in California and half the year in Maine. She is back to a small amount of teaching, on her own terms. She no longer forgets names or class plans.

LONG-TERM HEALTH CONCERNS

Breast Cancer

The most common concern women have about hormone replacement is the fear of breast cancer, and it's the main reason many women don't want anything to do with ERT, even when it could help them. Jerilynn Prior, M.D., founder and scientific director of the Centre for Menstrual Cycle and Ovulation Research (CeMCOR) in Vancouver, B.C., believes that progesterone might actually decrease the risk for invasive breast cancer because studies show it opposes the effects of estrogen.[68] Her controversial research shows that estrogen levels are significantly higher than normal during perimenopause.[69] To counterbalance these high levels of estrogen, Dr. Prior, also the author of *Estrogen's Storm Season: Stories of Perimenopause* (Centre for

Menstrual Cycle and Ovulation Research, 2005), prescribes progesterone to successfully treat hot flashes, low bone density, and menstrual problems.

I believe that if the estrogen and progesterone used in replacement were bioidentical as previously described, and if they were used at dosages tailored to an individual woman, we would not find an increase in breast cancer risk.

Dr. Isaac Schiff, chief of Vincent Memorial Obstetrics and Gynecology Service at Massachusetts General Hospital in Boston, keeps a breast cancer risk chart on his desk to help his patients see clearly what the estrogen–breast cancer statistics really mean for them personally. I have found this approach so helpful that I have reproduced the chart here. Risk of breast cancer must be kept in perspective.

TABLE 10

THE EFFECTS OF HRT ON BREAST CANCER RISK

Your Current Age	Probability of Breast Cancer Diagnosis This Year	
	With 5 years HRT	Without HRT
50–54	1 in 320	1 in 450
55–59	1 in 275	1 in 386
60–64	1 in 209	1 in 292
65–69	1 in 144	1 in 244

Source: Cancer Statistics Review 1973–1989, excerpted from the August 1995 issue of the Harvard Women's Health Watch, ©1995, President and Fellows of Harvard College.

As already mentioned, there is an association between excessive amounts of carbohydrates in the diet and breast cancer, so keep the amount of refined carbohydrates in your diet moderate.[70] Also, in a controlled trial of alcohol intake, women receiving oral Premarin and those on ERT had an average 300 percent increase in estradiol levels for five hours following ingestion of alcohol. Those not receiving hormone replacement showed no comparable increase. Women should consequently be counseled to limit alcohol intake when on oral hormone replacement therapy.[71]

The optimum approach for a woman with breast cancer concerns is either to avoid HRT or to use estriol, small amounts of progesterone, and botanicals, or to use the minimum effective dose of estradiol or estrone. (See Program to Promote Healthy Breast Tissue in chapter 10, "Breasts.")

Heart Disease

Heart disease is the leading killer of postmenopausal women. If you have any personal or family history of heart disease, understand that diet and lifestyle changes can reverse or greatly alleviate your risk of getting it with or without estrogen. Chief among the risk factors for heart disease is increased insulin resistance, which is present to some degree in 50 to 75 percent of women in this country. Problems with insulin and overconsumption of refined carbohydrates result in increased body fat and aberrations in lipid profile.[72] (See chapter 17.) An enormous amount of data exists on the link between nutrition and heart disease, particularly with regard to the ill effects of excess insulin and the benefits of antioxidants. A 1997 study reported in the *American Journal of Clinical Nutrition* demonstrated that a diet too high in carbohydrates and low in fat increased the risk of heart disease because of its adverse effects on lipids and insulin. The authors concluded that given their results, "it seems reasonable to question the wisdom of recommending that postmenopausal women consume low-fat, high-carbohydrate diets."[73] It has also been demonstrated that in individuals with stable angina (chest pain), a high-carbohydrate meal will induce cardiac ischemia during a treadmill test much more quickly than a high-fat meal.[74]

A lifestyle characterized by overconsumption of trans-fatty acids and refined carbohydrates, combined with inadequate exercise and protein and micronutrients sets the stage for cellular inflammation, which in turn creates a predisposition to hypertension, diabetes, and heart disease.[75] By contrast, a diet that contains fish oil has also been found to reduce the incidence of heart disease better than statin drugs in a number of studies. I'd recommend two servings per week of sardines, mackerel, salmon, or swordfish that is virtually mercury free[76] (such as products from Vital Choice Seafood; for more information, call Vital Choice at 800-608-4825.) If you are a vegetarian, high-quality flaxseed oil, ground flaxseed, hemp seed oil, or macadamia nuts or oil can be beneficial. (See Resources.) Anyone with a family history of diabetes, hypertension, or heart disease should follow the dietary guidelines in chapter 17.

Weight-bearing exercise can also be very helpful because it lowers insulin resistance dramatically. (See chapter 17.) It will help increase lean muscle, and because lean muscle mass has a higher metabolic rate than fat, it helps to burn excess body fat and thus lower the risk of heart disease. Women who perform such exercise live an average of six years longer than those who do not.

For those women who are already on hormone replacement of some type, including synthetic progestin in the form of Provera, Amen, Cycrin, or Prempro, I'd recommend a switch to natural progesterone. A study at the Oregon Regional Primate Center induced heart attacks, by injecting chemicals into several groups of monkeys whose ovaries had been removed to simulate menopause. They found that monkeys on Provera had an unrelenting constriction of their coronary arteries, cutting off blood flow. These monkeys would have died had treatment not been initiated. The chemical challenge produced the same effect in those monkeys not on any hormones at all. But in the monkeys on estrogen alone, and those on estrogen plus natural progesterone, blood flow was quickly restored with no treatment necessary. Similar effects have also been anecdotally reported in humans. Clearly, the take-home message is: get off Provera (or Prempro) if you are using it for HRT and substitute bioidentical progesterone. (In all fairness, the reanalysis of the data from the Women's Health Initiative [WHI] study and Nurses' Health Study showed a decreased risk of heart disease in women who started HRT within ten years of menopause, and the risk of heart disease was decreased by 11 percent even in those using estrogen plus synthetic progesterone. But the risk reduction was even better [44 percent] in women on estrogen alone—which may point to the adverse effect of the synthetic progestin.)

Some women experience heart palpitations in menopause, often related to emotions such as panic, fear, and depression, all of which raise adrenaline levels, which causes blood pressure and heart rate to increase. Biofeedback such as the HeartMath technique described earlier (see section on adrenals in this chapter) can help dramatically with this symptom. Saint-John's-wort may also be helpful (see section on mood swings and depression in this chapter). Regular expressions of joy and creativity are important for a healthy and functioning cardiovascular system and, in the end, are likely to be the best prevention. These emotions reduce levels of stress hormones. Louise Hay likens blood flow to the flow of joy throughout the body. The more pleasure and joy you take in life, the more freely the blood flows!

ALZHEIMER'S DISEASE

While the fuzzy thinking many women experience perimeno-pausally is not a symptom of Alzheimer's disease, it's important to understand what factors are associated with Alzheimer's, the most common cause of dementia—accounting for more than half of all cases. (Other forms of dementia are caused by hardening of the arteries in the brain and by the effect of chronic alcohol use and a nutrient-poor diet.) Currently, about 7 per 1,000 people between age sixty-five and sixty-nine have dementia (half with Alzheimer's). Between age eighty-five and eighty-nine, that number climbs to 118 per 1,000 (with almost 73 ascribed to Alzheimer's).[77] The total number of Americans with Alzheimer's, estimated at 4.5 million, has more than doubled since 1980 and is expected to reach between 11.3 and 16 million by 2050.[78]

While Alzheimer's is frequently portrayed as a disease targeting women more often than men, that's true only in data from Europe and Asia. U.S. data shows the incidence is split fairly equally among women and men.[79]

Millions of women have taken HRT in part to ward off dementia because estrogen was originally thought to be protective, yet data from the Women's Health Initiative Memory Study (WHIMS) showed that the risk of dementia in the estrogen-only HRT group was 49 percent higher than in women not taking hormones.[80] While the individual risk is small (among 10,000 women using hormones, 37 could be expected to develop dementia, compared to 25 in the no-hormone group—a mere 12 extra cases) and the risk was not deemed statistically significant, the data is still cause for some concern. As I've already said, I believe Premarin (the type of estrogen used in this study) to be the most problematic of all the choices out there. It is also true that estrogen, like birth control pills, increases the risk of blood clots. This is probably the reason for the dementia risk—small as it is. Given that a high glycemic index diet (which most Americans are on) also increases the risk of stroke, I'd highly recommend cleaning up your diet and taking antioxidants if you are on HRT.

While it's hard to predict exactly who will eventually be diagnosed with dementia, a long-term study of nuns showed that those with the highest cognitive function in early life were the least likely to develop Alzheimer's disease decades later.[81] Women who maintain normal memory and brain function throughout life tend to share a set of characteristics, which include:

~ Good health
~ Financial security
~ Above-average intelligence and education
~ Active personal interests
~ Sense of satisfaction and accomplishment in life

Dementia is not inevitable. Most women have a very good chance of preserving our memories as we grow older—and in fact may even improve them. Neuropsychological testing has shown that brain function in healthy older people remains normal throughout the eighth decade (which is as far along as it has currently been studied).

There is no question, however, that hormones have an effect on brain function. To date, there have been a few studies of women with mild to moderate Alzheimer's whose memory has improved initially on estrogen. And, in fact, estradiol (one type of natural estrogen) binds to the areas in the brain that are associated with memory and are affected by Alzheimer's disease: the cortex, the hippocampus, and the basal forebrain. Finally, both estrogen and progesterone have also been shown to enhance nerve cell branching.[82]

Brain function and memory preservation—and the acetylcholine levels associated with these functions—are also affected by a wide variety of other factors besides estrogen. For more information, see *The New Feminine Brain* (Free Press, 2005) by Mona Lisa Schulz, M.D., Ph.D.

Combat the Myths of Aging

Our society currently operates under the mistaken notion that it is normal to become senile, lose memory, and have a change of personality with age—and all of us have been around relatives and friends with Alzheimer's or other dementias and know what a toll this illness can take on everyone concerned.

Learn about normal brain development so you don't buy in to a self-fulfilling prophecy about memory decline with age. Here are the facts: When you are born, you have a full complement of nerve cells in your brain, which reaches its peak size at about age twenty, after which there is a gradual decline in size throughout the rest of your life. If bigger is better, that would mean that we reach peak wisdom and intelligence by age twenty, which is a completely ridiculous notion (this will immediately become obvious to you if you watch much MTV).

The key to appreciating and enhancing your brain function is to re-alize that normal loss of brain cells over time is not necessarily associ-ated with loss of function. In fact, studies have shown that throughout our lifetime, as we move from naiveté to wisdom, our brain function becomes molded along the lines of wisdom. Think of your brain as a tree that requires regular pruning if it is to acquire its optimal shape and function. Brain cell loss with aging is akin to pruning the nonessen-tial branches that may actually be interfering with optimal function by clouding consciousness and mental clarity. Complementing this process, the dendritic and axonal branching among brain cells actually increase with age as our capacity to make complex associations in-creases. What this means is that the older and more experienced you become, the more likely you are to lose inessential connections and cells in your brain but develop new connections that help you synthesize your experiences. This is how wisdom gets wired! By contrast, retarded adults do not appear to have this selective capacity as they age.[83]

An Alzheimer's Prevention Program

Protect yourself with antioxidants. Adequate antioxidant and vitamin intake helps prevent Alzheimer's since it reduces the amount of free-radical damage to brain tissue.[84] Free radicals are unstable molecules that are formed in our cell tissue by culprits like radiation, trans-fatty acids, and even oxygen. These free radicals combine with normal, healthy tissue and cause microscopic scarring and damage, which over time sets the stage for loss of tissue function and disease. Antioxidant vitamins, such as vitamin E, help quench these free radicals as soon as they are produced, thus helping to spare our brains, heart, blood ves-sels, and other tissues from their ill effects.

Make sure your diet is rich in vitamins C and E, selenium, and the B vitamins, including folic acid. In fact, vitamin E has been shown to slow the progression of already diagnosed Alzheimer's, but why wait? Another class of powerful antioxidants are the proanthocyanidins found in pine bark and grape pips. Since a great deal of brain health de-pends on minimizing free-radical damage, women should include a good antioxidant formula in their daily supplementation program.

Avoid smoking and excessive alcohol intake. Alcohol affects the basal forebrain—an area associated with memory. And cigarettes are well-known factors in causing cardiovascular disease and small blood vessel changes that decrease oxygen to your brain tissue.

Protect your brain acetylcholine levels. Avoid drugs that are known to decrease acetylcholine levels. Decreased acetylcholine is associated with memory loss and confusion. You'd be amazed at how many of these there are and how few doctors realize their adverse effect on brain function. Check the label of any medication used for sleep, colds, or allergies to see if it contains diphenhydramine (which is commonly sold under the name Benadryl). Examples are Tylenol PM, Excedrin PM, Actifed, Contac, and Tylenol Flu PM.

Estrogen, DHEA, and pregnenolone. Estrogen, DHEA, and pregnenolone (a steroid hormone related to progesterone) have been shown to encourage dendritic and axonal branching between brain cells—a process associated with enhanced memory.[85] This is one of the reasons why some women on estrogen report better mood and even memory. On the other hand, data from the Women's Health Initiative study suggests that Prempro actually increased the risk of dementia possibly because of the adverse effects of Prempro on blood flow in the brain (it's associated with increased risk of stroke). Again—this effect may have been because the HRT was used in older women who hadn't started HRT earlier. I'd also expect an adverse effect of hormones in smokers. It's ideal for memory when your body can be healed into producing its own steroids (like DHEA) naturally. (See Adrenal Restoration Program, page 555.) In some cases, however, a small dose of bioidentical hormones might be beneficial for memory.

Consume omega-3 fats. All of the cells of the central nervous system (the brain and spinal cord) are made from specific types of fat. The omega-3 class of fats is particularly important for healthy brain function. I recommend 1,000 to 5,000 mg of omega-3 fats daily. (See chapter 17.)

Engage in regular exercise. Studies have shown that exercise improves memory even in those who are already showing signs of dementia. Imagine what it does to prevent the problem!

Remain a lifelong learner. I can't stress enough how important this is. In fact, I feel that it's the most important factor of all for Alzheimer's prevention. To maintain and enhance your brain function and wisdom, you must remain interested in the ongoing process of life. You must be actively engaged in some form of pleasurable activity involving growth, development, and learning. Take classes, get together with friends, learn a new sport or activity, start a new career or business, or engage in volunteer work. Tone your brain cells and neural pathways with new ideas, new connections, and new thoughts every day. Make sure you're on the path toward becoming a wise woman of power—not a "little old lady."

DECIDING ON MENOPAUSAL TREATMENT

The Woman's Health Initiative data on Prempro changed the entire field of menopausal treatment overnight. Suddenly all the presumed benefits of HRT were replaced with doubt and fear. We moved from black and white to shades of gray. And at the end of the day, this is a good thing, though perhaps not as reassuring as the old "magic bullet" approach of the past.

Know this: when it comes to treatment for your menopausal symptoms, you really can't make a mistake. Think of the whole time as a grand transition in which you'll be flying by the seat of your pants and finding your own personal truth. Many women will look to their physicians for consultation and recommendations. Ideally their physicians will provide guidance while understanding that the person who is most familiar with her body and in touch with its responses is the woman herself, and she should therefore be encouraged to relate her experiences. All women going through this life transition need to heed their inner wisdom in deciding upon appropriate treatment.

If a woman is experiencing many menopausal symptoms, has tried dietary changes, supplementation, and exercise, and still has symptoms, I recommend a trial run of bioidentical hormones. After a three-month period on a starting dose your progress should be reevaluated. Remember, a woman's decision to begin HRT is not irreversible. Our bodies are constantly changing and evolving; therefore, prescriptions should be reviewed and updated regularly as hormone levels and life circumstances change. I recommend that women remake the decision about HRT on an annual basis depending upon how they feel. You have nothing to lose with this approach and a great deal to gain.

Getting Off HRT or Changing Types

Many women find that when one type of HRT doesn't work for them, another type will. In general, it is fine to switch from one type to another without any time lag in between. For example, you can take your Premarin one day, and start on natural estradiol the next.

If you want to *stop* HRT, however, do it very gradually. Usually this means taking one less tablet per week until you are off your estrogen completely. When you taper off slowly in this way, there is much less chance of having rebound hot flashes. Some women begin to use 2-percent progesterone cream and after one month or so gradually taper their estrogen so that they are just on the progesterone cream or herbal combination. This gives your body time to feel the benefits of the new regimen while slowly weaning it away from the old.

SELF-CARE DURING MENOPAUSE

When making your self-care choices during the menopausal transition, please keep the following principles in mind:

~ Your body was designed to be healthy for at least a hundred years and probably longer.

~ Dementia, osteoporosis, heart disease, and cancer are not inevitable—no matter what your mother or grandmother experienced.

~ The menopausal transition is a powerful, biologically driven opportunity to reevaluate all aspects of your life and your health.

~ There are a wide variety of treatments available to support you hormonally and otherwise as you go through the menopausal transition. You have the inner guidance you need to choose the ones that are best for you. This includes bioidentical hormones.

~ Women are designed to enjoy sexual pleasure for a lifetime. Sexual pleasure can be greatly enhanced after menopause.

~ Menopause is the springtime of the second half of your life.

~ The time and energy you are willing to invest in yourself now will pay off in spades for years to come.

MENOPAUSE AS A NEW BEGINNING

Many menopausal women have dreams of giving birth. These birth dreams are important—they signify that there is much within us that needs to come forth. In this culture, women who are about to go through menopause or who are already in it need more than ever to reach deep within themselves and give birth to what is waiting there to be expressed. We can no longer afford to let our culture silence the wisdom of the wise woman—the woman who contains her sacred blood.

Susan Weed writes, "The process of menopause—not the last menses, the last drop of blood, but the entire thirteen-year menopausal process—sets the stage for initiatory ritual the world 'round, just as menstruating women's natural needs/abilities became the basis for all other initiations.

"During the process of menopause each woman finds herself immersed in and creating the three classic stages of initiation: isolation, death, and rebirth... our female bodies insist on completeness, wholeness, truth, change. Much as any woman would like to deny her shadow-self, her body will not let her. Menopause brings the individual woman and thus the entire community face-to-face with the dark, the unknown."[86]

With or without the help of hormones, every woman will benefit if she enters menopause consciously, ready to gather the gifts available at this stage of life. What we have to lose is not nearly so valuable as what we have to gain: finding our own voices and the courage to speak our own truth. When women do this, they are truly irresistible in their power and beauty. I have noticed everywhere I go that more and more women over the age of fifty look better than ever before. As a culture, we are truly redefining what it means to truly ripen with wisdom.

Just a few short years ago, my mother began expressing her creativity and connection with animals through learning the art of carving them in stone. Up until then, she never considered herself creative or artistic at all... and she was too busy raising five children to discover her gifts in this area. Her work is beautiful and inspiring—and she, like so many others past menopause, has discovered aspects of herself that she didn't know existed. She also speaks up a great deal at town meetings and other forums that concern her. She is no longer afraid to tell the truth in a group or in her own family. She says, "I have nothing to lose, and I've come to see that people can often benefit by what I have to say."

At a recent family wedding, I led a Blessing Way ritual for my brother's fiancée to celebrate her upcoming wedding and to welcome her into our family. Seated in a circle around her were my oldest daughter, my niece, my sister, the mother of the bride, my sister-in-law, the bride's sister, and two of my mother's friends. The age range in that circle of women was sixteen to eighty-three. I felt blessed to have the wisdom of three strong, powerful, and capable older women available for all of us in this circle, but especially for my daughters. What a gift it is to have honest, straightforward, physically healthy women over the age of seventy in our lives. They give us hope, courage, and guidance for the path ahead.

As a culture, we've been too long without those powerful, honest wise women of old—too long without the images of their beauty, power, and strength. Welcome them back. Whether or not you know any of them now, remember that they are inside each of us, waiting to be born through the initiation of menopause.

Part Three

Women's Wisdom Program for Vibrant Health and Healing

There is great power inherent in the act of committing yourself to the process of creating vibrant health in all levels of your life. The moment you do, you will discover that guidance and information from many different sources become available to you. Commitment engages your will, the power to hold and direct conscious thought and feeling into its desired physical manifestation. Our power to do anything comes from the self-reflective nature of our minds—and our ability to change our thoughts and perceptions. Our biology responds accordingly. Making a commitment to vibrant health involves two steps: the first is admitting that healing is necessary, and the second is opening yourself to the information that you begin to attract following the commitment.

Goethe said it best:

Until one is committed, there is hesitancy, the chance to draw back, always ineffectiveness. Concerning all acts of initiative (and creation), there is one elementary truth the ignorance of which kills countless ideas and splendid plans: that the moment one definitely commits oneself, then Providence moves too. All sorts of things occur to help one that would never otherwise have occurred. A whole stream of events issues from the decision, raising in one's favour all manner of unforeseen incidents and meetings and material assistance which no man [or woman] could have dreamed would come his [or her] way. Whatever you can do or dream you can do, begin it. Boldness has genius, power, and magic in it. Begin it now.

Problem-solving, whether through drugs, surgery, or herbs, is entirely different from creating health. Creating vibrant health, on the other hand, requires a new way of thinking about and being in relationship with our bodies, our minds, our spirits, and our connection with the universe. It requires us to think of ourselves and our bodies as dynamic, ever-changing energy systems that respond to thought and emotion. Very few people maintain or regain health and wholeness until they make this shift.

Creating vibrant health means accepting that there are events in everyone's life that cannot be explained or changed, and at the same time realizing that each of us has conscious input into our state of health through choosing relationships, thoughts, foods, and activities that support and nourish us fully. Creating health is also based on the following eternal truth: acknowledging, feeling, and then releasing rage, guilt, loss, fear, anger, and grief is the key to all healing. Learning how to regularly feel and release these emotions and change the habitual thought patterns that accompany them lightens us up and returns us to vibrant health naturally. The following chapters will provide you with the information you need to do this work. If you apply this information wholeheartedly and with humor and compassion, your life will change and you will experience more freedom, joy, and vibrant health. Guaranteed.

15
Steps for Creating Vibrant Health

Te steps in this chapter will help you tune in to the inner guidance of your body, mind, and spirit. By going through this chapter mindfully, you will be practicing preventive medicine at its
best, whether or not you are currently being treated for anything. Use
a journal to write down your responses to these steps and record whatever material comes up for you. This will give you an accurate record
of where you are right now. I'd also recommend that you repeat this
process every few months as a way to see how far you've come. It will
be an affirmation of your own inner wisdom. I personally do this on
the equinoxes and solstices. Read your journal a year from now and
you'll see that you're not the same person!

IMAGINE YOUR FUTURE: CHANGE YOUR
CONSCIOUSNESS, CHANGE YOUR CELLS

Healing always involves releasing the past as we move into the future. If we don't release the past, we keep re-creating it—and it becomes the future. As we release, it's also crucial to have a powerful
vision of a hopeful and exciting future that draws us forward. For
years, I had my patients begin their health journeys by exploring their
pasts to find clues to how they were creating their present conditions.

Our cells keep replacing themselves daily, and we create a whole new body every seven years. So it is not really accurate to say that our pasts are locked in our bodies, though sometimes it seems that way. What is really going on is that the consciousness that is creating our cells is often locked in the past—and that consciousness keeps re-creating the same old patterns via old subconscious nervous system programming. If, however, we can change the consciousness that creates our cells, then our cells and lives improve automatically, because health and joy are our natural state. The easiest and fastest way to do this is to imagine your future self in as much detail as you possibly can. Doing this will assist you through any healing process you're currently involved in. So before you dive into the steps listed here, invite your future vision to accompany you on your journey. *If you were in optimal health, what would your life look like?*

This question may be answered in the form of an exercise, with a friend who fully supports you; in writing, without worrying about revising or spelling; or out loud to yourself as you look in a mirror.

Answer the following questions (have your friend ask you the questions one by one, or write for three to five minutes without stopping, or talk to your image in the mirror): If anything at all were possible, quickly, easily, and now, what would your life look like? Who would be in it? What would you be doing? Where would you be living? What would you feel like? What would you look like? How much money would you be making?

Don't think about these questions before you answer. Pretend you're a child, creating your life exactly as you want it, no holds barred. How would your life be? Your inner guidance knows exactly what your heart's desire is. When you open your mouth and remove the brakes—and get the judge out of your head for a minute—your inner guidance will come up with the right answers.

If you need help getting going, imagine back to when you were eleven. What did you love to do? Who were you? Who did you think you would be? Imagine yourself now, telling the world who you are—and who you are going to become. Speak it to your image in the mirror—tell it to a friend or to the wind. Call that eleven-year-old back, now. She's got something to tell you. Take her into the future with you and let her become everything she ever dreamed she would be.

After you have completed the first part of this exercise, imagine that it is one year from today. You have been able to create everything that you wanted, plus more. Everything that you dreamed could come true is now true. You are celebrating and looking back over this phenomenal year. You've created all of it almost magically, through the power of connecting with your inner guidance and wisdom. After you feel this scene fully, tell your partner (or your journal, or your image in the mirror) in detail about everything that you've created, share how excited you are, and invite her or him to celebrate with you. Keep talking for two to three minutes without censoring yourself. Just let it flow—like a child playing make-believe.[1] If you can't dream up any circumstances for the future, just imagine feeling joyous, light, and happy.

This exercise is extraordinarily simple and powerful. Part of the reason is that focused thought is what creates the reality around us. It has been said that if you can hold a thought or feeling for at least seventeen seconds without introducing a contradicting thought or emotion, then you'll see evidence of this thought manifest around you in the physical world, e.g., start thinking about and talking about blue glass, or white lilies, or something else that holds no particular "charge," and watch what happens. I have experienced this repeatedly. This exercise is so playful and fun that it's easy to reach and exceed the seventeen-second mark.[2] You can change the time intervals by dreaming up your future self one week from now, one year from now, or even at the end of your life. In each case, have your future self look back and take in everything that you've accomplished and healed. It's exhilarating and it will get you in touch with who you really are. I recommend repeating this experience at least four times per year.

Now, take this a step further. Pretend you are your future ideal self now. That's right. Envision yourself as a confident, fit, prosperous, magnetic, attractive woman right now. Lighten up. Play with this energy now. Call this future self to you now. As you go through the rest of this section, bring your future self along with you. Call her in and let your wisdom and joy help you as you explore your past. She—and your inner wisdom—will always be there for you. You don't have to do this alone.

STEP ONE: UNCOVER AND UPDATE YOUR LEGACY

You need only claim the events of your life to make yourself yours. When you truly possess all you have been and done, which takes some time, you are fierce with reality.

—Florida Scott-Maxwell

Every one of us inherits a specific legacy from our families that needs to be claimed and changed as needed. Legacy is defined as a huge amount of information about our own past and our family's past that affects our energy, health, and potential for change in each generation. It is unconsciously passed on in repeated behavior and consciously passed on in the form of advice. One woman pointed out, "Until I did this exercise, I never realized how much alcoholism was in my family. I also didn't see that my fibroid uterus started to grow right after I had that second abortion." Some women realize the significance of virtually every woman in their extended family having had a hysterectomy before the age of fifty—thus creating a self-fulfilling medical family prophecy around the uterus that has nothing to do with genetics and everything to do with belief!

Because conditions such as alcoholism and depression are often denied within a family system, it's important to address these areas directly, thus shining a light on areas we tend to downplay. ("I'm not really an alcoholic, I'm just a heavy social drinker.") Also, the emotional impact of a history that includes the premature death of a parent, loss of a beloved pet, or loss of a significant relationship is frequently denied. This, too, is often revealed in writing down the family history.

Lois, a forty-three-year-old woman with a history of early cervical cancer and pelvic endometriosis, said, "I was a battered wife five years ago and finally got out of that marriage, then my daughter was in a car accident and I had to take care of her for months. Then, this summer I was in another accident and sustained a whiplash injury. I seem to want to cry, but I keep pushing it down. It gets harder to do, though. Is this from early menopause?"

Going over Lois's history with her, it was easy to see that she had been through a very significant amount of change and loss in the past decade, which she'd tried to deal with by keeping everything in order, going to work daily, and appearing cheerful. She admitted that it seemed to be harder to keep her house in order these days, and that even though there was no current crisis, she still felt inefficient and emotional. In fact, her back pain from the whiplash was gone, her daughter was now in college, and her job was going quite well. What she realized she needed to do was acknowledge the losses she hadn't grieved and give herself the necessary time and space for this.

What Lois was experiencing was what I call Break Down to Breakthrough. She needed to feel what she was feeling. She took a week off from work and family, went to a small country inn, and spent the next week mostly in robe and slippers, reading, crying, drinking tea with the lady who runs the inn, and gradually getting back in touch with parts of herself and feelings that were long denied. When I next saw her, she looked fifteen years younger. "Now I know that those feelings you mentioned don't come up when you want them to," she said. "They come when they come. It took me three or four days of being quiet and by myself before I could really cry. But I also learned that I can get off by myself when I need to in order to do this for myself. My relationship with my husband [she had remarried] and daughter is better than ever. I learned that *when I take care of myself, everything else takes care of itself.*"

HEALTH INVENTORY: WHERE I AM NOW

It's helpful to fill out this form to get an idea of exactly what your health and life look like now. It is modified from the one I used for years in my practice.

Medical Status

General Health (circle one):   excellent   good   fair   poor

Medications (vitamins, prescription or otherwise): _____

_____

_____

Hospitalizations and Operations

Dates   Diagnosis/Operation

_____

_____

_____

Pregnancies *(including miscarriages and abortions)*

Dates   How far along   Sex   Weight   Problems

_____

_____

_____

Past or Current Medical Conditions *(circle those that apply)*

German measles	Varicose veins
Chicken pox	Phlebitis
Rubella	Clotting defects
Other childhood diseases	Bleeding tendencies
Heart trouble	Blood transfusion
High blood pressure	Diabetes
High cholesterol	Kidney trouble
Stroke	Rheumatic fever

Jaundice/hepatitis	Cancer
Epilepsy	Asthma
Arthritis	Chronic fatigue/Epstein-Barr
Colitis	Eating disorder
Fractures	Other

Habits

Dietary preferences/restrictions: _____

Sample of day's menu:

    Breakfast: _____

    Lunch: _____

    Dinner: _____

    Snacks: _____

Regular exercise (type, how often, how long): _____

_____

Tobacco use (how much currently, previous history): _____

_____

Alcohol use (how much, how often): _____

Caffeine use (how much): _____

Mood-altering substance use (i.e. marijuana, cocaine, etc.), past and present:

_____

Things I Do for Fun and Pleasure

Hobbies: _____

    Participatory sports: _____

    Musical/artistic endeavors: _____

    Group activities or clubs:_____

    Volunteer activities: _____

    Participation in religious/spiritual practice:_____

    Other: _____

Stresses

Family stresses: _____

Work stresses: _____

Personal stresses:_____

Family History

For each family member, note age (if still living), any important diseases (alcoholism, high blood pressure, cancer, diabetes, heart disease, osteoporosis, other addictions, other illnesses), and cause of death and age at death (if applicable).

Mother: _____

Father: _____

Sister(s): _____

Brother(s): _____

Maternal grandmother: _____

Paternal grandmother: _____

Maternal grandfather: _____

Paternal grandfather: _____

Paternal aunt(s): _____

Maternal aunt(s): _____

Maternal uncle(s):_____

Paternal uncle(s):_____

Gynecological History

Age at first period: _____

Any abnormal Pap smears: _____

    If yes, how were they treated? _____

Are you sexually active? _____

Do you have intercourse? _____

Do you have regular orgasms? _____

Do you know where your clitoris is?_____

Do you practice safe sex? _____

Are you trying to get pregnant? _____

Current birth control method (and how long): _____

    Any problems with it? _____

    Past birth control methods:_____

Normally (when not on hormonal methods of birth control), number of
    days from the start of one period to the start of the next: _____

Number of days of flow: _____

Amount of bleeding:_____

Amount of cramping:_____

Premenstrual symptoms (and when they start): _____

Any current changes in your normal pattern? _____

Any bleeding between periods?_____

Any unusual pelvic pain, pressure, or fullness? _____

Any unusual vaginal discharge or itching? _____

Any sexual concerns? _____

Any past history of tubal infection?_____

Any past history of sexually transmitted disease? _____

Did your mother take DES when she was pregnant with you? _____

Other:————————————————————————————————

Present Symptoms

General Physical
Fever or chills
Hot flashes
Unusual hair growth
Skin eruptions
Weight change

Abdomen
Bloating
Heartburn, indigestion
Cramps or pain
Nausea or vomiting
Change in bowel habits
Bloody or tarry stools
Diarrhea
Constipation
Hemorrhoids
Flatulence

Head
Headaches
Dizziness
Visual defects
Hearing defects
Sinus trouble
Fainting spells

Bladder
Frequent urination
Painful urination
Blood in urine
Inability to hold urine
Inability to empty bladder
Need to get up at night to urinate

Chest
Chest pain
Shortness of breath
Heart murmur
Mitral valve prolapse
Palpitations
Chronic cough
Coughing up blood
Wheezing

Breasts
Lumps
Bleeding
Discharge
Tenderness
Other concerns

Daily Living Profile

Indicate whether each statement does or does not describe part of your current life by circling "yes" or "no." This questionnaire is designed to increase your awareness of the effects of your lifestyle and stresses on your physical well-being. It is based on the one I used at Women to Women for years.

NEIGHBORHOOD

I like my neighborhood.	☐ yes	☐ no
My neighborhood is too noisy.	☐ yes	☐ no
My neighborhood is too crowded.	☐ yes	☐ no
My neighborhood is too quiet.	☐ yes	☐ no
I do not have enough friends/neighbors.	☐ yes	☐ no
It is a dangerous neighborhood in which to live.	☐ yes	☐ no
Having so many household tasks irritates me.	☐ yes	☐ no
The weather here bothers me.	☐ yes	☐ no

I'm new to this area.	☐ yes	☐ no

Other neighborhood problems (describe): _____

FAMILY

My family is a solid source of support.	☐ yes	☐ no
I am recently married.	☐ yes	☐ no
I am recently divorced or separated.	☐ yes	☐ no
I have recently moved or am planning to move.	☐ yes	☐ no
I am alone too much at home.	☐ yes	☐ no
I am concerned about my relationship with my partner.	☐ yes	☐ no
I am concerned about my relationship with another family member (parent, child, brother, sister).	☐ yes	☐ no
I feel I was raised in a dysfunctional environment.	☐ yes	☐ no
We have a new baby in our family.	☐ yes	☐ no
I or one of my family members is having legal problems.	☐ yes	☐ no
A family member or close friend recently died.	☐ yes	☐ no
Someone in my family has a serious illness.	☐ yes	☐ no
I am worried about one of my family members.	☐ yes	☐ no
Someone close to me drinks too much.	☐ yes	☐ no
One of my children has moved away from home recently.	☐ yes	☐ no
My partner has recently retired.	☐ yes	☐ no

Other concerns about home and family:

WORK

I like my work and find it fulfilling.	☐ yes	☐ no
I am bored with the work I do.	☐ yes	☐ no
Other people make too many demands on me.	☐ yes	☐ no
I have too little control over my own work.	☐ yes	☐ no
I am not satisfied with the work I do.	☐ yes	☐ no
I often feel overwhelmed by my responsibilities.	☐ yes	☐ no
I do not have enough time to finish my work.	☐ yes	☐ no
I just began a new job.	☐ yes	☐ no
I just lost my job.	☐ yes	☐ no
I don't get along with my boss/employees.	☐ yes	☐ no
I am having problems with people I work with.	☐ yes	☐ no

Other work-related concerns: _____

PERSONAL

My life is prosperous and fun.	☐ yes	☐ no
I enjoy many different kinds of friendships.	☐ yes	☐ no
I look forward to a bright future.	☐ yes	☐ no
I worry about money a great deal.	☐ yes	☐ no

I feel lonely.	☐ yes	☐ no
I am bored with my life.	☐ yes	☐ no
I am generally concerned about my health.	☐ yes	☐ no
I think a lot about dying.	☐ yes	☐ no
I have particular concerns relating to my religion.	☐ yes	☐ no

Other personal concerns: _____

_____

RESILIENCE

I sleep soundly each night, getting at least eight hours of restful sleep.	☐ yes	☐ no
I have difficulty falling asleep.	☐ yes	☐ no
I have difficulty staying asleep.	☐ yes	☐ no
I have difficulty staying awake.	☐ yes	☐ no
I feel tired when I wake up in the morning.	☐ yes	☐ no
My mood is steady and stable.	☐ yes	☐ no
I'm generally happy.	☐ yes	☐ no
I feel nervous most of the time.	☐ yes	☐ no
I often feel depressed.	☐ yes	☐ no
I worry a lot.	☐ yes	☐ no
I am ill frequently.	☐ yes	☐ no
I have considered committing suicide.	☐ yes	☐ no
I have some sexual problems.	☐ yes	☐ no
I sometimes feel weak or light-headed.	☐ yes	☐ no
I often have pains in my shoulder, neck, or back.	☐ yes	☐ no
I often feel like crying.	☐ yes	☐ no
I seek out whole, nutritious food.	☐ yes	☐ no
I enjoy good food and good company.	☐ yes	☐ no
I drink too much coffee.	☐ yes	☐ no
I smoke too much.	☐ yes	☐ no
I often drink too much alcohol.	☐ yes	☐ no
I eat more than I used to.	☐ yes	☐ no
I eat much less than I used to.	☐ yes	☐ no
I am concerned about my weight.	☐ yes	☐ no
I lose my temper more than I used to.	☐ yes	☐ no
I think counseling might help me.	☐ yes	☐ no

Other concerns: _____

After you've filled out this form, see if you can correlate your stressors with your symptoms—and then change them!

STEP TWO: SORT THROUGH YOUR BELIEFS

Commit yourself to setting aside some time to answer the following series of questions. You might want to do this with a friend or in a group. Your answers would make an excellent starting place for a personal journal that you can update regularly as new insights come to you. Writing your answers down is, in itself, a significant commitment of your time and energy toward creating health. You learn a great deal about yourself and your relationship with your body. *Note: this is health care that won't cost you a penny.*

Do you understand how inherited cultural attitudes toward our female physiological processes such as menstruation and menopause have contributed to the illnesses suffered by our female bodies? What are the thoughts that arise when you hear the words breast, menstruation, childbirth, vagina, vulva, menopause, *and so on?*

If you've grown up believing that your menstrual period is "the curse," for example, it's quite likely that your attitude toward your female physiology is less than optimal.

To what extent have you internalized negative cultural programming about the female body?

One of my patients became menopausal following chemotherapy for Hodgkin's disease at the age of twenty-seven. Though she had gone on estrogen replacement therapy for a few years, she eventually stopped it because "the thought of getting my periods back was chilling and repugnant to me," she said. I found her statement of disgust and its implications about her attitude toward her body equally chilling, but such attitudes are all too common. Luckily they can be changed.

Do you believe you can be healthy?

Women who have grown up in a household where the norm is to go to the doctor for sleeping pills, anxiety, headaches, and the common cold often internalize the belief that the human body is meant to suffer from all manner of ills and that there's a pill for every ill. Enjoying ill health is the norm for some people. The possibility of a sound body that isn't susceptible to every germ in the environment is inconceivable to them.

What challenges were part of your childhood?

Have you reviewed your childhood experiences to see how they may have contributed to your current perceptions and experiences? A childhood history of incest, chronic illness in a parent, unresolved losses such as a divorce in the family, or having a parent abandon the family are common occurrences that, if unresolved, can set the stage for later problems that have similar dynamics. Many women's fathers left them when they were children, and never returned. Other women have never talked openly about a parent's death. Though the impact of these events is as variable as our fingerprints, there is always an impact. How we name, express, and fully release emotions surrounding such losses can be a factor in our physical health. Recall that this information is directly related to the health of our first three chakras and the organs they comprise.

One of my patients, for example, developed panic attacks and severe PMS around her fortieth birthday, several months after her father was diagnosed with bowel cancer. Her mother had died suddenly from a reaction to penicillin when my patient was four years old. She went to live with an aunt with no explanation, and she was never given permission to speak about it or grieve her loss. She related that she was never really told what had happened to her mother, no one had cried, and that she got the idea that she was never supposed to mention it. Now with the possible loss of her father, all those long-buried emotions were working their way to the surface. This time she has the skills to express them in a healthy manner and release them over time.

What purpose does your illness serve? What does it mean to you?
A forty-two-year-old woman, recovering from a car accident, told me that there was no question that before the accident, the pace of her life was moving way too fast. To pay attention to her needs, she literally had to be forced to lie in bed and stare up at the ceiling for several months, as she was now. She regards this accident as a very positive turning point in her life. Leslie Kussman, a filmmaker who has multiple sclerosis, said that during one of her morning meditations it occurred to her that perhaps we need to rephrase the question from "What purpose does your illness serve?" to "What is the illness that will serve your purpose?"[3] *Illness is often the only socially acceptable form of Western meditation.* Our society is set up such that taking a nap or meditating in the middle of the day to recharge and renew ourselves is frowned upon as hedonistic or irresponsible, but getting the flu is a socially accepted way to rest.

Without slipping into self-blame, think back on the last time you had to miss work because of illness. Was the illness a satisfying break from your routine? What did you get out of it? What did you learn from it? Do you see any way that you could get the same rest without being sick? A young female doctor developed breast cancer while she was pregnant with her third child. As a result, she changed her diet, her work schedule, and her life. Two years later she told me, "My life has never been better. Every day is a joy. I'm glad I had cancer. It saved my life."

If you had only six months to live, would you stay at your current job? Would you stay with your current partner? Would it take a serious illness for you to begin making beneficial changes now?

Are you willing to be open to any messages that your symptoms or illness may have for you?

Before you begin working with this question, please note that a willingness to be open to the message is entirely different from a need to control and figure out the meaning of an illness exactly, especially while it is happening. The former is associated with vibrant health. The latter is just manipulating yourself and is part of our illusion of control. As they say in twelve-step programs, "Whying is dying." Being open to meaning means that you allow the illness to speak to you, often through the language of emotion, imagery, and pain. Your intellectual understanding of your situation may well come only after an illness is over with.

Back in the 1980s, when our culture was learning about the mind/body connection, people would actually ask questions like "Why are you needing to create cancer?" as though the intellect could figure that out through cause-and-effect thinking. These sorts of questions keep the intellect running in circles and take us away from our hearts—the place in the body that really heals us. Being open to meaning is an attitude, a process. It's "waiting with," not "waiting for." And it connects us with our soul's voice. Glanda Green, author of *Love without End* (Spirits, 2002), puts it beautifully. "The mind will seek to compensate for the discomforts of the heart. But the mind will never seek to cure or remove those discomforts."

When faced with an illness, what is your usual reaction?

Learning the meaning behind the illness is a process that doesn't lend itself to questions like "Why me, why now?" Evy McDonald writes, "Don't get caught in the tangling web of why. The search for the explanation and meaning of your illness can lead to frustration and depression and can paralyze your ability to make decisions and take action."

In the days of the ancient Greeks, a messenger would be sent to the leader with news of the current battle. If the news was bad, the messenger would be killed. Your task is not to kill the messenger of illness by ignoring it, complaining about it, or simply suppressing the symptoms. Your task is to examine your life with compassion and honesty while cultivating detachment—which simply means caring deeply from an objective place. From this place, identify those areas of your life that require harmony, fulfillment, and love.

What is preventing you from experiencing vibrant health?

"Waiting with" this question is a good meditation. Don't expect an answer to spring forth immediately, though it sometimes does. Back in the days when I had two small children and a busy practice, I repeatedly asked myself what changes I needed in my life and what I needed to do next. The answer that kept coming was simple: rest. You're burned out. Taking action on that insight took over a year. Why? Because at the time, I honestly believed that adequate rest was incompatible with my chosen life's work. It was, and always is, a process.

Some people never heal because they believe that if they were healed, they would be alone and abandoned. Being sick in this culture can be a very powerful way to get our needs met legitimately. Saying to someone, "Please hold me—I feel ill," is quite different from saying, "Please hold me—I want to be held because it feels good and I like it." The first sentence uses illness to justify the universal human need for closeness. The second sentence simply states the need clearly. Many people don't know that intimacy is possible without using our wounds to get it. We are brought up to be ashamed of our needs for touch, love, and companionship, so we learn very early to bond with each other via our wounds.

During my residency training, I was very proud of the way I had handled a certain woman's care, and I decided to tell one of my nurse colleagues who also knew this patient well and who could celebrate with me. When I told her, she said, "Don't break your arm patting yourself on the back." I was stunned. I had simply been expressing a natural human need to share my success with a colleague who would understand its implications. When I was growing up, my parents had always believed that each of us children needed his or her place in the sun. We were routinely recognized for our gifts and achievements, and we felt good about ourselves and each other when these were shared. (We still do this.) But my nurse colleague had obviously learned that it was not okay to "blow your own horn." Often, the only time good things are said about the life of another person is at their funeral. This is tragic. Each of us needs to accept that no matter how strong, independent, and healthy we become, we will always need others for companionship, celebration, and joyful living. And we need others who will reflect our worth back to us!

Do you take on everyone else's problems and put yourself last?

This is the classic dilemma for women. Feeling the need to be the healer and peacemaker for our entire family or place of work is a pattern that many of us learned in childhood as a way to get recognition. To create health, a woman must face this tendency squarely and commit to changing it.

Here's an example: When my children were ten and twelve, they complained repeatedly about one of my colleagues who is a good friend of mine. This woman helped with the research for this book and was a very entertaining companion for me during the process. My children perceived that my friend was taking up too much of my time and that I was not as available to them as they would have liked me to be. I noticed, however, that when Ann and Kate were playing with their friends, reading, or living their own lives fully, they ignored me for hours, even days on end. And during the many days and hours when my friend wasn't around, my children came and went as they pleased, focusing only on their own needs. They were not necessarily interested in my companionship if they had other things going on. They became extremely interested in me, however, the moment my entertaining friend walked in the door.

To deal with this situation, I initially spent hours listening to Ann's and Kate's complaints and trying to negotiate only *their* needs. Then I realized that, on an unconscious level, they didn't expect me to have any needs for friendship, laughs, and companionship *separate* from them. When I realized this, I let them know very clearly that I also had needs— individual needs that were as important (not *more* important—*as* important) as theirs. I came to see that I had to take a stand for my own needs as well as the needs of my children. Together, we began working on becoming conscious of the ways in which they, unconsciously, didn't expect me to have a life separate from them, and the ways in which I had been socialized to sacrifice my life for their needs.

When I became clear about this situation and what needed to happen, I had a dream about being given a red 1950s-style gas pump that pumped milk. The name painted on the pump was "The Mother." I had to keep the pump refrigerated so that the milk wouldn't spoil. I kept trying to think of who I was going to give the milk to. My family didn't need it—we don't drink milk. When I woke up, I realized that the pump represented me and that it was now time to let go of an obsolete kind of mothering (a 1950s gas pump that could service only one car—perform only one role—at a time).

Do you fully understand the workings of your female body and how intimately your thoughts and feelings are connected to your physical health?

Your body experiences every thought and sensation as a "physiological reality." By thinking of the taste and smell of chocolate, you trigger many of the same physical reactions as when you actually eat a piece. Our bodies are not static structures. The amount of sunlight shining on us in a day affects our physiology. The quality of the sounds we hear affects our physiology. The quality of the relationships we have with others affects our physiology. One woman said to me, "Oh, my breasts are being taken care of by Lahey Clinic!" Instead of believing that the Lahey Clinic is responsible for her breasts, she would be much better served by assuming responsibility for her breasts herself.

Many women don't understand not only how intimately our bodies are affected by our environments but also the basic anatomy of our bodies. Many who have had surgery don't know exactly what was taken out and what was left in. Yet knowing precisely where the organs in our bodies are is very reassuring. During my residency I once did an emergency appendectomy on a woman. She also required removal of her uterus and ovaries because of a life-threatening infection. Several days later, I learned that she thought her appendix was as big as a large melon and that now her entire lower abdomen was completely empty because we had removed it. I explained to her that her large and small intestine completely filled her lower abdomen despite the loss of her pelvic organs, which was very useful information for her in her recovery because it helped her feel that the loss was less overwhelming. Showing her drawings of her anatomy was also helpful—she learned that her appendix was smaller than her little finger.

I encourage women to get personal copies of all their records and go over them with a health care provider who can answer questions, particularly reports of any surgeries they have had, so that they know exactly what is going on inside their bodies, how things look, and what is left. When you go to the doctor, take a friend or a tape recorder. Ask questions. Be proactive. Keeping copies of her own records can also expedite a woman's health care if she is traveling or has to make an emergency-room visit.

Do you know where your organs are? If not, consider looking through an encyclopedia or standard anatomy guide. Get to know your body in health, not just in sickness! You also need to own all of it—even the parts that aren't considered socially acceptable!

What do you call your genitals? What was the name given to the female genitals in your family? Too many women were raised in families in which all the functions below the waist were considered shameful and not talked about. One friend said, "In my family, the area below the waist was referred to as 'down there.' It was kind of foggy. I didn't know what to call it. Likewise, women weren't supposed to pass gas!" At a recent meeting of the Association of Pre- and Perinatal Psychology and Health, renowned midwife Ina May Gaskin commented that women would be far better prepared for birth if they allowed themselves more humor and relaxation about bodily functions such as bowel movements and passing gas. I agree.

The first step in reclaiming your women's wisdom is naming and reclaiming all of you. Regena Thomashauer, author of *Mama Gena's School of Womanly Arts* (Simon & Schuster, 2002) and *Mama Gena's Owner's and Operator's Guide to Men* (Simon & Schuster, 2003), has spent years studying the goddess cultures of old Europe and has dedicated her life to helping women apply this knowledge in practical empowering ways in their daily lives. She uses the rather shocking word *pussy* to refer to the genitals. Many women find this offensive at first because of our cultural programming.

However, this friendly word can be used as a term of endearment that aptly describes a warm, fuzzy, and pleasurable area of the body. And it sure beats the other slang terms! Reading Regena Thomashauer's books will help you embrace not only this word, but also the power of your genital area!

Are you following your life's purpose?

Our bodies are designed to function best when we're involved in activities and work that feel exactly right to us and that bring us pleasure. Our health is enhanced when we engage in deeply creative work that is satisfying to us—not just because it pleases our boss, husband, or mother. This work can range from gardening to computer programming to welding.

Unfortunately, our culture doesn't believe that creativity is valuable for its own sake. To be considered worthwhile, an activity must be associated with tangible rewards or productivity. We consider the worth of an activity to be how much money is associated with it. For many people, going to work is more like "making a dying" than "making a living." People often put up with very unsatisfactory work environments because of the "benefits." I call this "dying for our benefits." Financial and gynecological health are intimately connected. The second-chakra area of the body (uterus, tubes, ovaries, lower back) is affected by financial stresses. Health in this area is created when we tap in to our ability to be creative and prosperous at the same time.

Becoming both creative and prosperous often involves as a first step a change in our attitudes toward money, self-worth, and work. We must be very clear on how our culture's belief in the zero-sum model affects us. For instance, many people believe, "If I am doing well, someone else has to suffer. There is only so much money to go around." Or vice versa: "If someone else is doing well, then there is no chance for me to do well also. There is no way to get ahead." Our personal finances are powerfully and directly affected by our beliefs about money. Poverty consciousness pervades our culture on every level. When we change our beliefs, we can change our income!

In their book, *Your Money or Your Life* (Viking, 1992), the late Joe Dominguez, a former Wall Street analyst, and coauthor Vicki Robin point out that for most people, money is the substance for which we exchange our life-energy.[4] Dominguez and Robin suggest that you figure out how many hours you have left in your life—your total life-energy. Then you calculate how much your work actually costs you in terms of your life-energy. If you work so many hours that you require expensive vacations and frequent illnesses to balance the energy drain of work, you may well find that your work is worth much less per hour than you are actually being paid, once you factor in the "hidden" costs of vacation and illness. Their program then helps you balance your relationship with money by determining how much fulfillment you get out of every purchase, compared with how much it has cost you in terms of your life-energy.

Your next step is to consciously make a decision to spend more money on the things or activities that bring you the most fulfillment and less money on the stuff that ultimately has no meaning. What happens is that eventually your expenditures decrease and the fulfillment that you derive from them increases. When you begin to look at money in this way, your entire relationship with it changes. You begin to see that it is not necessary to put off doing what you've always wanted to do until "later." Some of my greatest pleasures, such as walking on the beach, reading, and going to the movies, cost almost nothing. It need not cost you much money to begin living your life in a more fulfilling manner. By going through the Dominguez-Robin program myself back in the late 1980s, I realized that my free time was priceless to me and that I would never again be able to work in any job, regardless of high pay and good benefits, if the job didn't also fulfill my soul and give me ample time to create my life on my own terms.

At midlife when I went through an unexpected divorce, I was once again forced to come to terms with what I really valued. I had had a large fibroid removed from my uterus a couple years prior to the divorce—a sign that I had been leaking life-energy into a dead-end relationship. (Remember—the body never lies.) Overnight my income was cut in half and my expenses rose significantly. I also was faced with paying the vast majority of two private college tuitions for my daughters. There's nothing like a financial (or health) crisis to get our attention! Knowing about the connection between prosperity and thought, I read the classic *Think and Grow Rich* (Hawthorn Books, 1996; Aventine Press, 2004) by Napoleon Hill, all of Suze Orman's work, and also all of the financial advice from Robert Kiyosaki, author of *Rich Dad, Poor Dad* (Warner Business Books, 2000). (For more information, visit www.richdad.com.) Finally, I learned that financial literacy is crucial for all women. I got up to speed on the necessity of creating residual income (the kind that comes in regardless of whether you work or not). Residual income is the biggest difference between those who are prosperous and those who are struggling financially. I also learned how to reprogram my thinking about prosperity through the work of Catherine Ponder, author of *The Dynamic Laws of Prosperity* (Prentice-Hall, 1962), and Randy Gage. (For more information on Randy Gage and his ideas on prosperity, visit his website at www.randygage.com.) As I was going through my divorce, I happened to meet Suze Orman at the *Today* show. She told me that you can always see health problems start in someone's money situation first, because a balance sheet has no place to hide energy. Sooner or later that energy drain hits the body as a health problem. Suze is absolutely correct.

By applying the laws of prosperity in my own life (e.g., the Law of Circulation—if you want to receive, you have to learn to give, etc.). I eventually was able to create true financial abundance and also greatly improved health. This process was so empowering that I passed it on to my daughters so that they would not have to be dependent upon a man for financial security.

Have you designed your life in a way that fulfills both your innermost needs and your desire to be of service to others?

It is entirely possible to develop yourself fully, meet your innermost emotional needs, and at the same time work with others for the common good. Our culture has taught women just the opposite: that they must sacrifice themselves and their needs for the good of others. But you cannot quench the thirst of others when your own cup is always empty. Many studies have shown, for example, that women who sacrifice work they love and optimal self-development in order to nurture others are at risk for breast cancer. It is not the sacrifice alone that creates the health problem—it is the unexpressed resentment that results from it. When a woman doesn't believe that she has a right to self-development, she won't even allow herself to acknowledge her resentment. Her body wisdom must then bring it to her attention so that she can make a balance. The most prosperous people I know are also the most generous. They make the world a better place and also enjoy abundance themselves!

Do you regularly appreciate your strengths, gifts, talents, and accomplishments?

A large part of creating vibrant health—or anything else, including wealth—is giving ourselves credit for where we are now. Learning how to take in praise—to let ourselves really feel success and completion physically—is a skill that can be learned. A big reason why people get stuck and can't create better lives is that they don't give themselves credit for what they *have* created. This usually comes from the subconscious programming we received in childhood, e.g., "Money doesn't grow on trees," or "You'll never amount to anything." If you chronically skip this step of acknowledging your creations and continue to focus only on what you have *yet* to accomplish, then your subconscious hears only "You are not enough. You haven't done enough. There is so much more to do. You will never be enough," instead of "Good job. Look how far you've come."

Many women live with the following beliefs: there is too much work to do, I will never get it done, but I can't rest or have fun until it's done.

The classic double bind. This belief comes directly out of our cultural obsession with productivity and the belief that our worth depends upon what we can produce for others, whether this be children or goods and services. Operating under this belief system, we create more and more work that doesn't feel complete or fulfilling. Here's the truth. You'll never get it done. There's always more to do. The answer: build regular pleasure and appreciation into your schedule so you learn to feel good about yourself and your life right now! Remember optimal ovarian health requires that we acknowledge our creativity as an outward manifestation of our deepest inner need for self-expression. This creativity need not be measured in dollars or productivity to be a valuable contribution to our health and that of the others. When we allow others to exploit, judge, and control our innate gifts and talents, we put our health at risk.

One of my medical colleagues learned this lesson well when she developed an ovarian cyst while working on the faculty of a major medical center. Florence had originally gone to work in this center because she didn't believe that she had what it took to start her own practice using her creativity to the fullest. Following her ovarian removal, however, Florence knew intuitively that she needed to leave her workplace, that it was somehow dangerous for her to stay. In this work environment, others did not value her innate feminine creativity, and as a result she didn't value it herself when she was there. Florence knew that she was not yet strong enough to hold her own feminine viewpoint without at least some support from others, but the ovarian "sacrifice" really got her attention and mobilized her to make a change. She left the medical center and started her own highly successful practice. Only years later, after learning about ovarian wisdom and releasing her need to blame others, was she able to appreciate how profoundly she had put her creativity at risk in her original work setting.

Women's skills and voices need to be heard throughout all areas of endeavor: in industry, education, medicine, and other professions. Women must start by listening to themselves and hearing their own voices. Our self-development is a planetary priority. We have much to contribute but too often we are unsure of ourselves.

Think of one thing that you're proud of that you've accomplished today, this week, or this year. Feel your accomplishment(s) fully. Take it in, until it's more than just intellectual knowledge. Take yourself right into your heart. If we can't feel good about our skills and accomplishments, no one else can, either. Find a few friends you can brag with! Send each other e-mails regularly, bragging about how wonderful and skillful you are! (Note: women shoot themselves in the foot by complaining too much. It's a bad habit. Find friends who have the courage to consciously break it.)

STEP THREE: RESPECT AND RELEASE YOUR EMOTIONS

*Pain is the result of resistance to our natural state of well-being
and the more we pay attention to it, the more of it we attract.*
                                                                —Abraham

Emotions are a vital part of our inner guidance. Like our illnesses, our dreams, and our lives, our emotions are ours, and we must own them and pay attention to them. We must learn to feel our emotions, release our judgments about them, and be grateful for their guidance. They let us know how we are directing our thoughts and life-energy. Chronic anger or sadness, by the law of attraction, tends to attract situations to us that are filled with anger or sadness, e.g., you find yourself stuck in anger and then fall on the ice—or get pulled over for speeding. Daily doses of joy and appreciation of ourselves and others, on the other hand, tend to attract joy and appreciation into our lives.

Children automatically know how to feel their emotions and then let go. When they're hurt, they stop and cry. After just a short time, they're back playing again. Elisabeth Kübler-Ross points out that a child's natural anger and emotional outbursts last about fifteen seconds. Shaming or blaming the child for that anger, however, often blocks its natural release. The child's natural emotion may get stuck and become a form of self-pity that remains with the person for years! Kübler-Ross points out that people who weren't allowed a natural expression of anger in childhood are often "marinated in self-pity" as adults and are difficult to be around. This self-pity is the same thing as self-centeredness. It takes a great deal of energy to hold in our natural emotions. In fact, it's exhausting. If we haven't felt our feelings regularly during a period of personal crisis or change, we often have a backlog of sealed-off emotion stored up in our bodies.

Emotional suppression is a pattern that gets passed down from generation to generation. Many women have rage that's been held in check for decades. They hold in oceans of tears that are yet to be shed. One very overweight woman in my practice told me that her mother and grandmother had taught her how to gorge on chocolate whenever their husbands were out of town and they were feeling lonely. The fat on her hips, she told me, represented three generations of stagnated emotional energy held down with chocolate.

Emotional release, or what I've already called emotional incision and drainage, is an organic healing process that is completely natural and safe.[5] When I first went to an intensive workshop and sat with people who were doing deep process work, I felt as if I were on the labor and delivery floor at the hospital—standing by, allowing people to give birth to themselves. All of us have this ability within us. Dorothy's ruby slippers could get her home to Kansas all by herself—she just didn't know it. She thought she needed the wizard. Likewise, we all have the power to choose thoughts of appreciation and gratitude—and release old resentment and tears.

Making sounds is an important part of emotional release. Women naturally make deep primal sounds in labor. They help open the cervix and get the baby through the birth canal. Primal sounds are also part of lovemaking. Myron McClellan, a musician specializing in the healing power of sound, says that "singing is part of the emotional body's digestive system." Singing is one form of healing sound. Wailing or deep sobbing is another. These sounds are like grappling hooks that go through the body, cleaning out toxins and old debris. A woman recently wrote me, "I have taken several months of training in the martial arts simply to help release some of the tensions and muscular inabilities that I have felt in my body. An interesting by-product is that I have found my voice. In the process of learning tae kwon do, I had to be able to give a huge yell with the punches and the kicks that are part of the practice. I had never before in my life been able to make a noise with that much authority. As a child, I learned that if one didn't make noise, then one could possibly avoid aggravating or irritating one's abusers and, possibly, avoid abuse. I have carried that legacy with me for many years, even silencing my grief when my husband was killed. In other cultures women are traditionally taught to keen loudly to express grief, sorrow, and rage at death. I had never made that kind of sound, though I certainly have wanted and needed to do so. Not until now, six years after my husband's death, have I been able to make those sounds. They came, not only because of the karate, but as a result of the deep healings to my respiratory tract that I have been able to accomplish through macrobiotics and oriental medicine."

In many ways, the year or two *after* a traumatic experience are more difficult than the experience itself—possibly because we have support for crises in this culture but are then expected, both from within ourselves and from outside, to get on with it when it's over. But this can happen only once we've allowed ourselves to express and release our emotions fully.

A young woman who had recovered from Hodgkin's disease with the help of a bone marrow transplant a year before came to see me once. The chemotherapy had caused an early menopause, and we were working with estrogen replacement therapy to help her hot flashes. She was having problems with fatigue and weakness, but there was no sign that the cancer had returned. In going back over her history, she burst into tears in my office and told me that she never cried once during the year in which her diagnosis was made or during her entire chemotherapy experience. She had not allowed herself to experience her fear. She had simply gone through it as best she could.

A year later, there was no crisis in this woman's life. Her body was well, but she still didn't feel better. She didn't have the energy to exercise, and she didn't want to cook nourishing meals for herself. After sitting with this for a while, she realized that she needed time to process her recent experience emotionally.

When I first visited an acupuncturist, she told me that in Chinese medicine, emotions such as anger are viewed simply as *energy*. Many women have a problem with the direct expression of their anger and use it to manipulate others instead. But anger can be a powerful ally. When we feel angry, the anger is always related to something we need to acknowledge for ourselves. It is not necessarily about the situation or person that evoked it. It is always a sign that on some level we're not meeting a personal need that we may have. That's one of the reasons why anger is so often part of PMS.

All women must learn that no one can *make* us angry. Our anger is ours, and it is telling us something we need to know. Eleanor Roosevelt once said, "No one can make you feel inferior [or angry, or sad] without your permission." Anger is energy—our personal jet fuel. It is telling us that something needs adjustment in our lives. It is telling us that there is something we want that we don't yet know how to get. Next time you get angry, say to yourself, "Ah! My inner guidance is working. This is good. What is it I want here? What do I want to have happen here?" Anger is often an expression of the energy required to make that adjustment. This emotion is dangerous only if we deny it and stuff it in our bodies or lash out at someone else with it. Anger and all other "negative" emotions can serve us well when we don't turn them in on ourselves as depression or lash out with them against others. Next time you discover that you're angry (which might manifest as feeling jittery, having shaking hands, or being irritable), go off by yourself. Move around. Breathe. Yell. Love yourself for having the feeling. Then ask yourself, "What do I need?" Wait for an answer. Your anger at another may well be justified. But if you hang on to it overly long, the one who will be hurt the most is you. At the end of the day, you have to decide whether you want to be justified or healthy and happy! Let the anger pass. Ask for what you need with kindness. When you get it, say, "Thank you."

STEP FOUR: LEARN TO LISTEN TO YOUR BODY

Learning to listen to and respect your body is a process that requires patience and compassion. You can begin this process by paying attention to your body as you read through the following list. Go slowly and come back to it as needed.

~ Make note of those things in your life that are difficult, painful, joyful, and the like. As these things come up, notice your breathing, your heart rate, and your bodily sensations. What are they? Where are they?

~ Pay attention to what your body feels like. Do certain parts of you feel numb? Tired? Do you feel like crying? Do parts of you feel like crying? These feelings are your body's wisdom. They are part of your inner guidance system.

~ What is your image of yourself? How do you think you look to the world? To yourself? Through years of chronic dissatisfaction with their bodies and chronic dieting, many women develop an unrealistic image of themselves. Some feel much heavier than they actually are. But women who are in touch with their inner guidance will often appear taller and more imposing physically than their actual body size indicates. The way you feel about yourself creates an electromagnetic field of energy around you that broadcasts these feelings to the world and attracts your reality to you. Choose your signal consciously.

~ Notice how you routinely talk to your body. What happens when you look in the mirror each morning? Do you criticize your face, your legs, your hair? Do you routinely apologize to others for how you look? Or do you give your body positive messages, such as "Thank you very much for digesting last night's dinner without any conscious input from me"? Cultivate the link between your mouth and your ear—and the rest of you—so that you get used to hearing yourself. Barbara Hoberman Levine, in her book *Your Body Believes Every Word* (WordsWork Press, 2000), tells the story of a friend who always developed rectal pain during her period. Levine asked her if she thought of her period as a "pain in the ass." The woman gasped and admitted that that was exactly how she felt about it.

~ Pay attention to your thoughts and observe how they affect your body.

~ Notice what your body needs on a daily basis. Are you hungry? Do you have to go to the bathroom? Are you tired? Do you routinely ignore your body?

⁓ Understand that your health is at risk if you are constantly undermining certain parts or functions of your body. If someone at work has a cold, you automatically undermine your body's ability to stay healthy by obsessing about how many germs you've been exposed to. Instead, say to your body, "Don't worry—I know that you have the ability to stay healthy when I nourish and rest you optimally."

⁓ Notice what fears you hold about your body. Do you avoid touching your breasts because you are afraid of finding lumps? Instead, learn about breast anatomy and learn to touch your own with respect and love. You can transform and heal your entire relationship with them. The same goes for your genitals.

⁓ Notice whether there are parts of your body that you have disowned. What are they? Do you consider parts of yourself "unacceptable"? A patient of mine had frequent abdominal pain until she was thirty-five. In her family, she had learned that it was completely unacceptable for a woman to pass gas, even though it was okay for her father and her brothers. Thus, instead of allowing routine intestinal gas to leave her body as necessary, she literally held on to it, with resulting abdominal pain. Once she realized that she had disowned an entire natural body function, she learned how to allow this function and became free of abdominal pain. Note: farts are funny. Even Shakespeare knew that. Little children know it. Accept them and learn to laugh and let go!

⁓ When you experience a bodily sensation such as back pain, "a gut reaction," a headache, or abdominal pain, pay attention to it and see if you can pinpoint the emotional situation that may have triggered it. Niravi Payne teaches her clients a new vocabulary of symptom empowerment. For example, instead of "My stomach is hurting," say, "What is it I'm having trouble stomaching?" Emotions such as anger, or any other emotion that you may consider unacceptable or that you may find difficult to experience directly, will often affect your body instead. When a sensation arises in your body, stop what you are doing, lie down, breathe, and wait with your symptom, emotion, or feeling. You may be surprised at what other feelings or insights come up. John Sarno, M.D., a physical medicine and rehabilitation specialist at the Rusk Institute in New York, and author of *Mind Over Back Pain* (Berkeley Books, 1999) and *Healing Back Pain* (Warner Books, 1991), has a 75 to 85 percent success rate with treating back pain and other related conditions such as neck pain and fibromyalgia, all of which he refers to as TMS—tension myositis syndrome. He notes that the personality of those who tend to get this syndrome is characterized by being highly conscientious, responsible, and perfectionistic. (This is not the same as the type A personality, which is associated with hostility.) He teaches his patients how to make the pain go away by making the link between their emotions and their symptoms and by telling their brain that they've got the message—it's okay for the pain to go. The results are often astonishing! I had a friend who limped into one of Sarno's meetings with crippling sciatica, which she'd had for weeks. She walked out pain free!

~ Stand in front of a mirror regularly, and thank your body for all it has done for you. Notice what comes up when you do this. Write the following sentence down on a piece of paper and tape it to the mirror: "*I accept myself unconditionally right now.*" I've often written it on a prescription blank and handed it to my patient with the following instructions: "Say this sentence out loud to yourself in the mirror while gazing into your eyes. Do this twice per day for thirty days." You can learn to accept your body unconditionally right now, regardless of where you are starting. When you do this exercise, you will learn a great deal about the inner critics that live within you. Give them a name, such as Esmeralda or George, so that you won't take them so personally next time they put you or your body down. (Remember—they are just old subconscious and incorrect programs that got downloaded earlier in life. You can change them.) When you don't take their criticisms personally, you can tell them to be quiet. Or you can even choose to laugh at them. And guess what? They eventually lose their power over you and go away!

~ Remember always that 90 percent of your bodily functions take place without your conscious input. Who keeps your heart beating? Who metabolizes your food? Who tells you when you need to replenish your fluid intake by drinking water? Who heals your skin when you cut yourself? Who tells your ears to listen to beautiful music? Who tells your eyes to see beautiful sunsets? Acknowledge that your body is a miracle and that its natural state is health and joy.

STEP FIVE: LEARN TO RESPECT YOUR BODY

Almost all women in the United States have a body image distortion because of the millions of images of "perfect" airbrushed women that the media flash at us continually. We begin comparing ourselves with these icons of unattainable perfection even before puberty. Thus, we often relate to our bodies via negative comparisons: "My hips are too fat, my breasts are too small, my knees are ugly, my hair is too thin."

Consider the following:

~ Despite years of awareness that a "perfect," thin, model's body is often destructive to women (and men) on many levels, the desire to have this body is deeply embedded in our minds even though we know that the images, even of these women, are not "real."

~ The desire for what society believes is the "perfect body" is completely understandable. Respect yourself for being human and vulnerable to it. Know that you may be powerless over it. (By this, I mean that the desire rises up unbidden. You have no control over it.) But you *do* have control and power over what you choose to do with a thought or desire. This is why it is so important to begin to hear ourselves and our thoughts.

~ The culturally induced desire for a "perfect" body doesn't have to ruin your respect, caring, or love for the body you have. If you don't respect, care, and love the body you have, no one will or even *can*. Vow to treat yourself and your body with kindness, especially when put-downs and comparisons come up from deep inside.

~ Understand that your thoughts and beliefs about yourself send a powerful signal out into the universe that others can sense. In her book *Life Magic* (Miramax Books, 2005), Laura Bushnell suggests that you imagine a huge mirror in the sky above you. In red lipstick, write the following phrase on that mirror: "I am beautiful and irresistible." Over time, your body will respond to your thoughts. You will become what you affirm.

Articles in magazines have documented that most media personalities have had or will have plastic surgery at some point in their careers. The models of perfection who beam into our global living rooms every day set up a standard that is impossible for most to aspire to without resorting to measures such as surgery.[6] And there's nothing wrong with using surgery to look your best, either! But even then, the models on magazine covers routinely have several inches airbrushed from their thighs and buttocks and duct tape applied to various areas to pull them tight. They are human, after all, just as we all are—subject to the same wrinkles and sags as the rest of us. But their industry standards demand a certain image, and so they meet it by having the right genes to begin with, then use surgery and often a rigorous and disciplined lifestyle to maintain their looks. On a TV or movie set, someone follows them around the studio all day with a blow dryer. On some level, almost all women would look their very best (or at least their culturally determined best) if they devoted the same amount of time, energy, and money to their appearance as our cultural media icons do and had all their photo images professionally manipulated. We've all seen evidence of this on the popular makeover shows on television! The enduring appeal of makeovers is that they help us manifest on the outside how we feel inside! (Note: everyone has parts of her body that are problematic. To look your best, I recommend the book *What Not to Wear* [Riverhead Books, 2004] by Trinny Woodall and Susannah Constantine. It's very practical, helpful, and fun!)

The ancient arts of adornment are part of caring for ourselves. I applaud the increasing trend toward better self-care through regular massage, pedicures, manicures, and pampering. It's a step in the right direction!

Our approach to dressing, makeup, hair, and personal care can be well served by the wisdom of Dolly Parton, who said, "Find out who you are, then do it on purpose." If we can find out who we are on the inside, we can then express it on the outside. As Coco Chanel once said, "Adornment is never anything except a reflection of the heart."

On the other hand, if we're dissatisfied with ourselves when we're not wearing makeup or dressed in the latest fashion, we're not creating vibrant health or balance in our lives. We're in danger of what Anne Wilson Schaef calls "romance addiction"—always requiring our bodies, our homes, and our lives to look "just right," like a movie set. Some women's husbands have never seen them without makeup. Some still dress behind closed doors so that their partners won't see their bodies in broad daylight, when the imperfections catch the sunlight.

The next time a friend comes to the door unexpectedly, don't apologize for the way you or your house or apartment looks. Chances are theirs looks the same way. Just invite them in, and ignore the toilet paper or whatever else is sitting in the middle of the dining room table. They came to visit you, not your spotless kitchen or your perfect image. Notice what you learn from not apologizing.

STEP SIX: ACKNOWLEDGE A HIGHER POWER OR INNER WISDOM

There is an unseen force, a spiritual dimension, guiding our lives like a loving parent guiding its child.

—Pythia Peay

Our bodies are permeated and nourished by spiritual energy and guidance. Having faith and trust in this reality is crucial for lasting health and happiness. When a woman has faith in something greater than her intellect or her present circumstances, she is in touch with her inner source of power. Each of us has within us a divine spark. We are inherently a part of God/Goddess/Source. Jesus said that the kingdom of heaven is within, and we can make this spiritual connection through our inner guidance. We need go no further than ourselves to find it.

Learning to connect with our inner wisdom, our spirituality, is not difficult, but neither our intellect nor our ego can control either the connection or the results. The first step is to hold the intent to connect with divine guidance. The second step is to release our expectations of what will happen as a result. The third step is to wait for a response by being open to noticing the changes in the patterns of our lives that relate to the original intent.

Each of us has a guardian angel available for guidance. But we have to ask for guidance and be open to receiving it. Seeing the patterns, how all the parts connect, is a way of looking at life. This is the paradigm shift I mentioned at the beginning of this chapter. Understanding the big picture doesn't mean getting stuck in the particular moment. Gaining access to spiritual guidance means looking at the pattern of our lives over time. As David Spangler said, "Dreams, events, a book, the words of a friend: all of this might be one word from an angelic being."

About two years before I wrote the first edition of this, my first book, I was standing by my bed on a sunny Friday morning, getting ready for the day. I read through my favorite meditations, which I've written down in a small book made of handcrafted paper. I decided to say aloud a statement taken from Frances Scovel Shinn's book *The Game of Life and How to Play It*.[7] I spoke it out loud clearly with sincere intent: "Infinite spirit, give me a definite lead, reveal to me my perfect self-expression. Show me which talent I am to make use of now." That very afternoon I received a call from an acquaintance who is a literary agent. "I think it is time you wrote a book," he said. It wasn't until much later that day that I put those two events together. Sometimes the guidance comes easily and quickly. When it does, though, you sometimes have to go through the part of your intellect that tells you you're making it up and are crazy for believing this stuff.

Though each of us is part of a greater whole, we are also individuals. The unique part of this whole that we each embody must be expressed fully in order to create health, happiness, and spiritual growth for ourselves and others. The way to best express this divine part of ourselves is by becoming all of who we are. Our bodies direct us toward full personal expression by letting us know what feels good and "right" and what doesn't. Illness is often a sign that we are somehow off track from our life's purpose. That is why Bernie Siegel, M.D., says, "Illness is God's reset button."

Many doctors are open to this realm of mystery, too, but they don't dare to say anything. A highly skilled intuitive here in southern Maine once said to me, "Someday I'm going to have a cocktail party at my house and invite all the doctors in this area who've come to have readings. You will all stand around and be amazed at how many of you there are—and also at who is here."

When we invite the sacred into our lives by sincerely asking our inner wisdom, or higher power, or God for guidance in our lives, we're invoking great power. This can't be taken lightly. The reason people are cynical about this and make fun of it is that they are afraid. When you sincerely invite in the sacred (your inner guidance or spirit) to assist you with your life, you are granting permission for your life to change. Those areas of your life that no longer serve your highest purpose may start to disintegrate—and this can be frightening. Caroline Myss says, "Wiping out a marriage or a job is a day at the beach for an angel." Having been in both situations, I can attest to both the fear and the power inherent in this approach. The key to getting through it is being open to the greatness of your spirit.

Believing in angels, having your astrological chart done, or getting an intuitive reading doesn't excuse anyone from the work of healing and becoming whole. Remember that anything can be used addictively—even so-called spiritual pursuits. Too many people use their "spiritual practices" to avoid addressing the difficult areas of their lives. Using crystals, New Age music, and astrology or going to church twice a week while drinking four ounces of alcohol every night or being abusive to your children will not help you heal. Doing meditation faithfully twice a day and being beaten up by your husband every night will not keep you healthy. All the "spirituality" in the world won't do your human homework for you. Only you can take the action necessary to compose a vibrant life. As one of my twelve-step friends told me, "God moves mountains—bring a shovel."

To reconnect with their innate spirituality, many women have to get past years of religious abuse, particularly if they've been victimized by organized cults or patriarchal religions. God has too often been portrayed as a vengeful, righteous being, outside of human ability to understand or know, and so it's no wonder that being angry with God and struggling with the concept of a "higher power" or "inner wisdom" is a reality for so many. Some women are stuck at a very childlike stage in which they feel, "If there were a God, he would never have let this happen to me." One of my colleagues says, "If I make God something separate from me and outside of myself, then I get to accuse God of punishing me whenever my life doesn't go well."

We are all spiritual beings with all-knowing souls or Higher Powers. Connection with spirit is inherently part of being human. For centuries our culture has tried to control our inherent spirituality via religion. Though some women may gain access to their spirituality through organized religions, too many religions rely on static dogma and rules that serve to split us from our daily spirituality. Spirituality is free-flowing and ever-changing. Though it is clear that most religions were originally based on the immediate and profound spiritual insights of their founders, most organized religions today lack the flexibility and ongoing evolution necessary to truly be spiritually connected.

Partly in response to so many years of male-based religions, many women today are drawn to different aspects of the Great Goddess. As women, we need "a sexually affirming image of power and beauty as a focus for prayer and meditation," says Patricia Reis.[8] Having internalized God as male, we can find much-needed balance in the Goddess images that are now rising.

My mother is a dowser and frequently uses a pendulum for intuitive guidance. Others use runes, tarot cards, or Bible phrases. Spiritual guidance comes in all forms, so use the form that works best for you.

Regardless of what you believe about spirituality, it is important to bring a sense of the sacred into your everyday life. Spirituality pervades all that I do. My spirituality is not set aside for special days such as Christmas, nor do I practice it only in special buildings called churches, synagogues, or temples. My spirituality is every part of me. On some level I feel part of God/Goddess/All That Is—not separate from it. When I'm exercising, I'm in touch with my spirituality. When I'm writing, I'm very much in touch with my spirituality. I'm especially in touch with my spirituality when I'm assisting women in opening to their inner guidance system. This is because reaching out to another to help her heal and connect with her spirituality also helps me heal and connect with mine.

Like many women, I feel a deep spiritual connection with nature. Many people find peace and comfort in a special place, a place that they may have gone to as children to feel held close by the nurturing qualities of nature. Women often tell me about special trees, rocks, hills, or other places that connect them very strongly with their own spirituality. Time spent alone in a natural setting is often a catalyst for connection with your spirituality.

A powerful way to tune in to the natural world is to notice what phase the moon is in and see if this natural waxing and waning has any effect on your body, emotions, or perceptions.[9] Notice what effect the seasons have on you. Does the coming of autumn wake up your senses and find you braced for new beginnings—or does this happen for you in the spring? Find out when the equinoxes and solstices are. For centuries, people felt that more spiritual power was available to them at these times. All major religious holidays are held around these times. You don't have to study anything—just be aware of the moon and the rhythms of nature. I live on a tidal river and enjoy the changing water levels outside my window, knowing that, like my body, they're connected with the phases of the moon.

When I was growing up, my father used to go to church on Sundays because he liked the church and his family had always gone there. My mother, on the other hand, often went for a walk in the woods. "He has his church, I have mine," she said. Each woman must find her own spiritual center and her own inner guidance. And for each woman it will be different.

Regardless of whether we believe in angels, God, Jesus Christ, the human spirit, Buddha, the Blessed Mother, the Great Spirit, or the Goddess Gaia, being in tune with our spiritual resources is a vital healing force. Committing ourselves to remembering our spiritual selves and receiving guidance for our lives is part of creating vibrant health.

STEP SEVEN: RECLAIM THE FULLNESS OF YOUR MIND

Women need to know that they are capable of intelligent thought, and they need to know it right now.

—Adrienne Rich

The positive thing about writing is that you connect with yourself in the deepest way, and that's heaven. You get a chance to know who you are, to know what you think. You begin to have a relationship with your mind.

—Natalie Goldberg

If we are to reclaim the wisdom of our bodies, we must also reclaim our intellects, our minds, and our ability to think. Once we have experienced how intimately our thought and bodily symptoms are related and how intelligent we are, our thinking is less distracted by cultural hypnosis. We come to trust our inner voice. We question our assumptions more critically, thus freeing ourselves from the mental habits of a lifetime.

Journal writing, writing practice, and meditation are methods that many have used to successfully get in touch with their inner voices and get to know their minds. Proprioceptive writing (PW) taught me to trust my mind and inner wisdom. Originally developed by Linda Trichter Metcalf, Ph.D., author of *Writing the Mind Alive* (Ballantine Books, 2002), this writing process engages the intellect, the intuition, and the imagination simultaneously and is done to baroque music.[10] (Baroque music has been found to synchronize brain waves at about sixty cycles per second, a frequency associated with increased alpha brain waves and enhanced creativity.) (For more information on proprioceptive writing, see the website for the Proprioceptive Writing Center at www.pwriting.org.)

I learned through my writing that my thoughts have order, direction, and intelligence, and that these are all related to my well-being. More than that, my thoughts are deeply connected with my feeling self. I learned that I use words to express, create, and explore all the relationships and emotions that give my life meaning. When I was in junior high school, I had difficulty writing papers. My teachers told me that I wasn't sticking to the point and that my thoughts were too "scattered." I was taught that in order to succeed, I would need to organize my thoughts in a linear, cause-and-effect way, listing my points in order of importance, first to last. I needed to make only one point with every paragraph and then develop only that point before moving on to the next point. I was taught that ideas should come one at a time and that they should always have some concrete, obvious relationship to each other. (That was never obvious to me.) But my mind didn't work in a linear, nonemotional fashion then, and it doesn't work that way now.

When I write or think of a word or concept, my mind immediately goes in several directions at once—all of them rich with emotional content, and all of them related to each other equally, nonhierarchically, and nonlinearly. Thus, my natural thinking process is circular and multimodal, as it is for many women. If I write the word *bra,* for example, my mind goes off in all the following directions almost simultaneously: I think of a woman's relationship with her bra, how she purchased her first bra, what it was like for her, what that means about her relationship with her breasts, whether she's ever used an underwire bra, what her breasts mean in this culture, whether she was breast-fed, and so on.

If I simply wrote down my thoughts as I listened to them, at first they seemed random and without order. But as I continued the process, I saw that my thoughts were weaving a web of interconnected meaning that was going in a certain direction. My job was simply to go along for the ride and record what I heard or felt. I would always come back to my initial point of departure, but with a deeper understanding of my beliefs and wisdom.

Through writing I have come to see that every word that comes into my mind has meaning and that this meaning is connected to my entire being. I've come to appreciate that my ideas, thoughts, and wisdom come from all of me—my brain, my uterus, and my higher power—and that they may originate in any one of the numerous interconnected aspects of me. I have learned to trust my thoughts. Women's (and some men's) ways of knowing are not the logocentric left-brain approaches taught in our schools and universities. It's staggering to realize how many highly intelligent women feel that they are stupid because of this training.

To become free of thoughts and beliefs that don't serve you, you must first be able to hear them as they arise. Writing practice is a profound tool for learning how to hear ourselves and to appreciate the multimodal nature of our thoughts. Everyone has this ability. Listening to our thoughts teaches us that the way in which we talk to ourselves inside is exactly the way we will be perceived by others. We don't speak to others in a way that's any different from the ways in which we speak to ourselves inside our own heads. For years, the word *worthy* came up in my writing because on some deep level I didn't feel worthy. I spent hours asking myself what I meant by this word. Images of school, authorities, tests, and church always arose around this word. Eventually, my meditation on the word *worthy* led me to a breakthrough understanding of the original sin of being female. How could I have felt worthy, given my cultural programming?

If a word or phrase continually comes into your mind, it is important— it has meaning for you. Explore it. Write about it. Meditate on it. If a thought comes into your mind, learn to accept it without judgment. It will have meaning for you, no matter what it is. It is there for a reason. Linda Metcalf says, "There are no tourists in the mind."

To change the conditions of our lives outside, we must make a change inside. Proprioceptive writing is a tool to explore what is inside. After all, if we don't know where we are, how can we ever expect to get anywhere else? What I discovered within me were layers and layers of *shoulds, oughts,* and other impediment of my education and cultural indoctrination. Metcalf describes these as a "mangrove swamp, with all the roots twisted around each other."

Through weeks, months, and years of writing, I gained direct experience of my own indoctrination, and eventually came to hear my true self emerging—my own voice. But I also ran smack up against my guilt. This guilt seemed to be a part of who I was, neatly installed years before. (I also experienced how I had split spirituality from anything political. Now I know that we cannot separate the two.) Guilt is a fantastic tool for keeping women in their place. It is a form of internalized oppression and fear that serves to maintain the status quo. Guilt immobilizes us with "What will they think if..." messages. I realized that if I continued to wallow in my own guilt instead of examining its voice within me, I would forever be ineffective at doing the work I am best at—and which I love the most. How could this possibly help me, or anyone else? When I reclaimed my work as political and let go of guilt (mostly), I broke free from a set of health-destroying beliefs. It's an ongoing process.

My writing was vital in helping me break free from those parts of my life that no longer served me. However you do it, you, too, can learn to respect your intellect, your mind, and the fullness of your intelligence.

Dialogues with the Body: Listening to the Mind That Creates the Cells

I often ask women to carry out a dialogue with their bodily symptoms or with the organ that is giving them problems, through writing, meditation, or drawing. Sitting with your journal open while being receptive to your thoughts, ask your body what it needs or what it is trying to tell you.

One of my patients, who was experiencing heavy menstrual bleeding and a fibroid, asked her pelvis to speak to her. In her journal she wrote, "What is the wisdom you are trying to convey to me through my bleeding and my fibroid?" Over the next several days, she "waited with" this question for about ten minutes per day.

The answer that eventually came was, "Your periods are symbolic of the way you give yourself away too freely. The heavy bleeding represents your own life's blood draining away. You do the same thing in your relationship with your boyfriend. This is related to your relationship with your father."

Another patient told me, "You asked me to have a dialogue with my cervix. [She had had an abnormal Pap smear.] It's all about shame, it's all about deprivation, it's all about not being good enough. I think I need to listen some more."

Many fine publications have been written, and workshops offered, on how to do journal work, or other forms of introspective dialogue. I recommend Linda Trichter Metcalf and Tobin Simon's *Writing the Mind Alive* (Ballantine Books, 2002) and also Natalie Goldberg's books on writing practice, *Writing Down the Bones* (Shambhala, 1986) and *Wild Mind* (Bantam Books, 1990).

Working with Dreams: A Dream Incubation

The night dreams speak Wild Woman's Language. She is there broadcasting. All we have to do is take dictation.
—Clarissa Pinkola Estes

You can learn to work with your dreams actively and learn to consult them about specific problems in your life. The process of asking for a dream for guidance is known as dream incubation.[11] To do this effectively you must be willing to be 100 percent honest about the circumstances of your life. Here's how to do it.

Choose a night when you have some energy and focus to devote to the process. Spend ten to twenty minutes writing in your journal concerning the particular issue you want to focus on. Address the following questions within yourself, and be open to other input from your inner guidance:

What is the root cause of my problem?

What possible solutions come to mind about my problem right now?

Why aren't these solutions adequate?

How am I feeling right now as I work on this?

Does it feel safer to live with the problem than to resolve it?

What do I have to lose if I solve the problem now?

What do I have to gain if I solve the problem now?

Is there anything that my future self would like to tell me that could help?

Write down a one-line sentence or request that deals with the problem as directly and simply as possible, and keep your question gently in mind as you drift off to sleep. Have a paper, pen, and flashlight, or a tape recorder, handy at your bedside, and write down any dreams you remember. Sometimes insights will come to you at three A.M. or anytime you might awaken to go to the bathroom. If you don't write down at least the pertinent details of your dream, you are likely to forget it by morning. This process may take several nights before a clarifying dream arises.

Betty, one of my friends, found herself in a painful social situation in which she felt that two of her colleagues were blaming her for the fact that they were being passed over for job promotions. Betty is very bright and creative and is always able to come up with new approaches to her work that are fun, innovative, and productive. Her colleagues through the years have often been jealous of these abilities. Because she loves working with people and has great difficulty with interpersonal conflict, this latest situation was very painful for Betty. She contemplated quitting her job and moving across the country, even though her work was very fulfilling. When she became aware of the hostility of her colleagues in this current situation, the feeling this evoked in her was old and all too familiar. She had been unfairly "blackballed," "picked on," and "scapegoated" similarly by others. It had happened over and over again at other jobs and in several other settings, both personal and professional. Completely fed up with being thus victimized by others, she wanted to choose another way to live with her gifts and talents. She decided to do a dream incubation to ask for guidance in changing whatever unconscious patterns kept attracting situations in which she ended up as the victim of other people's inadequacies. After noting all the different situations in which she'd been victimized and allowing herself to feel fully how disgusted she was by the whole thing, she asked for a dream that would help her clarify her situation. She wrote, "Why do I keep re-creating situations in my life in which people pick on me?"

That night she had the following dream: A very good friend was seated to her left. The friend reached over to help a porcupine, and the porcupine shot its quills at her. Betty's friend took the quills and embedded them in Betty's arm—then looked in her face to see what her reaction would be. Betty simply sat there and allowed the quills to be painfully embedded in her arm. So now, the same friend took a handful of needles and pins and began sticking them in Betty's arm. Meanwhile, Betty continued to say nothing—simply sitting there with the pain of this. Finally, Betty decided to do something about her pain. She began taking the needles out herself. When she did this, a great deal of blood started pouring out of all the needle holes in her arm. Overwhelmed with the pain and the extent of the bleeding, Betty then decided to complain to her friend, telling her it was not okay to stick quills and needles in her arm.

Betty then looked to her right side and saw her mother, father, and sister all sitting there. She realized that throughout her childhood, these family members had insulted and physically beaten her. Betty had never complained and had never said anything. Instead, she fixed the pain herself and allowed herself to bleed. (Remember, blood is symbolic of family.)

When Betty awakened, she realized that she could no longer allow psychic, emotional, or other barbs to accumulate without saying anything. She knew that she had come to the point of "bleeding to death" from the accumulation of a lifetime of hurts that she had never acknowledged or complained about. Because of her upbringing, she had been led to believe that if she complained, she'd simply get beaten more. Now Betty realized that she had to stand up for herself at the first sign of discomfort in her relationships. She saw how deeply the victim mentality had been drummed into her in childhood. She had used her considerable gifts and talents to escape her family of origin—only to have the original family pattern recur in all her later relationships. Having become very clear about her part in creating victim situations by refusing to defend herself, Betty now speaks up for herself at the first sign of discomfort. She also realizes that if a colleague has problems with her abilities, this is not something that Betty has to fix. The colleague herself must deal with her own inner sense of jealousy and inadequacy to see what it is teaching her. Betty cannot do this for another.

STEP EIGHT: GET HELP

We do not believe in ourselves until someone reveals that deep inside us something is valuable, worth listening to, worthy of our trust, sacred to our touch. Once we believe in ourselves we can risk curiosity, wonder, spontaneous delight, or any experience that reveals the human spirit.

—e.e. cummings

Setting aside the time and money to go and talk with a skilled listener can be invaluable. This person may be a therapist, a minister, a life coach, or other trustworthy individual. These sessions can be a way to stop, reassess your life, and give yourself a much-needed focus on a regular basis. Many therapists have helped people begin to look at their lives differently and effect change. A good therapist should be like a midwife, standing by while someone gives birth to what's best in themselves.

When I was about fourteen and upset about something that I can't even remember now, my father told me how important it was to express what I was feeling and "get it off my chest." (The phrase "get it off your chest" is an accurate anatomic description of dealing with fourth-chakra issues, such as sadness, which tend to affect the shoulders, breast, and heart.) He told me, "I notice a tendency in you to clam up and not say what's going on. When you do this, you prevent others from helping you." It was good advice. We all can use a reassessment of our lives and a skilled listener on a regular basis. Support of this nature should be built into the culture. Community has been largely lost since the Industrial Revolution and the ensuing split between work, home, private, and public. In an ideal world it wouldn't be necessary for us to go to individual therapists or to create separate support groups for those with cancer, those suffering from loneliness, or even those who want to create health. Native cultures have lived for centuries without all the therapies that have evolved to fix a society whose basic worldview promotes the myth of the rugged individual who needs no one. No wonder so many people seek support from therapists!

My colleagues and I worked with a therapist regularly after starting our Women to Women health center to learn how to talk openly and honestly with one another—and to deal with emotions that women aren't supposed to have, like anger. Our therapist never tried to change or "fix" us. He simply provided a safe place for us to say what we needed to say to one another—without our thinking we had to take care of the feelings of the person we were angry with at the same time. In the early years of our practice, we honestly didn't know that we were capable of a perfectly functional relationship with each other even when we expressed our anger or disappointment. We had no skills for breaking through our old habits of "being nice." Having done extensive codependency (relationship addiction) recovery work we saw that those early therapy sessions were crucial for our ability to be honest with each other and with ourselves. As our self-awareness skills increased, we required many fewer sessions. Our group "therapy" (now called "team building" in the therapy profession) helped us create independence. We were able to take what we learned and internalize it, and we eventually learned to communicate among ourselves without an outside person assisting.

There are many different kinds of therapists. The entire field has been changing in response to evolving knowledge about addiction, recovery, and the influence of childhood trauma. Therapy is not something that should go on for years, in my view. When it does, it can become an addictive process in and of itself—not much different from the alcoholic-enabler duality. All relationships, therapeutic or otherwise, work best when the participants see each other as essentially whole beings with inner resources and strengths, though sometimes in temporary need of assistance.

Though individual therapy is often a first step for many women, group work of some kind, such as a twelve-step group or a skills training group, can be powerful in that this setting helps us see that our problems are shared by so many others. A member of Overeaters Anonymous once told me, "Addiction recovery is God's answer to community." Group work certainly is one answer that is helping millions. The practical wisdom contained in the twelve steps of Alcoholics Anonymous is a blueprint for how to live a life based on inner guidance. Many other twelve-step fellowships used AA's steps and simply take out the word *alcohol* or *alcoholic* if it's not applicable, substituting something more relevant. The program and the program's literature are still highly relevant and helpful. Groups help rid us of our "myth of terminal uniqueness," as a therapist friend calls it, while individual therapy for wounds such as incest can isolate a woman further because it "privatizes" what is in fact a cultural and even global problem. Part of the wounding of addictions, incest, or other sexual abuse is its hiddenness. Imagine the relief of participating in a group of women in which all of them are saying, "That happened to you, too? I always thought I was the only one!"

It has been my experience that women with histories of trauma recover most effectively in a type of therapy known as cognitive behavioral therapy. This form of therapy focuses not exclusively on the past trauma, but on helping people develop the skills necessary to live productive, healthy lives in the present. It is generally not helpful to spend a great deal of time revisiting the past, where it is too easy to get stuck in pain and immobility. Instead, women with trauma histories need to learn to develop the skills that they never developed in childhood. In cognitive behavioral therapy training, women learn to answer the following questions and then take effective, balanced action.

- ~ What am I feeling?

- ~ What is the purpose of this feeling?

- ~ What do I need to do for myself to deal effectively with this feeling?

I have seen more improvement in women's lives with this model than with most others. These skills are practical and helpful for everyone, not just those with histories of trauma because they reprogram old subconscious programming.

Many people with chronic or life-threatening illness also come together regularly to share not only their tears but also their joy and their laughter. This grassroots movement support group throughout the country has been a source of growth, comfort, and hope to many. I regularly refer people to support groups of all kinds in our community, and have participated myself. Dr. David Spiegel has clearly demonstrated that women with metastatic breast cancer who participated in a support group characterized by emotional openness and sharing lived twice as long as those who didn't participate.[12] If a drug had been shown to have this effect, you can bet it would be widely used. But to date, most women diagnosed with breast cancer are not encouraged to seek the health benefits of this group model.

For many women, it is important to spend time regularly in women-only settings. When we gather together as women, we each hold a piece of the whole story. Together we heal faster than we would if we remained isolated and separate, and group members hold up a mirror for us so that we can see ourselves more clearly.

In the early stages of self-awareness, women often don't tell the whole truth if there's even one man in the room. The same may be true for men. We've been socialized to tailor our conversations to accommodate the other gender. In order to become self-aware, we need environments in which we can truly be ourselves. For many, that means women-only settings until you can tell the truth about any given experience without changing your story to protect the men who are present. This process has taken me years to master.

Annie Rafter, a nurse-practitioner colleague, tells the following story: One summer she and a group of women friends crewed together on a sailboat and participated in races. They began to notice that if a man came on their boat, they automatically deferred to him—handing him the tiller or expecting him to chart the right course—before they even knew whether or not he was a good sailor.

Noticing this behavior in themselves, the women decided that for one season, they needed to sail with no men on the boat so that they could become a cohesive crew. So for that one season, they stuck by their agreement and learned to trust one another. By the next sailing season, it didn't matter who came on the boat—the women crew trusted themselves, one another, and their sailing skills. They no longer automatically deferred to men.

In the early days of Women to Women, we often referred back to Annie Rafter's story about "no men on the boat." Like her crew, we needed to learn to trust one another and to learn how to maintain that trust, no matter who came into the building. Back then, I found that working in a women-only environment gave me the time and space to talk out my problems in a way that simply didn't work with my husband. We women have been mistakenly taught that our mates should be our best friends and our primary source of emotional support. Occasionally this works, but not often. When we rely on men to support us emotionally, we often end up disappointed. I'd find that when I'd had my "process" time with other women, I didn't need my husband to be there for me to go over the details of my day and give me advice or support. When I went home, we met more as peers to share the events of our day in a way that was totally different from the way I shared them with one of my women friends. By having plenty of women-only time and support, I learned not to burden my primary male-female relationship with needs that probably weren't meant to be filled in that relationship in the first place.

Meetings and support help people to get out of denial. Twelve-step and other programs have helped millions of people recover inner strength and serenity—this should be the first step in moving on in their lives. In order to heal fully, however, each of us must get to a point in which we're not overly identified with our wounds. This is not easy, because "we learn the language of wounds as our first language and we use our wounds to create intimacy," as Caroline Myss says. People don't heal fully and move on with their lives as long as they continue to take what has happened to them too personally and identify themselves solely as victims. When a woman sees herself solely as a victim, she too often also becomes a perpetrator. She may lash out at anyone who dares to suggest that she has the inner wisdom to change. Be sensitive to when it's time to leave your group and move on. Be careful of your language. Though it may be appropriate to label yourself as an incest survivor or breast cancer survivor initially, eventually this identification with your wound may prevent you from becoming the healthy, whole person you were meant to be. At some point, you'll find that you'll be better served by something like "I am a woman who has experienced breast cancer or incest"—this expands your options, while the label "survivor" may limit them. Eventually we must take responsibility for our lives and stop laying blame for the conditions of our lives on everything from addictions and incest to the political system and the environment. Seeing our dysfunctional patterns, working on them, and letting them go is a process.

STEP NINE: WORK WITH YOUR BODY

For most of us, talking things out is simply not enough. "I know all of the things that happened to me as a child and with my husband," said one woman, "but talking about it just doesn't change a thing. I seem to be going in circles." When this happens, we often obsess and seem to spin our wheels. It's easy to get locked in to "thought addiction"—a kind of gerbil wheel in the brain that keeps us going around in circles.

Much of the information we need to heal is locked in our muscles and other body parts. Getting a good massage will often release old energy blockages and help us cry or get rid of chronic pain from "holding the world on our shoulders." There are many types of bodywork, ranging from polarity therapy to the Feldenkrais Method, that are beneficial. Bodywork can be divided into two different types: physical bodywork (like Rolfing, classical osteopathy, and massage) and energetic bodywork (like Reiki, acupuncture, and therapeutic touch). Though I will not be discussing these separately, I wanted to make this distinction.

Work on and with the body can be an opportunity for understanding and experiencing the unity of our bodymind. These therapies are often deeply relaxing and give our bodies a chance to rest and sleep, a time when much of the body's repair work goes on. Acupuncture works well for all kinds of problems that aren't easily treated through conventional means. I would like to see it and the many other kinds of physical and energetic bodywork used in conventional hospitals.

I've referred hundreds of patients for bodywork of different kinds over the years and am very gratified with the results. To help find the right body practice for you, I recommend Mirka Knaster's *Discovering the Body's Wisdom* (Bantam, 1996), a guide to more than fifty forms of bodywork that also explains beautifully how and why these approaches work. I personally get a full body massage once a week. I regard it as part of my general health maintenance program.

Schedule at least a shoulder or foot massage sometime this month. You can also trade massages with a friend. Eventually, work up to a full massage regularly.

STEP TEN: GATHER INFORMATION

Currently, more books of interest to women are available than at any other time in history. I recommend going to your bookstore or library and using your inner guidance to help you make a choice. Acknowledge that you have the wisdom to choose the right book at the right time. Just sit with the books for a while and look over a few titles. See which ones speak to you. Choose the ones that feel right and have appeal. You cannot make a mistake.

It is a powerful experience for women to begin to reclaim our forgotten history by reading about our bodies, menstruation, childbirth, and goddesses, all written from a woman's point of view. One of the greatest gifts of the feminist movement of the 1970s was the deconstructing of the patriarchal mindset, which was seen for centuries as "the truth" or "just the way it is." Ursula Le Guin points out that 50 percent of writers are women, but 90 percent of what we call "literature" has been written by men.

Books ranging from *Our Bodies, Ourselves,* by Boston Women's Health Book Collective, a book that heralded a much needed reevaluation of women's health care, to *The Chalice and the Blade* (Harper,

1990) and *Sacred Pleasure* (HarperSanFrancisco, 1995) by Riane Eisler have helped a whole generation of women rethink our history and how it has affected our lives.[13] Through the power of the pen, we receive support for our journey together.

The many new volumes on the mind/body connection are also of great help to women in reinforcing their own experience. *The Biology of Belief* (Elite Books, 2005) by Bruce Lipton, Ph.D., a cellular biologist and former research scientist at Stanford University School of Medicine, is particularly relevant and helpful as it documents the science of how thought and emotions affect cells in an easily understood manner that is both convincing and entertaining. (For more information on Dr. Lipton's work, see www.brucelipton.com.) Books are great companions for many otherwise isolated women who have not yet found each other or come together in communities. Reading and gathering information is a very nonthreatening first step on the journey to vibrant health. Many of my patients have spent years reading everything they could get their hands on before they felt ready to join a group or seek other support and sisterhood.

STEP ELEVEN: FORGIVE

We must let ourselves feel all the painful destruction we want to forgive rather than swallow it in denial. If we do not face it, we cannot choose to forgive it.
> —Kenneth McAll, *Healing the Family Tree*

Forgiveness frees us. It heals our bodies and our lives. It is simple but not easy. Forgiveness doesn't mean that what another person did to you was right or just. It simply means that you've decided to forgive and release the other person as a gift to yourself. It takes a great deal of energy to keep someone out of our hearts. When we forgive those who have hurt us, both of us are freed. Forgiveness and making amends are completely linked. Holding a grudge and maintaining hatred or resentment hurts *us* at least as much as the other person. Many times, the person who is hardest to forgive is yourself.

Forgiveness moves our energy to the heart area, the fourth chakra. When the body's energy moves there, we don't take our wounds so personally—and we can heal. Forgiveness is the initiation of the heart, and it is hands down the most powerful force for attracting vibrant health that I know. Fred Luskin, Ph.D., of the Stanford Forgiveness Project and author of *Forgive for Good* (HarperSanFrancisco, 2002), has demonstrated that forgiveness can improve the health and quality of life even in those who've experienced enormous wounding. After Dr. Luskin gave a week-long forgiveness training workshop for seventeen residents of Northern Ireland, each of whom had had a primary family member murdered in the violence there, symptoms of stress (such as dizziness, headaches, and stomachaches) decreased by 35 percent, depression dropped 20 percent, and anger dropped by 12 percent. In addition, participants' physical vitality (including energy level, appetite, sleep patterns, and general well-being) improved significantly.[14] (For more on forgiveness, including Dr. Luskin's Nine Steps to Forgiveness and information about his research, visit his website at www.learningtoforgive.com.)

Scientific studies have shown that when we think with our hearts by taking a moment to focus on someone or something that we love unconditionally—like a puppy or a young child—the rhythm of our hearts evens out and becomes healthier. Hormone levels change and normalize as well. When people are taught to think with their hearts regularly, they can even reverse heart disease and other stress-related conditions. The electromagnetic field of the heart is sixty times stronger than the electromagnetic field produced by the brain; to me, this means that every cell in our bodies—and in the bodies of those around us—can be positively influenced by the quality of our hearts when they are beating in synchrony with the energy of appreciation.[15]

When I think back on my breast abscess, I feel great compassion and forgiveness *for myself*. How could I have known what I was doing? I had no role models of women in OB/GYN for balance between work and motherhood. I have forgiven myself, and because of that I have also forgiven my colleagues at the time. It has taken years for me to come to grips with the concept of forgiveness. When I first wrote this chapter, I didn't even think of putting this crucial step in. When we forgive someone because we think it is the right thing to do, we're merely jumping through a socially acceptable hoop that changes nothing. Psychologist Alice Miller states that when children are asked to forgive abusive parents without first experiencing their emotions and their personal pain, the forgiveness becomes another weapon of silencing. Leaping to forgive under these circumstances is not really forgiveness—it is just another form of denial. Many women think that forgiving someone who hurt them is the same as saying that what happened to them was okay and that it didn't hurt them. Nothing could be further from the truth. Many women have been brainwashed into submission by the misunderstanding of forgiveness. To get to forgiveness, we first have to work through the painful experiences that require it. Forgiveness doesn't mean that what happened to us was okay. It simply means that we are no longer willing to allow that experience to adversely affect our lives. Forgiveness is something we do, ultimately, for ourselves.

I once saw a women with migraine headaches that were becoming increasingly severe. She also had chronic vaginitis, multiple allergies, and a host of other problems. A perfectionist, she routinely took on too much at her job. When she spoke, she formed her words in a careful and controlled way—and her face twitched in an exaggerated way. On her intake form, she noted that her father, maternal grandfather, paternal grandfather, three brothers, and all her uncles were alcoholics and that her mother had expected her to be an adult almost since birth. "I was never allowed to play. I had to keep the house neat," she wrote. She firmly believed that "none of these alcoholics had any effect on me during the time I was living at home." Her denial was very clearly in place, while her body was screaming to get her attention. Forgiveness of her parents would be ridiculous in her case. It would simply be used to build up another layer of intellectual armor. This woman first had to acknowledge that she was adversely affected by her parents' behavior. Forgiveness is completely premature when a woman doesn't even acknowledge that she has an emotional abscess, let alone that it needs to be drained.

True forgiveness, on the other hand, changes us at a core level. It changes our bodies. It is an experience of grace. As I write about this concept, I'm moved to tears by the holiness of what forgiveness really is. I experienced this profoundly a number of years ago when I was reported to the medical board in Maine by a general surgeon. One of this man's patients had come to me for a consultation. Three months before, she had gone to this surgeon because of abdominal pain, weight loss, and narrowing stool caliber. He had attempted a colonoscopy (a test in which a fiber-optic scope is put into the colon to examine the inside and check for conditions such as cancer), but he had been unable to get the instrument all the way up her colon. He told her that she would need to have surgery to remove part of her colon, since he was virtually certain she had a cancer that was causing her symptoms.

She had gone home, changed her diet completely to a macrobiotic approach, and over a three-month time period regained the weight she had lost, was free of abdominal pain, and had normal stools once again. All of this had taken place before she saw me. When I first saw her, she was healthy, vital, and committed to avoiding surgery. Since she was so much better, she wanted to know if I thought she still needed the surgery.

I told her that no one could be sure if she did or didn't have cancer without further testing. She had already taken a risk by not having the surgery earlier, but on the other hand, the actions she had taken had certainly reversed all the symptoms for which she had initially sought care. It was possible that she didn't have cancer and that her symptoms had been from diverticulitis (an infection of the colon that can mimic cancer) that was now healed. She decided to continue doing what she was doing with her diet, then have her colonoscopy repeated in a few months. After all, it was her body and she was feeling better than she had in years.

She understood that this decision was in direct conflict with what her surgeon suggested, but at this point he wasn't aware of her striking improvement. I felt sure that once he saw her, he'd agree to postpone her surgery and repeat her tests. Because I believe that people do best when they are cared for by a medical team that is informed, I sent a copy of our discussion to her surgeon.

As it turned out, he was furious with me for not "forcing" her to have surgery, and so he reported me to our state medical board. I had to submit a report of my end of the story and wait for the board to call me forward for a hearing. They met only every three months, so I had plenty of time to stew about this situation. I felt sure that a doctor-initiated complaint against me would be taken quite seriously, and I was terrified.

This event was the most difficult learning I'd experienced in my career. I had spent my whole life in the pursuit of good grades, respectability, and worthiness. I came from a family tradition of "good" doctors. Yet here was the manifestation of my worst fear: the authorities were going to say that I was a "bad" doctor, that I couldn't practice medicine in a way consistent with my own beliefs about healing, and worse, that my patients didn't have the choice with their own bodies, either! I worked with and felt my fear daily for weeks. If I could change how I felt on the inside, I knew, something would change in the world outside. This had always been part of my belief system. Now I had to put it to a very practical test.

Part of any healing is "letting go," relinquishing the illusion of control. For me, the letting-go was this conclusion: if I couldn't practice medicine in a way that was consistent with the healing power of the human body and individual free choice, then I would willingly give up my license. I was helped and supported during this process by colleagues and patients who told me that they'd accompany me to my hearing if necessary. Dr. Nancy Coyne, a local physician, told me that if I had to go, she'd make sure that the place was "packed with feminists" in support of me. For that, I will be forever grateful.

One day while doing my writing practice, I spontaneously began a letter to this surgeon who had reported me: Dear Dr. M., I know your fears. I know why you are upset... As I continued, I felt compassion for this man. I knew who he was. I felt him as a frightened man fighting for control—and I forgave him. As I continued writing, I felt the fear in my solar plexus lift for the first time in weeks. It was a physical feeling, not an intellectual exercise. And at the same time, I knew that everything would be all right, *regardless of the decision of the board.*

The next day, one of my colleagues who served on the board at the time saw me in the hospital and told me, "By the way, the board unanimously decided to drop your case. They felt that that surgeon was way out of line!" I never had to go before the board or plead my case in any way. They had upheld my patient's right to informed care, and my right to give it.

My ordeal was over. The most striking thing about this experience was the physical feeling of release in my solar plexus area when my fear finally healed and I felt compassion for my adversary. From this I learned that forgiveness is organic and that it is physical as well as spiritual and emotional. My intent had been to heal my own situation, not necessarily to forgive the surgeon. But I subsequently learned that the only way to heal the situation was to withdraw my energy from it and to forgive my accuser. I learned that forgiveness comes unbidden, by itself, when we are committed to vibrant health. To experience forgiveness, however, we must first make a commitment to healing and to making amends, when they are needed.

I never intended to feel compassion and forgiveness toward that surgeon. What I did want to do was get rid of the knot in my solar plexus. This I did by being willing to stay with the knot, to be in dialogue with it, and to learn from it. I believed at a deep level that I could learn from this experience, and that in fact I must learn from it, so that I wouldn't have to repeat it, in another way or another form.

Though I don't recommend being reported to a medical board for personal growth, it was one of the most freeing experiences of my life. I had faced one of my worst fears, stayed with it, and transformed it. The patient's tests were repeated at another hospital two months later. Her colon was perfectly normal, with no sign of a tumor. She had probably never had cancer in the first place, just an inflammation of the colon. She continues to be well. My former husband suggested that I report the surgeon to his board in Massachusetts and ask if it is the standard care in his state to remove a normal colon. I said, "No. The war needs to stop somewhere. It's stopping with me." I did, however, write Dr. M. a note with copies of the patient's normal tests and remarked, "Isn't the healing ability of the human body miraculous?"

Stephen Levine teaches us that the quality of forgiveness is miraculous for bringing balance. Most of us, he reminds us, have been given nothing in our training to work with resentment. Levine has given us the following meditation.[16]

> Close your eyes....
> For a moment just reflect on what the word *forgiveness* might really mean. What is forgiveness?
> And now, very gently—no force—just as an experiment in truth—just for a moment—allow the image of someone for whom you have much resentment—someone for whom you have anger and a sense of distance—let them just gently—gently, come into your mind—as an image, as a feeling.
> Maybe you feel them at the center of your chest as fear, as resistance. However they manifest in your mindbody, just invite them in very gently for this moment—for this experiment.
> And in your heart, silently say to them, "I forgive you.
> "I forgive you for whatever you have done in the past that caused me pain, intentionally or unintentionally.
> "However you have caused me pain, I forgive you."
> Speak gently to them in your heart with your own words—in your own way.

> In your heart, say to them, "I forgive you for whatever you may have done in the past, through your words, through your actions, through your thoughts that caused me pain, intentionally or unintentionally, I forgive you. I forgive you."
> Allow...Allow them to be touched...just for a moment at least...by your forgiveness.
> Allow forgiveness.
> It is so painful to hold someone out of your heart. How can you hold on to the pain, that resentment even a moment longer?
> Fear, doubt...let it go...and for this moment, touch them with your forgiveness.
> "I forgive you."
> Now let them go gently, let them leave quietly. Let them go with your blessing.

> Now picture someone who has great resentment for you. Feel them maybe in your chest, seeing them in your mind as an image—a sense of their being. Invite them gently in. Someone who has resentment, anger—someone who is unforgiving toward you.
> Let them into your heart.

And in your heart, say to them, "I ask your forgiveness, for whatever I may have done in the past that caused you pain, intentionally or unintentionally—through my words, through my actions, through my thoughts. However I caused you pain, I ask your forgiveness. I ask your forgiveness.
"Through my anger, my fear, my blindness, my laziness. However I caused you pain intentionally or unintentionally—I ask your forgiveness."

Let it be. Allow that forgiveness in. Allow yourself to be touched by their forgiveness. If the mind rises up with thoughts like self-indulgence or doubt, just see how profound our mercilessness is with ourselves and open to the forgiveness.
Allow yourself to be forgiven.
Allow yourself to be forgiven.
However I caused you pain, I ask for your forgiveness. Allow yourself to feel their forgiveness.
Let it be.
Let it be.
And gently ... gently ... let them go on their way in forgiveness for you—in blessings for you.

And turn to yourself in your own heart and say, "I forgive you" to you.
Whatever tries to block that—the mercilessness and fear.
Let it go.
Let it be touched by your forgiveness and your mercy.
And gently, in your heart, calling yourself by your own first name, say, "I forgive you" to you.
It is so painful to put yourself out of your heart.
Let yourself in. Allow yourself to be touched by this forgiveness.
Let the healing in.
Say, "I forgive you" to you.

Let that forgiveness be extended to the beings all around you.
May all beings forgive themselves.
May they discover joy.
May all beings be freed of suffering.
May all beings be at peace.
May all beings be healed.
May they be at one with their true nature.
May they be free from suffering.

May they be at peace.
Let that loving kindness, that forgiveness, extend to the whole planet—to
every level of existence, seen and unseen.
May all beings be freed of suffering.
May they know the power of forgiveness, of freedom, of peace.
May all beings seen and unseen, at every level of existence, may they
know their true being.
May they know their vastness—their infinite peacefulness.
May all beings be free.
May all beings be free.

STEP TWELVE: ACTIVELY PURSUE PLEASURE AND PURPOSE

*By pursuing your allurements, you help bind the universe together.
The unity of the world rests on the pursuit of passion.*
—Brian Swimme

When my elder daughter was nine, she reminded me how beautifully we are equipped with the innate capacity to live life fully, appreciating it as we go along. On Easter Sunday, she came bounding downstairs and exclaimed, "Don't you love it when you feel good, and you look good, and your room's clean, too?"

Watch children for a while, and you will begin to see what qualities you need to embody to wake up your soul and your immune system regularly. Most young children know exactly what they want. We are all born with an innate ability to know what we want. We are then socialized to believe that we can't have what we want, and so we gradually dismiss our innermost desires, our life's passion, to avoid disappointment. But I have come to the conclusion that feminine desire is the most powerful force for good on the planet.

David Ehrenfeld wrote in *The Arrogance of Humanism* (Oxford University Press, 1978),

> Our civilization is coming to equate the value of life with the mere avoidance of death. An empty and impossible goal, a fool's quest for nothingness, has been substituted for a delight in living and lies latent in all of us. When death is once again accepted as one of the many important parts of life, then life may recover its old thrill, and the efforts of good physicians will not be wasted.[17]

Get out a piece of paper and write on the top of it, "I desire..." or "I choose..." then write in what you want. For example, "I desire a strong, healthy body" or "I choose a strong healthy body." Notice that the word *desire* or *choose* feels effortless. You just have to allow it to come. This is the feminine receptive mode, so often lacking in our culture. Now write down exactly why you want what you want, so that you can literally feel the excitement generated by your enthusiasm. Remember: by the law of attraction, you attract your vibrational equivalent. It is the feeling and the vibration of the feeling that have the power to attract circumstances to you. In one example: "A healthy strong body makes me feel powerful and vibrant. I desire my body to be an instrument that is highly attuned to my needs. I desire a body that is a reflection of the beauty that is inside me. I choose a body that is capable of getting me where I want to go. I choose a body that has lots of energy and stamina so that I may enjoy my life more fully."

The positive emotional energy generated by this experience literally begins to draw the experience of health to you. Focus on and think often about what you desire, and you will be setting up an invisible magnetic field that begins to draw health to you, unless you keep blocking it with other thoughts such as "Well, I want it, but I'll never get it." (Review step one and see if your future self has anything to tell you here.) Your thoughts and your emotions need to line up on this one. You can't get around subconscious programming simply with affirmations. If you say you want a healthy body, but deep inside you don't feel that you are worthy of it or that illness is a punishment of some kind, you will be creating a mixed message, and your results won't be nearly as good.

Every day, spend just a few minutes focusing on appreciating what brings you pleasure now. Make appreciation a habit. Keep a gratitude journal. What you pay attention to expands. Spend time noticing what is working and what you like right now. You will never be able to feel happy or fulfilled in the future unless you can feel how that would feel right now. Over time this process will change every cell in your body.

For thirty consecutive nights, just before falling asleep, say to yourself, "I am peace. I am beauty. I am vibrantly healthful. I am prosperous." During sleep, the intellect is quieted and your inner guidance takes over. Your intent to attain or maintain pleasure and peace will be programmed into your bodymind as you sleep. Just try this and see what happens.

As you move through your day, use the power of intent to clear a path for yourself. Say, "I am Divinely irresistible to joy and freedom." Post affirmations at strategic places around your home and workplace to program your subconscious for more pleasure, health, and purpose. Take the time to really listen to good music and really take in beauty and pleasure.

Notice during each day how often your thoughts about what you want turn to the negative. Gently bring them back. Immaculée Ilibagiza, author of *Left to Tell* (Hay House, 2006), and whose story is told more fully in chapter 19, survived the Rwandan genocide by hiding for several months from the rebels. She faced unbelievable fear and deprivation each day. But every time a negative thought came into her mind (e.g., Who are you to think you should survive when everyone else is being murdered?), Immaculée, an ardent Catholic, referred to those negative thoughts as the voice of the devil. Then she'd pray for guidance and protection. Her faith and belief in good created miracles and saved her life. I've found her concept of the devil to be enormously helpful!

Make it a habit to concentrate on what is working in your life. Cultivate the habit of noticing what is good and appreciating it. A teacher named Abraham says, "Appreciation is the strongest emotion we have for attracting what we want."[18] When you look for people, places, and things to appreciate and learn to appreciate all of the aspects of your life that are working well, you'll attract more of what you like and less of what you don't. Start noticing little things, like how good the bedsheets feel on your toes at night or how good the pillow feels under your head.

I strongly recommend avoiding watching the news on television, hearing it on the radio, or reading about it in the papers for at least thirty days. Instead of waking up to the news or to people talking on the radio, wake up to music. When you do this, you will be removing a major impediment to tuning in to your inner guidance—negative information overload. Human beings were never designed to act as receiver sets for the bad news from around the entire planet. For most of us, our own daily lives and those of our families and coworkers offer quite enough opportunities for helping and healing. In this sphere we can make a difference. And if each of us took care of our immediate families, jobs, and communities, the planetary community would take care of itself. We cannot do this adequately if our thoughts are continually overwhelmed with bad news that we can do nothing about. Consciously avoid information overload until you can watch the news without feeling bad, scared, or agitated. Otherwise, you could be putting yourself at risk.

If you wake up to soft music or silence each morning, you will be better able to remember your dreams. Over time, you will notice that you don't miss much by avoiding the news. The culture being what it is, someone will always tell you what is going on "out there." You'll always find out what applies to you and what you need to know. But you'll have the advantage of a much more intimate relationship with yourself than most people have. I've been on a mostly news-free diet for over a decade. I cannot believe the difference it has made in my thoughts, dreams, and general state of well-being. Now, when I watch television or read the paper, I don't take it very seriously and I'm very selective. I have proved to myself, beyond any doubt, that my ability to create the life I want by selectively choosing what I will give my attention to is the most powerful creative force in my life.

Write down your lifetime goals. Over the past twenty years, I've written down my goals for the coming year every New Year's Eve and on my birthday. When my children were still at home, we did this as a family ceremony. When I look back, the amazing thing is that I've accomplished almost every one of my goals—even the ones I later forgot about. The very process of writing them down and thinking about them sets something magical into motion. The magical "something" is the power of intent—the power of our thoughts to create.

Get in the habit of noticing what you want—that is how you find your passion. Maybe you need to wear skirts that swing more, walk in the sun more, dig in the dirt more. When you allow yourself to feel more joy, your life will be filled with more abundance on all levels. I guarantee that somewhere inside you, you already know what it is you need and want. If anything at all were possible, how would you live your life?

You are now finished with the Woman's Wisdom Program for Creating Vibrant Health and Healing. Trust what you're feeling. Give yourself credit for staying with it. Here is a summary of the steps for your convenience:

STEPS FOR HEALING

Prepare for the Steps: Imagine Your Future

Step One: Uncover and Update Your Legacy

Step Two: Sort Through Your Beliefs

Step Three: Respect and Release Your Emotions

Step Four: Learn to Listen to Your Body

Step Five: Learn to Respect Your Body

Step Six: Acknowledge a Higher Power or Inner Wisdom

Step Seven: Reclaim the Fullness of Your Mind

Step Eight: Get Help

Step Nine: Work with Your Body

Step Ten: Gather Information

Step Eleven: Forgive

Step Twelve: Actively Pursue Pleasure and Purpose

I hope that going through this section has

~ Jogged some stuck places in you that needed readjustment
~ Reassured you that you are right on track
~ Touched your anger
~ Brought up tears
~ Made you laugh
~ Inspired you

That's what life is: growing, changing, moving, creating—every day.

Maybe you need to sing; maybe you need to run. Don't wait. This life is not an emergency, but it also doesn't offer any guarantees about going on forever. How do you want to feel? Imagine feeling that way often. What action do you need to take right now to live your life more fully? ... Got it?

Now take a step toward it!

Blessed be.

16
Getting the Most Out of
Your Medical Care

CHOOSING A HEALTH CARE PROVIDER

One of the most powerful tools for your healing is to develop a working partnership with a health care team in which all members respect the body's ability to heal and maintain health, and are willing to work together to facilitate this process.

Health care providers must be aware of how powerful their words are. The cloak of the shaman rests on their shoulders—whether they realize it or not. Their words have the power to heal or to destroy, because of the powerful impact of beliefs on the body, especially in a person who is vulnerable and afraid. Professionals' words must be truthful and at the same time chosen to support healing. As the late Norman Cousins wrote, "The doctor knows that it is the prescription slip itself, even more than what is written on it, that is often the vital ingredient for enabling a patient to get rid of whatever is ailing him. Drugs are not always necessary. Belief in recovery always is. And so the doctor may prescribe a placebo in cases where reassurance for the patient is far more useful than a famous-name pill three times per day."[1] The placebo effect is *physical*.[2] A very striking example of this (and there are many) was in a study reported in the *New England Journal of Medicine* in 2002 of people with severe knee pain. Bruce Moseley, M.D., an orthopedic surgeon from Baylor College of Medicine in Houston, wanted to know just what part of his surgery was the most effective. He divided the study patients into three groups. One group had arthroscopic surgery in which the cartilage was shaved. Another group had the knee flushed out to remove material thought to cause inflammation. The third group was put to sleep and the standard incisions were made in their knees, but no surgery was done. The results were amazing. The first two groups who actually received surgery improved. But the truly shocking finding was that the third group—who had no surgery—improved just as much! (I've seen this same thing happen with intractable pelvic pain and laparoscopy. The very act of doing something—along with the patients' belief in the procedure—often effected a cure even though I didn't do much to the pelvis!)[3]

The effect of working with a healer you trust and believe in is a *physical* part of healing, as much a part of your healing as the mode of treatment you actually choose. People have described their doctor's words as burning right into their souls. You must choose a health care provider carefully and deliberately.

One of the most common questions I'm asked is "Is there a doctor like you in New York?" or California, or elsewhere. Many patients value an approach that honors their inner wisdom, acknowledges the message an illness holds, and combines western medicine with other modalities. A new "third line" of health care providers who are open to this approach is rapidly emerging. Everywhere I go, I meet doctors and medical students who are interested in and actively practicing what is now known as complementary or integrative medicine: the coming together of the best of both worlds—conventional allopathic and so-called alternative medicine, which acknowledges the body as an energy system. Many other health care practitioners trained in different disciplines also share this approach.

There are scores of deeply committed, caring physicians practicing in the United States and around the world who don't necessarily call themselves holistic. The vast majority of family practice physicians I know are inherently holistically oriented and open to new ideas. This is because family medicine training emphasizes the importance of the family system to health. This orientation quite naturally leads to an openness to explore hidden aspects of illness and the mind/body connection.

The doctor you're working with now may well be open to your ideas about your illness and may be willing to follow along with your new path. Here are some steps to help you find the right health care practitioner for you.

1. *Getting the right referral.* When seeking a specialist or other type of health care provider, there are two kinds of referrals to consider:

those from satisfied patients (or clients) and those from other medical colleagues. If a health care provider works with alternative medicine, he or she might or might not work within the mainstream medical community. For this reason, your family physician may not know of a good acupuncturist or massage therapist. But that does not mean that there aren't any. Often the best health care providers are found through word of mouth—women talking to other women. So ask your friends whom they see and why. And when it comes to doctors in your area, see if you can find a nurse who has worked with the local doctors at your favorite hospital to give you a recommendation.

If you're looking for an alternative health care practitioner, a good place to start other than friends is your local health food store. Many times the staff at these places knows who is available in your area. They may also have a bulletin of listings available. And more and more, alternative practitioners are teaching classes at Y's, high schools, colleges, and adult education programs around the country. Taking a yoga, massage, tai chi, or other class is a very good way to find out who is doing what in your area, because those interested in complementary medicine tend to know one another. Of course, the Web has revolutionized networking to the point where you need only type in the word "acupuncturist" to find someone in your area. Still, the best referrals are from someone who knows the practitioner personally.

2. *Credentials.* Board certification is evidence that a doctor has passed a number of qualifying exams that measure competence to practice in his or her chosen field. Having been through the process, I can attest to the rigor involved. Of course you'll want to know a specialist's training—and most good ones have this information readily available in their practice brochures. Credentialing varies widely in the alternative health care field and in some cases is not yet in place, though this is changing rapidly. The American Holistic Medical Association now has a new specialty board to certify holistically trained physicians using the same rigorous criteria that other specialties have employed. (For more information, visit the AHMA's website at www.holisticmedicine.org.)

3. *Is it a fit?* A health care provider can have all the credentials in the world and still be the wrong person for you. So, having checked out all their credentials with your intellect, you'll ultimately have to trust your heart and your gut before you let someone care for you or operate on you, no matter how highly they've been recommended to you. When my daughter needed oral surgery, I knew before I met him that the oral surgeon had impeccable credentials. But I was not willing to allow him to do anything to my daughter until I had had a chance to ex-

perience his interpersonal skills and what I've come to call his "healer quotient." If they hadn't been there, I would have left the office—and so should you.

4. *Assessing "healer quotient."* Does your health care provider feel like a healer? Do you leave the office feeling reassured and uplifted? Do you feel like you're in good hands?

Over my many years in medicine, I've found that true healers work everywhere, regardless of the tools they use. (This can include the custodial staff at the hospital, by the way!) Though I already knew this, the lesson was brought home to me in a big way when my husband and I went to a gifted intuitive in Vermont for a reading. This woman told my husband that he had a great deal of healing energy in his hands and asked him whether or not he did any healing work with them. He said that he didn't, and she suggested to him that he might consider looking into massage or chiropractic. Later, as we were driving home and he was thinking about the reading, he said to me, "Do you suppose that orthopedic surgery counts as doing healing work with my hands?" Then we both laughed, because my husband—as well as much of our culture—has assumed that "healing" was not part of mainstream medicine. He assumed that because he's a pretty mainstream orthopedic surgeon and quite skeptical of much of alternative medicine that he must not be a healer—that healers are those people who use herbs and massage. How wrong he was. My heart is continually warmed by the caring, compassion, and true healing that I see happening every day, regardless of the setting.

On the other hand, when your health care provider is aloof, trying to be objective—giving only facts—only the intellect of the patient gets taken care of, and that is not enough. I once had a patient with breast cancer who told her doctor, "Coping with the cancer is no problem, but recovering from my visits with you takes me about two weeks." She was referring to his detached manner and her perception that he didn't care. She didn't expect a miracle, but she longed for some reassurance and an occasional touch. After she conveyed this to him, their relationship improved. This improvement often happens when you give your doctor or other health care provider a chance.

Another acquaintance of mine found herself very tearful following a medically necessary hysterectomy when she was in her thirties and hadn't had children. When she told her surgeon about it, he replied, "Well, we can't have that!" What she was longing for was simply for him to tell her that her response was normal and expected. One of my patients came in for a checkup and complained about her doctor in

Boston. "She doesn't think she can take care of me without filling the pages with all these little numbers," she said. "I know she's a good technician, but I don't feel heard."

One of my friends told me that while her doctor was looking at her ovaries via a sonogram during a failed cycle of IVF, he remarked, "What do you have growing in there? Grass?" She complained about this to the head of the hospital's OB/GYN department. His response? "Oh, Brenda, quit being so sensitive. Your doctor felt bad and was trying to make light of it." There's not much "light" about a failed IVF cycle that just cost you $10,000!

Unfortunately, I continue to hear too many stories like these and I realize how much we, as a society, need to open our hearts to one another. Unfortunately, fixing a patient through the manipulation of blood chemistry or the repair of broken bones is the main focus of allopathic health education. This has been what medical students get graded on—not how well they communicate with the patient. Though this is changing in medical schools today, most doctors now in practice were taught the skills of curing, not caring.

The average OB/GYN in this country has also been sued for alleged malpractice at least twice. I am no exception. The emotional toll of this experience is heavy and has served, unfortunately, to put doctors and patients at odds. And it's getting worse—a testimony to the need for the heart and the intellect to work in partnership in all of us! It makes some physicians less willing to go against the standard treatment used in their communities, even when better and safer ones have been shown to work. One of the ways to get around this is for women to include a signed statement in their medical chart releasing the physician from any potential litigation should they choose alternatives to standard conventional care. (Malpractice insurance now costs many OB/GYNs more than $100,000 per year.) Though this is not an ironclad guarantee against a lawsuit, it helps many physicians feel more comfortable with approaches that weren't covered in medical school. If we are to get to a partnership between doctors and patients, we have to start from where we are, and both sides have to be honest about their needs and fears.

Because of my willingness to avoid surgery, I've had the experience of watching conditions such as ovarian cysts go away with such things as emotional and dietary change. I've learned many things about the female body that were not included in my training. My general optimism, coupled with the courage and forthrightness of my patients, has allowed us both to collect a body of clinical information that many gynecologists wouldn't necessarily see. This is only possible, however, with patients who are truly willing to take responsibility for themselves and their choices. To create health we must all step out of the "blame" model. Still, it's important to be informed. A recent ten-year survey of government statistics concluded that iatrogenic illness (e.g., adverse drug reactions, poor surgical outcomes, etc., that are caused unintentionally by the actions of health care providers) is the leading cause of death in the U.S. and that adverse reactions to prescription drugs account for more than 300,000 deaths per year![4]

5. *Holding up your end of the health care partnership*. I know how tempting it is to want someone to intuit exactly what is going on with you and to give you the precise prescription that will cure you no matter what your problem. Each of us harbors this childhood fantasy of finding a doctor whose advice we can unquestioningly follow without fear of side effects or a bad outcome. The bad news is that this outer authority simply does not exist. And the good news is that each of us has a still, small voice within—our inner guidance and authority—that will unfailingly guide us where we need to go. The hard part is learning to take information from outside of yourself and then run it by your inner wisdom before making a decision or taking action. Changes in the medical system will come about as all of us begin to take responsibility for the part of the problem we're creating. (After all, the vast majority of health problems are related to lifestyle choices.) In the meantime, although medical training and the mindset it often engenders can be frustrating, it's good to have a competent doctor on your side when you need her or him.

It's all too easy to get swept along with the tide, especially when you're in a situation in which an authority who you assume knows more than you is at the helm. And besides, women have been taught for years not to make waves or rock the boat. When one of my friends had surgery, I asked her if she had talked with her anesthesiologist beforehand and asked her or him to use healing statements (see the section on how to prepare for surgery) when she would be going under and coming out of anesthesia. She said to me, "No. I was too embarrassed." Her statement summarizes a huge problem in health care: women are too often afraid to ask for what they need.

Take someone with you who will help you speak up if you find yourself getting caught like a deer in the headlights. (When I was a teenager I used to have dreams about walking down the aisle to get married, then turning to the congregation and telling them I had made

a mistake but we could have a party anyway.) But stopping any culturally ingrained tide requires a great deal of courage and self-trust. The
reason why it's so difficult and requires such strength is that most of us
have been brought up to be afraid of being wrong or making a mistake.
That's why it is so much easier to transfer responsibility for our health
onto someone else rather than assume it ourselves. Blaming someone
else for our problems is a default setting for many. But ultimately the
rewards of trusting yourself and knowing that you have the ability to
get your needs met are much more satisfying than any fleeting relief
that comes from forgoing responsibility for yourself and transferring it
to someone else.

Understand that different physicians often have very different training and interests. As a physician who "walks between the worlds," I see
the good that's done by a variety of approaches. The patient herself
must become her own authority and understand how to get information from various sources. If the patients could understand the amount
of disagreement even among the OB/GYNs in a small city such as
Portland, Maine, about how to treat a certain condition, they would
appreciate how vital their own input is in creating an optimal outcome.

On a very practical level, it's important for you to go to your health
care practitioner fully prepared with a list of questions that he or she
can reasonably answer in the time allotted to you. And be aware that
you may need to schedule another appointment if your situation is unusually complex.

6. *Utilizing the law of attraction.* In part 1, I mentioned the law of
attraction. Basically, this powerful law of the universe states that we attract to ourselves that which is like ourselves. This means that how you
really feel deep inside determines what kind of experience you are likely
to attract to yourself. For instance, if you believe that you will be
able to get your needs met in any given situation, you will most likely
attract to yourself what you need. There are no exceptions to the law
of attraction, so please begin to make note of it in your daily life.

Having said that, I also acknowledge that far too many women's
health care needs have not been met well in the medical offices of this
country. The end result of this—and women's waking up to it—has
been a backlog of mistrust of health care professionals, particularly
doctors, that tends to color the relationship between health care
provider and patient from the outset. And, because of the law of attraction, this can create a kind of downward spiral that serves no one.

So before going to a new doctor, please ask yourself the following
questions and answer them honestly:

~ In general, do I trust doctors? Do I feel that doctors, for instance, charge too much money and are just in this business to get rich?

~ Do I believe that doctors won't listen to me no matter how I state my concerns?

~ Do I believe that drugs and surgery are inherently bad and that it's always better to treat illnesses with alternatives to these modalities?

~ Am I afraid, ashamed, or embarrassed to ask my doctor to be a partner with me in my health care decisions?

~ Am I really willing to trust my inner guidance, even if it's different from what my doctor suggests?

~ Am I willing to suggest a compromise position with my doctor so that I can have the advantages of her or his care while taking some responsibility myself?

If you've answered honestly, you may have uncovered some of the beliefs that are keeping you from having a fulfilling and satisfying relationship with a good health care provider.

To turn this situation around, I'd like you to think about the fact that there are literally thousands of different health care providers practicing in the United States and around the world who can help you help yourself. I'd like you to spend a moment or two each day visualizing how great it will be to have a health care team you trust, feel safe with, and feel empowered by. Feel how exhilarating it is to know that no matter where you travel, you have the ability, through your thoughts and feelings, to be able to attract just the circumstances you need for healing.

7. *Acknowledging the power to choose.* Over the years I've heard many patients tell me that they couldn't take a supplement or get a massage, or whatever it was, because their insurance wouldn't pay for it. Almost invariably, the health of these people has not been as good as the ones who say things like "I don't care what it takes, I'll find a way to get what I need. Where there's a will, there's a way. I'm not sure how I'm going to do this, but I know I can work it out." Please think for a moment about what it means when you tell yourself that you can't do something for your health because of the rules and regulations that a bunch of insurance executives have come up with. Whom are you giving your power to?

I have come to see that one of the leading causes of chronic ill health in this country is the belief that your insurance—or the government, or someone else besides you—is responsible for your health care choices. Culturally, we need a big shift in consciousness around this issue. In my view, we should abolish the term "health insurance" and call it what it ought to be called, which is "crisis insurance." The business of creating health and staying healthy is your responsibility, and because none of us is perfect at this, we need a backup in case of catastrophic illness or an accident. That's what our disease-care insurance should be for. So, for now, while the entire old system is breaking down, I suggest that you get the highest possible deductible that you can afford and then put the amount of your deductible away in a money market account if needed. Health savings accounts are becoming increasingly common but they have a long way to go. Then, with the considerable savings that you aren't putting into the pockets of the insurance executives, you could afford all kinds of good food, gym memberships, or massages. These suggestions might sound overly simplistic—and in some cases they are. But for many others, they are a ticket to true health care choice and freedom, in contrast to the sheep mentality that is so prevalent and disempowering. (I'm also aware of the plight of those with no health insurance. And I'm dismayed by the ever-increasing cost of health insurance. But until we as a nation start addressing lifestyle issues, we'll continue to have to pay the enormous cost of bailing people out of situations that could have been prevented in the first place!)

In conclusion, though I don't deny that there are problems with today's medical system, I also know that we are moving toward a time of unprecedented choices and ways to create health daily in our lives. Why not be a recipient of the health care of the future, starting today? You can do this by working with a great paradox: you have to create health yourself, but you don't have to do it alone.

Please acknowledge your power to create health in your life daily, and understand that healing often comes to us through our connection with others.[5]

Do You Need a Female Doctor?

Though I worked for years in an all-woman setting, there are scores of male physicians who are compassionate and highly skilled. Many women physicians and patients will tell you that going to a woman is no guarantee that you'll be treated better than you would be by a man. Sometimes you'll be treated very poorly. The reasons for this are many. To succeed in medical school, women often devalue their own knowing and try to become distant and objective—like some of their male or female role models.

A male physician who is a real healer can do at least as much to help women as a female physician could—sometimes more. If a woman is an incest survivor, for example, and has the mistaken idea that she can't trust men, her entire worldview could be nicely healed by a caring interaction with a male physician who demonstrates to her that not all men are dangerous. One of my patients had been operated on for endometriosis during her teenage years. She was left with a pelvis full of scar tissue and had become infertile. I referred her to an infertility surgeon who was not only highly skilled as a surgeon but also an extraordinarily caring man. My patient told me later that having a man help her heal her pelvis was very precious to her. As she put it, "A man wounded me as a child and set up the conditions that led to my pelvic problems. It is a big healing for me to have a man assist me in healing this part of my body."

Women who think that only women are really healers and that only men can be skilled surgeons miss out on a great deal that could help them. At this time in history, we need some women-only places to heal, but true healing goes way beyond whether we are male or female. Each of us has the capacity to wound one another. We also have the capacity to heal.

CHOOSING A TREATMENT: FROM SURGERY TO ACUPUNCTURE

If you are sick, treat the critical symptoms first, by whatever means are the most appropriate for you. Look for insights later. Conventional medicine is unparalleled in its ability to deal with emergencies and severe symptoms. Though there are many alternative treatments in addition to drugs and surgery, conventional medicine is sometimes necessary and helpful.

To approach illness without using the diagnostic tools of modern medicine where they are appropriate is as dualistic and harmful to patients as saying to someone with arthritis, "We've completed your tests. You have arthritis. It is a lifelong chronic debilitating disease, and you might as well learn to live with it"—without exploring nutrition, work stress, or lifestyle. Because mystery is a constant part of life, we can never be sure how anything will turn out; we can never be sure that a medical condition is hopeless because there are well-documented spontaneous remissions from just about everything!

Once a thorough assessment of a patient's situation has been made and she has been informed of the standard recommended treatments for her situation—like hysterectomy for a large fibroid uterus—then the patient herself must decide what "feels" right. For one, the choice will be a hysterectomy. Another with the same problem might be more comfortable with dietary change, castor oil packs, or myomectomy. The internet has helped women become far better informed about their options.

Once a treatment program has been recommended to you, regardless of what it is, let the information "sink in" for a few days or more. See if it feels right in your body. If it doesn't, give it more thought, get another opinion, ask for a dream, or turn it over to your inner guidance. If surgery has been recommended, I'm a very big fan of second and even third opinions. Very few conditions are such an emergency that you have to make a decision on the spot. If you sit with a decision for a while, you'll be much more trusting of your instincts if a real emergency does occur.

Which Treatment Is Best?

How a woman chooses to treat a condition will depend on her own needs at the time. I say this while acknowledging the power of the medical-pharmaceutical industry to sway public opinion and the cultural biases I've already explored. (See chapter 1.)

People often have prejudgments about treatments. Those who are oriented toward natural therapies sometimes see surgery or the use of drugs as a failure, and the use of vitamins for the same problem as a triumph. To those who are more familiar with conventional drugs and surgery, the very notion that an herb or dietary change could help seems preposterous. I teach women that there are many choices and they need not exclude entire categories that could help them—either conventional or alternative.

Eating brown rice, tofu, and vegetables is appropriate for some women who want to decrease symptoms related to excess estrogen, for example, while taking a progesterone preparation is the best option for others with the same problem. Sometimes a woman needs both. Many women are confused about these points and need to understand that they have options.

A thirty-eight-year-old artist came in for her annual checkup once. She had been trying to decide whether to go on Prozac, an antidepressant, for her periodic depressions. Philosophically she didn't like the idea, but her condition wasn't getting any better. She had had an intuitive reading with a well-respected person in our area who had encouraged her to try the drug. She finally decided that the only way to know whether the drug would help was to give it a trial. She released her judgment and started to take it.

When I saw her three months later, she said that she was feeling wonderful and that the drug seemed to be a "missing link" for her. "I can't believe how my life has changed around," she reported. "Now the universe seems to be providing for me. My artwork is selling well, and I am much more creative. I'm also claiming my power and energy as my own and am not nearly so worried about what other people think or whether I'm better than or worse than anyone else [as an artist]. I have more energy than I've ever had before." Taking the drug became a turning point for her, but before she could accept it, she had to release her prejudgment about it. Though the drug definitely helped, she didn't ignore the issues from her past—childhood sexual abuse—that were core issues in her depression. She told me, "One of the most helpful things about coming to you was to tell you about my intuitive reading and to tailor my medical care around how I was feeling about that information. That you were willing to listen to all the different parts of my story is precious to me."

Six months later, she stopped taking Prozac because she felt that it was creating "an artificial euphoria" that didn't feel right to her. What had worked well at one point was no longer appropriate. She continues to feel well, powerful, and creative without the drug. (Interestingly, the data on antidepressants versus placebos shows that placebos are just as effective! That means that antidepressants work because we all believe in them!)[6]

There are many ways to heal. The right way for you is the way that feels best for you at a particular time. We must learn to see ourselves as processes—changing and growing over time. *Eventually, any externally imposed guidelines for how to become well must be consistent with our own inner guidance system. Eventually, we must learn to support ourselves through self-respect—not through restrictive regimens filled with "shoulds" and "oughts" that feel punitive.*

Externally imposed regimens such as dietary improvement are often a first step in healing. These regimens often help women feel good enough to get on with their real work of finding out both about their deepest woundings and about what is most nourishing in life that will help them heal their wounds. These two quests go hand in hand. We can't skip over the parts of our lives that hurt or are disturbing in an attempt to "follow our bliss." But when we commit to following our bliss, the healing of our wounds begins spontaneously.

Analysis Can Cause Paralysis

We are running around looking for knowledge, but we are drowning in information.

—Karl-Hendrick Robert

Information-gathering is only a first step in creating health. Many people, equating techniques, medicines, and even vitamins with health, stop at this level. I've seen women with a variety of different conditions go to scores of health care practitioners of all types but come no closer to healing than they were before. Often, the more facts they have, the more confused they become. This information dilemma is common and can immobilize us.

Some people can get paralyzed by looking at a menu and trying to decide what to eat: "Well, I want the chicken, but we're having chicken tomorrow, and besides, I'm not sure if it will have too much fat in it, and whether or not I like the sauce. What do you think, Mark? Should I have the chicken?" and so on.

Another example is the following: in people who are tying to heal a condition with diet, there's a time when trying to control the amount and quality of everything they put into their mouths dominates their lives: "How many greens should I have? One cup or a half cup? Should they be cooked? How about my bowel movements—should they sink or float? If they sink, does it mean I should add bran? What about water—two glasses or three? And is it okay to have an orange? How many? One a day or two?" This is an example of taking the dualistic model and transferring it to everything we do.

It is simply not possible to know and understand everything. This approach becomes very problematic when we are dealing with a living, breathing, ever-changing human body.

Estrogen replacement therapy is a common situation in which women can work themselves into a real frenzy if they rely on intellect alone. No amount of studies on estrogen replacement, calcium intake, or exercise will ever be able to take into account all the variables that affect a woman's life around menopause.

Sometimes we have to take a step back from our intellect and laugh at it, running around in circles, chasing its tail. Writer Natalie Goldberg calls this "monkey mind." Regardless of what the issue is, once you've read all the books and consulted all the experts, only your inner guidance, of which the intellect is only a part, can give you the right answer.

CREATING HEALTH THROUGH SURGERY

At some point in their lives, many women are faced with the prospect of surgery. Thirty million people in the United States have surgery each year, and 70 percent of them are women.[7] I've watched many women put their lives on hold for months or even years while trying to cure "naturally" a condition that is very amenable to conservative, organ-sparing surgery. Surgery to repair the pelvis is totally different from surgery to remove everything in the pelvis. Surgery should always be considered along with other healing modalities. I like to help heal the negativity often associated with surgery by renaming the experience Creating Health Through Surgery. Surgery can be approached as a healing ceremony. Jeanne Achterberg and Barbara Dossey give full instructions for how to do this in their book *Rituals of Healing* (Bantam Books, 1994).

The Second Opinion

Before having an elective surgery, get a second opinion if you have any doubts whatsoever. I've seen countless women for second opinions regarding hysterectomy. The second opinion gives women time to think about their decision, and it exposes them to the vast differences in thinking that exist within the medical profession about treating a particular problem. Some women see as many as five or six different specialists before they decide on a course of action. Ultimately, they have to tune in to their inner guidance to come up with the best answer for them, since no doctor can provide it.

Often when I've rendered a second opinion, I've agreed with the referring surgeon's rationale for the hysterectomy; heavy, irregular bleeding that has resulted in anemia, for example, is a conventional reason for hysterectomy, though there are many ways to treat the problem besides surgery. If surgery feels like the right solution to the woman, however, she should go with that. If, on the other hand, she is open to alternatives such as dietary change, she should give those a try. The main thing to be aware of is that there are often many different choices—all of which have merit!

Women who have taken the time to read and gather information embark upon a chosen course of therapy or a surgical procedure from a place of strength and knowledge, not because some authority figure said they should! This is a great place to be! No one should ever have elective surgery if they feel they don't have permission to speak up, disagree, or get more information.

Surgery Is Not Failure but a Healing Opportunity

Too often, women think they've failed if they require surgery for their problem. This is an example of dualistic, black and white thinking. One woman with a fourteen-week-size fibroid uterus said to me through tears, "I'm so ashamed. I keep thinking that I should have been able to prevent this or at least to have made it go away by myself." Further questioning revealed that she had the type of family background in which she had repeatedly heard the phrase "Don't cry, or I'll give you something to cry about." She felt shamed for asking for help and for having needs. She realized that her fibroid was connected to grieving for the childhood she had never had.

Gail, whose ovarian cyst healing was covered in chapter 7, said, "As a good 'New Age person,' surgery was my last resort. With classic New Age hubris, I felt I should have been able to heal myself, and if I chose surgery, I was a failure. So I tried a gamut of holistic approaches—acupuncture, herbs, castor oil packs, working with a friend who is a channel, and visualization. All of these methods were helpful and were surely healing on certain levels. But I realized that this cyst was too dense, both physically and spiritually, to be melted even by acupuncture needles. It needed to be cut out."

Another patient of mine, June, had a persistent ovarian cyst and very much wanted to avoid surgery. She spent three months doing visualizations, emotional cleansing, and dietary change to heal her cyst. I told June that I felt that surgery was her best option. Her cyst was large—ten centimeters—and had failed to go away on its own after three months. Though she wanted to believe that the cyst was gone and that she could avoid surgery, she had had the following dream: "I went to get my car from the repair shop, and it wasn't ready yet. This dream recurred several times. I started to wonder if the cyst was indeed gone. I never had felt that the cyst posed any real danger to me, but even though I felt that I had completed my work"—she had developed a great deal of clarity about what the cyst represented in her life and had experienced a great deal of grieving and sadness about this—"I wondered if maybe the cyst was still there. I rarely admitted that thought to myself at all, choosing instead to think positively that it must be gone because I had completed what I thought was my healing work."

A few weeks before her scheduled surgery, June had dinner with a woman she had just met who was fascinated with myths, dream work, and art therapy as tools to help people heal themselves. "When she heard about my car dreams," June later wrote, "she started to push hard. She asked if I knew what was wrong with my car. She said I should have found out what was broken and called in a specialist to tell me how to fix it." This was to be done in dream state. "She was horrified that I was going to let someone take my ovary without trying harder to keep it. The implication was that if I did not try things her way, I wasn't trying hard enough. I answered her questions seriously. The questions felt so heroic, so guilt ridden.[8] I am responsible, and this cyst must be what I want. After I left her place, I felt dirty, sort of emotionally raped. Later I realized that searching endlessly for a nonsurgical cure is addictive, that I could keep the cyst and be addicted to the process, or I could just let it go and be done with it."

An Opportunity to Heal Old Fears

For many women, particularly those who are drawn to natural methods of healing, surgery is terrifying. My patient Gail, after her cyst surgery, said, "That cyst helped me uncover several powerful patterns I hadn't been aware of. My terror around my body, disease, doctors, and hospitals was a result of my mother's long mysterious heart disease, which led to her death. Throughout parts of my childhood she was in and out of hospitals, never seeming to get better, and the doctors never seeming to know what was wrong with her. What caused even more suffering on my part was the feelings everyone in my family was experiencing around her illness that were never discussed."

Many women have transformed their fears of the hospital and surgery, however, by using such experiences as a "spiritual initiation"—a time to face their fears and walk through them, as well as a chance to reverse old patterns that no longer serve them. Gail wrote, "As I contemplated my upcoming surgery it was absolutely clear to me that I had a wonderful opportunity to confront my childhood terror of hospitals and all they represented. I could experience that my story was totally different from my mother's story. I learned some wonderful lessons. Reversing my family pattern, I shared my fears and concerns with my husband and dear friends and asked for their support. Their outpouring of love and support was a precious gift that I shall treasure for a long time."

Giving yourself permission to let another individual help you can be a profoundly healing experience. When surgery is the best treatment choice, surrendering to the skills of the anesthesiologist, your surgeon, your nurses, and your inner guidance can be a true growth experience. If you received the message in childhood that your physical and emotional needs for support and comfort don't deserve to be met, asking for support during surgery or a hospitalization is an opportunity to reverse this message.

Healing energy is available in hospitals. The nurses and staff can be seen as healing angels. The people who work in hospitals—whether they be nurses, nursing assistants, or orderlies—are often in these settings because they are naturally drawn to healing. When you stop fighting those who are there to help, it's quite a relief.

Take a friend or family member to the preoperative visit if you're having surgery. Your friend can then accompany you to the hospital to meet the anesthesiologist and go through the pre-op phase in the hospital setting. After surgery, these friends or others can provide support at home through cooking, cleaning, or backrubs. Women must learn how to ask for this support. Getting it is a skill. Sometimes we need help learning this.

June wrote the following about getting support: "On my way home after finding out that I needed surgery, I knew I could not be alone that whole weekend, so I stopped at my friend Carol's house. I think Carol became afraid when she saw how depressed I looked. She delivered a strong lecture about how important I am to my son, and to her, and to many other people. I never had acknowledged my importance to any of those people except my son. She made a very strong case for going forward and letting myself be supported by my friends. She told me that I was to recover at her house so that I wouldn't have to cook or shop, or do any other of those details for myself. She helped me immeasurably."

In preparation for her surgery, June went to see a hypnotist and had three sessions. Her hypnotist produced two tapes for her to use—one to prepare her for a healthy experience and a quick recovery, and a second to help her move on afterward. She used these tapes many times during the next two weeks prior to surgery.[9] She also began work with a physician who understood and taught Chi Kung. (Chi Kung is an ancient Chinese art that teaches us to circulate our life-energy through movement, massage, and the breath.)

How to Prepare for Surgery (or Chemotherapy) and Heal Faster

Here are some scientifically proven ways to approach your surgical procedure consciously, learn from it, and heal quickly. Having done surgery for years, I can assure you that nothing is more gratifying to a surgeon than having a patient who will work with her or him in partnership—each trusting the input of the other—so that optimal results can be obtained.

Peggy Huddleston, M.S., a colleague of mine, has written a remarkable step-by-step guide to help people everywhere get the most out of their surgical experiences. Her book and the program it outlines are being used in hospitals all over the country. The techniques that Peggy uses have succeeded in helping many of my patients and thousands of people around the world achieve the following benefits:

- Feel calmer before surgery (or chemo)
- Have less pain after surgery (or chemo)
- Use less pain medication
- Strengthen the immune system
- Save money on medical bills (a study in California reported that patients who prepared for abdominal surgery with specific instructions left the hospital 1.5 days earlier and saved $1,200 per person in hospitalization)[10]

Whether you're having a minor outpatient procedure or a major operation, this approach can help you. And by the way, these techniques can also be used to help you get through radiation and/or chemotherapy.

Step one: relax to feel peaceful. Eighty-five percent of all medical problems are associated with unresolved tension and stress held in the body. This chronic response to tension results in a cascade of physiologic changes that can and do affect your health adversely. What's the antidote? Learn the skill of deep relaxation and practice it often so that you know you can call up a deep sense of peace at will. Learning deep relaxation is easy and there are a number of different ways to do it. For the purpose of preparing for surgery, I'd recommend using a tape or CD prepared specifically for this purpose. (I particularly recommend the tapes and CDs from www.healthjourneys.com and www.healfaster.com, as well as the Surgical Support series developed

by The Monroe Institute and available at www.hemi-sync.com.)
Don't be surprised if, when you are first starting to learn to relax,
strong emotions emerge, such as sadness, anger, or whatever. Feel
them fully, cry as long as you need to, don't hold back—allow whatever you feel to wash through you. Welcome those intense emotions.
They've probably been waiting within you for a long time trying to
get expressed.

Studies have shown that relaxation improves the immune system,
calms the central nervous system, and often cures tension headache, migraine, hypertension, and anxiety, as well as helping you prepare for
your surgery. Many hospitals now offer "prepare for surgery" programs as well.

Step two: visualize your healing. Visualize your ideal surgical outcome.
Imagine as vividly as you can that your operation is now over and you
are comfortable, filled with peace, and healthy in every respect. Feel
yourself surrounded by healing light, or sound, or a feeling of deep
peace. The more you can imagine an ideal outcome in great detail, the
faster you will heal. Your intuitive wisdom will provide you with the
images that seem most healing. Visualize, visualize, visualize: five times
a day for five minutes each time is more effective than one twenty-five-
minute session.

Step three: organize a support group. Surgery is a wonderful time to
reach out for support. Make sure that someone will be with you when
you arrive for your surgery, will visit you daily while you're in the hospital, if necessary, and will help you at home for as long as you require
that assistance. (For abdominal surgery, that's at least two weeks.)
Many women simply don't realize how vulnerable they may feel post-
op, so prepare for this so you can be in a healing cocoon as long as
needed. This will allow you to receive the caring and loving thoughts
of your friends and family. This aspect of preparing for surgery can be
especially healing for those of you who feel that "to get anything done
right, I have to do it myself." You will have the opportunity to allow
others to give to you and provide for you. You'll learn skills of receiving, which for many women is a major challenge.

When you're in the hospital and/or after you're home, I'd recommend having at least one Reiki, therapeutic touch, or massage session.
A daily treatment for the first two or three days would be ideal. Both
Reiki and therapeutic touch are energy medicine treatments that are
completely safe and have been shown scientifically to speed the healing
process. Ask your doctor or nurse if they know anyone who is trained

in these therapies—many health care professionals and lay individuals are trained in these modalities. (To find a Reiki practitioner, visit www. reikialliance.org; to find a therapeutic touch practitioner, visit www. therapeutic-touch.org.)

Step four: use healing statements. There are four healing statements that you'll want your surgeon or anesthesiologist to say to you during your operation. Research has shown that these statements are associated with having less pain, fewer complications, and faster healing. Make three copies of these statements; give one to your surgeon and one to your anesthesiologist, and tape one on your hospital gown so it's visible as you go into surgery. Do not let any embarrassment prevent you from asking your doctors to do this for you. Believe me, most doctors have gone into medicine because they want to be healers. Ask them to do their job. I've never once seen a surgeon or anesthesiologist scoff at a patient's request for these statements. If they do, go to someone else. If your consciousness isn't safe with them, then your body won't feel safe, either—and your healing won't be as rapid as it otherwise could be.

Here are the statements:

AS I AM GOING UNDER ANESTHESIA, PLEASE SAY:

1. "Following this operation, you will feel comfortable and you will heal very well." (Repeat five times.)

After saying the statements, please put on my earphones and start my tape player.

AT THE CONCLUSION OF THE SURGERY, PLEASE SAY:

2. "Your operation has gone very well." (Repeat five times.)

3. "Following this operation, you will be hungry for ———. You will be thirsty and you will urinate easily." (Repeat five times.)

4. "Following this operation, ———." (Ask your surgeon to fill this in with recommendations for recovery, such as "You will be able to exercise and be back to full activity within four weeks," and so on. And add some of your own goals. If you're currently a smoker, you might also ask that your anesthesiologist add the following: "You will be a nonsmoker who detests the taste of cigarettes" or "You will be free of the desire to smoke." Anecdotally, I've seen this work.)

As you prepare your CD or tape player for surgery, adjust the volume so that you can barely hear the music. Then stick some tape on the volume control so that it can't be increased. When you are under anesthesia, the tiny tissues involved in hearing will be very relaxed and any sound will be amplified. You don't want to risk damaging your hearing by playing a tape or CD too loudly during this vulnerable time.

Choose the kind of music you enjoy the most. Mozart is a popular choice, since his music has been found to enhance immune response. Adagio movements are especially good. But anything you love will work, including country western!

Step five: meet your anesthesiologist. You will be entrusting your consciousness to this doctor, so you'll want to meet him or her before surgery. In these days of same-day surgery, it is common to meet your anesthesiologist just before your actual procedure, but with some effort on your part, it's still possible to work with his or her schedule as well as your own. A study at Harvard showed that meeting your anesthesiologist well before surgery significantly decreased patients' preoperative anxiety. Ask your surgeon to arrange this for you. This is no time to worry about "making waves." Your doctors will remember you and give you more individualized care if you've established yourself as someone who asks respectfully to have their total being taken care of during surgery.

Step six: use supplements to speed healing. Supplements that have been shown to speed healing are the following:

~ *Vitamin A.* The suggested dose is 25,000 IU daily (unless you are pregnant). Numerous studies have shown the beneficial effects of vitamin A on healing after surgery. It also helps boost the immune system. Start one week before surgery and continue three to four weeks thereafter.

~ *Bromelain.* This supplement, derived from pineapple, helps prevent bruising and also relieves the swelling associated with surgery. Take 1,000 mg per day starting several days before surgery and continuing for about two weeks postoperatively.

~ *Vitamin C.* Two thousand mg per day. Vitamin C is essential for collagen synthesis, which is part of normal wound healing. Your need for it will increase after your surgery. Start at least a month before your procedure and continue for one month postoperatively.

~ *Zinc, Magnesium, B complex.* These supplements have been shown to promote wound healing. The recommended dose is zinc picolinate, 100 mg; magnesium, 800 mg; and B complex, about 50 mg of each.

~ *Vitamin E.* Postoperatively, apply vitamin E oil (d-alpha tocopherol) onto the incision daily as soon as the surgical dressing is removed (if your surgeon agrees that there is no contraindication to this). This speeds healing and decreases scarring. Some women prefer aloe vera gel, calendula ointment, or other herbal treatments for this purpose.

~ *Homeopathy.* Take Arnica Montana 30X, three or four pellets twice per day (dissolved under the tongue) on the day before surgery and also as soon before surgery as possible. You can take these just before being wheeled into the operating room. Then take them as soon as possible once you get into the recovery room. Your anesthesiologist can help with this, or you can wait until you're back in your room. Take the same dose daily for a week following surgery. Arnica is very good at preventing ill effects from any kind of physical trauma. Many other homeopathic remedies are available that can be used for specific types of surgery. Consult with a trained practitioner.

~ *Herbs.* The Chinese herb known as Yunnan Paiyo is excellent for promoting wound healing and enhancing the ability of blood to clot. Many of my patients have used this successfully to speed their recovery from surgery. It results in decreased swelling and bruising. Dose is one tablet four times per day for one week prior to surgery, and continuing one month postoperatively. Start as soon after surgery as you can take things by mouth.

Because the thought of surgery is so terrifying for many people, it can be used as a sort of wake-up call—a time to reprioritize your life. If you honestly approach it with an open mind and an open heart, and go through the steps above sincerely—with a sense of surrendering yourself to the process—you may actually heal on your own and find that your surgery will no longer be necessary. I've witnessed this several times in my practice, and Peggy Huddleston gives some examples of this in her book. But don't go through the steps to avoid surgery that may truly be necessary. The key to healing on all levels is that you must proceed with complete willingness to go through with the procedure if necessary. In twelve-step programs they refer to this as "letting go, and letting God." It can work miracles.

Understand that this surgery is a choice. If you want to cancel at the last minute because you've rethought the whole thing or it suddenly feels wrong, then go ahead and cancel it. There are two times when a woman needs to grant herself full permission to change her mind: one is at the altar before her wedding, and another is before having elective surgery. (This doesn't apply to life-saving surgery in emergencies.)

Four to six weeks before major surgery such as a hysterectomy or myomectomy, donate two units of your own blood (unless you're too anemic) in case there is any risk of blood loss requiring transfusion. The needle used by the Red Cross for blood donation is large. I suggest you ask your doctor for a prescription for EMLA, a transdermal anesthetic cream that is applied to the antecubital fossa of the arm (the area where the blood is drawn) one hour before your blood will be drawn and covered with a plastic bandage known as Tegaderm. It makes the procedure painless.

Notice and acknowledge whatever feelings arise after surgery. When a part of your body is removed or when the integrity of your body surface is marred through an incision of any kind, you may need to grieve the loss of your former state.[11] None of us likes surgical scars on our body. It matters little whether you ever did or ever will wear a bikini. We *all* care about how our bodies look.

Old memories may surface after surgery that have been stored in the tissue itself. Surgery has the potential to bring cellular memory to conscious awareness. Incest or other abuse memories may arise in the recovery room or in the days or weeks following surgery. These memories won't surface until you're ready to deal with them, so you need not worry about this. The body's wisdom about when to release information is exquisite.

Acknowledging grief and loss is only one part of creating a healthy surgery. Another equally important step is looking forward to a life free from the problem that required surgery. Think of the surgical loss as a cutting away of the old so that there is space for the new to grow.

Allowing yourself to feel emotions connected with surgical removal of tissue is important. Caroline Myss teaches: "When you pull cell tissue out before any of the data has been finalized, the body gets out of synchronicity." Many people have most of their energy tied up in the past and very little available in the present for healing. When an organ or cell tissue is removed and the body messages associated with it are not acknowledged or processed, then part of our energy will remain in the past like an unpaid account—a part of our personal unfinished business. So if any emotions or other data surface before or after surgery, feel them fully and let them work their way through your system.

When one of my patients had her fibroids removed, she wanted to be awake during the procedure, so she was given a spinal anesthetic. It turned out that she had severe adenomyosis, a benign condition in which the endometrial glands inside the uterus grow in the uterine wall, causing excessive bleeding. A hysterectomy was the optimal treatment for this. Her doctor gave her the choice of stopping the operation and leaving the uterus in, since there was no malignancy.

She had been chronically anemic from her condition and experienced some pain. She had tried dietary change and acupuncture without much success. As a mother of three relatively young children her time for taking optimal care of herself was limited, and so she wouldn't have time to prepare again for a further surgery. She realized that it was time she let go of trying to save her uterus.

Before the uterine removal began, she asked the staff to hold up a mirror for her so that she could see her uterus. She then thanked it for providing her with three healthy children, blessed it and *herself* for trying to preserve it, then said goodbye. Only then did her surgeon begin the hysterectomy. She later told me that the process of letting go and being able to thank her uterus was a key part of her healing. She ended up feeling empowered by this surgery, not devastated.

June, who had the ovarian cyst, also had a spinal and was awake during her surgery. "The operation took less than an hour," she wrote. "I had a spinal block so that I could be fully aware during the surgery. I had a mirror hooked up so that I could watch. It was fabulous. My body is healthy-looking and young for my age [forty-two]. Being able to see the very good condition of my body did me a lot of good. I had lost a lot of confidence in my ability to assess what was going on in my body. [This was because she hadn't realized that her cyst was growing larger. She couldn't feel it.] This showed me what was right about it. My body is in good shape, and the cyst was just not something dangerous that could bring me to the point of surgery. The cyst was almost as large as a softball, but instead of being inside my ovary, it was just on the outside wall. Chris said my ovary looked perfect, and asked me if I wanted to try to save it. She did."

June had prepared a dedication for her left ovary that she could say at the time we removed it. I had a copy in my pocket ready to read in case she was unable to do so. I planned to have one of the operating room staff people read it to her when the time came. She had written the following to make closure around the sacrifice of her ovary:

Thank you, ovary, for helping me become aware of my anger
—my misplaced love
—my disappointment in men
—and my conflicts

As you leave my body I pass through this stage of holding on to anger,
disappointment, and conflict.
And I pass into a life of feminine creativity and beauty.

The vacuum that forms in your absence becomes the feminine vessel
—It fills with healing.
—It connects with my Qi (life-energy).
And it provides beauty and creativity for the rest of my life.

As it turned out, we didn't have to remove the ovary. I was able to remove the cyst and then repair the ovary. The scrub nurse handed her the cyst, which she wanted to touch and feel, still warm from her body. She later wrote: "When Chris gave me the cyst to bless, I had a hard time. The dedication that I wrote and had memorized was to my ovary, not my cyst. And I was so ecstatic that she could save my ovary, I almost didn't care. I recited the relevant parts and left the rest out. I'm not sure it made much sense, but I wasn't performing so it doesn't matter."

Postoperatively, June's friend Carol spent the day and evening with her. June wrote, "She was so supportive and caring. I am so glad she was there. On her way out, she gave me permission to cry. And I did. It was great."

After two and a half weeks of recovery at Carol's house, June's body yielded yet another piece of healing information. She wrote: "Finally I made it home. I still had one more related realization to make and feel. One night I was touching the numbness above the incision, feeling unspeakably sad about the loss of feeling, when I started to cry. Chris had said that if this should happen, to stay with it and explore the feelings. I was crying about the feeling that no man has ever loved me for being the person I really am. Suddenly I realized I was crying about my father. The only two men who have ever loved me for the real me are my cousin and my father. And it was my father who was always there for me. I had never grieved this loss when he died. So I did."

Another patient of mine, a highly intuitive artist, had a hysterectomy for a large fibroid uterus when she was about forty-four. She had visualized the energy in her pelvis and fibroids as very erratic and unhealthy. Postoperatively in the recovery room, she told me that she realized that the static energy in her pelvis was gone. In its place she sensed an even spiral of healthy energy, a vortex in her pelvis. This surgery was a healing for her.

But I Had Surgery Years Ago
and Didn't Know About This

If you've had surgery in the past, reading through this chapter may cause you to feel sad for missing the opportunity to be more fully involved in your healing process. (Stay with this feeling—it is not too late.) Many women who have had hysterectomies had few choices available to them for alternative treatments. The choices for treatment that I've mentioned were not nearly so available even a decade ago as they are now. Each year anesthesia becomes safer, and the techniques to preserve pelvic organs have improved—largely through infertility surgery techniques.

It is natural for women who have had unavoidable surgery in the past to feel some loss, especially now that things have changed. I can't prevent you from feeling grief over events that are past and organs that have been removed. I do know, however, that it's never too late to grieve properly and fully over your loss, if this comes up for you. If you are feeling sad now, stop reading, lie down, and see what comes up. Stay with your emotions or whatever you are feeling in your body. This is the way you heal—this is the way you process data in your body and bring all of your cells into the present. Remember, part of what keeps us stuck in our lives is thinking that we should have known years ago what we now know—and beating ourselves up for not knowing it at the time.

Removing an organ doesn't necessarily heal the energy blockage associated with the problem in the first place, though it can be a step in the right direction. Some women, years after surgery, still have energetic attachments to tissue that was removed and have not grieved fully. This attachment can still be read in their energy field. The electromagnetic field of the body contains a pattern of the whole, even after a physical part is gone.

Our healing ability is not limited by time or space. We can heal our past at any time, even fifty years later. Our past waits in our bodies until we're ready. Learning about the female energy system in the body can bring up delayed feelings that a woman never dealt with at the time of her hysterectomy or other surgery. Better late than never. That's the nice thing about understanding energy and medicine. Healing on the energetic level is always a possibility, regardless of what has gone on at the purely physical level and regardless of how long ago it happened. So if you have had or are having surgery, know that this, too, can be part of creating health. Stay with whatever comes up, and plan to make your surgery a healing opportunity.

Many health care options and choices are available to you. Know that there is no one monolithic "right" way to care for your body. Most important, I hope I have encouraged you to listen to your inner guidance when choosing partners in health care. Albert Schweitzer once said, "It's a trade secret, but I'll tell you anyway. All healing is self-healing."

17
Nourishing Ourselves with Food

If women are truly to enjoy food, it must become one of life's freely experienced sensuous pleasures. By eating well, women take care of themselves on the most basic level.

—Dr. Karen Johnson

Eating healthy, high-quality food is one of the simplest and most powerful ways to create health on a daily basis. Since we women do most of the food shopping and preparation in this country, we can have a significant impact on our and our family's health when we improve our diets. Individual food choices also affect the health of our planet overall.

Our bodies evolved over millennia to assimilate foods that are found in the natural world. Therefore, we function at our best when we eat these natural foods much of the time, not imitations. In the process of improving our diets, we all have an opportunity to increase our respect for our own bodies, as well as the body of the planet as a whole, through nourishing ourselves optimally with high-quality food. Optimal nourishment involves eating the right amount and type of protein, fat, and carbohydrates. And it also involves understanding that your body's metabolic processes are profoundly influenced by the following seven factors:

- Your emotional state, including past or present stressors
- Genetic heritage
- Macronutrient intake (proteins, fats, carbohydrates)
- Micronutrient intake (vitamins and minerals)

~ Exercise habits
~ Environment and timing
~ Food *chi* (food energetics)

Nourishing yourself optimally means paying attention to each of these areas, which I will cover in the steps that follow. (See figure 17, page 712.)

CREATING OPTIMAL BODY COMPOSITION
AND VIBRANT HEALTH

Reaching optimal body composition and vibrant health through the right food choices happens in both your mind and body simultaneously. I've spent more than forty years studying nutrition and its effects on women's bodies, minds, and spirits—both personally and professionally. My interest began in childhood. I was raised on organic food and my parents studied the work of Adelle Davis, author of *Let's Eat Right to Keep Fit* (Harcourt, Brace, 1954) and Robert Rodale. But eating whole grain bread, homemade yogurt, and seven-grain cereal as a child didn't prevent me from feeling the need to go on my first weight loss diet at the age of twelve. I had read in a fashion magazine that a girl of my height (5'3") should weigh 115 pounds, a weight I could never maintain no matter how much I starved myself. (My natural weight by the eighth grade was 125 pounds—heavier than most of the girls in my class at that time.) Thus began a personal war with my size and weight that lasted through my forties when I finally learned the secrets of lifelong weight maintenance and health that I share with you here. Being born with a body that my parents termed "solid," having had to work consciously at controlling my weight for most of my life, and having worked with thousands of women with the same problem, I can assure you that I know what works and what doesn't.

Though I had grown up knowing about the healing power of food, it wasn't until I met Michio Kushi, the founder of the American macrobiotic movement, that I really saw, up close and personal, how effective diet was at reversing chronic disease. At the end of my residency training in Boston in 1980, I met Michio and sat with him while he used techniques similar to those of Traditional Chinese Medicine (TCM) to diagnose and treat everything from heart disease to cancer in people who came from all over the world. Because they came with their medical records, I could easily see that they'd gone through the gauntlet of western medicine and had exhausted its ability to help. Macrobiotics was their last hope. In those who followed Michio's dietary recommendations, the changes I witnessed in the ensuing months were nothing short of miraculous. In those who were willing to make changes, a simple diet of whole grains, beans, and vegetables helped heal heart disease, cancer, and other diseases as well. It also produced such striking changes in people's faces that they were often barely recognizable two months later when they'd come back for follow-up. I was so impressed with these results that I realized I had to incorporate this approach in my medical practice when possible. And I also knew I had to adopt it myself. I read everything I could get my hands on about the health benefits of vegetarian diets. I also took cooking classes and became a very proficient macrobiotic cook. My daughters were "imprinted" with this diet, which is what I ate when I was pregnant with them and also what I served up until they were about ten years old. Now in their twenties, they remember their childhood "comfort" foods as being brown rice and miso soup.

Though macrobiotics was not the panacea I had originally hoped it would be, it was a great start for discovering how powerful food is for healing. A mostly vegetarian diet rich in whole grains, beans, and vegetables became the cornerstone of my approach to PMS, endometriosis, menstrual cramps, and other women's health problems for years. And for those who followed it, this approach resulted in vast health improvements compared to their former dietary habits. I've now refined my approach considerably and have discovered the key to lifelong weight loss and vibrant health through proper diet. If you follow the steps I've listed below, I guarantee you that you'll lose weight for good, keep it off, and never have to buy another diet book or go on another "diet" again. Simple. Not easy.

Know this: it's possible to achieve a healthy, vital body that has the right amount of body fat and also looks wonderful. You can begin to move toward this right now. Read through this section and commit to doing as much of it as you can right now, even if that means simply taking a walk once a week, enjoying your breakfast more slowly, or starting a vitamin supplement. Each step you take will make it that much easier to begin the next one. Take the parts that work for you now, and leave the rest.

Be easy with yourself and integrate these steps to nourishment comfortably. When you change your attitude about self-nourishment, your body composition and body image will also be transformed. You'll have much more success in maintaining the health of your body if you take the time to integrate your new behavior into your overall self-concept. Research has shown that people who have been obese their whole lives, for instance, and then lose weight quickly often continue to have a distorted body image and literally can't see what they really look like even after their size is normal.[1]

Step One: Understand That Self-Respect and Self-Acceptance Are the Cornerstones of Permanent Health and Weight Loss

Regardless of how you feel right now, the first step toward optimal health is deciding to respect the body you have. It's a big stretch for many women to love their bodies if they are overweight, sick, or have been abused. But everyone can learn to stop talking to her body abusively. Would you talk to a small child or loved one in the way you routinely talk to yourself about your body? Probably not. Look deeply into your eyes in the mirror and tell yourself out loud, "I respect you and I will take care of you today." A commitment to body respect is an essential step toward feeling and looking your best. Women who like themselves are irresistible and fun to be around, regardless of their size. It's also important to remember that respecting yourself will actually help you reach your optimal size. That's because the feelings associated with self-respect create a metabolic milieu in your body that is conducive to optimal fat burning. By contrast, the metabolic processes associated with unresolved emotional stress tend to keep excess body fat firmly in place. This is because of the effects of the stress hormones cortisol and adrenaline, which drastically affect metabolism.

Excess fat is not a health hazard in all women. This observation is supported by a study done by Dr. Margaret Mackensie, a social anthropologist who works in Western Samoa, where body fat is *not* considered undesirable in any way. Dr. Mackensie showed that the fat women have no more or different health problems than the rest of the community.[2]

There is no doubt, however, that for many overweight women, excess fat represents armor against pain they've avoided experiencing. The pain of sexual abuse and incest is an especially common root cause of overeating behavior. It's not surprising that the huge 1998 ACE (Adverse Childhood Experiences) study, which has documented the dramatic adult health consequences of childhood abuse and dysfunction, was initially triggered by observations made in the mid-1980s in the obesity program at Kaiser Permanente's Department of Preventive Medicine in San Diego.[3] This program had a very high dropout rate—

and, surprisingly, the people dropping out were successfully losing weight! Detailed life interviews of almost two hundred such individuals unexpectedly revealed that childhood abuse was remarkably common and antedated the onset of their obesity. Many patients spoke openly about this. Obesity was not their problem: it was their protective solution to problems that they had previously never discussed with anyone. For example, a woman who gained 105 pounds in the year after being raped said, "Overweight is overlooked. And that is exactly what I need to be." Another of my patients, whose father was an alcoholic, once told me, "Whenever I'm upset, I eat pastry. As it goes down, I can almost feel myself stuffing down the sad feelings as well!" Here's the truth. The end result of family dysfunction—whether it is a depressed mother who is unable to show her love for you, or an uncle who sexually molested you—is the same. You make a decision that you are not lovable or worthy as a result of how you are treated. And you use food or other addictions to keep from feeling the pain of how bad this belief makes you feel! When fat is used as armor against the world or to protect one from unwanted sexual advances, it is indeed a health risk, since it has become symbolic of an unlived life—dreams in storage.[4]

Back in the early 1980s, I found that every case of severe PMS I saw was in a woman who had come from an alcoholic home or was currently residing in one. This kind of observation and others like it were what prompted me to write this book in the first place! My original work was based on my observations in a small town in Maine. Since that time, I have found that women's experiences are the same the world over.

Step Two: Stop Dieting for Good. Eat for Vibrant Health Instead

Having tried everything from Atkins, to macrobiotics, to the Zone diet, I can assure you that there is a kernel of truth in every one of them. But every "diet" out there is doomed to eventual failure unless you understand what kinds of foods our bodies were designed to function best with and then begin to enjoy them fully to create vibrant health. I know I'm not telling you anything you don't already know.

Studies have shown that weight loss and regain and the "diet mentality" have negative health consequences independent of one's actual weight.[5] And only a very small percentage of women achieve permanent weight loss by dieting, despite the multibillion-dollar diet industry.

We need to look honestly at our behavior around this and commit to change. You want to make slow and permanent changes in your eating that become a way of life—not be on a "diet."

DO YOU HAVE THE "DIET MENTALITY"?

- Do you avoid eating all day so that you can binge at dinner?
- When you're standing before a buffet, do you routinely tell yourself that you can't have what you really want?
- Do you weigh yourself several times throughout the day?
- If you step on the scale and weigh a pound or more than usual, do you routinely beat yourself up for it? Do you let it ruin your day and influence what you eat?
- Do you allow yourself to get so hungry that you gulp whatever is available, rarely even tasting it?
- Do you say, "I'll eat this now, but I'll start on a diet on Monday," or after New Year's?
- Do you routinely drink coffee or caffeinated diet drinks during the day as a substitute for food?
- Do you know the calorie count of almost every food?

If you answered yes to any of these questions, you probably have inherited the "diet mentality." Bob Schwartz, Ph.D., author of *Diets Don't Work* (Breakthru Publications, 1996), did a study of people who had no problems with their weight or with their food intake to determine whether the "diet mentality" could be created by food restriction. The study subjects were placed on weight-loss diets to lose ten pounds each. In the process of dieting to lose weight, many of these formerly "diet-free" individuals actually developed a "diet mentality." They became obsessed with food, often for the first time ever. After losing the required ten pounds, many gained back not only the weight that they had lost but an additional five pounds besides. These additional five pounds were even harder to lose than the original ten had been. By the very process of food restriction and dieting, these formerly thin people had been transformed into people with a weight problem.

After reading about his study, I finally understood why I had been fighting the same ten to fifteen pounds since I was thirteen. My very first diet had firmly implanted the "diet mentality"—and my body had responded rebelliously with a physiologic "starvation response" mechanism that decreased metabolic rate, thus making each later attempt at restriction that much more difficult.[6] (I didn't yet know about the blood sugar/inflammation connection—see below.) I vowed then and there to stop, and I didn't weigh myself (except for an insurance physical) for six years. During that time, I began breaking free from a destructive cycle of body abuse started many years before. I, like so many, had allowed the number on a bathroom scale to tell me that I was good or bad and allowed it to determine the entire quality of my day. If I weighed less than 125 (or whatever my ideal was at the time), it was a good day; if I weighed more than that, it was a bad day.

Most women cannot reach the stage of eating to nourish themselves fully until they've made some progress in the areas I listed above. Eventually, though, you will be motivated to eat high-quality foods; as you regularly tap in to your inner guidance about food, you will find that the foods that are good for you and the foods you want to eat will become the same. Be patient.

A thirty-nine-year-old artist improved her diet to help heal her chronic vaginitis. She said to me, "I feel lighter when I eat this way—and cleaner. My nose doesn't run all the time. And I've lost eight pounds since I last saw you. I don't feel deprived at all. I know that I can eat whatever I want. You told me to eat only whole foods and to experiment after avoiding all dairy foods for one month. So I went back to eating cheese after about one month, but I found that I didn't like the way it felt in my body. I stopped eating it, and I feel better. *Increasingly, what I want is also what makes me feel best.* This isn't a punishment—it's just a different way of looking at things. It's a complete change of philosophy for me."

This patient underwent a paradigm shift in the way she looked at food. Weight loss was a side effect. She changed her diet to create health—not to lose weight. By changing her diet to create health, she not only lost weight but eventually came to the point where the food she wanted the most was also the food that made her feel the best. She is now in tune with the wisdom of her body, and her former war against herself is over.

Nutritional improvement and regular exercise are powerful ways to create health. Most women are amazed by how much better they feel when they eliminate most refined foods, excess sugar, and caffeine from their diets. The link between diet and the health of female organs is impressive. A recent study in Italy, for example, found a direct association between breast cancer risk and the consumption of sweet foods with a high-glycemic index.[7] Our trans-fatty-acid-rich, refined-carbohydrate-rich, fiber-poor, nutrient-poor diet and its effects on blood sugar is part of the reason that breast cancer, endometriosis, and uterine fibroids are on the increase, affecting millions of women. Sixty percent of all cancers in females (breast, ovary, and uterus) are diet-related.[8] Both benign and malignant conditions of the ovary, breast, and uterus are related to estrogen levels that are too high.[9] This is because a diet too high in refined carbohydrates raises blood sugar. High blood sugar results in increased levels of metabolically active circulating estrogens because the high triglyceride levels produced by a high-refined-carbohydrate diet displaces estrogen from steroid-binding globulins, which render it metabolically inactive. A diet high in a variety of vegetable fibers can lower a woman's estrogen levels, therefore decreasing her risk of breast cancer. Vegetable fibers change the metabolism of estrogen in the bowel; less is available for absorption into the bloodstream and more is excreted.

Women who start their menstrual cycles (undergo menarche) earlier and their menopause later are at greater risk for breast cancer. American women's menarche is characteristically early (at age twelve or thirteen) and their menopause late.[10] But women who follow low-fat, primarily vegetarian diets, such as the Chinese and the !Kung, typically start their menstrual periods at age sixteen or seventeen. These women also begin menopause earlier. Their breast cancer rates are very low.[11] However, the same was true for hunter-gatherer societies in which the diets were rich in meat and fat, but relatively low in carbohydrates. It is also clear that high levels of physical activity, common among women in the groups just mentioned, also contribute to balancing hormones and to lowering an individual's percentage of body fat.

Step Three: Understand the Blood Sugar/ Inflammation Connection

To understand how we as a culture got to where we are now in terms of the foods we're eating and the problems so many of us are having with them, it helps to go back in time. Our species adapted to a Paleolithic hunter-gatherer diet for more than a hundred thousand years before agriculture was widely adopted. That diet consisted of lots of wild bitter greens rich in pharmacologically active plant chemicals that have well-documented anti-inflammatory and other properties. They also contained wild fruits and berries in season, as well as wild meats from game that ate the same wild foods. Archaeological evidence shows that hunter-gatherers paid special attention to consuming the nutrient-rich organ meats such as the brain, the kidneys, the liver, and the heart. Concentrated sweets, other than occasional honey, were simply not available. And though there were a few wild grains in the diet, these bore almost no resemblance to the modern corn, rice, and wheat that are staple foods today. One of the most important things to remember when deciding what is healthy to eat is this: we still have the metabolisms and physiologies of the Paleolithic hunter-gatherers![12]

Agriculture was introduced about ten thousand years ago, a mere blip on the screen of evolutionary time. To put this in perspective, for 99.8 percent of our time on Earth as *Homo sapiens,* we ate exclusively wild foods.[13] Selective breeding practices since that time have increased the starch and sugar content of fruits, vegetables, and grains as well as markedly changed the biochemical composition of the meat we eat. And in the last sixty years, scores of chemical additives and nonfoods such as trans-fats and preservatives have been added that our Stone Age metabolisms simply weren't designed to cope with. Soil depletion and the addition of nitrate-based fertilizers after WWII (in response to the need to get rid of the stockpiles of nitrates used for bombs) have further changed the food supply. Overnutrition, excess weight, and elevated blood sugar and blood fats are now the norm as food quantity has far outstripped food quality in most of the developed world. According to Joseph Mercola, D. O., author of *The No-Grain Diet* (Dutton, 2003), the average American is now eating sixty pounds more grain and thirty pounds more sweeteners per year than we did twenty-five years ago.[14] (For more information, visit Dr. Mercola's website at www.mercola.com.) Grains, starches, and sugars—and everything made from them (all of which raise blood sugar and lead to addictive eating)—are the real culprits when it comes to excess weight. It's little wonder that the resources of our health care system are being crushed under the weight of the chronic diseases that are the result of this profound shift in the human diet. But that doesn't mean it's impossible to eat a healthy diet these days. In fact, it's getting easier and easier. Here's all you need to know.

Stable Blood Sugar Is the Answer

The most important key to lifelong weight maintenance and vibrant health is knowing how to keep your blood sugar stable. Pure and simple. Stable blood sugar results from eating the right amount of protein, the right kind of carbohydrates, and the right kinds and amounts of fats at the right time. Stable blood sugar throughout the day is also the key to preventing or reversing the diseases that are associated with cellular inflammation. (Note: most of the vast changes in the hunter-gatherer diet that we evolved with are associated with chronic disruptions in blood sugar as their final common pathway!)

It has taken me more than forty-five years of research and clinical experience to figure this out. Back in the late 1980s and early 1990s, like many health conscious people, I was still eating a mostly grain-based, low-fat diet. And I was gaining weight. And at about four P.M. to five P.M., I would come home from work famished and stand in front of the fridge and begin my evening "grazing," which didn't end until I went to bed hours later. I craved sweets and had a difficult time controlling my appetite. My patients complained about the same thing. We also noticed that our waistlines seemed to be disappearing when we hit forty. What had gone wrong with the low-fat, high-complex-carbohydrate, vegetarian diet that so much research said should be keeping us healthy and slim?

At about this time, the popular Zone diet of Barry Sears, Ph.D., came out, followed by the work of family physicians Mary Dan Eades, M.D., and Michael Eades, M.D., authors of *Protein Power* (Bantam Books, 1996) and colleagues of Sears's. I read the research that their books were based on. It made sense. Too many carbs raise insulin levels, which makes the body store excess calories as fat. And enough protein increases glucagon, which jump-starts the body into burning fat. Moreover, the right kinds of fats in small amounts are necessary building blocks for the cellular hormones that fight inflammation and create optimal cellular metabolism (these are known as eicosanoids, and the inflammatory cytokines and prostaglandins are part of this group; see section on fats, below).

Based on this research, I dutifully added more protein to my diet and cut way back on grains, fruits, and sweets. (I didn't want to, though, and it was hard. As a friend said to me, once, "I never met a carb I didn't like!") Impressed with my newfound energy and a decrease in sugar cravings, I suggested the same to my patients. We felt better, but my cravings were not gone. And I simply couldn't seem to give up my refined carbs. Besides, my medical intuitive friend Mona Lisa Schulz, M.D., Ph.D., kept reminding me that the path of deprivation was not healthy for me. (And she was right.)

I was still having a hard time losing weight, however. So like thousands of others, I decided to carry things a step further. If carbs were bad, why not eliminate them completely for a week or two to see if I'd lose weight? So I went on the Atkins induction program. But that didn't work either. Though I ate less than 20 grams of carbs per day, my body absolutely refused to go into ketosis, the state in which your body begins to use fat for energy and ketone bodies are eliminated in the urine. My body was holding on to its fat for dear life, it seemed. When I called the late Robert Atkins, M.D., to discuss this with him, he couldn't explain it except to say, "Well, you're menopausal." That explanation didn't work for me. I also didn't like eating all that meat and bacon. It had felt infinitely better to eat more fruits, vegetables, and grains. But my weight had crept up to an all-time high of 148. (I weighed 150 when I was at the end of my pregnancies!)

The Missing Link: Glycemic Stress and Insulin Resistance

Finally I was introduced to the work of Ray Strand, M.D., author of *Healthy for Life: Developing Healthy Lifestyles That Have a Side Effect of Permanent Fat Loss* (Real Life Press, 2005), a family doctor who, like me, had spent more than twenty-five years seeing the same people and watching them slowly but surely develop expanding waistlines, high cholesterol, high blood pressure, cancer, hypertension, etc. Dr. Strand's research documents the fact that conditions known as glycemic stress and insulin abuse begin in childhood and are the result of eating a diet that is far too high in nutrient-poor refined foods that raise blood sugar (and insulin levels) too quickly. This is true even in those who will never get diabetes. Unfortunately, high-glycemic foods are the "comfort" foods most people crave, including macaroni, white bread, cookies, cakes, and bagels. Eating too many high-glycemic foods on a daily basis results in glycemic stress/inflammation of the blood vessels because of the free-radical damage that ensues when blood sugar is too high. Over time, the blood vessel lining thickens, making it more and more difficult for the insulin to get out and into the cells. As Dr. Strand points out, insulin resistance actually begins in the blood vessels of the skeletal muscles, the place where blood sugar is designed to be burned most efficiently. This process—which begins in childhood—sets the stage for hardening of the arteries and also full-blown insulin resistance. (For more information, visit Dr. Strand's website at www. releasingfat.com.)

Glycemic stress and insulin abuse are the start of the long, steady march to full-blown insulin resistance or metabolic syndrome (also known as Syndrome X—see table on p. 700). Depending upon your genetics, metabolic syndrome either results in diabetes or heart disease or both. (My grandparents on both sides of the family died of cardiovascular disease. And all of them had a sweet tooth.) Just about every cell in our bodies is affected by insulin abuse, which also results in the production of excess inflammatory chemicals—the basis for all chronic disease, including headaches and insomnia! No wonder Kenneth Cooper, M.D., once said, "We die not so much of a particular disease, as from our entire lives." No kidding. Finally I knew why I had had sweet cravings my entire life, why my HDL cholesterol had been dangerously low when I was in my thirties, and why I was having so much trouble losing weight at midlife. It was all that high-glycemic food. (Many vegetarians eat way too many sweets, pastas, and breads, which results in high blood sugar. I was no exception.) The link between glycemic stress, insulin abuse, and cellular inflammation is why everything from headaches to PMS and high blood pressure often improve when you eat to stabilize your blood sugar.

Over time, as blood sugar levels continue to be too high, the insulin receptors on the cells actually lose their ability to respond to high blood sugar. The wrong kinds of dietary fats also change the insulin receptors on the cell membrane itself, thus contributing to the problem. Micronutrient deficiencies such as too little chromium also contribute to the problem. (See micronutrients, below.) Over time, the pancreas simply loses its ability to produce insulin and the cells lose their sensitivity to it! Type 2 diabetes is the result. But there's more. It has recently been discovered that fat cells themselves produce inflammatory chemicals, which is another reason why obesity is a risk factor for cancer. Body fat is loaded with insulin receptors. The fatter you get, the more insulin it takes to get blood sugar into your cells. And because insulin is a storage hormone, the higher its levels, the harder it is for the body to release fat as fuel. Insulin actually locks fat in place!

Stages of Insulin Resistance

1. Glycemic stress: Eating too many foods with a high-glycemic load leading to blood vessel inflammation. Many individuals at this stage actually experience hypoglycemia in which their blood sugar becomes too low after a high-glycemic meal. This is particularly likely after eating a high-glycemic meal combined with caffeine (the standard American breakfast of a doughnut or bagel and cup of coffee!).

SIGNS OF INSULIN ABUSE AND EARLY GLYCEMIC STRESS

Carbohydrate cravings and uncontrollable hunger (the munchies)
Emotional eating
Nighttime eating
Slowly expanding waistline

Increasing resistance to weight loss

Fatigue and possibly shaky weakness following a meal

2. Beginning of insulin resistance: Beta cells of the pancreas are stimulated to produce more insulin to get it across the thickened blood vessel walls. High insulin levels result in high triglycerides, abnormal estrogen metabolism, low HDL cholesterol, high blood sugar, cardiovascular disease, and increased risk of diabetes. Once insulin levels are raised, a chain reaction is triggered that results in so many metabolic changes, it can't be stopped without significant lifestyle changes. (When I was a macrobiotic vegetarian—and also eating too much bread!—my HDL cholesterol was a dangerous 35. I was only thirty-two years old. Now it is at a healthy 70!) Muscles are the first place to become insulin resistant. Once they do, however, blood sugar (glucose) gets redirected to your fat cells, primarily in your abdomen. That means that when you eat a high-glycemic meal, it goes right to your tummy and seems to bypass your muscles entirely! (Over time, skeletal muscles also become marbled with fat.) This is the stage at which you and your doctor should be looking for signs of insulin resistance (high triglycerides and low HDL are often the first signs of glycemic stress and early insulin resistance). The sooner you change your diet, the better. You'll then be able to reverse and prevent all kinds of problems, and also reach your normal weight.

SIGNS OF EARLY INSULIN RESISTANCE

Nighttime eating

Central weight gain (expanding waistline)

Slow weight gain without change in diet

Low HDL cholesterol

Increased triglycerides

Heartburn

Increased fatigue following a high-glycemic meal or snack

Menstrual irregularities

Hypoglycemia

Craving sugar and high-glycemic carbohydrates

Insomnia

3. Full-blown metabolic syndrome: Inexorably, if diet and lifestyle aren't changed, insulin resistance leads to full-blown metabolic syndrome in which high blood pressure, high cholesterol, obesity, increased fibrinogen in the blood (a clotting factor), and a whole host of other problems results.

INSULIN RESISTANCE (SYNDROME X OR METABOLIC SYNDROME) CONTRIBUTES TO:

Type 2 diabetes

Increased levels of fibrinogen (increased blood clotting)

Central obesity (apple-shaped figure)

High blood pressure

Abnormal cholesterol levels

Sleep apnea

Cardiovascular disease, including stroke

Heavy menstrual periods

Most forms of polycystic ovary disease

Anovulation and fertility problems

Hirsutism

Male pattern baldness

Breast, colon, and other cancers

Depression

Dementia

Given the high prevalence of insulin abuse and glycemic stress, I can guarantee you that there's no way you can learn to trust your body's instincts around food until you go on a program that stabilizes your blood sugar and resets your metabolism. You simply have to eliminate all refined carbohydrates; and eat low-glycemic-index carbs; and eat the right amount of protein, healthy fats, and micronutrients. This requires a significant reeducation for most people. Though there are many ways to do this (e.g., Ann Louise Gittleman's *Fat Flush Plan,* Adele Puhn's *Midlife Miracle Diet,* Mercola's *No-Grain Diet,* Diana Schwarzbein's *The Schwarzbein Principle,* etc.), I have personally found that the USANA five-day Reset program (see www.usana.com, and from the products menu, click on Macro-optimizers and then on Reset) is the easiest and most effective way to decrease food cravings and reset your metabolism. Once you've finished this five-day program, you'll know what it feels like to be free of cravings and have stable blood sugar. You may also notice that you sleep better and have a lot more energy. You will notice that a wide variety of health problems improve considerably when you get your blood sugar and insulin under control.

Once you have reset your metabolism, you are in a much better position to continue eating for health. The Reset program of preprepared shakes, pharmaceutical grade vitamins and minerals, and nutrition bars supplemented with fruits and vegetables has been clinically proven to stabilize blood sugar and insulin levels, lower cholesterol, increase energy, decrease cravings, and promote weight loss (the average person usually loses about five pounds in five days—mostly from losing the excess fluid that is so common when insulin levels are too high). Because the Reset program has been scientifically formulated to reset the body's metabolism quickly and easily, it's a very convenient and practical way for most people to experience what it feels like to have a normal metabolism with stable blood sugar. What is particularly remarkable is that the first fat to go is that which is around the abdomen, typically the most "stubborn" fat to get rid of. The reason for this, notes Dr. Strand, is that when you begin to reverse insulin resistance and glycemic stress, the body automatically starts to release its stored fat, particularly the fat around the abdomen that is so metabolically active and difficult to lose on conventional low-calorie and low-fat diets.

What to Eat

Your diet should consist of 80 to 90 percent low-glycemic-index foods, high-quality fats (see below), and lots of low-glycemic fruits and vegetables. Some people can tolerate grains and other can't. Eliminating ALL grains from the diet for one month or so can work wonders. Then add a few back and see how you do. The same is true with having a small amount of high-glycemic foods. (I eat dessert regularly, including chocolate. But I've gotten to the point where I know what "enough" feels like. And it's not much. Believe me, that took years!)

Breakfast: Breakfast is the most important meal of your day because it sets the stage for your blood sugar for the rest of the day. If a person hasn't eaten a blood-sugar-stabilizing breakfast, she will feel the effects of this at what I call "arsenic hour" (about four to five P.M., when stress hormone levels are at their peak and when all the stresses of the day seem to accumulate at once). If you haven't eaten a decent breakfast, you will tip right over into wanting to eat the wallpaper off the wall at this point.

Your breakfast must contain some protein, healthy fat, and low-glycemic-index carbohydrates. If you don't have time to cook, many shakes and bars on the market make this easy. If you do, then a couple of omega-3-rich eggs, some berries, and a cup of tea make a good breakfast. Another of my favorites is slow-cooked oatmeal with a scoop of soy protein powder in it. (Note: all "instant" foods have a much higher glycemic index. Instant oatmeal is no exception.)

Lunch: Lean protein in the form of fish, chicken, meat, or vegetarian alternatives such as tofu. Include lots of low-glycemic-index vegetables such as bok choy, kale, salad greens, etc. Note: vegetables like carrots have a relatively high-glycemic index, but their glycemic load (the total amount of sugar in them) is low. They are fine! Other alternatives include bean or lentil soup and a salad, etc.

Dinner: Same as lunch.

For snacks, choose fruits and cheese, various low-glycemic nutritional bars, or a small handful of nuts.

A Note About Timing

Far too many women make the mistake of "saving up" their calories for dinner by starving themselves during the day. This pattern inevitably leads to erratic blood sugar and is a setup for weight problems, too. It has been scientifically demonstrated that people who ate 2,000 calories' worth of food in the morning lost about two pounds of weight per week, while those who consumed this amount of calories after six P.M. gained weight.[15] It's ideal to wait for three hours after eating before going to bed, though this will not work for everyone.

Controlling Blood Sugar Is Not a "Diet," It's a Lifelong Job

Learning to control your blood sugar and cravings is a lifelong job for the 75 percent of the population (like me) who are prone to excess consumption of refined carbohydrates. There are times that you will slip off the bandwagon. But then you get right back on. Don't expect carbs to stop "singing" to you. They won't. And depending upon your recovery around sugar addiction, you may or may not be able to tolerate some dessert now and then. For example, I recently went to New York City for a holiday weekend with my daughters. We went to a French restaurant for breakfast, where I felt compelled to order the basket of croissant and rolls because they looked so good. After enjoying these refined carbohydrates thoroughly, I later "paid" the price. I got so tired from rebound low blood sugar that resulted from eating all that bread that I felt like lying down on the sidewalk to take a nap! (And this was in November so it was cold.) It took me a total of twenty-four hours to fully recover from the metabolic effect of eating two rolls and two croissants—even though I also had a protein-rich omelet, which should theoretically have helped prevent the blood sugar swings! (Protein eaten at the same meal as refined carbs helps blood sugar remain stable.) Once you really feel the effect of excess high-glycemic food on your blood sugar, you can never go back to mindless eating again!

Craving high-glycemic carbs is not a character flaw and it's not because of lack of willpower. We were designed to crave foods that put on weight quickly—which are invariably foods with a high-glycemic index. The simple truth is that for the vast majority of human history, it was a survival advantage to be able to gain weight quickly during times of plenty in order to make it during lean times. It's interesting to note that those with the most recent hunter-gatherer ancestors (e.g., Native Americans, Inuits) have the most trouble with high-glycemic foods and also grains. (Note: about 25 percent of people, usually but not always Caucasians, are what I call genetic celebrities, who appear to be able to eat anything they want and never gain a pound. Interestingly, however, these individuals really don't crave refined carbohydrates like the rest of us. Many don't even like chocolate! Imagine.)

Step Four: Be Completely Honest About the Food/Emotion Connection

Guilt is one of the worst foods for the intestines.
        —Bill Tims, former macrobiotic counselor

Many women gain weight when they are upset and lose weight easily when they are happy or newly in love. The tendency to eat when emotionally upset can cause you first to retain fluids and then to add body fat, partly because of the action of the hormone cortisol, which is secreted in greater amounts when you are under what you perceive as inescapable stress. Cortisol is a steroid, and if you've ever taken steroids or seen someone balloon up on prednisone, you know what I'm talking about. Scientific studies have shown that unexpressed and unresolved emotional stress results in changes in metabolism that inhibit fat breakdown—

comparable to what happens on prednisone. Eating fat-laden, refined-carbohydrate foods while under stress not only results in excess fat storage, but also sets the stage for many other illnesses in your body.[16] I once gave a party for my daughter after her first formal dance. This required staying up until three A.M. following a hectic day of preparation. Though I ate my usual amount of food, I gained two and a half pounds, which took four days to go away. The same thing happened to one of my friends who was helping me out at the time. I've experienced this pattern repeatedly. On the other hand, I've also gone on vacations where I've eaten more than usual and have actually lost weight because there was no stress. Many women have this same experience in France and Italy, where eating well is a stress-free, pleasurable ritual.

Excess fat and fluid can also be our body's armor against feeling what we don't want to feel. I have seen women release emotions held for a long time and literally lose five or more pounds overnight from a good crying (or laughing) session. Many of you have also experienced the fact that when you are in love you don't need to eat much because you feel so full of life-energy. This life-energy is always available to us whenever we are doing work we love—even when we're not "in love" with another person. This is yet another reason to follow your heart as a way to create health in your life.

Look honestly at how you use food and how much of it you really eat. Include when, why, and how. If you really want to make peace with food, for two weeks or more write down everything you eat, where you ate it, and how you were feeling at the time. This exercise breaks through denial and will help you come to terms with how well you nourish yourself with food. My clinical experience has taught me that those women who write down what they eat in order to get clear with themselves have a much better chance of successfully changing their health.

If you eat primarily for emotional comfort, you may not want to give that up right now. That's okay. One of my patients who was obese until the age of twenty-one told me that she always knew she would lose weight once she moved away from home and stopped caring for her mentally ill mother and younger siblings. Though her parents took her to doctor after doctor and she was put on a series of diets, she knew that she required food to keep from feeling the pain of her circumstances. Once these changed, she lost weight.

We cannot apply *any* information about improving nutrition until we've looked squarely at our issues around food and have committed to making peace with them. For that reason, please go through the steps to healing in chapter 15 before or at the same time as you decide to improve your nutrition.

If your compulsive overeating is out of control, you will have to follow a structured eating plan such as that of Overeaters Anonymous. Such a plan works as an external control system as you learn what your internal triggers to overeating are. Many women have not yet established the link between their emotional pain and how they are using food to control it. Others may have so much stress in their lives that their immune and metabolic systems are adversely affected. For these women, even small amounts of sugary sweets, yeasty foods, or salty or fatty foods set off binge eating. Most women will fall into one of two broad categories: those who binge on fat-laden sweets such as ice cream and those who binge on salty, fat-laden foods such as potato chips. For these women, sugary or salty fat-laden food is like alcohol to an alcoholic. Sugar-addicted women have told me that once they start, they become light-headed, feel drunk and disoriented, and develop an insatiable desire to eat more and more sugary foods. (The same thing can apply to fatty and salty binge food.) When women avoid these "trigger foods," their eating returns to normal. Food cravings also lessen considerably when you eat a diet that is adequate in protein and fat and low in refined carbohydrates. (See Step Ten: Rehabilitate Your Metabolism, page 717.) Once a woman has dealt with the emotional causes of overeating and has also improved her diet to reduce cravings, she will often no longer require a food plan as an "external authority." She will know what to eat and when.

Nothing Says Loving
Taking nourishment just for ourselves and not to please others is uncommon for women. Women are socialized to interact with others and demonstrate our love for them through shopping for, preparing, serving, and cleaning up food every day. When relationships at home or at work are not completely fulfilling and nourishing, women (and men) try to fill the hole we feel at our center with food—a hole that no amount of food will fill. Because of the massive cultural forces that keep us stuck in a pattern of eating to fill our inner emptiness, your attempts to improve your diet will be sabotaged until you become aware intellectually and emotionally of why you overeat, or don't eat, or eat only food low in nutrient value. Only we ourselves can take the first step toward breaking free of these influences. When enough women do this, the culture, too, will change.

Dietary improvement and exercise programs are doomed to failure unless they're accompanied by a great deal of self-love, humor, and personal flexibility. Any hint of self-blame when you eat ice cream is a personal setup for failure, and it is also a form of self-abuse. One of my patients who was using a macrobiotic diet to heal her fibroids learned that when she said, "I love and respect myself," her cravings resolved. The better she felt about herself, the more she felt like eating in a healthy way.

Eat in Good Company

Just about everyone who has ever improved her lifestyle knows one thing: when you begin to adopt healthier habits, you're bound to have friends and family members who will try to sabotage your efforts. This is because your desire for better health (or anything else) will hold up a mirror to them and make them question their own behavior, which they may not want to change. So you're perceived as a threat. Expect this. Resistance to change is normal. Make every effort to spend time with people who are on the same lifestyle path as you and with whom you can find support for the inevitable times when you feel as though a hot fudge sundae is the solution to your problems!

Nourishment is not just the food that we put in our mouths. It is also the environment around us: the people we're with, the sunlight and starlight from the skies, and the color of our walls. These things affect how food is metabolized in our bodies. You need to reevaluate any friendships you have that support unhealthy eating. If you always spend time with those who use eating to suppress their emotions or as their only form of entertainment you will quite literally feel and act heavier around these people—and you are apt to gain excess fat. You may need to make some new friendships. On the other hand, when you eat with people who enjoy food fully and without any guilt, you may well find that you feel more satisfied than in the past.

I have noticed that I eat much less when I go out to eat than when I'm at home. The entire process of being served and having to wait between courses results in a very different digestive process and an enhanced sense of well-being.

Step Five: Update Your Cultural Programming

Food and emotions are very deeply linked in human beings for reasons far older than our current obsession with thinness. For centuries, the human race was able to survive because we ate the things that our tribes said were okay to eat. We avoided the poisonous berries and ate what Mother said was safe. Food has always been an essential part of the daily ritual of living, and the foods we were fed in childhood have left a very deep impression on us. At an unconscious and conscious level, they *help us feel safe* and cared for.

Women's role as traditional mothers—providing the "tribal foods"—is out of date. Women need no longer think of themselves as the sole providers of food for their clans, but these roles are still deeply ingrained nonetheless and so are the tribal food choices that go along with them. A number of vegetarian patients of mine have mothers who *still* present roast beef as a special meal when they come home. For these mothers, a roast is symbolic of love and caring. The conditioning that says a woman should serve abundant rich food to her family to ensure their survival runs very deep. We must become conscious of these patterns now. What once ensured our survival is killing us.

Susie Orbach's *Fat Is a Feminist Issue* (Galahad Books, 1997) documents how tied up with food women are because it is our cultural imperative to feed everybody. Though my mother was way ahead of her time in many areas, she was still a product of her culture when it came to food preparation. As soon as the breakfast dishes were cleared, my father would say to her, "What's for lunch?" She used to tell me not to ask my father anything important or controversial until after he had eaten his dinner, which taught me that my job was to feed men, because a hungry man was supposedly unpredictable. At the end of the afternoon, around the time my father came home from work, my mother used to set the table even if she hadn't started dinner, so that my father would *think* that dinner was under way and that she had been busily preparing it for him for hours. A physician friend of mine said that *her* mother used to begin frying onions just before her father arrived home. The house would smell as if dinner were cooking, even though it hadn't been started. Her father would say, "Smells great, honey!" Then she'd start the meal, having already produced the illusion that the meal preparation was long since under way.

Both my mother and my friend's mother were operating under the 1950s and 1960s imperative that the woman's job was to feed the breadwinner when he came home, regardless of her own needs or her own schedule. This imperative to feed hungry men also operates in the sexual arena, I believe. Women have been brought up to believe that men have "sexual needs" that a woman must fulfill. It's *her* job and *her* duty to satisfy his sexual appetite as well as his nutritional appetite. If she doesn't do well enough, he's justified in seeking fulfillment for those *male* needs outside the home. Despite the fact that nobody ever died from lack of an orgasm, the cultural mythology of the past several centuries has been that if a man isn't happy in his marriage, it is the woman's fault. My grandfather left my grandmother, I was told, partly because she wasn't "woman enough" for him. (We can only guess what that means.)

Many women have told me how when they were young their

dinnertimes were orchestrated around their father's arrival home. If he was late, they waited one or two hours, while the mother tried to keep the food appetizing and calm the hungry children into waiting so that they could all sit down to a "proper" family meal. Mary Catherine Bateson's book *Composing a Life* (Grove Press, 2001) documents that the presence of a man in a household increases the workload significantly—not because he leaves that many more dirty socks around but because of the *expectations* that he has of those around him and that *those around him have of themselves*. "Women are taught to deny themselves for the sake for the marriage," she writes; "men are taught that the marriage exists to support them."[17] We have the power to change this situation and also create happy relationships with men—first by noticing how we ourselves perpetuate old outmoded patterns.

Many women have told me how much easier life is when their husband is gone on a trip and they don't have to arrange their eating, cleaning up, and recreation schedules around his. Having been indoctrinated for a lifetime that their worth is tied up with cooking for men, many women *don't cook for themselves at all* when there's no man to please. Deep inside they've learned that only *he* is worth the effort, not themselves. And they've resented this in silence for years.

Many men's nutritional and emotional needs have been met by women since birth. When they marry, their wives often take over where their mothers left off. When a man cooks or takes care of the children, it's not culturally expected, and so it is almost always regarded as a gift, as something extra that he does for the family. When a woman tells me that she cooks three separate dinners every night because of all the various preferences in her house, I immediately prescribe for her a book or meeting on codependency. Cooking three separate meals for people who don't appreciate the effort—and who in fact pass negative judgment upon it—is a classic relationship addiction. (If, on the other hand, she's well rewarded for her efforts, loves to cook, and she and her family have all agreed on the arrangement, no problem.)

My mother and thousands of other women employed strategies like cooking onions to give the illusion that dinner was cooking in order to survive—and then they passed these subtle dishonesties down to us. Only in the last decade or so have I become aware of how far I've come in my own deprogramming from these early messages. In the past when I was home and my husband was not, I was very aware of my personal programming that the house should be picked up before he arrived home from work and that dinner should be started, even though we both worked full-time. I also sometimes got resentful when my husband would innocently ask me, "What are we doing for dinner?" I used to think that he was *making* me plan the meals, shop for food, and pre-pare the meals. He didn't understand why I became irritable. For a while, neither did I. Then it became clear to me that I was automati-cally assuming that feeding him was my responsibility, even though we both worked long hours at the same job!

Once I became conscious of my programming (which I brought into my marriage as surely as I brought my hopes and dreams), I didn't blame him for *the fact that I felt compelled to* cook and clean against my wishes. I also started to change my behavior. For example, I didn't necessarily pick up unless I wanted to. At the same time, he also began to take a look at his programming—with some help from me. He came to see that he *expected* me to do the jobs that his mother had always done. Once both of us made conscious our unconscious expectations about food, cooking, and cleaning, our relationship improved in this area. (In most relationships the unspoken *shoulds* and *oughts* for both members need to be articulated—I don't pretend that this is easy.)

I encourage you to review some of the subtle and not-so-subtle ways in which you have been conditioned. You cannot make any di-etary improvement until you've mapped out your personal food mine-field (from childhood to the present) and have honestly examined your assumptions about being the chief cook and bottle-washer or that you cannot take the time to prepare and enjoy good food for yourself. Especially now that the majority of women are working outside of the home, our expectations of ourselves about food preparation need con-siderable updating from our mothers' day.

Ask yourself the following questions:

- ⌐ Do you feel personally responsible for thinking about, shopping for, and preparing the family meals?
- ⌐ If the refrigerator is empty when family members are hungry, do you feel guilty? Inadequate?
- ⌐ Have you ever discussed this with your spouse? Your children? Your other loved ones?
- ⌐ Do you enjoy preparing food?
- ⌐ Do you prepare delicious meals for yourself even when you're alone? If the answer is no, do you make healthy choices when you eat out or when others prepare food for you?

For me, a vacation is not worth it if I have to cook three meals a day. We once rented a cabin on an island nearby, and it seemed that all I did was cook and clean up. The kids were looking for snacks constantly but weren't old enough to get them for themselves. I was not relaxed at the end of that week—I was angry. Vacation cooking can be fun, however, when the activity is shared with others.

My mother once remarked, "I'm not surprised retirees like to eat out so often. Many of those women have had to prepare three meals a day for over forty years. No wonder they're sick of it." And although the food on airplanes is not always healthy, I sometimes prefer being served by someone else rather than carrying healthy food with me. I believe this stems from being a mother and having to serve others while excluding myself for so long. I enjoy being served and not having to clean up afterward. I also find that I eat less, but feel more satisfied, when I eat out and am served by someone else. Now that I'm single and my daughters have left home, I eat out nearly every day at restaurants that serve organic food. This nourishes me at all levels and is well worth the expense.

The women's movement of the late 1960s gave unprecedented numbers of women the impetus and means to support themselves financially for the first time. As a result, we no longer have to marry for economic survival. This makes true partnerships between men and women a far more viable proposition. To get to this, however, we have to change our conditioning. When you do, you'll find that many men will knock themselves out to please you if you value yourself, know what you want, and ask for what you want without anger, guilt, or self-doubt.

Step Six: Make Peace with Weight

Excess weight is dreams in storage. There's a myth that we can store up time. Primitive cultures store up for the winter. We store up time in our hips.

—Paulanne Balch, M.D.

Countless women over the years have asked me, "How much should I weigh?" Though all of us have been weighed and measured since birth and compared with the cultural ideal, each individual woman has a natural weight at which her body will stay, for the most part, if she is eating according to physical need and exercising regularly. A woman's weight will often fluctuate by two to four pounds in any given week, and it will also vary with her monthly cycle or annual cycle. This fluctuation is almost always due to changes in fluid levels, not fat or muscle, and is normal. A woman's natural, healthy weight may not match the weight tables of any insurance company or doctor's office, and it may not be related at all to clothing size. (See table 11.)

Weight as a measure of health doesn't address body composition and is therefore misleading and ambiguous. The concept of "ideal" body weight is not only extremely destructive for many women, but also an obsolete way of thinking about health. A much more meaningful measure is your percentage of body fat, which I will cover on page 716, and also body mass index (BMI). To determine your BMI, simply find your height and weight on table 11. A BMI of 24 or less is considered ideal, while a BMI of 30 or above is defined as obese and carries an increased risk of death and disease. BMIs between 25 and 29, though not ideal, do not necessarily increase health risk.

TABLE 11
USDA SUGGESTED WEIGHTS FOR ADULTS

Height[1]	Weights in Pounds[2] 19–34 years	>35 years
5'0"	97–128	108–138
5'1"	101–132	111–143
5'2"	104–137	115–148
5'3"	107–141	119–152
5'4"	111–146	122–157
5'5"	114–150	126–162
5'6"	118–155	130–167
5'7"	121–160	134–172
5'8"	125–164	138–178
5'9"	129–169	142–183
5'10"	132–174	146–188
5'11"	136–179	151–194
6'0"	140–184	155–199

1. Height is without shoes.

2. Weight is without clothes. The higher weights generally apply to men, who tend to have more muscle and bone than women. The lower weights more often apply to women, who have less muscle and bone.

Adapted from the U.S. Department of Agriculture and U.S. Department of Health and Human Services, *Nutrition and Your Health: Dietary Guidelines for Americans,* 3rd edition (Washington, D.C.: U.S. Government Printing Office, 1990).

FIGURE 17: BODY MASS INDEX CHART

Height (Feet and Inches)

Weight (Pounds)	5'0"	5'1"	5'2"	5'3"	5'4"	5'5"	5'6"	5'7"	5'8"	5'9"	5'10"	5'11"	6'0"	6'1"	6'2"	6'3"	6'4"
100	20	19	18	18	17	17	16	16	15	15	14	14	14	13	13	12	12
105	21	20	19	19	18	17	17	16	16	16	15	15	14	14	13	13	13
110	21	21	20	19	19	18	18	17	17	16	16	15	15	15	14	14	13
115	22	22	21	20	20	19	19	18	17	17	17	16	16	15	15	14	14
120	23	23	22	21	21	20	19	19	18	18	17	17	16	16	15	15	15
125	24	24	23	22	21	21	20	20	19	18	18	17	17	16	16	16	15
130	25	25	24	23	22	22	21	20	20	19	19	18	18	17	17	16	16
135	26	26	25	24	23	22	22	21	21	20	19	19	18	18	17	17	16
140	27	26	26	25	24	23	23	22	21	21	20	20	19	18	18	17	17
145	28	27	27	26	25	24	23	23	22	21	21	20	20	19	19	18	18
150	29	28	27	27	26	25	24	23	23	22	22	21	20	20	19	19	18
155	30	29	28	27	27	26	25	24	24	23	22	22	21	20	20	19	19
160	31	30	29	28	27	27	26	25	24	24	23	22	22	21	21	20	19
165	32	31	30	29	28	27	27	26	25	24	24	23	22	22	21	21	20
170	33	32	31	30	29	28	27	27	26	25	24	24	23	22	22	21	21
175	34	33	32	31	30	29	28	27	27	26	25	24	24	23	22	22	21
180	35	34	33	32	31	30	29	28	27	27	26	25	24	24	23	22	22
185	36	35	34	33	32	31	30	29	28	27	27	26	25	24	24	23	23
190	37	36	35	34	33	32	31	30	29	28	27	26	26	25	24	24	23
195	38	37	36	35	33	32	31	31	30	29	28	27	26	26	25	24	24
200	39	38	37	35	34	33	32	31	30	30	29	28	27	26	26	25	24
205	40	39	37	36	35	34	33	32	31	30	29	29	28	27	26	26	25
210	41	40	38	37	36	35	34	33	32	31	30	29	28	28	27	26	26
215	42	41	39	38	37	36	35	34	33	32	31	30	29	28	28	27	26
220	43	42	40	39	38	37	36	34	33	32	32	31	30	29	28	27	27
225	44	43	41	40	39	37	36	35	34	33	32	31	31	30	29	28	27
230	45	43	42	41	39	38	37	36	35	34	33	32	31	30	30	29	28
235	46	44	43	42	40	39	38	37	36	35	34	33	32	31	30	29	29
240	47	45	44	43	41	40	39	38	36	35	34	33	33	32	31	30	29
245	48	46	45	43	42	41	40	38	37	36	35	34	33	32	31	31	30
250	49	47	46	44	43	42	40	39	38	37	36	35	34	33	32	31	30

☐ Underweight ▨ Weight Appropriate ☐ Overweight ▨ Obese

Nevertheless, almost all women (myself included) have been brainwashed at some point in their lives about what they should weigh. So each of us lives our life, usually beginning in adolescence, with an ideal weight etched deeply in our brain. This ideal weight is almost invariably five to ten pounds less than what we really weigh.

If we are to constantly judge ourselves by the ideals of our media, we will always be at war with our bodies. The average Miss America's weight dropped from 134 pounds in 1954 to 117 pounds in 1980. The ideal fashion model twenty-five years ago weighed 8 percent less than the average American woman at that time, but today, the ideal fashion model weighs 25 percent less than the average American woman.[18] Thus, the current media image of the "ideal" body is unachievable for most women—unless they take laxatives daily, are anorexic, or use exercise addictively as a form of weight control.

Magazines written for teenage girls are full of dieting and weight information that simply serves to hook young women into a lifetime obsession with weight and food that keeps their energy and their power tied up until they finally find the courage and the guidance to get off this road to nowhere, freeing up enormous creative energy in the process. The statistics on eating disorders speak for themselves. Currently, 1 percent of the female population has full-blown anorexia nervosa.[19] Bulimia, which consists of binge eating, self-induced vomiting, laxative use, diuretic use, or exercise to try to lose weight, is present in up to 20 percent of college students. It occurs mostly in young women age thirty or younger. Less than 5 percent of cases are in males.[20] Even so, most bulimics don't lose excessive weight but weigh slightly more than they would like to.

The medical profession reinforces these addictive behaviors by serving as "weight police," having women weigh in and admonishing them to lose weight year after year without addressing the complexities of self-nourishment for women. Because until recently most doctors have been men, their internal image of the "ideal" female is influenced heavily by the media. The male experience of weight management is often used as a model for women. One of my colleagues was an oarsman in college on the lightweight crew. His weight has always been about 160 pounds, and he's six feet tall. When his weight was a bit higher than the limit for crew the week before a race, he simply stopped eating desserts for a few days and ran a little more. Weight management was always easy for him—it wasn't a "moral" issue at all. He also came from a family of people whom I refer to as "genetically gifted"— none of them tended toward overweight, even at midlife. He and his family clearly metabolized carbohydrates into energy with great efficiency. My colleague's approach to weight issues is the norm in the medical community: losing weight, women are told, is simply a matter of self-discipline and willpower. Therefore, if you can't get your body where you want it (or where society thinks it should be), you are weak and have no self-control.

I personally decided at about the age of fifteen that my ideal weight for my height should be 115 pounds. I made this decision based on reading teen magazines in which it was written that for a person five feet three inches tall, that figure was ideal. Then I spent the next twenty years trying to achieve that figure—which I did only once, during college, as a result of erratic eating and food restriction. Later, after having two children, I reluctantly adjusted up to a new "ideal" of 125 pounds—another elusive goal I also couldn't manage to reach despite exercise and dietary adjustment. It took me till I was forty-seven years old to realize that at a healthy percentage of body fat and with the large frame size I have, my weight was fine at 137 to 140 pounds, which is where it stayed until five years after menopause when it fell to about 132—the result of eating far more low-glycemic foods, no longer having to cook meals for others and having the time to exercise more. Up until this year, I, like so many of my patients, had been fighting with my body's natural and healthy size for the better part of my adult life. I am thankful that behavior has finally drawn to a close for me—and for many other women as well. To signify my newfound self-acceptance, I actually put my correct weight on my driver's license renewal form several years ago, allowing the elusive 125 to slip into history. I did this as an act of reclaiming my personal power, and I encourage more women to do the same.

Most women have bodies that are meant to be larger than the cultural ideal. Women's bodies have more fat on them than men's, nature's way of ensuring that the energy needs of childbearing and lactation will be met even during times of famine. The much larger amount of testosterone men's bodies produce contributes to a leaner body for men and a much higher metabolic rate than women have. Men also have proportionately more muscle than women, which is another factor that leads to a higher metabolic rate. Since cultural expectations of women are that we can never be too thin, and since being thin is associated with self-control, a lifelong struggle with food and body weight is a cultural norm. Our bodies and their weight are the barometers by which society measures how good we are, how attractive we are, how worthy we are.

How much self-control and body abuse must women go through before it dawns on us that there is something deeply wrong with our entire approach to the "weight problem"? Willpower and self-control are exactly the opposite of what we need. We need to see media images of normal, healthy women who are strong and lean but not anorexic. Oprah Winfrey is a good example of this, and I applaud her. But as it turns out, even women with culturally "perfect" bodies tell me that they're not happy with themselves. Regardless of our body size, self-respect and self-acceptance are the starting points for making peace with our size. We must know that we have the power to get off the weight treadmill and start enjoying our lives, no matter where we are not. When it comes to our bodies, we would be wise to heed the advice of Louise Hay, who teaches that changes in our lives (and our bodies) that are loved into existence are permanent, while the changes that happen through self-abuse and denial will always be transient. I find it fascinating that I, and many other women my age (fifty plus) now like our bodies more than we ever did in our twenties—this is great reason for celebration! Healing one's body image is definitely possible regardless of the cultural messages!

Step Seven: Determine Your Body Frame Size

To reach optimal health and your optimal body composition, you may need to rehabilitate how you have been programmed to think about your size. To determine whether your frame size is small, medium, or large, take your thumb and third finger and encircle your opposite wrist with them right at the point where you would normally wear a watch or bracelet. If the tips of your fingers overlap, you have a small frame. If they just meet, you have a medium frame. If your thumb and third finger don't touch, you have a large frame. Finger length has nothing to do with this—your finger length will be proportionate to your wrist size. Studies have shown that large frame size in and of itself is often associated with repeated unnecessary and unsuccessful attempts at dieting. So if you have a large frame, bless it and get on with your life. You will probably never weigh 115 pounds and there's no reason to think that you ever should—in fact, it's dangerous. Though I've told you that weight is an obsolete measure of health, I do want to help you heal from your past misconceptions about the subject. Take a look at the USDA suggested weights in table 11 for adults— both men and women—as well as the BMI chart. You'll see that, depending upon your frame size, there's a very large range that is perfectly acceptable and healthy.

Step Eight: Find Out if You're Fit or Fat

Excess body fat is not just unsightly but also a serious health risk. But weight itself is truly a meaningless measure of health. Why? Because lean body mass weighs much more than fat. Muscles are 80 percent water, while fat is only 5 to 10 percent water. Muscle is over eight times heavier than the equivalent amount of fat.[21] An individual can be at "normal" weight, or even less than that, and be overfat. Others may weigh far more than they "should" according to the weight tables, yet be at an ideal body fat percentage. Some women will actually gain weight when they start to increase their lean body mass, but at the same time they will lose inches. This is because six pounds of fat takes up almost a gallon of space.

One of my patients, whom I'll call Mildred, was a former marathon runner who had believed for years that she was shaped "like a knockwurst." Although Mildred wore a size 8, exercised regularly, and looked wonderful in her clothes, I could not convince her that she should stop trying to get down to 125 pounds. Her friends always thought she weighed a lot less than she did because she had a very significant amount of lean muscle mass. It wasn't until we measured Mildred's body composition—which revealed that her body fat percentage was only 25 percent—that it finally began to dawn on her that her weight range of 136–140 pounds was both healthy and in the ideal range.

Get your body fat measured. It's one of the most helpful steps you can take to break out of the "I weigh too much" tyranny. You can do this at many doctors' offices, or at almost any fitness center or Y. Brookstone and other stores also sell devices that measure body fat. A healthy percentage of body fat for women ranges from 18 to 28 percent. Currently, the average American woman's body fat is 33 percent.[22]

For the sake of comparison, female competitive runners' average body fat is 18 percent, while anorexic women may be as low as 10 percent—so low that their bodies must consume their internal organs as fuel. On the other hand, a healthy body fat percentage for men is 15 percent, and competitive male athletes may be as low as 3 or 4 percent. Body fat percentage is one area where it can be deadly to imitate men, however, because a woman's normal hormonal cycle can be interrupted at body fat percentages lower than 17 to 18 percent. (This is the level of body fat required to have "washboard" abs or a "six-pack"—it is altogether too low for many women and girls.)

If your body fat is currently in a healthy range, congratulate yourself and keep on doing what you're doing. If it is too high, know that by reducing it, you will not only look and feel better, but you will also be lowering your risk for high blood pressure, high cholesterol, adult onset diabetes, heart disease, and fluid retention. In fact, increasing your lean body mass and decreasing your body fat percentage is one of the best treatments for these conditions if you already have them.

Step Nine: Retrain Your Eyes

We're all aware that the cultural icons of beauty—today's super-models—seem thinner than almost anyone we know or see regularly. We also know that the images in magazines are airbrushed and manipulated so much that even the supermodels don't look like themselves. How can any of us feel attractive at a healthy body fat percentage when all the supermodels must be about 18 percent body fat or less?

The answer is that we all have to retrain our eyes to see the beauty inherent in a healthy woman with a healthy body composition, whose image is not an airbrushed, computer-enhanced, quasi-anorexic body that looks something like that of an adolescent boy with big breasts. Once you start looking for it, you'll see this kind of beauty everywhere!

Step Ten: Rehabilitate Your Metabolism

Exercise. As women age, muscle mass is often replaced by fat because of lack of exercise. Exercise reverses this fat gain/muscle loss trend no matter at what age you start. Women who exercise regularly can look forward on average to twenty more years of productive living than those who don't. Regular exercise also decreases insulin resistance, which helps your body burn carbohydrates more efficiently, making fat storage much less likely. Because glycemic stress begins in skeletal muscles, regular exercise helps prevent it. The best way to increase your lean muscle mass is by doing weight-bearing exercise regularly. Miriam Nelson, Ph.D., has shown that a weight-training program that exercises all the major muscle groups for forty minutes twice a week helps women lose excess fat and gain significant muscle mass—thus resulting in a higher metabolic rate and ability to burn calories effectively.[23]

Aerobic exercise also increases your metabolic rate. Anything over twelve minutes per day at your target heart rate will be effective. (See chapter 18.) Try for twenty to thirty minutes three times per week of aerobic exercise and two sessions of weight training per week. The more exercise you do, the faster your metabolism speeds up. Fast walking works very well, as do stair climbing, bike riding, treadmills, and similar forms of exercise. (Watch it—exercise taken to extremes can also be a form of addiction.) The increase in metabolic rate lasts for up to twenty-four hours after exercise is finished.

Eat the right carbohydrates. It has been my clinical experience that families in which there are several alcoholics also invariably have members who are addicted to sugar, even if they are not prone to excessive alcohol intake themselves. These addictions tend to flip-flop. Any veteran of Alcoholics Anonymous will tell you that sugary snacks are a staple at meetings, as individuals substitute sugar for alcohol.

This observation has been confirmed by the work of Kathleen DesMaisons, Ph.D., a specialist in nutrition and addiction and author of *Potatoes Not Prozac* (Simon & Schuster, 1999), who was able to achieve a 90 percent success rate in rehabilitating repeat-offender drunk drivers by teaching them how to eat in order to stabilize their blood sugar and brain chemistry. Her research, which matches my clinical experience, revealed that individuals who crave either alcohol or sugar—or both—have an increased need (probably inborn) for the brain chemicals serotonin, dopamine, and beta endorphin. (Many such people are also highly creative. It's no secret that some of our greatest writers have been alcoholics.) The key to gaining control over their addictive, and often destructive, eating or drinking behaviors is for them to learn to balance their brain chemicals by understanding the food-mood connection.

Dr. DesMaisons has a simple test to help you decide whether you're sugar-sensitive. Here it is: When you were a kid and went out with your family on summer nights for ice cream, what part of the trip do you remember most? The car, the feel of the night air, your family members, or the ice cream itself? If ice cream comes first in your recollections, you're probably sugar-sensitive.

We know that having enough of the brain chemical serotonin is key to feeling calm and focused, which is why antidepressants such as Prozac, Paxil, and Zoloft, all of which enhance serotonin, have become so popular. The weight-loss drugs "fen-phen" and Redux, now removed from the market because of their dangerous side effects, also boosted serotonin. Luckily, you can learn how to enhance and balance your own serotonin without help from drugs.

Serotonin is manufactured in the brain from the amino acid tryptophan, which is found in protein. In order for tryptophan to enter your brain from the bloodstream, your body requires insulin—which means you need to eat some carbohydrates as well. You want just enough in-sulin to do the job, but not so much that you get rebound low blood sugar. If you are prone to seasonal affective disorder (SAD) or other forms of depression, you will crave carbohydrates more than most peo-ple in order to boost your serotonin to adequate levels.

There's a reason we call refined carbohydrate foods "comfort foods." Macaroni and cheese, garlic mashed potatoes with plenty of butter, french fries, pancakes, waffles, cakes, and cookies all raise blood sugar quickly, thus increasing our levels of beta-endorphin, a natural, morphinelike substance in the blood. There's a new over-the-counter PMS medication called PMS Escape that contains almost nothing ex-cept pure sugar! It's designed to elevate mood. You'd be better off hav-ing some chocolate! Unfortunately, what goes up must come down. And continually eating "comfort foods" eventually wreaks havoc with just about every system in the body, leading to cellular inflammation and chronic degenerative disease. So much for long-term comfort! Happily there are other ways to boost your serotonin and balance your brain chemicals. Exercise, natural light, and meditation are all good.

The bottom line is this: growing up in an alcoholic or other dys-functional family (which I've come to see is the majority of us) is stress-ful. The imprint of that stress continues to affect how we feel about ourselves. We use food as a drug to soothe us. Sugar addiction, whether or not you are from an alcoholic family, is an addiction like any other. It needs to be treated like one. Most alcoholics finally begin to recover when they realize that they can't control their drinking on their own. In other words, they admit they are "powerless" over the addiction. And then they invoke their Higher Power (which can be thought of as our soul) to help them. This is what the twelve-step program is all about—letting go and letting God. The best book on sugar addiction and recovery I have ever read is *Holy Hunger: A Memoir of Desire* (A. A. Knopf, 1999), by Margaret Bullitt-Jonas, a brilliant Episcopal priest. She never touches sugar, is at peace with food, and writes the fol-lowing words of wisdom: "The first step in the long process of recov-ery, and the foundation of a food addict's subsequent well-being, is putting down the fork, putting down the food, one day at a time. No insight into self, however subtle; no analysis of the dynamics of addiction, however accurate; no understanding of the nature of desire, however sophisticated or enlightening—none of these fine things can substitute for action. The healing of addiction depends, first and foremost, not on what we know, nor on what we feel, but on what we do—a fact that remains as stubbornly true of 'old timers' as it does for newcomers."[24]

Get enough protein. What is "enough protein"? Well, experts disagree. Some feel that all we need is about thirty grams per day; others suggest higher amounts. Though some Americans get more protein than they need, others—and that includes a lot of women—don't get enough to feel their best. This is one area in which I've changed my mind over the past decade based on newer research and both clinical and personal experience.

I, like many, used to think that it was possible for everybody to get all the protein they required for optimal health from grains, beans, and vegetables. Now I realize that while a diet high in complex carbohydrates from whole foods is great for some—the metabolically gifted, who have no problem with insulin—it is not the answer for everyone. I used to erroneously believe that a diet rich in protein and fat was invariably associated with an increased risk of losing calcium in the urine, thus increasing the risk of osteoporosis. However, a review of the current literature has shown that this is simply not always true.[25] It depends on the quality of the protein and fat. And also how much insulin is hanging around.

Whether you choose to improve your diet on your own or follow the recommendations in one of the many books on diet and nutrition, make sure you are getting an amount of protein every day that is adequate to maintain (or build) your lean body mass—the part of you that burns fat most efficiently. (Not every diet proclaimed to be "high-protein" will provide sufficient amounts of protein.) (See table 12 to determine the appropriate amount of protein.)

TABLE 12
CALCULATING YOUR DAILY PROTEIN REQUIREMENT

To determine the daily protein amount required to preserve your lean body mass (LBM), you must first measure your percentage of body fat. (See page 716.) I'll use Mildred, the former marathoner, as an example. She weighs 138 pounds and has a body fat measurement of 25 percent.

1. Multiply your weight in pounds by your percentage of body fat expressed as a decimal. This tells you the weight of your body fat. (For Mildred: 138 × .25 = 34 pounds)

2. Subtract the weight of your body fat from your total weight. This tells you your lean body mass. (For Mildred: 138 - 34 = 104 LBM)

3. Now multiply your LBM by the cofactor that best describes you:
   Sedentary (you do no physical exercise whatsoever): you need 0.5 grams of protein per pound of lean body mass. Multiply your LBM by 0.5

Moderately active (you do twenty to thirty minutes of exercise, two to three times per week): you need 0.6 grams of protein per pound of lean body mass. Multiply your LBM by 0.6.

Active (you participate in organized physical activity for more than thirty minutes, three to five times per week): you need 0.7 grams of protein per pound of lean body mass. Multiple your LBM by 0.7.

Very active (you participate in vigorous physical activity lasting an hour or more, five or more times per week): you need 0.8 grams of protein per pound of lean body mass. Multiply your LBM by 0.8.

Athlete (you are a competitive athlete in training doing twice-daily heavy workouts for an hour or more): you need 0.9 grams of protein per pound of lean body mass. Multiply your LBM by 0.9.

Mildred has an LBM of 104 pounds and is moderately active. Therefore, her daily protein requirement is 62 grams—considerably less than when she was training for marathons.

Source: This method for calculating protein requirements is based on *Protein Power* (Bantam, 1996) by Drs. Michael and Mary Dan Eades.

As you can see, the terms "high-protein" and "low-protein" are completely meaningless when your dietary approach is individualized.

There is no question that some individuals are very sensitive to arachidonic acid (AA), which is found in all animal products—especially organ meats, red meat, and egg yolks. In fact, this sensitivity to AA is what causes most of the problems that have been commonly attributed to saturated fat and cholesterol. Arachidonic acid is higher in the modern meat supply than in the past because the grain that is fed to livestock results in the same eicosanoid imbalance in animals as it does in humans—that is, it results in more inflammatory chemicals than is healthy. Ph.D. T. Colin Campbell's famous China study, the most comprehensive large study ever undertaken of the relationship between diet and disease, has shown beyond a shadow of a doubt that the Western penchant for too much animal protein and not enough plant food is deadly. (See *The China Study* [BenBella Books, 2005] by T. Colin Campbell.) The symptoms of arachidonic acid sensitivity are the following: chronic fatigue, poor and restless sleep, grogginess upon awakening, brittle hair, brittle nails, dry and flaking skin, minor rashes, and arthritis. It seems clear that some of the health advantages we've attributed to a vegetarian diet are simply the result of lowering the AA content of the diet! To find out if you are susceptible to AA, eliminate all red meat and egg yolks from your diet for one month. Then eat a meal of steak and eggs and see if your symptoms return. To avoid excess AA, eat only low-fat meat (AA is mostly stored in animal fat), or switch to wild game or free-range livestock, which has much lower levels of AA. Look for free-range chickens and the eggs from them in your health food store. Excess consumption of carbohydrates (particularly refined ones) also increases AA levels.

It's not necessary to eat meat in order to increase your protein intake, however. Many vegetarian protein powders including those made from whole soy are now available. The nutritional quality of soy protein has been studied in depth. Studies have shown that nitrogen balance, digestibility, and protein utilization are similar between beef and soy proteins.[26] Other studies show that soy protein can support nitrogen balance[27] and provides adequate amounts of the amino acid methionine, which is important for growth and development.[28] Recent studies have reported that nitrogen absorption, protein digestibility, biological value, and net utilization of soy protein are similar to those of milk protein.[29]

The high digestibility of soy protein, the content and bioavailability of its amino acids, and its nitrogen content make soy protein a high-quality protein. Based on protein digestibility calculations, soy protein achieves a score of 1.0, the highest score possible and on par with other high-quality proteins like egg white and milk proteins. Therefore, the addition of soy to the diet is a good way to meet your protein nutritional requirements.

It is also possible to get adequate protein from veggie burgers, tofu, seitan, and tempeh. Eggs, whey powder, soy powder, and milk products are good sources of protein if you're not sensitive to them. Most women do better with some animal food in their diets. Though I appreciate the sentiments of animal-rights activists and the environmental impact of the current meat production industry, I don't feel that it is healthful or necessary for everyone to become a vegetarian. There is no question, however, that the vast majority of the population needs more fruits, vegetables, and whole grains! Organic methods of producing animal food that respect the soil, the water, and the animal itself can overcome the environmental concerns posed by the meat industry. You can now buy meat from animals raised without chemicals and antibiotics; this meat tends to be leaner and has smaller amounts of pesticide residues in it. The effects of low-fat beef on blood cholesterol and other lipids are no different from those of fish and chicken.[30] The problem with most commercially produced beef is that it is heavily marbled with fat as a result of being fed too much grain. So it has the same inflammatory chemical imbalance that many humans have.

Eat the right kinds of fats. Our bodies can produce most fatty acids from the carbohydrates that we eat. However, there are two fatty acids known as essential fatty acids that our bodies cannot produce and which we must therefore get in our diets. These two acids are linoleic acid (LA), an omega-6 fatty acid, and a-linolenic acid (LNA), an omega-3 fatty acid. LNA is the starting material for the biosynthesis of eicosapentaenoic acid (EPA) and docosahexaenoic acid (DHA), two important polyunsaturated fatty acids. LNA, EPA, and DHA are the main members of the omega-3 family of fatty acids.

The essential fatty acids are also converted in our bodies into two important classes of eicosanoids—leukotrienes and prostaglandins. These later compounds are hormonelike substances that influence a huge number of metabolic processes. An overabundance of the wrong kinds of eicosanoids leads to—you guessed it—cellular inflammation. Eating enough omega-3 fats (1,000–5,000 mg per day) helps prevent cellular inflammation, which is what causes menstrual cramps, joint pain, breast pain, PMS, and a host of other problems.[31] (Note: virtually every pharmaceutical drug on the market, such as Celebrex and Advil (ibuprofen), works in part by suppressing cellular inflammation from free radical damage and imbalanced eicosanoids such as leukotrienes and prostaglandins.)

Omega-3 fats (found in fish, dark green leafy vegetables, flaxseed, and sea algae) are essential for the optimal functioning of every cell membrane in the body. As a result, getting enough of this nutrient is highly beneficial to your immune system, cardiovascular system, brain, and eyes. A deficiency in omega-3 fats can lead to dry skin, cracked nails, brittle hair, fatigue, depression, memory problems, hormone imbalances, achy joints, arthritis, and a poor immune system. Hundreds of studies have shown the health benefits of increasing your intake of omega-3 fats (from fish, flax, egg yolks, and macadamia nuts, as well as fish oil, flaxseed oil, hemp seed oil, and macadamia nut oil) while also decreasing refined carbohydrates, saturated fats, trans fats, and omega-6 fats (found in most seed oils such as corn, canola, peanut, and safflower oils).

A body of evidence suggests that our current epidemic of heart disease began in the last seventy years, when partially hydrogenated fats (trans-fatty acids), the foods containing them, and refined foods devoid of antioxidant vitamins were introduced into the mainstream diet. Trans fats are not found in nature, so our bodies haven't evolved to deal with them. Produced instead by a chemical process in which hydrogen is added to naturally occurring polyunsaturated fat at extremely high temperatures, these fats are solid at room temperature and have an extremely long shelf life (making them useful for margarine, as well as just about every processed food product you can think of, including cookies, crackers, baked goods, and even baby formula). Processed foods containing trans fats often replace foods in which naturally occurring essential fatty acids are found, such as almost all unprocessed nuts, grains, and many vegetables.

BENEFITS OF "GOOD" FATS

~ Omega-3 fatty acids (in the form of fish oil supplements) lower cholesterol better than the statin drugs.[32] Several prospective cohort studies have found an inverse association between fish consumption and risk of cardiovascular disease.[33] Essential fatty acids also decrease hardening of the arteries by reducing the "stickiness" of blood cells, so they cling less to artery walls.[34]

~ Other studies have shown that the essential fatty acids can moderate the cancer-causing effects of radiation and certain chemicals because of their ability to balance inflammatory chemicals.[35] The right dietary oils may also help inhibit the development of breast and other forms of cancer by regulating immune system function in the body.[36]

~ Omega-3 fats (particularly DHA) support brain function. Studies have shown that sufficient amounts of DHA for infants and babies in utero have been linked to higher IQs, while deficiencies have been associated with learning disabilities such as attention deficit/hyperactivity disorders (ADD, ADHD) and dyslexia.

~ DHA can stabilize your moods. Deficiencies are a contributing factor to depression, postpartum depression, preeclampsia, and various postmenopausal conditions.

~ Fish oil supplements have been shown to be effective in supporting healthy joints.[37]

~ Essential fatty acids can lessen the symptoms of autoimmune diseases. Multiple sclerosis patients in one study who remained on a diet high in naturally occurring essential fatty acids and low in saturated fats had only minimal disability for as long as thirty years. But for patients who discontinued this therapeutic diet, their disease was reactivated and their symptoms increased dramatically.[38]

RISKS OF "BAD" FATS

~ Partially hydrogenated fats are associated with higher cancer rates than are saturated fats.[39]

⁓ These artificial fats inhibit normal fatty acid metabolism in our bodies, decrease HDL (the good cholesterol), and increase LDL (the bad stuff), increasing the chance for heart disease.

⁓ Excess trans-fatty acids (as well as sugar, cortisol, alcohol, and inadequate levels of magnesium, zinc, vitamin B_3, vitamin B_6, and vitamin C) inhibit the conversion of essential fatty acids to cellular hormones that are needed for the optimal health of the female body. This can result in water weight gain (edema), increased blood clot formation, arthritis, and increased uterine cramps and pelvic pain.[40]

⁓ Diets that are high in saturated fat, trans fats, and omega-6 fats have been found to significantly alter insulin efficiency and glucose response and to contribute to insulin resistance. These types of fats have also been found to increase the accumulation of storage triglyceride in skeletal muscles (leading to marbling). Marbling of skeletal muscles leads directly to insulin resistance in these muscles and it also reroutes triglycerides directly to abdominal fat storage sites. In order to burn glucose effectively, the cellular membrane must be flexible. Cell membranes are comprised of the kind of fat we eat. The more "unsaturated" a cell membrane, the better glucose is utilized and the better our overall health. (Remember, the cell membrane is the "brain" of the cell—and it must be flexible and be comprised of the right fats in order to function optimally. The more saturated and "stiff" the membrane, and the more trans fats are incorporated into it, the more deleterious the effect on insulin efficiency and other cell functions as well.)

In conclusion, fat is not the enemy it has been made out to be in the last forty years or so. When sugar and insulin levels are kept normal and the diet is adequate in the right balance of omega-3 and omega-6 fats and micronutrients, then there's no need to worry about the impact of your fat intake on overall health. (By the way, olive oil is an omega-9 fat, which has a neutral effect.) You can safely use some butter and some saturated fat in your diet, too. But everyone needs to severely limit her intake of "sweet fats" such as doughnuts, pastries, macaroni and cheese, etc.

Calories Count but Don't Count Them!

Though calories do count in a broad general way (it's possible to overeat nearly anything and your body will figure out a way to store the excess as fat!), using the calorie counts of foods to determine what to eat is obsolete. Using only the calorie count of a food as a basis for whether or not to eat it completely ignores how food is metabolized in the body for optimal health. Though you may be able to lose weight on 1,200 calories a day from bread and pasta, your body won't be able to build the lean muscle mass you need to burn fat efficiently, and your body—in response to the insulin levels generated to metabolize the starch—will tend to go into conservation mode.

Step Eleven: Take Nutritional Supplements

The Role of Micronutrients

For over two decades, I've recommended nutritional supplements to my patients, friends, and family, and I have taken them regularly myself. During this time, I've seen tremendous results. For example, women on a good supplementation program almost never have colds. They also report fewer aches and pains or other symptoms from hormonal imbalances and recover more quickly from surgery and other stressful events.

Vitamins and minerals can help do all of the following:

- Enhance your immune system[41]
- Reduce oxidative stress and damage from free radicals
- Support healthy brain function
- Protect your cardiovascular system
- Lessen joint pain and enhance the health of your bones and joints
- Promote radiant skin and prevent wrinkling
- Increase your metabolism and help stabilize blood sugar
- Support your vision

Nutritional supplements bridge the gap between adequate and optimal nutrition. And this is what really makes a difference. Today, we're living longer, and we all want to be active and healthy into our seventies, eighties, and even nineties. Receiving the right amount of nutrients from food sources and nutritional supplements can help everyone achieve this goal. The Recommended Dietary Allowances (RDA) were first established in 1941 by the Food and Nutrition Board (FNB) and have been updated only a few times in the last sixty years. At the time, the board looked at large populations to determine how to prevent diseases due to gross vitamin deficiencies. Based on their studies, the FNB set the RDA for vitamin C at 60 mg—the amount needed every day to prevent scurvy—and determined the RDA for vitamin D to be 400 IUs (international units)—the amount required to prevent rickets. While it seems obvious that those levels are antiquated by today's standards, many still hold on to the belief that you can get all the nutrition you need from a healthy diet. Although you were meant to get the nutrients your body needs from what you eat, it's nearly impossible to do so to-day—even if you eat a diet of whole foods with lots of organic fruits and vegetables. That's because over the last fifty years, the soil has been depleted of nutrients—especially minerals—due to overfarming, chem-ical fertilization, and other practices. As a result, the nutritional value of many foods has declined. In addition, our fruits and vegetables are rarely eaten straight from the garden. Instead, they're picked, shipped, and stored—losing nutrients along the way. (One of the reasons that the food tastes so good in Italy and France is that it's picked at the height of freshness and eaten very soon thereafter!)

Nowadays, we're also exposed to many more environmental haz-ards, including pollution, pesticides, and chemicals in cleaning prod-ucts. Your body must detoxify these assaults—and it requires the right nutrients to get the job done properly. Toxins that remain in the body can cause a variety of health problems and lead to DNA damage. When the DNA in your cells is altered, your risk of chronic degenerative dis-eases (such as heart disease, certain cancers, arthritis, macular degener-ation, osteoporosis, and Alzheimer's) increases significantly. Recent studies have shown that taking the right multinutrients can protect you from this type of cellular damage.[42] Although the RDA classifications are still used as the basis for nutritional supplements (not to mention being upheld by many mainstream medical organizations), the empha-sis at the FNB has changed over the last few years. They're now look-ing at nutrition as a way to reduce the risk of chronic disease, as opposed to just preventing vitamin and mineral deficiencies. Focusing on optimal versus adequate nutrition is a giant step in the right direc-tion, since there can be a huge difference between the two.

Four Basic Categories

A good supplement provides nutritional support in four basic cate-gories: antioxidants, omega-3 fats, B vitamins, and minerals. (See the table on page 745 for a list of important nutrients from each category.) Providing specific information for every vitamin or mineral on this list would take an entire library, but I will cover the basics.

Antioxidants. Sometimes referred to as "antiagers," antioxidants help protect the body at the cellular level by ridding it of free radicals. Free radicals are unstable molecules that are released when you eat poorly, are under considerable amounts of stress, and are exposed to environmental pollutants, as well as through normal body functions. Smoking of all kinds (including marijuana), drinking alcohol, taking drugs, drinking caffeine, and eating high-glycemic foods are all stressful for the body and produce free radical damage. If left unchecked, free radicals can damage cell membranes and change the way DNA is expressed, thus accelerating aging and putting your health at risk. The most common antioxidants are vitamins A, C, and E, although there are many others, including glutathione, coenzyme Q10, and alpha lipoic acid. One of my all-time favorites is OPC. Often called pycnogenol, it's made from grape seeds or pine bark. Many people have taken it successfully to reduce arthritis symptoms because of its anti-inflammatory properties. And since OPC enhances the suppleness of collagen throughout the body, it's also good for hair, skin, and nails. Antioxidants work together synergistically—thus OPC also boosts the body's vitamin E levels, which can thwart free radical damage, such as oxidation of LDL (good) cholesterol. (See below for a note on vitamin E.) This in turn helps protect the cardiovascular system and boost the immune system. For those who have inflammation problems, start off with approximately 1 mg of OPC per pound of body weight in divided doses throughout the day. For example: A 140-pound woman would start with about 140 mg of OPC (40–50 mg, three times per day with meals) for two weeks to load the tissues. (Tablet size varies, so shoot for a daily loading dose that's within 20–30 mg of your total weight in pounds.) After that, you can reduce the dose to 30–90 mg per day. Take more or less depending upon the amount your body requires. (Many brands of OPCs are available at natural food stores. I use Proflavanol brand from USANA Health Sciences.)

Vitamin E Is Safe and Important!

A recent study presented at the American Heart Association meeting in New Orleans by Edgar Miller III, M.D., Ph.D., and co-workers received a totally overblown amount of publicity and scared people into thinking that vitamin E isn't safe. Just the opposite is true. Dr. Miller's study, which was a meta-analysis of previous studies—many of which were small and dissimilar—suggested that high-dose vitamin E supplementation may increase mortality in adults.[43] Many studies that could have been included in the analysis were eliminated because total mortality rates were low. And many of the studies that were included were conducted with older adults who already had advanced chronic degenerative disease. In other words, most studies that Dr. Miller included were not conducted on normal, healthy adults. And he left out many of the studies showing the most benefit for vitamin E! Many of the studies were small, involving fewer than a thousand people. More important, only the smaller studies showed significant adverse effects. None of the larger (and therefore more powerful) studies, involving several thousand subjects each, showed a statistically significant impact on mortality of vitamin E supplementation. Moreover, the researchers' secondary analysis showed that differences in death rates were statistically insignificant, and that at the highest dose, risk of death was actually lower!

Here's the bottom line. Years of clinical research have shown that vitamin E supplementation is effective and safe.[44] For example, the famous Nurses' Health Study, which involved thousands of women over many years, showed that vitamin E from supplementation (but not from food) reduced the risk of heart attack by 30 percent.[45] In the Iowa women's study, it was associated with a significant reduction in bowel cancer.[46] Vitamin E has also been shown to reduce the risk of dementia.[47] And a recent study from Tufts showed that this powerful antioxidant slows the development of cataracts.[48] Vitamin E should be part of a comprehensive supplementation program.

Omega-3 Fats (see above under fats)
B-Complex Vitamins. The right levels of B vitamins can bolster your energy level and stamina. Women who take birth control pills or hormone replacement, who are under a lot of stress, or who experience hormonal changes are likely to require additional B vitamins. The liver needs this nutrient to metabolize hormones. When estrogen isn't metabolized properly, too much of it stays in the bloodstream, especially in relation to progesterone levels, resulting in estrogen dominance. Estrogen dominance leads to an imbalance of the neurotransmitters—norepinephrine, serotonin, and dopamine—which makes you prone to anxiety, nervous tension, and PMS symptoms. In addition, B vitamins support the adrenal glands, which are often strained during stressful periods.[49]

Over the past ten years, we've learned a lot about the benefits of folic acid, one of the B vitamins. It can support cardiovascular health by lowering homocysteine levels,[50] and it's also one of the B's that helps metabolize hormones in the liver. (Many individuals are genetically predisposed to having high homocysteine levels, an independent risk factor for heart disease. Taking enough folic acid (800–1,000 mcg a day) effectively metabolizes homocysteine and eliminates risk.)[51] Perhaps more important, 800 mcg a day can help prevent birth defects, such as cleft lip and spina bifida, when taken before conception. Because they work synergistically, it's important to take folic acid with the other B vitamins. Along this same line, a recent study has shown that taking multivitamins prior to conception significantly reduced the risk of prematurity. It also enhances fertility![52]

Minerals. A variety of minerals, but especially calcium and magnesium, are typically associated with bone health, but they're responsible for so much more. Magnesium, for example, can mitigate neuromuscular pain, lessen the severity and frequency of migraines, and keep your heart healthy. (See The Wonders of Magnesium, below.) Further, copper and selenium support the immune system; chromium and vanadium can help stabilize blood sugar; and manganese can boost the antioxidant process. Of course, calcium is needed for strong bones, but it doesn't act effectively on its own. It needs to be taken along with all the bone-building minerals, including magnesium, boron, zinc, manganese, and copper. Enough vitamin D must also be present. Most menstruating women need iron. Craving ice is a sign of deficiency. I know—I used to have this symptom! The usual amount of iron to take is 30 mg per day, and this is especially important during pregnancy. The mineral chromium has been found to increase the metabolic rate. Chromium is in short supply in nine out of ten American diets, and it is absolutely essential for normal insulin function.[53] Ingestion of 200 mcg of chromium daily has been shown to support optimal blood sugar.[54] Sometimes it is necessary to increase chromium up to 1,000 mcg per day in problem cases. Look for it in the form of chromium polynicotinate.

Dairy foods and the calcium question. My siblings and I didn't drink milk growing up and my children didn't drink it, either. When my sister once told a pediatrician friend that my children didn't drink milk, her response was, "They'll die." This is not a scientific evaluation. It is pure emotion, and a typical response.

My children were breast-fed until almost age two. Human milk, a living, dynamic food, is designed for the optimal growth and development of baby humans. Cow's milk, very different in composition from human milk, is designed for the optimal growth and development of baby cattle. Children are bigger today than they used to be. Cow's milk produces rapid growth in children, just as it does in cattle. This is one of the reasons why the American children of relatively small immigrants are so much bigger than their parents. In this country we associate bigger with better.[55]

But conventionally produced milk can be a problem food for many children and adults. Frank Oski, M.D., former chief of pediatrics at Johns Hopkins Medical School, published a great little book entitled *Don't Drink Your Milk* (Mollica Press, 1983), which documented the link between dairy foods and allergy, eczema, bed-wetting, and ear infections in children.[56] Countless children are needlessly treated with antibiotics for repeated ear infections that would go away if they were taken off dairy foods. Dr. Oski's honesty about the adverse health effects of dairy foods is a much-appreciated contribution. Since you will find so little cultural support for removing conventionally produced milk from the diet of your children, it is helpful to have good information.

Over the years, I have seen many problems associated with dairy foods: benign breast conditions, chronic vaginal discharge, acne, menstrual cramps, fibroids, chronic intestinal upset, and increased pain from endometriosis. Consumption of dairy foods has been implicated in both breast and ovarian cancers.[57] I can't help but think that there might be some correlation between overstimulation of the cow's mammary glands, through the use of certain hormones intended to increase milk production, and subsequent overstimulation of our own. Nursing babies as well as their mothers are affected by what the mothers eat. They sometimes develop symptoms of cow's milk allergy when their mothers are consuming a lot of cow's milk.

Like most Americans, I was taught that milk was necessary for getting enough calcium, even though three-quarters of the world's population manages to maintain health without drinking milk after infancy. (Many do, however, consume other kinds of dairy foods, usually fermented forms, such as cheese and yogurt, often made from sheep's or goat's milk.) Stopping dairy foods or substituting organically produced dairy foods often improves menstrual cramps, endometriosis pain, allergies, sinusitis, and even recurrent vaginitis. Because an entire generation of baby boomers has been raised on cow's milk instead of human milk, the cow at some deep level is now associated with "mother" and "nourishment." The very notion of eliminating dairy products causes heart palpitations in some people; they cannot conceive of living without milk.

On the other hand, dairy foods produced organically, without bovine growth hormone and antibiotics, have a very different effect on the body. Some of my patients with GYN problems related to dairy have had complete remission of these problems when they have switched to organically produced milk products, which are now widely available. One of my newsletter subscribers in Indiana even went so far as

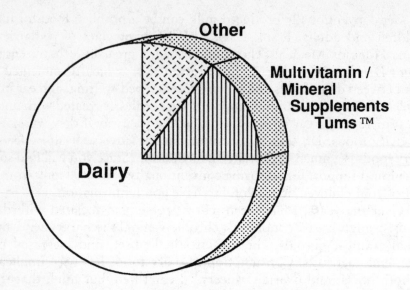

FIGURE 18: CONVENTIONAL AMERICAN APPROACH
TO CALCIUM INTAKE

to buy a milk cow for her family's milk supply. They have no health problems at all. On the other hand, some people continue to have an allergic-type reaction even to organic cow's milk.

People often wonder, "If I don't drink milk, where will I get my calcium?" Though milk is generally a good source of calcium, there are nondairy sources as well—for example, dark green leafy vegetables such as kale, collard greens, and broccoli. Most of the world's population, including inhabitants of China, which has almost no breast cancer and no osteoporosis in rural areas, gets its calcium from greens. Studies also show that while the Chinese consume only half the calcium of Americans, osteoporosis is uncommon in China despite an average life expectancy of seventy years—only five years less than ours.[58]

African Bantu women eat no dairy foods, but they consume 150 to 400 mg of calcium daily through the foods they do eat. This is half the amount of calcium consumed by the average American woman. Yet osteoporosis is essentially unknown among the 10 percent of female Bantus who reach more than sixty years of age. Genetic protection was considered the reason but has been ruled out. When relatives of these same Bantu people migrate to more affluent societies and adopt rich diets, osteoporosis and diseases of the teeth become more common.[59]

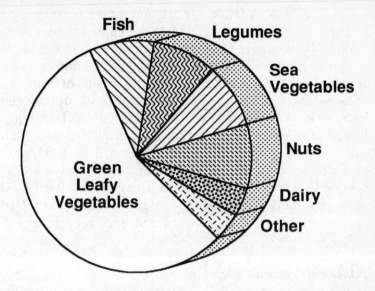

FIGURE 19: BALANCED APPROACH TO CALCIUM INTAKE

GREEN LEAFY VEGETABLES	NUTS	FISH	SEA VEGETABLES
Collard greens; wild greens (lamb's-quarters, wild onions); broccoli; kale; beet greens; bok choy; mustard greens; watercress; rhubarb stems; parsley; dandelion greens	Almonds; sunflower seeds; Brazil nuts; hazelnuts; sesame seeds	Sardines; salmon; oysters	Hijiki; wakame; kombu (kelp); agar-agar (Kanteen flakes); dulse

LEGUMES	DAIRY	OTHER
Tofu, firm; tempeh; garbanzo beans (chickpeas); black beans; pinto beans; corn tortillas	Milk (skim, whole); cheese; ice milk; nonfat yogurt; cottage cheese	Mineral waters (Perrier, Mendocino, San Pellegrino, Apollinaris, Contexeville); molasses; orange juice (calcium fortified); calcium rich herb infusions

The current recommended daily allowance (RDA) for calcium in the United States is 1,200 mg a day for women age twenty-five and older. Fully 50 percent of American women do not consume this RDA and are thus at increased risk for osteoporosis. The current World Health

Organization recommendation for calcium intake is 400 mg per day—one-third the amount recommended in the United States. For most of the world this is adequate. The average Chinese, who has a very low risk of osteoporosis, consumes 544 mg of calcium each day.[60]

The calcium supplement and dairy industries have been so effective at offering us an osteoporosis "fix" that we think we can reduce the complexity of bone physiology to a formula as simple as taking calcium pills. But bone is affected by a whole host of factors (see chapter 14), and bone health is profoundly affected by our daily food and exercise choices. Caffeine, alcohol, sugar, and tobacco also have a negative effect on bone health and contribute to osteoporosis. With lifestyle improvement on all levels, our bones would stay healthy on relatively less calcium, as long as we also exercised, cut back on refined foods, and got enough vitamin D.

Update on Vitamin D

The most recent research reveals that calcium is virtually useless without enough vitamin D, which plays a crucial role in maintaining bone health. Studies now show that women with osteoporosis typically have less vitamin D in their systems than women with healthy bones. In fact, the former RDA of this vitamin (400 IU per day) is not even half the amount that is actually necessary to maintain optimal bone health! I recommend taking at least 1,000 IU of vitamin D per day.[61] Note that a fifteen- to thirty-minute sunbath without sunscreen will provide 300 to 350 units of vitamin D, but most people don't get outside enough and leave too little skin exposed to the sun when they do. For the average Caucasian living in the United States, exposing the hands, face, and arms for fifteen to twenty minutes to midmorning or late-afternoon sun three days a week provides sufficient vitamin D during the months of March through October. After that an eight- to ten-minute sunbath in a tanning booth once a week will provide you with adequate vitamin D. Women with darker skin have a lower risk for osteoporosis, and all women near the equator will have an easier time meeting their vitamin D needs from sunlight. I also recommend that you get your vitamin D level checked as a baseline. According to leading vitamin D expert Michael Holick, M.D., Ph.D., Chief of Endocrinology, Metabolism and Nutrition at Boston University School of Medicine, blood levels of vitamin D should be at least 20 ng/mL, and preferably 30–50 ng/mL.[62] Those are adequate levels; the ideal level is 100 ng/ml.

The famous Women's Health Initiative Study on calcium and vitamin D supplementation showed that women who took both calcium and vitamin D experienced a 29 percent reduction in the risk of hip fracture over a period of seven years as compared to the placebo group, but no decrease in vertebral fractures. Study participants took 1,000 mg of calcium per day and only 400 IU of vitamin D, which most experts believe is not a high enough dose. The risk of kidney stones was also increased in those who took the calcium, a risk that would probably have been greatly reduced by including adequate magnesium to balance the calcium. The other limitation to the study was the fact that most women didn't start taking the supplement until they were over sixty years old—after many had probably already lost considerable bone mass.[63]

Bones are made of much more than calcium.[64] Magnesium is in much shorter supply than calcium in our diets because of poor dietary choices (refined grains and too few dark green leafy vegetables), soil depletion from erosion, and overuse of chemical fertilizers instead of organic farming methods. (See The Wonders of Magnesium, below.)

Television advertising promotes the use of antacids (e.g., Tums) because of their calcium content. But antacids like Tums (calcium carbonate) decrease the acidity of the stomach, which can lead to decreased absorption of calcium, since hydrochloric acid in the stomach is necessary for assimilation of calcium.[65] Given that studies have shown that about 40 percent of postmenopausal women are already deficient in stomach acid, using an antacid such as Tums to supplement calcium doesn't make sense. In addition, it has been shown that people with insufficient stomach acid can absorb only about 4 percent of an oral dose of calcium as calcium carbonate, while a person with normal stomach acid can absorb about 22 percent. Those with low stomach acid secretion need a soluble, ionized form of calcium such as calcium citrate, succinate, malate, aspartate, or fumarate.[66] Also, the strong alkaline nature of carbonate combined with the calcium that is absorbed can set the stage for kidney stones, especially if milk products are a regular part of the diet. Calcium citrate can act as a good antacid if you need one, even though it isn't marketed as such.

Colas and root beer also contribute to osteoporosis, because the coloring agent and the phosphorus used in these drinks interfere with calcium metabolism.[67] Depression is also a significant contributor to osteoporosis because high levels of epinephrine and cortisol, produced by the adrenal glands in greater quantities in depressed individuals, can increase calcium loss in the urine and also cause breakdown of bone.[68]

The best approach to building bone health is a holistic one in which we look at all the dietary, environmental, and genetic factors related to osteoporosis development and improve those areas in which we have some control. (See chapter 14.) Note the following points about calcium sources:

~ The nutritional content of food is dependent upon where the food was grown, when it was harvested, the quality of the soil, and so on.

~ There can be wide variation in the mineral content of foods, depending upon soil mineralization.

~ Organically grown vegetables have higher nutritional content.

~ The figures presented in table 14 represent average amounts of calcium found in the foods that were analyzed at the time of data collection.

~ Calcium is only one of the minerals needed for optimal nutrition.

~ Nondairy sources of calcium are particularly rich in the other minerals needed for health. Some argue that plant oxalates, found in spinach and some other greens, interfere with calcium absorption. The same argument has been used for phytates in grain. Newer data suggest that this absorption issue has been highly overemphasized and is not very significant.

TABLE 13
HIGH-CALCIUM FOODS[69]

Food	Amount	Calcium (mg)
Green Leafy Vegetables		
(cooked, unless specified)		
collard greens	1 cup	300
wild greens	1 cup	350
(lamb's-quarters,		
wild onions)		
broccoli	1 cup	150
kale	1 cup	179
spinach	1 cup	278
turnip greens	1 cup	229
beet greens	1 cup	165
bok choy	1 cup	200
mustard greens	1 cup`	150
rhubarb	1 cup	348
watercress (raw)	1 cup	53
parsley (raw)	1 cup	122
dandelion greens	1 cup	147

Food	Amount	Calcium (mg)
Sea Vegetables (cooked, unless specified)		
hijiki	1 cup	610
wakame	1 cup	520
kombu (kelp)	1 cup	305
agar-agar	1 cup (dry flakes)	400
(kanteen flakes)	16 tablespoons	
used as a thickener for		
sauces, etc.		
dulse	1 cup (dry)	567
Fish (bones: the major source of calcium in fish)		
sardines (with bones)	3½ ounce can (drained)	300
salmon (canned)	1 cup	431
oysters, raw	1 cup	226
Bean and Legumes		
tofu, firm	4 ounces	80–150
tempeh	4 ounces	172
garbanzo beans	1 cup (cooked)	150
(chickpeas)		
black beans	1 cup (cooked)	135
pinto beans	1 cup (cooked)	128
tortillas, corn	2	120
Nuts and Seeds		
sesame seeds	3 tablespoons	300
(must be ground for		
absorption)		
almonds	1 cup	300
sunflower seeds	1 cup (hulled)	174
Brazil nuts	1 cup	260
hazelnuts	1 cup	282
Other Sources		
blackstrap molasses	1 tablespoon	137
orange juice calcium	1 cup	210
fortified (Minute Maid)		
Mineral Waters		
Perrier	1 liter	140
Mendocino	1 liter	380
San Pellegrino	1 liter	200
Apollinaris	1 liter	91
Contexeville	1 liter	451

Food	Amount	Calcium (mg)
Dairy		
milk		
skim	1 cup	300
whole	1 cup	288
cheese (American, Swiss, cheddar)	1½ ounces	300
ice milk	1 cup	204
nonfat yogurt	1 cup	294
cottage cheese (low fat)	1 cup	150

CALCIUM-RICH HERB INFUSIONS

OLD "SOUR PUSS" MINERAL MIX . . . À LA SUSUN WEED.[70]

(1 tablespoon supplies 15–200 mg calcium)

Choose one or more of the following herbs (these grow all over the United States and are very easy to identify):

Yellow Dock (*Rumex*) leaves/roots;
Dandelion (*Taraxacum*) leaves/roots;
Plantain (*Plantago*) leaves;
Nettle (*Urtica*) leaves;
Raspberry (*Rubus*) leaves/canes/berries;
Mugwort (*Artemisia vulgaris*) leaves;
Comfrey (*Symphytum*) leaves/flower stalks;
Red Clover (*Trifolium pratense*) blossoms;
Clean eggshells/bones

Fill a quart/liter jar with fresh herbs. Pour apple cider vinegar over herbs until jar is full. (Vinegar dissolves calcium and other minerals and holds them in solution.) Cover with a plastic lid and let sit for six weeks. To use: Pour on your salad, put on your beans, add to soup, or dilute 1 tablespoon in 1 cup of water and add 1 tablespoon of blackstrap molasses, which adds 137 mg of calcium.

BONNY BONY BREW

(1 cup contributes 300 mg calcium)

Nettle (*Urtica dioica*): 1 ounce/30 g dry
Horsetail (*Equisetum arvense*): 1 tablespoon/2 g dry
Sage (*Salvia officinalis*): 1 tablespoon/2 g dry

Crush sage between palms and drop into quart/liter container with other two herbs. Fill with boiling water, cap tightly, and let brew for four hours. Strain. Red clover, oatstraw, or raspberry may be substituted for the nettles.

Note: think of herbs as mineral-rich dark green leafy vegetables. These recipes are very easy ways to add minerals and other nutrients to your diet.

THE WONDERS OF MAGNESIUM

Magnesium requires its own section because it is so often overlooked and is so important for women's health. I was first introduced to the wonders of magnesium during my obstetrical training where I saw, up close and personal, how effective magnesium sulfate was in preventing seizures and restoring normal blood pressure in pregnant women suffering from toxemia. Years later, I often gave my patients magnesium intravenously (along with a series of other vitamins) as part of an IV mix known as Meyer's formula. I found that this mixture frequently relieved muscular pain and also helped speed healing from surgery, sprained ankles, and so on. It also appeared to boost immunity, which is why I often had a colleague give me an IV of it myself when I was coming down with something. Worked like a charm!

An astounding number of studies have documented the effectiveness of IV magnesium in helping prevent cardiac damage and even death following a heart attack. The reason for this is that 40 to 60 percent of sudden deaths from heart attack are the result of spasm in the arteries, not blockage from clots or arrhythmias![71] And magnesium helps coronary artery muscles (and all other muscles) relax!

Most of us don't require intravenous magnesium, of course. We can get all the benefits we need just by making sure that we get enough of it in our diets or through supplements. Here's what everyone needs to know about getting optimal benefits from this essential (but often overlooked) mineral!

Why We Need Enough Magnesium

Magnesium is essential for the functioning of hundreds of different enzymes in the body, particularly those that produce, transport, store, and utilize energy. Magnesium is essential for the following:

~ Protein synthesis. DNA and RNA in our cells require magnesium for cell growth and development.

~ Sparking of the electrical signals that must travel throughout the miles of nerves in our bodies (including our brain, heart, and other organs)

~ Normal blood pressure, vascular tone, transmission of nerve cell signals, and blood flow

~ Functioning of all nerves and muscles

~ Release and binding of adequate amounts of serotonin in the brain

In short, living with suboptimal levels of magnesium is like trying to operate a machine with the power turned off.

The Magnesium/Calcium Connection

Though the role of calcium has received an enormous amount of attention, very few people realize that without its partner—magnesium—calcium doesn't serve the body nearly as well as it should. In fact, too much calcium can actually impede magnesium's uptake and function, creating further imbalance. When it comes to building healthy bones, magnesium is as important as calcium and vitamin D!

Magnesium and calcium are designed to work together. For example, magnesium controls the entry of calcium into each and every cell—a physiological event that happens every time a nerve cell fires. Without adequate magnesium (which is also a natural calcium channel blocker) too much calcium gets inside the cell. This can result in muscle cramping, blood vessel constriction, migraine headache, and even feelings of anxiety.[72]

Magnesium also keeps calcium dissolved in the blood so that it won't produce kidney stones. In fact, taking calcium without magnesium for osteoporosis can actually promote kidney stone formation!

Magnesium Deficiency on the Rise!

In 1997, the National Academy of Sciences found that most Americans are deficient in magnesium.[73] There are a number of reasons for this:

~ **Food processing depletes magnesium:** And the vast majority of Americans eat mostly processed foods. When wheat is refined into white flour, 80 percent of the magnesium in the bran is lost; 98 percent is lost when molasses is refined into sugar. Similarly, magnesium is leached out of vegetables boiled in water or frozen. Additives such as aspartame and MSG, as well as alcohol, also deplete magnesium stores.

~ **Indigestion and antacid use:** Insufficient stomach acid impedes magnesium absorption. Unfortunately, a refined-food diet is a potent recipe for indigestion. Antacids, the number-one over-the-counter consumer drug in the U.S., further deplete hydrochloric acid in the stomach.

~ **Farming practices:** Magnesium and other minerals have been depleted from much of the soil that we grow produce in today.

~ **Medications:** Many drugs including common diuretics, birth control pills, insulin, tetracycline and other antibiotics, and cortisone cause the body to waste magnesium.

Selected Foods Rich in Magnesium
(In mg per 100 grams [3 ½ ounce] servings)

~ *Kelp 760*
~ *Wheat bran 490*
~ *Wheat germ 336*
~ *Molasses 258*
~ *Dulse 220*
~ *Almonds 270*
~ *Peanuts 175*
~ *Collard greens 57*
~ *Cooked beans 37*
~ *Tofu 111*
~ *Millet 162*

In general, organically grown whole grains and vegetables are rich in magnesium. So is good quality sea salt and sea vegetables.

The Impact of Magnesium Deficiency

The following is a partial list of health conditions associated with magnesium deficiency. These conditions may be helped by increasing magnesium intake:

~ **Anxiety and panic attacks:** Magnesium helps keep adrenal stress hormones under control and also helps maintain normal brain function. In her book *The Miracle of Magnesium* (Ballantine Books, 2003), Carolyn Dean, M.D., N.D., points out that the rate of depression has gone up every decade since WWII. It's quite possible that this is related to magnesium depletion.

~ **Asthma:** Magnesium helps relax the muscles of the bronchioles in the lungs.

~ **Constipation:** Magnesium helps keep bowels regular by maintaining normal bowel muscle function. Milk of magnesia has been used for decades to help constipation.

~ **Diabetes:** Magnesium helps insulin transport glucose into the cell. Without this, glucose builds up in tissue, causing glycemic stress and damage.

~ **Heart disease:** Magnesium deficiency is common in those with heart disease. It's an effective treatment for heart attacks and cardiac arrhythmias.

~ **Hypertension:** Without adequate magnesium, blood vessels constrict and blood pressure increases.

~ **Insomnia:** Magnesium helps regulate melatonin, a hormone essential for normal sleep and wakefulness cycles.

~ **Nerve problems:** Magnesium helps eliminate peripheral nerve disturbances that can lead to migraines, leg and foot cramps, gastrointestinal cramps, and so on.

~ **Osteoporosis:** Without magnesium, calcium may actually contribute to osteoporosis.

Supplementing with Magnesium

The ratio of calcium to magnesium in the diet for the majority of human history was 1:1, a ratio that's considered optimal. Anywhere from 1:1 to 2:1 is adequate (for example, 800 mg of calcium to 400 mg of magnesium). Unfortunately, today's diets contain an average of ten times more calcium than magnesium.

In addition to eating a nutritious diet, I recommend that you use supplements that contain magnesium. (I do this myself, especially when traveling, dealing with the stress of deadlines, etc.) There's considerable variation among individuals as to the ideal amount of magnesium to take. Here's what I recommend: keep your calcium intake between 800–1,400 mg per day, adding enough magnesium to balance it. For example, if you take 1,000 mg of calcium per day, you need at least 500–800 mg of magnesium.

Magnesium comes in many forms. Magnesium oxide or chloride is fine, as is chelated magnesium. Capsules usually contain 250–500 mg of magnesium. You can also use a calcium/magnesium supplement. Experiment with levels. If you're healthy, start with 200 mg of magnesium twice a day. If you have any of the conditions mentioned above, you may want to start higher: 500 mg twice a day. You'll know when you've reached your limit—you'll develop loose stools. It's best, of course, to take your magnesium in divided doses throughout the day. You can take it either on an empty stomach or with meals. You can also add Epsom salts to your baths—Epsom salt is magnesium sulfate. It's absorbed through the skin and will help replenish magnesium stores. (A great excuse to read a good book in the tub!) And there is also the transdermal magnesium formulated by Norm Shealy, M.D., Ph.D. (See the nutritional section of the Adrenal Restoration Program for a Healthier Menopause in chapter 14.)

If you want to learn more (and I think that everyone should), I recommend that you read Dr. Dean's *The Miracle of Magnesium*. Quite frankly, this book should be in everyone's home library. The information could surely save your—or a loved one's—life!

Getting Started. When starting a supplementation program, a well-rounded approach is best. Some people mistakenly think that vitamins should be taken to treat a medical condition. For example, they read that vitamin E can help reduce the occurrence of breast cysts and their painful symptoms, so they take a bunch of vitamin E. This method equates to conventional medicine's practice of writing a prescription for a pharmaceutical drug to suppress your symptoms. Instead, start with a good foundation and add other supplements according to your individual needs. But take care not to distort the foundation—think of it this way: adding a little extra sugar to a cake may not change it significantly, but adding a whole lot will throw everything else out of proportion. Please understand that optimal supplementation requires at least four to five tablets or capsules per day. In other words, the "one-a-day" mentality is inadequate—you can't get optimal supplementation from one pill a day. (See Resources.)

Once you've found a balanced approach, stick with it for at least three months before switching to another product or adding additional supplements. Sometimes the results are dramatic; more often they're not so remarkable in the first few weeks. But over a period of six weeks to three months (sometimes up to six months), you'll notice that you've had fewer colds and that you just feel better as some of your minor complaints lessen or go away altogether. You may also experience more vitality and a better ability to "go with the flow." Often when you're feeling good, it's hard to remember how far you've come. Here's a tip for measuring your progress. Make a list of your complaints when you start your supplementation program and then review this list every three weeks. This is a great way to chart your advancement.

Tips for Choosing a Supplement

Take the quiz on the benefits of supplementation from the Council for Responsible Nutrition at www.crnusa.org/benefits. I also recommend that you take the well-designed free health assessment on the Usana website (www.usana.com) for specific recommendations based on your current lifestyle. Also consider the following tips:

~ Pick a high-quality supplement from a manufacturer that follows Good Manufacturing Practices (GMP). They use pharmaceutical-grade (as opposed to food-grade) ingredients to ensure quality and efficacy.

~ Good supplements cost money. Like organic produce, more expensive products represent the real price of high-quality nutrients.

~ Folic acid is an expensive ingredient. If your multivitamin contains 800 mcg of this nutrient (instead of 400 mcg), this is often an indication that the manufacturer isn't skimping on other ingredients in their product.

~ A formula with a combination of antioxidants, such as rutin, bioflavonoids, grape-seed extract, and olive extract, is often more effective than a product containing only one or two antioxidants.

~ Make sure that your supplement has both natural vitamin E (d-tocopherol as opposed to dl-tocopherol) and tocotrienols. These are all part of the vitamin E family—and you get the most benefit when they're all present.

~ Always take a vitamin B-complex, as opposed to just one or two of the Bs.

~ Choose chelated minerals only. These are wrapped in an amino acid when manufactured to ensure proper absorption.

~ If you're taking a well-balanced formula, you don't have to worry about megadosing.

Remember that supplements are not a substitute for a diet of whole, organic foods. The quality of the food you eat is still the cornerstone of good health! But more and more, research is clearly showing that a commitment to supplementing, day in and day out for your entire life, can make an amazing difference in your health. And remember the old saying "An ounce of prevention is worth a pound of cure."

Recommended Supplement Dosages

Here is my list of recommended daily supplements for adults. There really isn't that much difference between the nutritional needs of men and women (except for iron) unless a woman is pregnant or nursing. So these recommendations can also be used for the men in your life.

TABLE 14
RECOMMENDED DAILY SUPPLEMENTATION

Vitamins	
Vitamin C	1,000–5,000 mg
Vitamin D_3	800–5,000 IU
Vitamin A (as beta-carotene)	25,000 IU
Vitamin E (as mixed tocopherols)	400–800 IU
Glutathione	2–10 mg
Alpha lipoic acid	10–100 mg
Coenzyme Q10	10–100 mg
(total of 1,000–5,000 mg)	

Omega-3 Fat	
DHA	200–2,500 mg
EPA	500–2,500 mg

B Complex Vitamins	(total of 1,000–5,000 mg)
Thiamine (B_1)	8–100 mg
Riboflavin (B_2)	9–50 mg
Niacin (B_3)	20–100 mg

Pantothenic acid (B$_5$)	15–400 mg
Pyridoxine (B$_6$)	10–100 mg
Cobalamin (B$_{12}$)	20–250 mcg
Folic acid	400–800 mcg
Biotin	40–500 mcg
Inositol	10–500 mg
Choline	10–100 mg

Minerals (should be bound as amino acid chelates for optimal absorption)

Calcium	500–1,200 mg
Magnesium	400–1,000 mg
Potassium	200–500 mg
Zinc	6–50 mg
Manganese	1–15 mg
Boron	2–9 mg
Copper	1–2 mg
Iron	15–30 mg
Chromium	100–400 mcg
Selenium	50–200 mcg
Molybdenum	10–20 mcg
Vanadium	50–100 mcg
Trace minerals from marine sources	

OTHER COMMON CONCERNS

Can Diet Help Irritable Bowel Syndrome and Other Digestive Problems?

Many women have taken numerous courses of antibiotics for acne, urinary tract infections, and upper respiratory infections. Chronic use of antibiotics kills the normal bowel flora that are necessary for a healthy, functioning colon—a place in the body in which essential bacteria play an important role in nutrient absorption and manufacture. In addition, chronic use of aspirin and other nonsteroidal anti-inflammatory medicines—such as ibuprofen (the active ingredient in Advil) and acetaminophen (the active ingredient in Tylenol)—has also been shown to affect both the stomach's and the intestines' physiological function. (One-half to two-thirds of patients who use nonsteroidal anti-inflammatory medicine chronically show evidence of inflammation of the small intestine.)[74] More than 56,000 emergency-room visits per year are due to acetaminophen overdoses; 100 die annually from overdosing on this drug, which is also the leading cause of liver failure in the country.[75]

Because of our national penchant to overuse antibiotics and aspirin (and other nonsteroidal anti-inflammatory medicines), to eat a refined-food diet, and to have a high-stress lifestyle, many women have digestive difficulties, such as chronic constipation, excess gas, frequent diarrhea, and lower abdominal distress. All of these conditions may result from an imbalance in normal intestinal bacteria, intestinal parasites of various kinds, overgrowth of intestinal yeast, and an increase of intestinal permeability (leaky gut syndrome). These conditions are collectively known as intestinal dysbiosis. Intestinal dysbiosis is often related to and may result in chronic vaginitis, migraines, arthritis, autoimmune diseases, and food allergy.

This problem is diagnosed either clinically, from symptoms such as chronic gas or diarrhea, or by sending stool cultures to a lab that specializes in this testing. Intestinal parasites are often diagnosed as well. As with nearly every other disease, chronic cellular inflammation is caused in part by a diet too high in refined carbohydrates and too low in nutrients, fiber, and omega-3 fats. So the first step—and often the only one necessary—is to follow the dietary guidelines outlined in this chapter. Additional supplements such as acidophilus and bifido bacteria, digestive enzymes, and hydrochloric acid also often help restore normal bowel flora and get the yeast under control. A yeast-free diet is also prescribed for some, but it has been my repeated experience that this type of rigorous dietary restriction is not necessary once your metabolism, emotions, and food choices become optimal. Once they do, the yeast—and often parasites as well, if present—will go away by themselves.

Another very common related problem, irritable bowel syndrome, often responds well to both dietary change and enteric-coated peppermint. It is available in natural food stores. I have prescribed the Mentharil brand with good success.[76]

What About Food Allergies?

Many women are sensitive to certain foods, which can result in symptoms ranging from intestinal distress to weight gain. Common culprits are dairy foods, wheat and other gluten-containing products, corn, and food additives. Intestinal dysbiosis is often accompanied by food allergies.[77] There are a number of ways to diagnose these, the most common being a blood test known as an I_gG Elisa assay. This test should be ordered by a physician familiar with this type of testing and should be performed by a lab that specializes in it.[78] A special diet is then prescribed based on the results. Rather than go through all that, however, I recommend that you just eliminate all grain and dairy products for a week and eat mostly lean proteins, fruits, and vegetables. You'll be amazed by how much better you feel. Another convenient alternative is the USANA Reset program. (See page 699.)

Women with multiple food allergies that are resistant to simple dietary change often have a history of abuse of some type, or they are continuing to live in dysfunctional relationships or to stay in overly stressful jobs. When this is the case, dietary change alone won't address the problem over the long term. There is a dramatic synergy between lifestyle choices, stress, and the parts of the immune system that maintain bowel and vaginal health.[79] Supporting your body nutritionally while you learn to support yourself emotionally and psychologically can help enormously. Studies have shown that this normalizes immune system response. I refer to it as "replenishing the soil."

The Nambudripad Allergy Elimination Technique, known as NAET, is a very effective method of clearing allergies of all types, including those to foods. NAET was developed by Dr. Devi Nambudripad, an acupuncturist and chiropractor who discovered through personal and clinical experience that allergies are often associated with certain physical, emotional, and nutritional patterns, all of which require reprogramming in order for them to be eliminated. Her technique uses acupuncture or acupressure "clearing" of the pattern as well as temporary elimination of the allergen until the pattern is cleared. I have referred many patients to practitioners trained in NAET, and I highly recommend this revolutionary approach. (For more information, visit www.naet.com.)

Do I Have to Give Up Caffeine?

Caffeine is a very popular drug worldwide, perhaps the most popular. The average American drinks some thirty-two gallons of caffeinated soft drinks and twenty-eight gallons of coffee a year, and more than a thousand proprietary drugs list caffeine as an ingredient. Ninety-five percent of pregnant women consume caffeine during their pregnancies.[80] I personally love coffee but now drink decaf, having grown increasingly sensitive to the effects of caffeine over the years.

Caffeine stimulates the central nervous system and affects the heart, skeletal muscles, kidneys, and adrenals. Because of the boost of adrenaline that comes from caffeine, it is associated with increased mental acuity initially. However, it may also result in rebound confusion once the effect has subsided. Caffeine also results in an increase in blood sugar followed by a rather sudden drop. When it's combined with a sweet pastry or other "white" food such as a bagel, the blood sugar drop is even worse—and is a setup for out-of-control cravings later in the day. In some women caffeine is a factor in breast pain and cysts. An occasional woman is so sensitive to it that one piece of chocolate (which contains both caffeine and theobromine, a related substance) will cause breast tenderness premenstrually during the month in which she eats that chocolate. Caffeine has also been implicated in cellular inflammation.

However, studies done since 2000 have shown that coffee, like wine, is not harmful in moderation. Once again, you need to consult your own body wisdom.

Sleep disorders often disappear when people stop using caffeine—and so does urinary frequency. Some studies have shown that the effects of caffeine on females may vary according to the level of estrogen in their system.[81] Even decaffeinated coffee can be a breast and bladder irritant for some.

Here's a test to see if you're addicted to caffeine: go without it for three days. If you get a headache, you are addicted. If you don't, it probably doesn't affect you much. Withdrawal from caffeine takes only two or three days. The headache and the fatigue that accompany this withdrawal, however, can be quite debilitating. I recommend that women plan to withdraw over a weekend, or whenever they have time to rest and nurture themselves in other ways. During caffeine withdrawal, drink plenty of water and drink three to four cups of chamomile tea per day. This tea is considered a "nervine" (nerve tonic) and helps maintain alertness. Many of my patients noted that their tolerance to caffeine decreased over the years. Those who have stopped caffeine and try it again often notice that the drug affects them quite dramatically.

Eliminating caffeine may be a step in the right direction for you. Certainly you will want to do this if you are planning a pregnancy.

Can I Have Diet Soft Drinks or Other Foods with Aspartame?

Aspartame is a combination of two naturally occurring amino acids (aspartic acid and glutamic acid) that can be toxic when combined.

These amino acids trigger nerve cells to fire, and although some nerve cell firing is needed for alertness, too much overstimulates them and causes them to release free radicals. This causes brain cell death. Aspartame consumption has been linked to headache, blurry vision, slurred speech, and memory loss. Some people are particularly susceptible to the toxic effects of aspartame. They include people who have the following conditions (or family histories of these conditions): neuropsychiatric challenges including depression, anxiety attacks, obsessive-compulsive symptoms, manic-depression, or schizophrenia; a history of head injury; blurred vision; memory loss; chronic fatigue syndrome or fibromyalgia; tinnitus (ringing in the ears); spasms, shooting pains, or numbness; attention deficit disorder or hyperactivity disorder; spinal-cord injury; multiple sclerosis; Lou Gehrig's disease; migraine headaches; spinal disc problems; Parkinson's disease; or Alzheimer's disease. As with everything, I believe that a small amount of aspartame is okay for most people. Many are reporting adverse effects from Splenda (sucralose) as well. Again, I feel that it's safe in moderation. Stevia, which is an all-natural sweetener from the stevia plant, is without a doubt the safest sweetener.

Can I Drink Alcohol?

Excessive alcohol consumption is associated with increased risk of breast cancer, menstrual irregularities, osteoporosis, and birth defects. I ask women who drink alcohol regularly to become conscious of why and how they are using alcohol. If they feel the need to have two drinks every single night "to relax" (whether at home or out), I seriously question that behavior. Meditation, listening to music, making love, or taking a long bath are good alternatives.

I point out that two drinks of alcohol per night effectively wipe out rapid eye movement (REM) sleep, the type of sleep associated with dreaming. Dreaming is part of your inner guidance system. Why wipe it out with alcohol? Having two drinks per night also increases the risk of breast cancer. In the Nurses' Health Study, for example, researchers found that the risk of breast cancer was 60 percent higher in those who had one or more drinks per day compared to those who didn't drink.[82]

The amount of alcohol a woman takes in has very little to do with whether she has a problem with alcohol. What determines an alcoholic is her relationship to alcohol. One of my patients realized that she felt much more comfortable when she had her bottle of sherry by her bedside. She rarely drank it, but she realized that if it wasn't there, she'd feel agitated. For that reason, she checked out a few Alcoholics Anonymous meetings and found that she did indeed have a tendency toward alcoholism. (Note: alcohol abuse is common and begins early. The latest data from the University of Michigan's "Monitoring the Future" study shows that 32 percent of twelfth graders get drunk once a month. This gets worse in college.)

Many women hold the "cocktail hour" as a sacred ritual. When I suggest that they drink spring water or sparkling cider as an alternative, in order to see what effect the alcohol is having on them, the reaction I get gives me a few clues about their relationship to alcohol. One woman said, "But my husband and I look forward to this hour. We have such fun we often forget to eat dinner." (!) Another said that she couldn't substitute a nonalcoholic drink for herself because if she did, "everyone else would start to look stupid." (Hmmmmm.)

Please be good to yourself. Examine your relationship to alcohol and make adjustments if necessary. If you feel you can't go without your evening wine or cocktail, you have a problem.

Note also that when you take in enough B vitamins, decrease sugar, and increase protein, you may find that your craving for alcohol decreases.

CAGE SCREEN FOR DIAGNOSIS OF ALCOHOLISM

Doctors typically use the following screening tool to diagnose alcoholism (two or three positive responses indicates a high suspicion, while four positive responses is considered diagnostic).[83] Have you ever:

C Thought you should CUT back on your drinking?

A Felt ANNOYED by people criticizing your drinking?

G Felt GUILTY or bad about your drinking?

E Had a morning EYE-OPENER to relieve hangover or nerves?

Drink More Water

Research by the late Fereydoon Batmanghelidj, M.D., author of *Your Body's Many Cries for Water* (Global Health Solutions, 1995), indicates that most pain and sickness that we experience is actually the result of chronic dehydration. For many of us, he believed, the caffeine and sugar in many of the beverages we drink (including coffee, tea, soda, and juice) actually deplete the body's water supply because they draw water from the body's reserves as well as cause us to lose our natural thirst for water. (For more information, visit Dr. Batmanghelidj's website at www.watercure.com.) The chronic dehydration that results commonly leads to fatigue (particularly in midafternoon), as well as conditions including dyspepsia (heartburn), arthritic pain, back pain, headache (including migraine), colitis pain and associated constipation, pain from angina (from the heart), and leg pain (when walking). One of my long-time colleagues, an internationally known expert in food and healing, told me that her chronically splitting fingernail problem healed with one month of starting to drink more water! I recommend drinking spring or filtered water because in many places, tap water is not pure enough. Drink half your body weight in ounces per day. If you weigh 140 pounds, for example, you need to drink 70 ounces of water each day.

A WORD ABOUT SMOKING

I know I should stop smoking...
I don't lecture smokers because they generally want to quit anyway. Sometimes a few facts help them to make the decision:

~ Tobacco companies have targeted adolescent girls as their number-one market for cigarettes because this group has been found to have the lowest self-esteem and is therefore the most likely to start smoking as a result of peer pressure. In fact, the monthly rate of cigarette smoking for eighth-grade girls rose by more than 40 percent between 1991 and 1996, thanks in part to the effectiveness of the tobacco companies' advertising combined with girls' vulnerability...not to mention the desire to be thin! (Fortunately, that number has steadily declined since then, with the rate for 2005 less than half the rate for 1996.)[84]

~ While the number of teens who smoke has declined recently (in 1996, 49 percent of eighth graders reported having tried smoking, compared to 26 percent in 2005), the number is still unacceptably high. The latest data from the Monitoring the Future study shows that one in eleven eighth graders and one in four twelfth graders reported smoking in the last month.[85]

~ While the leading cause of death among all Americans remains heart disease, cancer is the leading cause of death among women ages forty through seventy-nine—and the leading cause of cancer deaths for women is lung cancer, according to Action on Smoking and Health. (For more information, visit www.ash.com.)

~ People who smoke are up to four times more likely to suffer blindness later in life from age-related macular degeneration (AMD) than nonsmokers, according to a 2004 study published in the *British Medical Journal.*

~ Tobacco kills more *nonsmokers* each year than AIDS, illicit drugs, and teenage drinking.

~ Tobacco costs the American public $100 billion each year.[86]

~ One out of every six deaths in the United States is related to tobacco.

~ Smoking increases the risk of stroke by 300 percent.

~ More Americans die each year from tobacco than from fires, car accidents, illegal drugs, murders, and AIDS combined.

~ Tobacco kills more people in two days than crack and cocaine kill in a year.[87]

~ Tobacco companies know that once hooked, females are less likely to quit than males. (More nurses *start* smoking during training than any other profession.)

~ Cigarettes are more addictive than heroin because taking smoke into the lungs immediately produces a profound drug effect in the brain. It's like mainlining the most addictive substance in the world. Some kids are hooked after only one cigarette.

~ More than four thousand chemicals, including two hundred known poisons such as DDT, arsenic, formaldehyde, and carbon monoxide, are housed in tobacco.

Smoking and Specific Women's Health Problems

The power of addiction and denial is nowhere more striking than the case of a pregnant patient who, despite a history of infertility, continues to smoke throughout her pregnancy. Consider the following data:

~ Smokers have a miscarriage rate that is twice as high as that of nonsmokers. These miscarriages are often of genetically normal fetuses.

~ Infants whose mothers smoke run double the risk of dying of sudden infant death syndrome (SIDS).[88]

~ Smoking in pregnancy is the number one cause of low-birth

weight babies, who have a much higher death rate than normal-weight babies. Part of this is because smoking markedly increases the risk of prematurity.

~ The children of smoking parents have many more respiratory illnesses (such as asthma) per year than those of nonsmokers.

~ Smokers are at increased risk for cervical cancer, vulvar cancer, and abnormal Pap smear, possibly because smoking depletes vitamins C and A and beta-carotene, antioxidants that are somewhat protective against cancer.[89] Smoking literally poisons the ovaries.

~ Smoking ages the skin more quickly than normal.

~ Lung cancer has now passed breast cancer as the number one cancer killer of women. (You have come a long way, baby!)

~ Smokers are at increased risk for osteoporosis, premature aging, and heart disease.

Dr. Andrew Weil points out that there are tobacco leaves carved on the pillars of the Capitol in Washington, D.C.—testimony to the entwined interests of the government and the tobacco companies. Since the handwriting is on the wall for smoking in the United States, however, tobacco growers are now targeting the almost limitless market overseas in such places as China.

How to Quit Smoking
~ Know that every attempt at quitting increases your chances of success next time. Give yourself credit for trying. Remember that fifty million Americans have successfully become smoke-free.

~ For now, when you smoke, try to become very conscious of your smoking. Go outside, breathe in deeply, and pay attention to your lungs.

~ Ask your lungs for permission to smoke. Check in with this part of your body and see how it feels.

~ When you smoke, just smoke. Try to get as much pleasure from the cigarette as possible. The idea here, as with food, is to change your consciousness around smoking. Doing so will stop the "robot" approach that is the basis for this habit.

~ When you decide to quit, keep a smoking log for a week in which you write down where you smoked, when, who you were with, and how you feel. This will help you identify your smoking "triggers."

~ Develop a list of alternative behaviors to smoking that you can have ready at your "trigger times." These may include taking five deep breaths, going for a short walk in the fresh air, eating some strongly flavored hard candy such as cinnamon, or drinking a glass of water.

~ Understand that when you stop smoking you won't just be giving up cigarettes, you'll also be giving up your identity as a smoker. That means that your entire social network, which is so often organized around smoking, will undergo changes. Because so many women are relational in nature, this part of smoking cessation may be the hardest part. When I look at the groups of smokers hanging around outside nonsmoking buildings these days, I see how bonded smokers, who may have nothing else in common, have become during their smoking breaks. One of my newsletter readers wrote, "The only reason I wanted to quit smoking was that I never knew where I could smoke anymore and I wanted to be considerate of others who are sensitive to smoke."

~ Prepare to feel fully. All addictions numb feelings. Smoking in particular shuts down the energy of your heart and makes it difficult to feel the depth of your passion and joy—even if it does temporarily help you feel less grief, anxiety, or anger. One newsletter subscriber who successfully quit said, "I felt that smoking was numbing me in a certain way and that if feelings or parts of myself were numbed then they were unavailable to me. I was ready to quit when I became unwilling to live any longer with missing parts or inaccessible feelings because they were numbed or smoke-screened. It took me a while to get there, but at that point it became more important to have all of me available to myself in life than to smoke."

~ Don't worry about weight gain. This is not an inevitable consequence of smoking cessation. The only reason women gain weight is that they are substituting one addiction for another. (The dictum to be thin is so great that many smokers would rather risk lung cancer and death than risk being overweight. A few very honest smokers have told me this.)

~ Get support. You can find a support group or smoking cessation program through almost any hospital. For referrals to local groups, you can also call the American Lung Association 800-586-4872; www.lungusa.org or the American Cancer Society 800-227-2345; www.cancer.org. Smokers Anonymous, a twelve-step program, is available through AA (look in the yellow pages). Another good resource is Nicotine Anonymous (NicA) 415-750-0328; www.nicotine-anonymous.org. Also see the extensive information at The Foundation for a Smokefree America's website at www.anti-smoking.org.

⁓ Try hypnosis. I've been sending smokers for hypnosis for years—often with very good results.

⁓ Use acupuncture. Acupuncture and Traditional Chinese Medicine are known to be of benefit in helping with withdrawal from cigarettes and other addictive substances. In New York City, the March of Dimes and Columbia-Presbyterian Hospital advocate acupuncture-based treatment for addicted clients. One three-year study involving 2,282 cases demonstrated that acupuncture had a 90 percent success rate in a nicotine detoxification program.[90] Generally it only takes one treatment. An added benefit is that acupuncture lessens your chance of gaining weight after you stop.

What about pharmacological help? Some women have been helped by nicotine gum or the nicotine patch; both are available over the counter and have been heavily promoted as a way to "taper off" smoking. The short-term success rate of each is comparable, and both work better when combined with psychological support. The data on long-term outcomes are mixed. My own preference is for the programs listed above. You want to get rid of nicotine in your system as soon as possible, and these simply draw out the process. If you do try them, follow the package directions precisely, or you could actually overdose on nicotine.

APPRECIATE THE ENERGY OF FOOD

Years of clinical practice have convinced me that the energy of food has emotional and psychological consequences. Foods aren't broken down completely into anonymous fats, carbohydrates, and proteins when they're digested—they retain some of their original energy.[91] Like humans, food is more than the sum of its parts. It is affected by the way it is raised, processed, handled, and cooked. In short, food has its own unique energy field, *prana,* or *chi.* In ancient monasteries, only the most enlightened monks were allowed to cook and handle the food, because it was felt that their energy field affected the food.

On a recent trip to Italy, I was simply amazed at how good the locally grown food tasted. There is, of course, a rich food tradition there. Food is locally grown on mineral-rich soils, harvested at the peak of freshness, and enjoyed in season among family and friends. Eating there versus gulping fast food in the United States are two entirely different experiences.

A number of studies have documented the link between food, behavior, and mood. Studies on schoolchildren and the observations of many parents have supported the fact that foods that are low in nutrients and high in sugar, caffeine, and food additives sometimes produce erratic behavior. Alexander Schauss has documented the link between diet, crime, and delinquency, showing the connection between diets high in sugar and preservatives and subsequent erratic behavior.[92] On the other hand, if you were sitting on a beach in Hawaii reading novels, you could eat almost anything you wanted and suffer few ill effects—even from foods that usually give you problems (provided, of course, that you like Hawaii and the beach). But when you're under stress, hurried, or unhappy, digestion and food assimilation are adversely affected because of the adverse effect of stress hormones on insulin, blood sugar, and digestive function. This link is important to understand.

Digestion, absorption, and assimilation of our food are also dependent upon our state of consciousness. So if you're eating brown rice and vegetables out of guilt or as a way to beat yourself up, chances are they won't have nearly the beneficial effects that they're capable of providing.

A now-famous study on heart and blood vessel disease was conducted at Ohio State University on rabbits. These rabbits were all genetically bred to develop atherosclerosis (hardening of the arteries) and coronary artery disease. The investigators fed the rabbits an atherogenic diet to speed up the disease process. At the end of the study, when the rabbits were sacrificed, the researchers found that more than 15 percent of the rabbits had almost no coronary artery disease—their arteries were clean. After much head-scratching, they discovered that the bunnies with the clean arteries were the ones whose cages were at waist level. The female graduate student who fed the rabbits used to take these ones out of their cages and pet and play with them a while before their feeding.[93] This study has been repeated several times, mostly because no one could believe it initially, but the results were the same. Studies like this fly in the face of what we normally believe is going on. My advice: if you're going to eat doughnuts, get a massage—or pray over them first.

Another example of the effect of consciousness on how food is assimilated in the body is the fact that people with multiple personality disorder can be very allergic to a food while they are in one personality; yet the same food doesn't affect them a bit when they are in another personality—in the exact same body. Clearly, more is going on with food and nourishment than simply fat, carbohydrates, proteins, vitamins, and calories. When all is said and done, diet is only one factor in creating health, albeit a very powerful one. According to numerous investigators, dietary patterns that are associated with low cancer and heart disease risk are usually present in those individuals who have other lifestyle factors that are associated with a low risk of cancer. These include less consumption of alcohol and fast food, more exercise, and an optimistic worldview.

Commit to the joy and pleasure of eating whole organic food most of the time. But also understand that your consciousness around a food can change that food's effect on your body. For me, the pleasure of eating out at a restaurant where I can relax and be served almost always outweighs the damage of any partially hydrogenated fat in the salad dressing or on the fish. Melvin Morse's study of long-term survivors of near-death experiences showed that they eat better than controls and in general take better care of themselves. They do this not to avoid dying but because, as a result of their near-death experience, they value their lives more than ever before. Eating well is a way of valuing and nourishing ourselves.[94]

The late comedian George Burns, who lived until he was one hundred, once said, "If I had known I was going to live so long, I'd have taken better care of myself." Part of George Burns's longevity secret was his sense of humor. Don't lose yours—and don't eat without it! Keep food in perspective.

18
The Power of Movement

Our body creates our soul as much as our soul creates our body.
—David Spangler

Physical exercise or regular movement of some kind is a vital part of creating health, which is why the new USDA food pyramid has exercise as its base! Our bodies were designed to move, stretch, and run. It feels wonderful to have a strong, flexible body—including a strong heart for endurance. Exercise needs to be part of your commitment to yourself. It's easy to put off exercising until the house is clean, more work is done, or you've gone through the mail. But each of us needs to develop the discipline to do it anyway. The endless household and work duties will always be there, even after you're dead. Think of it this way: given that exercise adds an average of seven years to your life, you're *saving* time by exercising.

If we wait to take care of ourselves until everything else is done, there will never be time for exercise. If we don't create exercise time, we'll never have it. Exercise is an essential part of weight control. Though I have a family history of heart disease, I don't exercise because I'm afraid of heart disease. I do it because it feels good and my body loves it! The old feminist adage "How you do it is what you get" applies to exercise just as it does to any other area of life. Getting to this point took me more than forty years. First I had to overcome the "no pain, no gain" legacy that I grew up with.

OUR CULTURAL INHERITANCE

Many women have to heal their early perceptions of themselves and their physical capabilities before they can become comfortable with physical activities. Schools and the culture tend to confuse sports skills with fitness. Being good at batting a ball and being physically fit are not necessarily related. Many girls end up feeling bad about their physical prowess simply because they're not "good" at sports, especially during the middle-school years, when there is such a wide variation in development. John Douillard, author of *Body, Mind, and Sport* (Crown, 1994) and a pioneer in the field of fitness and consciousness, cites a Louis Harris poll that discloses that upward of 50 percent of Americans experience their first major failure in life in sports! The reason many girls don't have the skills to succeed in sports is that no one ever taught them. One of my friends who was a pro baseball player told me that when boys are first learning to throw, they also throw "just like a girl." Boys learn to "throw like a boy" from practicing over and over again with those who are more skilled than they. It's part of their cultural heritage.

Are you someone who was never picked for the school softball team? Did you feel you had to quit playing sports with the boys when you started to grow breasts? Check to see if your history and any messages you received as a girl are preventing you from enjoying physical activity now. If they are, bring them to consciousness so you can experience them fully, and then let them go. Brian Swimme, Ph.D., physicist and author of *The Universe Is a Green Dragon* (Bear, 1985), said it best: "To exercise actually means to bring into action. When we exercise, we bring into action our ancestral memories. Our bodies remember that we lived in trees and forests. We need to crawl and climb and run if we are to develop our intellectual, emotional, and spiritual capacities...We tend to think of exercise as losing weight, as trimming off the fat. But to exercise is to enable the body to remember its past, so that it can stretch out with all its intertwined powers of being and thought and reflection."[1]

Many of the bodily changes we associate with aging have nothing to do with aging per se. Decreased muscle mass and increased fat may be normal in this culture, but these conditions are not necessarily natural—and we needn't expect them. They are caused by inactivity and the cumulative effects of glycemic stress and insulin resistance, accompanied by a mindset that expects us to grow weaker as we age. As we have seen, the physical condition of sixty-year-old Tarahumara runners was better than that of the twenty-year-olds. I can relate. I am actually more flexible and fit now than when I was in my twenties!

Unfortunately, our own "tribe" collectively believes that we are supposed to fall apart when we age. We have no culturally supported tradition that teaches us that we can improve with age. Though countless exceptions to this rule exist, we still suffer under the collective delusion about what happens to our bodies with age.

BENEFITS OF EXERCISE

Joanne Cannon, a wellness educator, defines physical prowess as "the ability to meet the physical demands of one's day, plus one emergency." I like that definition because it is so individualized. Feeling strong and capable is an essential ingredient to building health. Studies show that women who are moderately physically active enjoy the following benefits more than sedentary women.[2]

~ Lower overall cancer rates and better immune system function (more white blood cells and increased levels of immunoglobulins)[3]

~ Decreased risk of breast cancer (women who exercise at least four hours per week have been shown to have a 37 percent reduction in risk for breast cancer)[4]

~ A life expectancy that is on average seven years longer;[5] a recent study in the *New England Journal of Medicine* showed that asymptomatic women who weren't fit had twice the risk of death of those who were fit[6]

~ Significant reduction in heart attack and stroke risk secondary to beneficial effect of exercise on blood vessel function[7]

~ Less depression and anxiety, and better mental efficiency and speed (higher IQ scores are associated with exercise in some studies)[8]

~ Improved cognitive function in middle age and beyond[9]

~ More relaxation, more assertiveness, more spontaneity and enthusiasm; a better attitude about their bodies and better self-acceptance[10]

~ Stronger bones, increased bone thickness, increased bone mass, and increased ability of the bone to resist mechanical stress and fracture[11]

~ More restful sleep[12]

~ Higher self-esteem[13]

Another benefit of physical exercise is that it increases insulin sensitivity and can therefore prevent glycemic stress, insulin resistance, and non-insulin-dependent diabetes.[14] Remember from chapter 17 that insulin resistance begins in skeletal muscles. Regular exercise is an essential part of controlling blood sugar and weight. It is also energizing. If you're always tired, it may be because you don't move enough. (But sometimes it's because you need to rest. You'll have to check this out for yourself.) For women with PMS, exercise often alleviates symptoms.[15] And pregnant women who exercise moderately have decreased constipation, hemorrhoids, varicose vein complications, and morning sickness.[16]

Even women who are disabled or confined to a wheelchair can benefit from strengthening their upper bodies and increasing their cardiovascular fitness.

Exercise and Intuition

The mind pervades the body. Moving your body rhythmically and repetitively helps you tap in to your intuition, and more of your mind becomes available to you—the mind in your legs, your heart, and in your biceps. Exercising is a necessary process for fully digesting thoughts. Raising your heartbeat brings into play more of yourself. Your body wakes up—and so does your mind. During your workouts insights arise spontaneously. When you don't do it, you eventually find that your body craves it!

Studies have shown that repetitive movement increases alpha waves in the brain—and the alpha state is associated with enhanced intuition. Exercising hard is the perfect balance for the mental activity so often required in modern life.

People have very different approaches to exercise and physical activity. Each of us has an innate sense of what feels right for our bodies. As a scholar in a family of "jocks," I've had to find my own truth about what works best for me. You will need to find yours, too. Your truth will not necessarily be what any outside authority tells you is "the right way to do it." And different approaches to exercise work best at different times in people's lives. For some, a twenty-minute walk three times a week is all that is necessary. For others, aerobics, weight training, or dancing feels the best. Above all, exercise and body movement should be joyful and fun.

Ways to Move the Body

Aerobic Exercise and Target Heart Rate

Back in the 1960s, the concept of aerobic exercise was a revolutionary breakthrough in exercise physiology. Exercising aerobically keeps the heart, lungs, and entire cardiovascular system in good shape. It also burns off excess fat. Aerobic activity is defined as exercise in which the heart rate is elevated for fifteen to twenty minutes into what is called "the target zone."

To calculate your target rate:

1. Subtract your age from 220.

2. Subtract your resting heart rate (beats per minute) from this figure.

3. Multiply the remainder by your "exercise quotient." This is 0.6 for a beginner or 0.8 for an advanced exerciser.

4. Add your resting heart rate to the figure from step 3. This number is your target heart rate in beats per minute. You can divide by 6 to find out your heart rate for a ten-second interval.

Example: Your age is thirty-two. Your resting heart rate is 60, and you are a beginner. Hence: 220–32 = 188. 188–60 = 128. 128 × 0.6 = 76.8. 76.8 + 60 = 136.8. Your target heart rate is 137 beats per minute or 23 beats for a ten-second interval.

Most experts agree that twenty minutes of aerobic-type exercise three times a week is adequate for cardiovascular fitness.

Rethinking the Target Heart Rate and Everything Else

John Douillard, D.C., Ph.D., director of the Invincible Athlete program in Boulder, Colorado, has found that the target heart rate and most other "fitness truths" don't necessarily apply to individuals who breathe fully through their noses while exercising and consciously tune in to what their bodies are comfortable with. When you learn how to do this, you can easily go through a workout with a heart rate and breathing rate that are much slower and more comfortable than expected. Dr. Douillard's insights have revolutionized the way I approach all sports and exercise and have enhanced my enjoyment of physical activity immeasurably. (For more information, see Dr. Douillard's website at www.lifespa.com.)

Take a moment right now and take three slow, deep breaths through your mouth. When you are finished, stop for a moment and take three full, deep breaths through your nose, allowing the air to go all the way down to the lower lobes of your lungs. Notice which type of breathing gives you the fullest amount of air in your lungs. The nose breathing wins by a mile, even though it may seem harder at first. Infants normally breathe through their noses, and so do all animals. (Have you even seen a racehorse breathing through its mouth?) In fact, mouth breathing is a sign of stress. Nose breathing is associated with both parasympathetic and sympathethic balance in the body and feels very meditative; it enhances the balance between the right and left hemispheres of the brain. When you train yourself to breathe through your nose during exercise, your lungs become much more efficient and you can achieve higher levels of fitness than ever before with much less effort.

Consider also the larger implications for our lives. We breathe twenty-eight thousand times a day. If our breaths are shallow, taken in through our mouth, and confined mostly to the upper lobes of our lungs, our body gets the message that we're facing an emergency. Heart rate increases; the body chemicals associated with stress increase. The majority of illnesses are stress-related, and we can choose to decrease or increase stress every time we breathe. When we learn how to breathe fully through our nose, aerating our lower lungs and allowing our rib cage a full expansion, our body relaxes and we experience a sense of peace. Paradoxically, our body also operates much more efficiently. Just breathing properly has the potential to cure sinusitis, chronic colds, and even asthma. I've had more than one woman tell me that when she adopted nose breathing, she was able to get rid of her asthma attacks! I'm convinced that everyone should adopt this method of breathing not only for exercise, but for daily living.

In all traditional sports and fitness training, the coach (or leader) is the mind and the athlete is the body. (You've probably experienced this in exercise classes.) As a result, most of us are trained to exercise by tuning out our bodies. (When my daughter was running track in high school, and if she finished a run feeling good and energized, her coach told her that she wasn't working hard enough!) The dictum is "Just do it" ... but don't feel it! There is evidence of this in every gym I've ever been in: people use loud music or TV programs as a way to avoid feeling their body's response to exercise. It hurts too much, and rather than feel that, it's easier to either avoid exercise entirely or just get through it by distracting yourself.

But once you start breathing properly and enjoying the meditative state that results, you'll find yourself tuning in to and respecting your body's ability more than ever. You'll realize clearly that the old adage "No pain, no gain" is physiologically incorrect. And you'll also discover that exercise, sports, or any workout becomes a very personal time of tuning in and getting strong. What was once a chore becomes a joy. Now, instead of a forced march to the standards of someone else, my exercise or sports time is just between me and me. That doesn't mean that I don't strive for improvement. I do. I also work with a Pilates teacher regularly, which is a big help.

Aerobics and Weight Training

Aerobic exercise plus weight training is more effective than aerobics alone because the weight training increases the amount of muscle in the body relative to fat and does so much more effectively than aerobics alone.[17] This is a relatively new understanding.

Studies show that as we age, we create an average of one and a half pounds of fat per year. We also lose a half pound of muscle each year if we don't exercise regularly. Muscle loss results in fat gain. Weight training prevents the muscle loss that too often accompanies aging. Aerobic weight training produces more muscle gain on an average than aerobics alone. It also shapes muscles, resulting in a healthier appearance. The increase in muscle strength that comes with weight training is very beneficial to women, who are often weak in their upper bodies. (Older women break their hips not only because of osteoporosis but because of muscle weakness and decreased strength, which makes them more susceptible to falling.)

Aerobic exercise combined with weight training results in more fat loss and produces more muscle gain compared to aerobics alone. The reason this is so important is that one pound of muscle requires 30 to 50 calories a day just to stay alive. One pound of fat requires fewer calories for maintenance. Remember—fat is covered with insulin receptors that tend to "lock" it into place while muscle helps burn fat. People with more muscle have higher metabolic rates. This is one reason that overweight women with lots of body fat often maintain their weight even when eating relatively little. To change their metabolic rate, they need to increase their physical activity and also reduce or eliminate high-glycemic-index carbs! This results in the body resetting its metabolism and releasing fat easier.

It is well known that bone mineral content increases with physical activity.[18] Putting "vertical vectors of force" on bones through weight-bearing exercise such as walking, jogging, biking, weight training, or stair climbing sets up a mini electrical current in the bone, known as a piezoelectric effect. Yoga and Pilates also do this. This current actually draws in calcium and other minerals we need for bone density and strength. Dr. Miriam Nelson has been able to demonstrate significant gains in bone density in postmenopausal women who did two forty-minute sessions of weight training twice a week. None of the women were on estrogen replacement. A wonderful side effect of this training was that as the women in the program increased their self-confidence and strength, they also felt more empowered in the world and tended to go out more and get involved in life.[19]

Gentle Approaches to the Body

Fitness involves more than strength and endurance. It also must include flexibility and proper alignment. The effects of gravity over time and buckling under to life's stresses quite literally wear us down. Our muscles, flexibility, and alignment deteriorate over time unless we become aware of this and do something to counteract it. Yoga, the Feldenkrais Method, Pilates, and the Alexander Technique work, and other body-realigning techniques are a wonderful way to relax, stretch, and gently stimulate the muscles and internal organs. They also help maintain the body in proper alignment to gravity and keep the spine and joints supple. I've seen women totally transform their bodies with Pilates, myself included. My Pilates experience more than any other exercise has convinced me that it's possible to grow stronger, more fit, and more flexible with age—not the opposite.

Martial Arts

Martial arts training such as aikido or tai chi combines the body, mind, and spirit very consciously. This approach also increases strength, endurance, and flexibility simultaneously. Studies of individuals who do tai chi regularly, for example, have found that tai chi modifies their biological function via their nervous and hormonal systems. It has been shown to be effective in the treatment of heart disease, hypertension, insomnia, asthma, and osteoporosis. It decreases depression, tension, anger, fatigue, confusion, and anxiety.[20] A more recent study of two hundred people over the age of seventy found that tai chi decreased the risk of falls—a major factor in hip fracture.[21]

When I was in college, I got a green belt in jujitsu. Though that's not a high ranking, I did have to spar with a couple of big guys from Cleveland Heights in order to earn it. From that, I learned that I have the strength and the will to fight someone in self-defense if I need to. Studies of men who rape show that they tend to go after women who seem the most vulnerable. The self-confidence and resulting self-confident stance that come from knowing you can fight for yourself is conveyed in the energy field around you and is one way to decrease your chances of being raped. Martial arts can also help you discover your voice.[22]

EXERCISE AND ADDICTION

Just about anything can be used addictively, and exercise is no exception. The call to use physical activity as a way to disconnect from and to conquer nature (and our feelings) saturates our culture. For example, an ad for a well-known running shoe reads:

> *Trees should duck*
> *Rocks, cower.*
> *Anything soft and low*
> *Should learn what is hard.*
> *We have come into the mountains*
> *Because they*
> *Would not come*
> *To us.*
> *And then*
> *We move*
> *Them.*

Some people have actually had to go to rehab for running addiction. Several years ago, I visited a popular spa to give some lectures. One of the women in the group spent three hours per morning on a treadmill, worked out with a personal trainer most of each afternoon, and then went out every evening to buy alcohol, which she'd imbibe until drunk! Though she looked good, I knew that at the rate she was going, her health and beauty were both in jeopardy! When we use exercise to run away from the stress in our lives or to disconnect from our deepest selves, it is no different from the addictive use of Valium. (It may be a healthier choice initially, but it is still an addiction.)

Our society's attitude toward exercise as a fix is illustrated perfectly by an article that appeared in *Longevity* magazine in May 1991 (just before "swimsuit season"). The article was entitled "The Quickest Fixes: Emergency Diet/Shape-Up Strategies from 8 Famous Bodies."[23] In the top left-hand corner was the line "30 Days to Summer." (This serves to hook you into the crisis-intervention mode for "cellulite management.")

Celebrities and their nearly impossible routines were featured. When I read this article, I couldn't believe what I was reading. How many women have personal trainers—or have the time to work out even an hour a day? Presenting this information on celebrity women to ordinary mortals and expecting women to meet their standards is ridiculous. Celebrity women make careers out of having perfect bodies. It's part of their work. They don't accomplish this in addition to raising a family by themselves and holding down another job. You don't have to be a drug and alcohol counselor to see the language and process of addiction in this article and hundreds more like it. Celebrity women fall prey to the same addictive tendencies as the rest of the culture—"I just do it harder," said one of them in the *Longevity* article, when asked what kind of exercise she does when she needs to shed a few pounds fast.

Unfortunately, many women do use exercise as a fix to run away from stress or as a way to keep their weight down. While exercise does accomplish both of these goals, you'll never establish a healthy relationship with exercise and your body if you do the exercise strictly for stress and/or weight control.

EXERCISE, AMENORRHEA, AND BONE LOSS

Studies have repeatedly shown that female athletes whose menstrual cycles have stopped suffer from premature bone loss.[24] In the past, I feared that this data would be used to scare women away from choosing to use their bodies as fully and powerfully as men. (By the way, having a baby uses your body as fully and powerfully as any athletic event I can think of, but we can't do this routine every week!)

Follow-up studies have shown that many women athletes stop having periods for the same reason as women who go on stringent diets or become anorexic: they don't eat enough, and their total body fat drops to a level that is too low. This results in loss of periods (amenorrhea) and early osteoporosis.[25] In one study, when women who had developed amenorrhea from exercise ate 500 to 700 calories more per day, their periods returned. (Most competitive women runners won't do this.)

One of my friends, a former competitive bodybuilder, told me that competitors in women's body building actually look forward to losing their periods and consider it a sign of adequate training. Competitive runners have told me the same thing. Hormonal shutdown of this nature is actually a training goal! Clearly, this is a sign of unhealthy behavior. It's not surprising that drug use in the form of anabolic steroids is the norm rather than the exception in high-level competitions. The same cultural norms apply to bodybuilding as anywhere else. My bodybuilder friend was told that she'd have a better chance of winning if she dyed her hair blond and got breast implants. She said that the body-building ideal is "a Barbie doll with muscles."

Studies indicate that women marathon runners who exercise to the point of becoming amenorrheic often have bone densities comparable to those of osteoporotic women who are much older. There is no definite point at which running may begin to have deleterious effects on a woman's body, although in competitive runners it appears to begin at about fifty miles of training per week.

Still another reason these women become amenorrheic is that, as studies have shown, leanness *combined* with chronic concern about becoming overweight is associated with brain changes that lead to disturbed menstrual cycles.[26] Women athletes are just as influenced by the cultural desire to be thin as other women. For that reason, their caloric intake is often lower than it has to be for the level of activity in which they participate. Eating disorders are just as common in athletic women as they are in nonathletic women, but athletic women sometimes use the training as a form of weight control. They exercise heavily—then they don't eat. This is no different from other forms of anorexia.

Since resumption of menses can take some time, progesterone therapy to help restore bone mass is often helpful. Once ovulatory periods have resumed, bone mineral density also begins to improve.[27]

Not all women are at risk for losing their periods from extreme amounts of exercise. In a study by Nancy Lane, M.D., amenorrhea from excessive exercise was primarily a problem of young, childless women. After a woman has had children, she is less likely to develop this problem because childbearing appears to make her hormonal system difficult to suppress via extreme exercise. Her monthly cycling becomes harder to turn off. That's why women runners in their thirties and forties who've had children rarely become amenorrheic.[28] I believe that there's another reason why women who have had children are at less risk for exercise-induced amenorrhea: they are much less likely to maintain ruthless competitiveness, and this shift is associated with an opening of the heart that changes body chemistry. Having a child changes a woman in very fundamental ways—emotionally, psychologically, physically, and spiritually. Her priorities about what's really important change.

MY EXERCISE STORY: MAKING PEACE

I grew up, as I've mentioned, in an atmosphere teeming with physical activity and exercise. Most of it was outgoing and energetic, like jogging and skiing. Even on Christmas Day, to my chagrin, my parents and siblings would race out the door to hit the slopes. Though my mother did yoga and I learned the basic postures in the eighth grade, this was done not as an inner meditation with attention to breathing but as a humorous competition to see who could actually get their bodies into the postures. We especially liked doing yoga headstands—they looked impressive.

My sister regarded my meditative stretching or muscle toning as a sissy approach. When not on the racing circuit, she was out running up our back hill with ski poles doing dry-land training. Every family vacation was camping or hiking; most of the hiking had a "race to the summit" feeling, and I didn't even pretend to be interested. I enjoyed being out in nature, but not as a competitive event.

My ski-racer sister now does yoga and tai chi regularly, paying attention to her breathing and inner feelings. After years of pushing and multiple injuries, she no longer approaches fitness in the old, abusive way. For years, she couldn't even look at a Nautilus or other weight machine—right about the same time that I got into weight training very enthusiastically. Now we both enjoy yoga and dance as well as some weight training and aerobic activity. Our paths have crossed as both of us have reached a balanced approach to physical activity.

When I was in medical school and residency, I jogged for twenty to thirty minutes three to four times a week and did a bit of yoga for balance. Unfortunately, I was chasing the elusive "runner's high" in those days. Looking back on those years, what I remember most is how wonderful it felt to be out in the sunshine and fresh air after all those hours of being confined inside a hospital. I looked forward to my runs for that reason, but also wanted to get my thirty aerobics points for the week. To accomplish this, I ran in place even at stoplights. I wish I had been more aware of the air and the light—and less aware of how far I was running or how high my pulse rate was. I didn't know then that running is best done for the enjoyment of the process. I was doing it to get something—not because of enjoying the process (classic addictive behavior).

During my pregnancies I did prenatal yoga. I found, like many pregnant women, that jogging just felt awful. I've never returned to it. After the children were born and while they were little (below age four), I occasionally went for a walk, but that was about it for a few years. (I don't remember much from those years—it's a blur of diapers and fatigue.) When I came home at the end of the day, I couldn't bring myself to go out the door to exercise. The children seemed to need my attention too much. Learning to balance my needs and theirs took a while. They're only little once, and my instincts told me that being with them as much as I could was crucial.

As the children grew older, though, I bought a NordicTrack and set it up in front of the television. I did twenty minutes of this three times a week or so while watching *Entertainment Tonight* or other such fare or listening to music. During the first few months my children whined, complained, and constantly asked me to get them a drink, tie their shoes, or do something that would focus my attention completely on them. Pointing out to them that they could color or play right in the same room with me and that I wasn't going to leave them to exercise worked. The children understood. When I was clear about my needs, without feeling guilty about them, I found that even young children would cooperate for short periods of time. I also promised them that when I finished I would play with them, or in some other way give them the attention they needed. This worked well for a number of years. Later I added weight training three to four times a week and a walk or twenty to thirty minutes on a treadmill or elliptical trainer in between times. As I already mentioned, once I incorporated the breathing and consciousness approach of Dr. Douillard, exercise took on a whole new meaning.

Our whole approach to fitness and sports needs to be completely revamped if lifetime fitness is our goal. Individual sports or activities that teenagers enjoy long after they've finished school need to be added to every school's physical fitness curriculum. And they need to be taught how to tune in to their bodies' wisdom in middle school. (Dr. Douillard has documented how effective this has been in the schools where it has been done.) Though tennis, yoga, dance, and martial arts are often available at the college level, I'd like to see them in elementary schools.

This past Christmas, I went back to my childhood home for my mother's eightieth birthday party. It was the first time I'd been there at Christmastime in thirty years. The whole family had come full circle with exercise and sports! Not one person got up to go skiing on Christmas morning. Instead, we all sat around and ate breakfast. I had finally manifested my ideal Christmas morning!

GETTING STARTED

Step one: choose an exercise program. It is just as healthy to discard the concept of the "ideal" amount of exercise as it is to discard the concept of the "ideal" weight. When people ask me what exercise program is best, I reply, "The one that you'll actually do." Women can find joy and fitness by participating in a very wide variety of activities, ranging from yoga, tai chi, and dance to teaching Outward Bound courses.

Try this: Recall a time in childhood when you were outside playing—skipping, jumping rope, or throwing a ball just for fun. Or perhaps you remember dancing—twirling around till you fell on the ground dizzy. Play with this memory in your mind for a while, and feel how it felt. Smell how it smelled. Feel the sun or wind on your face. Feel how good it felt to move your body with joy and energy, stretching it to its full capacity.

When you are ready, bring yourself back into the present. Begin moving your body the way you used to. See how it feels now. Be in your body. Enjoy it, appreciate it—experiment with moving it. Did any type of movement come to mind as something that felt really good? What was it? How could you incorporate that into your life now?

Step two: *make a commitment to move your body.* Commit to moving your body in some way or in some form three to five times a week for twenty to thirty minutes. Make exercise as simple as possible for yourself. For me, that used to mean keeping the NordicTrack all set up in the family room and keeping my weights arranged on the floor, ready to go—I didn't have to do any elaborate setup. I didn't worry about leaving it out all the time: after all, the house was for me to live in, not to look perfect in case company came. Sometimes I used to go to a gym, especially when traveling. Most of the time, I like to be home. Now that the children are gone, I have a room I've converted into an exercise studio.

Commit to doing an exercise program for one month. Within that time your body will probably come to look forward to exercise.

If you drop out for a while, let yourself know that you will get back to it when you can. Don't spend a minute beating yourself up.

Step three: *learn how to breathe through your nose.* Go slowly. Learn the Salute to the Sun and go through it to learn how to pace your breath. (For full instructions, see the book *Body, Mind, and Sport* [Three Rivers Press, 2001] by John Douillard, D.C., Ph.D. The postures can also be found in many yoga texts or videos.) Don't exert yourself beyond the level at which you can comfortably keep your breathing steady through your nose. If you're already a regular exerciser, you'll notice that it will probably take you three weeks or more to get back to your former level of achievement while breathing properly. Take your time. Once you've trained your body to use oxygen efficiently, you'll find that you'll soon be running farther—or walking faster—with less exertion than you ever dreamed possible. Your rib cage will also become much more flexible and your breathing more efficient.

Step four: watch out for self-sabotage. One of the most common reasons that women stop exercising is that they do too much too soon (addictive behavior). Having been out of shape for three years, they vow that they'll run three miles a day for a week and get in shape fast. A much better approach is to do less each day than you are capable of—at least for a while. This will give your body the message that it can trust you to take care of it and not push it to exhaustion. Your body will get the idea that exercise is fun! Dogs love to go for their walks—and we would be just as enthusiastic if we followed our instincts as well as animals do.

If you never push yourself, on the other hand, and always do less than is expected or needed, then you need to push past your current limit. It's good to know your body is capable of the long haul when necessary. Don't ever use exercise as a way to beat your body into submission or to punish it for not looking perfect. (Anne Wilson Schaef once said that she thinks addiction to self-abuse is probably the most common addiction in our culture, and I would agree.)

Be aware of using exercise as a way to run away from your feelings or as a way to decrease stress. Though exercise can blow off steam, if it's used primarily for this purpose it can become a "fix" anytime you feel stressed; you'll use exercise to medicate your emotional pain. It's much better to deal with the source of the stress than to use exercise as a fix. On the other hand, a ten- to fifteen-minute brisk walk will often elevate your mood and help you put things in perspective. It also helps the body get rid of the effects of stress hormones that often trigger overeating.

If you hate your exercise program and have to manipulate or force yourself into doing it, you'll just build up resistance. You'll eventually quit or manage to get injured, or you'll make the exercise program into an external authority controlling you—and you'll sabotage yourself to get out of doing it. So make sure you're doing something you like!

Step five: enjoy yourself. One of my patients, an art teacher in her forties, started going to a gym for weight lifting. She had a great time pumping iron. Newly divorced and on her own, her muscle strengthening reflected the strengthening she was doing in other areas of her life as well. She began to look and feel wonderful—and powerful. She was living proof that exercise releases naturally occurring substances called endorphins, which are related to morphine and the other opiates. It naturally produces a feeling of well-being.

So give physical activity a try. If, as David Spangler says, "our body creates our soul as much as our soul creates our body," maybe your soul could use a better set of biceps!

19

Healing Ourselves, Healing Our World

If you bring forth what is within you,
What you bring forth will save you.
If you do not bring forth what is within you,
What you do not bring forth will destroy you.
—Jesus, in *The Gospel According to Thomas*

All of us must acknowledge our female heritage and then have
the courage to transform it in order to create lives of vibrant
health and joy. We carry in our own bodies not only our own
pain but that of our mothers and grandmothers, however unconsciously. Hatred of the body is very deep in most women—generations
deep. Most of us had mothers who were brought up to distrust their
own bodies and the processes of their bodies. So had their mothers,
grandmothers, and great-grandmothers before them.

From time to time I have had the very vivid experience of entering
a place inside myself that I call "the pain of women." The first time it
happened, at an intensive with Anne Wilson Schaef, I felt my consciousness going backward in time, as layers and layers and centuries
and centuries of denial peeled away. My entry into this process was
when Anne said to me, "You're so tired," and then suggested I lie down
on a mat to see "what comes up." Having a woman, a mentor at that
time, acknowledge my tiredness instead of demanding more sacrifice
was one of the most profound experiences of my life. At first, as she sat

with me and told me to stay with myself, I felt how strongly my body resisted feeling what I was feeling. I experienced how good I was at pushing down my tears and getting on with whatever I had to do. But eventually, as Anne suggested that I simply stay with myself, I felt my consciousness go backward through all the times when I had never rested: when I'd had my children, during residency, during medical school, during college, during high school. Backward, backward, through my childhood—"Don't ask for a lighter pack, ask for a stronger back," I heard my mother say. And I wept for myself and for that part of me that so needed rest. When I had finished crying all the tears that I had never cried for myself, I began to weep for my mother— for all the times that she had not been allowed to feel or to rest, for all the pain of her own childhood, for all the times she was up all night with a sick child, for the endless grief of losing two children.

And when that was over, I felt my grandmother's grief, raised by her twelve-year-old sister after her own mother had died in childbirth. When that was complete, I went backward further still—until I was wailing for all women, for all the pain, for all the labors unattended, for all the injustice, for so many thousands of years. What had started as very personal became universal: not my pain, but *the* pain.

When it was over, several hours later, I knew exactly why I was on the Earth and what my mission was: to work toward transforming this collective pain into joy. I knew in a flash that there are no mistakes, that I had been destined to become an obstetrician/gynecologist, and that no other path would have served as well. I knew why I had cried so many years before in medical school, when I had first witnessed the birth of a baby: I had tapped in to the field of women's experience—including all of the pain and fear. Seeing the birth had brought up emotions for me that I had no words for back in 1973. I only knew that I had been moved beyond all reason by this birth and that there was no other specialty in medicine for me except the care of women. But I put those emotions down then, instead of experiencing them fully, as I did on so many other occasions. Two days after this experience I got my period, confirmation for me that our deepest material often comes to consciousness premenstrually—the time when the veil between the worlds of the conscious and unconscious is thinner.

About a week later, I was relating my experience of this deep process to my mother over the phone. When I had finished, she was silent for a long time. Then she said, "I was sexually abused. I remember the room, I remember the smell of his pipe. I can see it as though it were happening now. It was old Bill, the man who rented a room from my mother. He told me never to tell anyone. I felt dirty. I was eight years old."

My mother, who was sixty-three at that time, had not remembered this part of her history before that moment. Somehow I had broken into the family memory bank with my process—and the contents were easier for her to access as well. A few months prior to this, she had been having a recurrent dream in which there were horrid growths on her body. She'd awaken in terror. She now knew that these dreams were related to her long-suppressed abuse; the growths on her skin were symbolic of material coming up to consciousness "just under the surface"—ugly material, horrid material.

Mom was alone in her cabin when I called and she remembered her abuse. I asked her if she would be all right after we hung up. She said she would but that she'd call back if she needed support. I suggested that she be willing to stay with that which was "not acceptable." She prayed for guidance and let herself experience the sickening feeling that had surfaced with the sexual abuse memory. She then went to bed. Her loft window was open—it was a warm autumn night—and she later told me that three blue lights came in the window, followed by a large gleaming sphere of white light. The next thing she knew, it was morning. She awakened feeling profoundly at peace, knowing that she had had an experience of grace.

OUR MOTHERS: OUR CELLS

Our memories are stored up in our bodies. Incest memories often surface after a uterine biopsy, and sadness often arises after pelvic surgery, all for a reason. We carry our personal history in the tissue that our consciousness co-creates. It remains there like data banks until we transform it. But we carry much more than what is simply personal. On some level, we carry everyone and everything—the collective—all there within and around our very cells.

It's known that mitochondrial DNA, the DNA that carries out the daily activities of the cytoplasm of the cells, is inherited strictly through the maternal line. The entire human race can be traced back to a group of females in Africa.[1] This fact lends biological credence to my experiences and those of my patients who've entered into realms of experience that don't fit logical thinking. Sometimes body symptoms are the doorway not only into our own individual pain but into the collective pain of others. Insights from quantum physics have now proved that the consciousness of one of us affects all of us.

An old Sufi saying captures the essence of what this means and what each of us must do with it:

Overcome any bitterness that may have come to you because you
were not up to the magnitude of the pain that was entrusted to
you.

Like the mother of the world who carries the pain of the world
in her heart, each one of us is part of her heart and therefore en-
dowed with a certain measure of cosmic pain. You are sharing the
totality of that pain.

You are called upon to meet it in joy instead of self-pity. The
secret is to offer your heart as a vehicle to transform cosmic suffering into joy.

Stephen Levine taught me that the work we do to let go of our suffering diminishes the suffering of the whole universe. When we have
room in our hearts for our own pain, we have room for the pain of
others and our compassion helps lighten the suffering of others.

A RITUAL OF RECLAIMING

Years ago, Brenda, a close friend from childhood, decided that
she'd like to have her IUD removed in order to get pregnant. She'd been
using IUDs for contraception for almost eighteen years with no problem, but now, at the age of forty, she had met a man with whom she
wanted to share her life and have children. Because this decision was a
major turning point in her life, she wanted someone close to her to
share it. So she asked me to remove the IUD while she was here visiting in Maine.

We decided to do a simple ceremony prior to the procedure—to
bring intent and consciousness to the process of removing the IUD and
inviting in a child. So on a glorious Sunday afternoon in autumn, with
the trees ablaze with color, we went over to Women to Women, set up
a circle of cloth on the carpet in my office, picked a geranium from an
office plant, and gathered a few seashells to place in our circle. We filled
a shell with water, lit some candles, and then sitting around our small
circle, we acknowledged the forces of nature, God, and the mysteries of
life, and we invited them to be present with us.

We called Brenda's fiancé on the phone (he was at work in another
state at the time). I asked each of them to speak about their fears and
hopes for a child, which they did. The fiancé had already had a child
many years before, but he was eager for a chance to participate more
fully in the process this time. His support and love for Brenda were very

evident and clear as he spoke; he had no doubts about his willingness to participate in parenthood. His commitment to support her was strong and inspiring. Their relationship felt like the very embodiment of the masculine at its best when it is in full support of the feminine.

Brenda herself, though eager to have a baby, voiced a concern that she wouldn't know how to give birth. Despite her fear, she was ready to proceed with the IUD removal. We said goodbye to her fiancé, promising to call back as soon as we had completed the procedure.

Now we moved into one of my exam rooms, and I placed a small amount of local anesthetic in the cervix. Once Brenda felt ready, I asked her to cough while I pulled out the IUD. (Coughing while something is going into or coming out of the cervix often interferes with pain pathways and thus makes the procedure more comfortable.)

I told her that she would feel the visceral sense of her uterus as the IUD was pulled out and that this would be a good time for her to tune in to the information stored in there. I told her that the body holds memories and that these sometimes come to the surface during an office procedure such as an endometrial biopsy or an IUD removal. I explained that I would be taking some time after the procedure to "put her energy field back together" by placing my hands over the uterus. Her job was to simply pay attention to any thoughts or feelings that came up.

The IUD came out with no difficulty. I then took Brenda's heels out of the stirrups, had her lie flat, and then ran my hands over her body from head to toe several times, doing therapeutic touch. When finished, I laid my hands over her lower abdomen. She began to cry and laugh at the same time as her body released the tension and the emotional charge associated with this sort of procedure. I encouraged her to do whatever she had to do for herself. And I reminded her to simply stay with whatever was coming up.

After crying for a bit, Brenda closed her eyes and then began to laugh. She spoke of being in a forest, with light shining down through the tall trees. She described herself as being young, too young. Then she became frightened again. At this time, I didn't know exactly what was going on, but I simply remained with my hands over her lower abdomen. She told me that having my hands there felt good and she wanted me to keep them there.

She continued to recount being a young girl, alone in the woods. She was pregnant there, without the support of anyone. Her body began to go through what looked like labor. She kept saying, "It's too soon. I don't know how to do this." She began to go through contractions and then pushing. (I've sat with enough women in labor to know what a laboring woman's body goes through.) After about ten minutes she looked down at what sounded like a thirty-week-size stillborn when she described it. And she asked me, "What is that white rope-like thing going into my vagina?" She was describing the umbilical cord. I told her what it was and said that she'd have to deliver the placenta. Her body then went into another contraction and went through the motions of pushing out a placenta. Brenda had never seen a thirty-week premature baby, a placenta, or a white translucent umbilical cord, but she was able to describe them perfectly—but with the curiosity of a young girl who didn't know exactly what was happening to her, not a worldly forty-year-old.

At this point, the energetic labor and delivery complete, Brenda began to laugh and also to chant, "O-ne-an-ta, O-ne-an-ta." It sounded like a Native American language. During this time she said, "I know the whole language." I wish I had had a tape recorder—we might have figured out what language it was.

We stayed in the exam room a while longer while Brenda returned to the twentieth century and stretched her legs. Both of us were amazed by what had just happened. I reminded her that her body did in fact know how to give birth—she had just gone through it, though not on what we'd conventionally call a physical level. Nevertheless, her body now "knew" or "remembered" what labor and delivery were like, and her fear of the process was gone. We returned to my office, sang a lullaby together, and blew out the candles. When she was ready, she called her fiancé and related the experience.

Brenda had tapped in to the collective unconscious, had gained access to some ancient memory that still lived on in her cells. It was an extraordinary experience. I believe that in taking out her IUD and allowing her process to unfold, we were able to heal something deep, on a level that is available to all of us but that we rarely allow ourselves to touch or acknowledge.

Martha, when she had her stomach pain described in chapter 2, did the same thing. *Our bodies contain information that is beyond our intellectual mind's capacity to understand. We are much more than we think we are.* And when we acknowledge and then release our pain, our bodies and our lives become joyous and healthy. Martha has never had stomach pain again. And Brenda conceived three months after I removed the IUD, and gave birth to a healthy son. The work we do to transform our pain into joy heals the whole world.

CONQUERING OUR FEAR OF OUR SHAMAN PAST

In the Middle Ages, it is estimated that up to nine million women, many of them midwives and healers, were burned as witches. This witch craze, fueled by the Catholic Church, lasted for hundreds of years and has been well documented by others.[2] It's not uncommon for women who are reclaiming their power or speaking their personal truths to have terrifying dreams of being burned. I have heard this countless times in my work. The burning times have been suppressed for centuries but are now surfacing in our consciousness to be cleared and transformed so that the feminine and masculine energies can move into true partnership within each of us and men and women can co-create as equals. When I first wrote about this fear of our past, I had no idea how powerfully I, too, carried it. Only after the book was published and I started having nightmares about being murdered every night for a week did I see how prophetic my own words were.

When a woman enters into the work of healing her body and speaking her truth, she must break through the collective field of fear and pain that is all around us and has been for the past five thousand years of dominator society. It is a field filled with the fear of rape, of beating, of abandonment.

Rupert Sheldrake, Ph.D., a British biologist, posits that all the knowledge of the Earth's past exists all around us as electromagnetic fields of information, or "morphogenic fields."[3] Jung called it the collective unconscious. Quantum physics calls it the "unified field." When an athlete first breaks a world record, Dr. Sheldrake notes he or she often has to work for years to do it and is often told that it can't be done—that it is not humanly possible. It was once felt, for example, that no one would ever be able to run a mile in under four minutes. But once Roger Bannister did it, athletes all over the world were able to do it, too. The same is true for many other athletic feats. Dr. Sheldrake explains that the morphogenic field around this world record is changed by the first person who breaks it, thus making it easier for others to equal that performance by tapping in to the new morphogenic field. (For more information, see Dr. Sheldrake's website at www. sheldrake.org.)

Women all over the planet are finding the courage to break through the collective morphogenic field of shame, fear, and pain. One of my patients recently went home to tell her father what it was like to grow up in a household in which he had sexually abused her sisters and herself for years. She stood there and told all of it, not to change him but to break the years of silence. She later told me, "I am ready to go on national television with my father's name. He not only ruined my girlhood, but also has abused almost every girl in my neighborhood!" She finally had found the courage to feel her anger and pain. This is a first step toward transformation. True forgiveness can't come until a woman does this step. Another one of my patients had a mastectomy. When she was casually asked how she was doing, she graciously said, even to a male colleague who didn't know about it, "I am healing very beautifully from my mastectomy. You do know I had one, don't you?" Both of these women are breaking the silence—releasing the secrets that keep all of us trapped. They are saying, "No more!" All over the world, women like this are changing the morphogenic field of fear and silence. From Africa, where women are speaking out about female genital mutilation, to India, where selective abortion of females is being addressed, to the U.S., where we no longer tolerate intimate violence—silence is everywhere being broken and healing abounds!

Breaking the silence takes courage. I know of no woman who has tapped her inner source of power without going through an almost palpable veil of fear, often feeling as though her very life would be threatened by telling the truth. The journalist Vivian Gornick says, "For a woman, coming off fear is like an addict coming off drugs." I don't know any way around this fear except to name it and then go through it with the help of others who've also experienced it and come out on the other side. Millions of women healers and wise women, and the men who have supported them, have been killed for telling the truth. It is little wonder, given the collective history of women, that we have been afraid. When we deny this fear or discount its presence in others, we only give it more power. Experiencing the fear we collectively hold is a very important step toward healing—we need not judge it in others or in ourselves.

But as each of us acknowledges, feels, and moves through her fear, it becomes that much easier for the next woman to heal and the next one after her, just as when a world record is broken. We are changing the morphogenic field together, as thousands of women the world over break through their fields of fear at the same time. The first women who told the truth about their incest were accused of making it up. Now, when a woman remembers and speaks—no matter what the in-dignity she has suffered—support, books, the internet, and meetings are available for her. She need no longer feel alone, like she's crazy or the only one this has happened to.

And then, the magic starts. As you allow the life-force to guide your life, the exhilaration comes. Once you break through this fear and begin living your life according to your inner wisdom, you find you have everything you need to create a life for yourself that is based on free-dom, joy, and opportunity. I have seen this repeatedly and have experienced it myself. So take heart. There is great hope, joy, and love—all around us, all the time—when we clear ourselves of past habits, change our thinking, and embrace our power.

In 1993 I wrote the following: "I often think of myself as standing on the shoulders of all the strong women who came before me and being supported by them, women who had the courage to speak their truths even in the face of great opposition. I reassure myself with the thought, 'They can't burn me this time. There are too many of us this time. This time I am safe.' " Now, in 2006, I am happy to report that not only am I safe, I am freer and happier than I have ever been. My life is full of more abundance, more love, and more joy than I ever dreamed possible. I look back on where I was in 1993, and I smile with compassion for who I was then. And I want you to know that I see my own journey reflected daily in the lives of women the world over.

OUR DREAMS: EARTH'S DREAMS

Women are rising like yeast all over the planet.

—Sonia Johnson

As we heal, through feeling our grief and our joy, the Earth heals. Part of the rise of the feminine that I see happening all over the world is the strengthening of ties between women. Gwendolyn, one of the women we met earlier, said that as a result of her healing, "What has come into my life are beautiful female relationships. This never happened before because I put so much energy into men. Now a sisterhood is starting to happen. When you take the time to tune in to yourself and your needs, the sisterhood starts happening." I see it growing stronger and more powerful every day.

I couldn't do the work I do without the support of my sisters throughout the country. My women friends and colleagues sustain me. I feel supported and blessed. Brian Swimme, Ph.D., once wrote that we humans are the space where the Earth dreams through us. Our heart's desire is the desire of the Earth—it is what She is asking you to do. The dominator system has told us that "if it doesn't hurt, it is not worth doing—no pain, no gain." But often just the opposite is true. If what you are doing gives you no joy, no pleasure, no sense of purpose, no sense of fulfillment, it is not worth doing. Your state of health is the barometer of this. Your cells know what you need to do—listen!

Every cell in your body responds to your inner dreams and to plea-sure. All children know this. Joy and pleasure are necessary for your health and for that of our planet. The dreams the Earth dreams through you are different from the ones She dreams through me. But I need to hear your dreams, and you need to hear mine—otherwise we don't have the whole story. The dominator system has had a vested interest in keeping us from hearing each other for centuries. But our time has come. Let's listen to one another.

Personal Healing Is Planetary Healing

For all of written history, the Earth and the natural world have been viewed as feminine, with "virgin resources" to be "exploited." What happens to individual women and what happens to our planet are linked. Our personal and collective degradation of nature, women, and the feminine is drawing to a close, one person at a time.

Outmoded Newtonian science will not save us because it is obso-lete. It lacks the voice of intuition, the feminine voice, the voice that speaks from our bodies. We require balance now. We require embodied wisdom that is filtered through all of us—including what the mind of our bodies and our inner guidance is telling us.

I recall a cover of *Ms.* magazine showing a crowd of women with the headline *RAGE + WOMEN = POWER*.[4] This message made me uncomfortable until I saw the potential embedded in it. The anger and rage of silenced women, when used as fuel for positive change, is in-deed power. But it must be power from within, power that is fully grounded and centered—not rage directed *against* someone or some-thing. Rage *transformed* is power. Rage transformed is *strength*. It can be likened to fire—fire can destroy your house, or it can cook your din-ner. It all depends on how you use it!

To name your work "political," especially when it comes to your body and to things that are womanly, is an act of power. If you are a mother, believe me, your work is political. If you are a nurse, a child care worker, or anything else—your work is political. If you're healing a fibroid tumor or remembering your incest, you are doing political work. Breast-feeding is political.

How refreshing to see our body's healing as political. Let us give it the importance that it deserves! Gloria Steinem once said, "Any woman who is up off her ass is part of the women's movement." I like that a lot—it leaves room for a wide range of interpretations. We have many choices. No one but you gets to define your healing or your politics for you. Do you need to take six weeks off from work to heal from pelvic surgery? Think of it as political. And then when you've learned from it, see if you can channel future energy outward from your body into work that is positive and life affirming. Or if you need to take six weeks off just to enjoy and get in touch with yourself, that, too, is political!

In the epilogue to her book on her recovery from breast cancer, *A Burst of Light* (Firebrand Books, 1998), poet Audre Lorde writes, "I had to examine in my dreams as well as in my immune function tests the devastating effects of overextension. Overextending myself is not stretching myself. I had to accept how difficult it is to monitor the difference. Caring for myself is not self-indulgence, it is self-preservation, and that is an act of political warfare."[5]

In a political system that has not represented womanly values, each woman must represent herself and become a lobbyist for her own needs. Caring for yourself as well as you possibly can, *whether or not* you are sick, is indeed an act of political warfare.

Physician, Heal Thyself—Revisited

My inner guidance came to me through the mind of my uterus while I was in the process of writing the original edition of this book. I was diagnosed with a fibroid tumor that made my uterus about thirteen-week size. I had no symptoms. I had been eating an essentially dairy-free, low-fat diet for years. (I didn't know then that my intake of bread and high-glycemic foods was probably contributing to the problem.) At first I was saddened and didn't want anyone to know about it. I grieved for the loss of my "normal" uterus. When my colleague Annie Rafter did my pelvic exam and told me about the fibroid, the first thought that flashed through my mind was, "I better get this book finished, because I'm sure this growth is related to it."[6] I felt intuitively that it had started to grow in the early stages of my writing process, two years before. I also thought, "Damn, I've been hanging around too many women with fibroids. Maybe I caught one."[7]

I felt as though I had done something wrong, as though I had somehow failed. I was reminded that our emotions don't always match our level of intellectual development. I was humbled. Later that night, as I lay in my bed, I put my hands over my lower abdomen and said to my uterus, "Okay, now I have to take my own medicine and tune in to what you're telling me." My uterus gave me the following message: "This fibroid is a reminder that you need to learn how to move energy through your body more efficiently. If you take care of yourself now and pay attention, you'll avoid more serious problems in the future. This is also a wonderful opportunity to teach other women by example. Remember, the work you're doing with others applies to you. You've always believed that it is possible to dematerialize fibroids. Here's your chance." I meditated on creativity and what was needing to be birthed through me.

The next day I began a regimen of castor oil packs, and I started a course of acupuncture, something I'd been wanting to do as a general preventive measure for a long time. My acupuncturist told me that my kidney and triple warmed meridians were very low and had been for some time. This was related to overwork and stress and adrenal exhaustion. I was reminded of a chronic energy pattern called, in Oriental medicine, "stuck blood" or "stuck *chi,*" on the right side of my body. My previous migraine headaches had been on my right side; Caroline Myss had once diagnosed energy leaking out of my right hip, manifesting as a hip problem on the right; my breast abscess had been on the right; and now I had a fibroid on the right side of my uterus. All were on the right side of my body—the "masculine" or yang side—and all were related in an energy sense. What that meant to me was that it had been important to develop a strong foundation for my work and to take it out into the world—that was my "masculine" task. Up until the late 1980s I had been afraid of doing so fully because of my perception that the world wasn't ready to hear it and that it would be dangerous for me. Hence, the repeated "wounds" on my right side. The fibroid was simply the latest manifestation—and a timely one at that, given my life's work with women. And despite an ongoing recovery from relationship addiction, I realized how much I still wanted the approval of others, and I finally understood how powerless I am over what people will think of me. It became clear that the fibroid was about more than the book and the depleted acupuncture meridians. After several months of acupuncture and castor oil packs, it seemed to get larger, not smaller. My learning had to go much deeper. What did I need to learn?

I knew that fibroids are related to pouring your creativity into dead-end relationships or jobs. I assumed that mine was related to my work. I realized that my entire relationship with my office and with my profession needed to change—that I was in bondage to an obsolete form. While my heart wanted to write, lecture, and teach women a whole new way of being in relationship with their bodies, my intellectual sense of responsibility dictated that I continue to practice medicine in the way I had been trained: see patients, do surgery, and do my share of emergency calls like everybody else (my relationship addiction in yet another guise!). I realized that I needed more freedom. I needed to change my practice to teach more of the material in this book. I needed to be responsible to my deepest dreams and my innermost wisdom.

Women's health will never change substantially unless large groups of women begin to reclaim the wisdom of their bodies collectively. For me to do this meant letting go of being "the doctor" to the hundreds of women I'd enjoyed working with so much over the years. I didn't want to leave the practice of medicine—I wanted to transform it. I knew that I could no longer do primary care with all of its cultural assumptions, assumptions that were chaining me to limits that I could no longer tolerate.

I wanted to reinvent the practice of medicine in a whole new way. I realized at a deeper level than ever before that one-on-one health care, though valuable, tends to isolate each woman's problem and doesn't allow physicians the time necessary to educate a woman fully about all the issues that can affect her body and how she has the power to transform them. So I began to move toward teaching women in groups how to create health on a daily basis.

I wrote a letter to my patients that said, "I am not leaving the practice of medicine. I am redefining it and expanding into new areas that are critical to truly improving women's health over the long term." I told them that disease screening (which my training had prepared me for) and creating health (where my heart was taking me) were two different things. I needed to concentrate on a new form now. In my letter I asked my patients to consider the following questions. I ask you to do the same.

⁓ What would it be like if you reclaimed the wisdom of your body and learned how to trust its messages?

⁓ What would your life be like if you no longer feared germs or cancer?

⁓ How would your life be different if your body were your friend and ally?

⁓ How would your life be different if you learned how to love and respect your body as though it were your own precious creation, as valuable as a beloved friend or child? How would you treat yourself differently?

⁓ What would it be like to know, in the deepest part of you, that every part of your anatomy and each process of your female body contained wisdom and power?

These are the kinds of questions that women all over the world are now asking themselves—and, I'm thrilled to report, are finding answers to... answers that are transforming their lives and the lives of everyone they touch.

Though I was sure that the fibroid would start to shrink once I finished this book, that wasn't the case. It persisted and tended to wax and wane in size. I asked it to teach me. I had dialogues with it. I tried to love it. I then realized that my relationship to work was only one part of my life. I had to reevaluate every relationship I was in, including those with my husband and immediate family. I saw yet another pattern emerging: I tended to put my emotional and creative needs on hold until the needs of my husband and children were met. I allowed them to interrupt me in my home office and during my work, and I didn't set clear boundaries. My husband and I especially had to begin the process of renegotiating every part of our relationship, since my success made him feel "less than."

I also uncovered the deep belief that if I truly moved into my full potential, those closest to me would feel threatened and left behind. As a result of this, I felt responsible to help others become all that they could be as well, so that they could move ahead with me. (Or sometimes I felt the need to make myself "less than," so that I wouldn't be threatening.)

Just before Christmas 1996, the fibroid got bigger. An ultrasound documented that it was causing backup of urine in my left kidney. I found that I had gradually adjusted my life (and my wardrobe) around my fibroid. Though my periods were never a problem, and I had no symptoms, I simply got tired of having a protruding abdomen. I decided that it was time to let go of my dream of dematerializing my fibroid. I saw that I, too, had a belief that it was "good" to use "natural" methods to shrink the fibroid, but "bad" to seek the help I had so often offered to others. I had run headlong into my own addictive thinking. So I decided to schedule surgery—the path I had tried to avoid (and therefore energized) for four years. I called a trusted pelvic surgeon, a man to whom I have referred many patients, and made an appointment in which we scheduled the fibroid removal. I told almost no one, deciding that it would be best for me to contain my energies, thoughts, and feelings about this. I also started on a GnRH agonist (Synarel) to shrink the fibroid so that the incision would be smaller. (By now the fibroid had reached the size of a very large cantaloupe.) I experienced hot flashes on the Synarel and decided that for me, at least, these were not "power surges"—they were uncomfortable, sweaty disturbances in my day. But other than that, I had no problems, and the fibroid shrank nicely.

My surgery time arrived. I asked both my surgeon and my anesthesiologist to say the four healing statements to me. (See the section on surgery in chapter 16.) And in addition to the four healing statements, I asked the anesthesiologist to say the following and repeat it several times: "When you awaken, you will have released the emotional pattern associated with this fibroid." My surgery went well; there was only one large fibroid on the right side of the uterus, embedded in the wall; my recovery was easy, with very little pain; and I left the hospital the day after surgery. For the next three weeks I took naps, had acupuncture, watched movies, and rested. The surgery and recovery were a peak experience for me in many ways. I had faced something I had tried to avoid—the healing path of surgery—and in facing and moving through it I had found care, compassion, skill, and great healing there for me. Though I had wanted to write someday that I had dematerialized my fibroid in a blinding flash of insight, I came to see that in my case that wasn't to be, and my attachment to that as an "ideal" and "superior" path was just a case of spiritual materialism. (I still know it's possible, however, for women to dematerialize fibroids; I've seen it.)

Looking back on what I originally wrote about that fibroid in 1993 and again in 1998 with the first revision, I have to laugh at myself. I wrote about "carrying the creations" of others, needing to change my work, and on and on. I see now that I was circling around and around the real issue but was blind to it because I didn't want to go there. I didn't want to change the very thing that most needed change. My marriage. The thing that was right in front of my eyes. This is so often the case. Be careful what you ask for, the saying goes, because you'll probably get it! Sure enough, once my surgery was completed, those magic words that were whispered to me during anesthesia—"When you awaken, you will have released the emotional pattern that led to this condition"—began to work their magic. My marriage of twenty-four years ended in 1999, about a year and a half later. Like everything else in life of significance, this was a process, not an event. And as so often happens in life, I wasn't interested in taking this particular dose of healing medicine. I wanted to be married until death do us part. But the price was getting too high. And my body wouldn't let me forget it. I knew too much. If you don't pay attention the first time, you get hit by a bigger hammer. A fibroid today. Breast cancer tomorrow.

*   *   *

My fibroid, like all the conditions in our bodies, was a great teacher. Through it, I learned up close and personal that you can't create anything for another person, only for yourself. I also learned that when we face our worst fears and work through them, the process transforms us in miraculous and unpredictable ways. You can't take another person where he or she doesn't want to go, no matter how skillful, loving, and compassionate you are! But you can take yourself where you've been afraid to go. Personal growth and fulfillment are inside jobs. Ultimately each of us must tap in to the Source of creativity, wellness, and joy that is our birthright. Each of us has that ability. It gets strengthened through intent, faith, and the courage to choose pleasure over pain. And it never fails. My divorce forced me to grow in ways that I never dreamed possible. It forced me to take dominion over my life and my finances in ways I never would have otherwise. It forced me to really trust myself on all levels for the first time in my life. Though enormously painful at the time, I now feel nothing but gratitude! It made me into a wise woman.

We can't create a new world if we believe that we must remain small and ineffective on any level in order for others to love us or for them to feel safe around us. When we dim our light so that others appear to shine brighter, the whole world gets darker. I have had to apply this learning to all of my relationships, on all levels, from my marriage, to my friendships, to those with entire institutions such as hospitals and financial institutions. The issues in each situation, large or small, are always the same. And they boil down to the same fear: will I be loved if I become everything I was meant to be? Let me be the first to report to you from the front lines of this process. The answer is a resounding YES! But this love must begin with yourself first. When you become more loving toward yourself, more loving toward your body and its processes, and more appreciative of yourself, your vibration changes. Your point of attraction changes. If you wait for someone else to make the first move here, you'll be stuck in the painful, powerless, victim mode—complete with all its longing, pining, and health problems— endlessly. I've been there. It's hell. But when you have the courage to say "yes" to yourself, "yes" to your soul, and "yes" to life, and begin to realize that you deserve a heavenly, wonderful life right now, then fulfillment beyond your wildest dreams will start coming your way. And the world will open up to you in ways that you never before dreamed possible. Old, outmoded ways of being and living, and old, outmoded relationships will fall away. And this can be very painful.

Just think of it as the natural process of labor through which you are birthing your new self—a self that reflects who you really are and who you were always meant to be. It's always worth it.

MAKING THE WORLD SAFE FOR WOMEN: START WITH YOURSELF

If we are ever to create safety in the outside world for ourselves, we must first create safety for ourselves *right in our own bodies*. If, as we undress for bed, we look in the mirror and beat ourselves up for our breast size or our cellulite, we are not walking our walk. *We are not safe with ourselves.* If we can't create a safe space *within ourselves* for our own bodies—their shape, their size, their natural functions, and their weight—if we are forever putting down our own flesh and blood, starving our bodies, and giving them adverse messages, how can we ever expect anyone else to create health for us on the outside? Even if they did, we'd still be carting around our own internal terrorist!

The truth is that we can change only ourselves, not anyone or anything else. This is such good news and such a relief! After centuries of being told that someone else could, should, and would take care of us, we just became what they wanted us to become and did what they wanted us to do. But now we have the chance to take care of ourselves—together. We can create fulfilling lives on our own terms. A past Boston Women's Fund brochure said it best: "The people we've been waiting for are us." Aren't you energized just reading that? We can start saving ourselves now. We can start living our own lives now. This is the starting point for true partnership and communion with others—including men.

When we change ourselves *inside* by allowing ourselves to experience and own our long-suppressed emotions and woundings *as well as* our hopes and dreams for ourselves, our families, and our planet, the conditions of our lives change on the *outside*. Working for social changes must go hand in hand with the willingness to heal within ourselves all the internalized messages of blame, self-doubt, and self-hatred that are encoded in our very cells. Otherwise, our actions originate out of unhealthy places within us and simply re-create polarization and pain. Being led by the Spirit means living in tune with our inner guidance. Listen quietly. What do you need to do next? Perhaps just being still for a moment is the best way to heal or to serve. Perhaps there's nothing you need to do right now. There is no one "right way" to heal your body. The same goes for any area of life. You must find the way yourself. Emerson once wrote, "The essence of heroism is self-trust." Self-trust is more than the essence of heroism. It is also the basis for trusting our intuition and the healing voice of our cells. Sorting out the genuine messages from our innermost selves (and cells) is no small task. It is indeed the work of heroes.

It takes courage to learn to respect yourself and your body, regardless of how wounded you've been, regardless of your current weight, regardless of who you married or what your sexual preference is. I recently met a true hero who is the very embodiment of my message: when you change conditions inside yourself, the conditions outside yourself change in response. This hero is named Immaculée Ilibagiza (author of *Left to Tell* [Hay House, 2006], about the Rwandan holocaust), a beautiful woman with peace and divinity shining out of every pore. During the Rwandan genocide, Immaculée, along with seven other women, was forced to hide in a small bathroom for three months. Her entire family was murdered. Her weight dropped to sixty-five pounds, she was covered with lice, and she couldn't move or talk for fear of being discovered and killed by her former friends and neighbors, who repeatedly came to the door, demanding her death. Despite conditions of unimaginable suffering, she reached deep into herself with faith and conviction and found the living presence of God in her heart. By tapping in to this Source, she manifested miraculous events that saved her life and allowed her to eventually create a joyous life despite the loss of her family and country. Meeting this woman and reading her story has taken my faith to a new level. If she was able to face what she faced and not only survive, but thrive, the rest of us can do the same.

Whatever you call the inner power that Immaculée tapped in to— God, Goddess, Source, the Universe, or your Higher Power—know that it lives in each and every cell in your body. It is the one thing that we can count on always. The women whose stories I've shared with you are ordinary women; they are healing women. They have all tapped in to this source of goodness and miracles. Their stories are the stories of transforming pain into joy. These women are my heroes.

Self-healing is a highly personal and individual process. Self-healing requires personal disarmament, refusing to be at war any longer with a part of your body or your life that's trying to tell you something. Let war end with you. One of my patients, a fifteen-year member of Alcoholics Anonymous, summed this up beautifully: "Each morning I pray for willingness to do whatever it is I must do. *And I also pray to remain teachable.* There have been times in my life when no one could teach me anything. I thought I knew it all. I never want to be there again." Commit to creating heaven on Earth for yourself. Know that it takes great courage to be as happy and fulfilled as you can be. It takes great courage to resist the voices of doubt and fear that inevitably crop up in our minds and hearts when we decide to become as magnificent as we really are. Be courageous anyway.

Commit to living your dreams—one day at a time. This is the process that is required to create vibrant health in our families, our communities, and our planet. May you go forth now, to take a nap, to embrace a child, to feel the sun on your face, or to eat a good meal slowly, knowing deep within you that the next step for healing and living joyfully is already there, waiting for you to listen to it, waiting to be born into the world—through you, dear woman.

Resources

This resource section is updated with subsequent printings of this book. For the most up-to-date information, visit Dr. Northrup's website at www.drnorthrup.com.

Christiane Northrup, M.D., F.A.C.O.G.
P.O. Box 1999
Yarmouth, ME 04096
www.drnorthrup.com

Dr. Northrup welcomes your letters, although she is unable to answer your questions personally. She addresses many of her readers' questions on her website and in her bimonthly newsletter.

MEDICAL AND EDUCATIONAL LITERATURE FOR WOMEN
The Wisdom of Menopause: Creating Physical and Emotional Health and Healing During the Change (Bantam, 2006).

In Dr. Northrup's second book, she shows women how they can make menopause a time of personal empowerment and positive energy—emerging wiser, healthier, and stronger in both mind and body. The "change" is not simply a collection of physical symptoms to be "fixed," this book explains, but a mind/body revolution that brings the greatest opportunity for growth since adolescence. Dr. Northrup outlines how the choices a woman makes now—from the quality of her relationships to the quality of her diet—have the power to secure her health and well-being for the rest of her life.

Mother-Daughter Wisdom: Understanding the Crucial Link Between Mothers, Daughters, and Health (Bantam, 2005).

Dr. Northrup's latest book explains how the mother-daughter relationship sets the stage for our state of health and well-being for our entire lives. Because our mothers are our first and most powerful female role models, our most deeply ingrained beliefs about ourselves as women come from them. And our behavior in relationships—with food, with our children, with our mates, and with ourselves—is a reflection of those beliefs. In this book, Dr. Northrup shows how once we understand our mother-daughter bonds, we can rebuild our own health, whatever our age, and create a lasting positive legacy for the next generation.

Women's Health Wisdom Monthly E-Letter

Through her monthly e-letter, Dr. Northrup provides a forum for discussing safe, effective, and natural solutions to women's health problems. With her characteristic compassion, she presents the most up-to-date information on topics from help for hot flashes to choosing the best foods for your body. She also answers readers' health questions, shares personal success stories from readers, and recommends further reading. E-letter subscribers also have access to a wide range of products and services designed to help women live their lives more fully and healthfully. Available at www.drnorthrup.com.

The Dr. Christiane Northrup Newsletter

Dr. Northrup's monthly newsletter covers topics ranging from sexuality and menopause to the link between financial and physical health. In each issue, Dr. Northrup includes articles, recommended reading, and helpful tips so you can get to know your body, nurture your soul, and discover that "true health comes from within." Dr. Northup also answers readers' questions and offers guest columns by well-known authors, including Louise Hay, Terah Kathryn Collins, and Caroline Myss, Ph.D. Available at www.drnorthrup.com or through Hay House (800-654-5126 or 760-431-7695; www.hayhouse.com).

HEALING CARDS

Women's Bodies, Women's Wisdom Healing Cards: A 50-Card Deck and Guidebook.

The Women's Bodies, Women's Wisdom Healing Cards were created by Christiane Northrup, M.D., to help women reach clarity, fulfillment, and success in each of five major life areas: fertility and creativity, partnership, nurturance and self-care, self-expression, and the development of an enlightened heart and mind. The deck comes with a 72-page instruction booklet that offers a variety of practical ways to access intuitive, grounded information on a number of issues. Available from Hay House (800-654-5126 or 760-431-7695; www.hayhouse.com) or www.drnorthrup.com.

AUDIOTAPES

Dr. Northrup's audiotape programs are all available through www.drnorthrup.com or through Hay House (800-654-5126; www.hayhouse.com).

Mother-Daughter Wisdom: Creating a Legacy of Physical and Emotional Health

Dr. Northrup narrates an abridged version of her latest book, *Mother-Daughter Wisdom,* discussing the bonds passed from generation to generation that shape our physical, mental, and spiritual well-being.

Intuitive Listening—How Intuition Talks Through Your Body. Six-CD audio program by Christiane Northrup, M.D., and Mona Lisa Schulz, M.D., Ph.D.

Drs. Northrup and Schulz help you tune in to your inner guidance by understanding the language your body talks. The program covers immune-system health, endocrine-system and hormonal health, digestive health, the structural system, and the brain and mind.

Igniting Intuition: Unearthing Body Genius—Six Ways to Create Health, Happiness, and Almost Everything Else in Your Life. Six-tape audio program by Christiane Northrup, M.D., and Mona Lisa Schulz, M.D., Ph.D.

Dr. Northrup and Dr. Schulz teach you powerful, energizing, and life-changing tools for personal growth—how to use your body's own unique intuitive language to help you heal body, mind, and soul. With over thirty years of combined medical practice between them, Drs. Northrup and Schulz describe the seven emotional centers that are associated with the major organ systems in the body, and show how both good health and illness communicate information you can use to change your life. With wit and wisdom, they teach you how to recognize the patterns associated with disease so that you can change the conditions of the cells themselves by changing your thoughts, your relationships, and your activities.

Igniting Intuition. Two-tape audio program by Christiane Northrup, M.D., and Mona Lisa Schulz, M.D., Ph.D.

Drs. Schulz and Northrup explore the basics of how intuition is wired in the body and brain.

General Resources

Holistic Health Care Organizations

American Holistic Medical Association (505-292-7788; www.holisticmedicine.org)

The AHMA (founded in 1978) is an organization of licensed medical doctors (M.D.s), doctors of osteopathic medicine (D.O.s), and medical students studying for those degrees. Physicians from every specialty are represented. The AMHA website contains both an online physician referral directory as well as a guide to choosing a holistic practitioner.

Citizens for Health (612-879-7585; www.citizens.org)

Citizens for Health was formed by a group of ordinary people who believe that good health is a right, not a benefit that should be determined by government or based on economic or social status. This idea grew into a movement and is now a national and international network of thousands of individuals, young and old, at every level of society, who want to exercise their right to make informed choices regarding their health care.

Homeopathy

National Center for Homeopathy (877-624-0613 or 703-548-7790; www.homeopathic.org)

The NCH website has a wealth of information and resources, including an interactive directory to help you find a homeopath in your area.

Formulary Pharmacies

International Academy of Compounding Pharmacists (IACP) (800-927-4227 or 281-933-8400; www.iacprx.org)

IACP (formerly known as Professionals and Patients for Customized Care, or P2C2) is a nonprofit organization made up of more than 1,300 compounding pharmacists nationwide. The IACP website has a locator feature that can help you find a compounding pharmacy in your area.

Diagnostic Laboratories

Genova Diagnostics (800-522-4762 or 828-253-0621; www.gdx.net)

Genova Diagnostics offers hormone testing, as well as a wide range of other functional testing for bowel health, cardiovascular health, and more. Collection kits, articles, abstracts, and other publications regarding test methodology, clinical applications, and patient aids are available.

Botanicals and Herbs

Emerson Ecologics (800-654-4432 or 603-656-9778; www.emersonecologics.com)

Emerson Ecologics provides high quality nutritional supplements, antioxidants, vitamins, minerals, herbs, standardized herbal extracts, green foods, and essential fatty acids from the world's leading manufacturers of professional supplements.

Quality Life Herbs (207-842-4929; www.qualitylifeherbs.com)

My personal acupuncturist, Fern Tsao, and her daughter Maureen, both experts in the use of Chinese herbs, now distribute Chinese herbs internationally. All the herbs mentioned in *Women's Bodies, Women's Wisdom,* as well as numerous others, are available through mail order from Quality Life Herbs. Their products meet the highest standards possible for effectiveness and quality. I have referred patients to Fern for many years with excellent results in a wide variety of conditions.

Multivitamin-Mineral Supplements

USANA (888-950-9595 or 905-264-9863; www.usana.com)

USANA makes a superior line of nutritional supplements using pharmaceutical-grade ingredients. Other brands I recommend include Verified Quality, available through Emerson Ecologics (800-654-4432 or 603-656-9778; www.emersonecologics.com).

Chapter 1: The Patriarchal Myth: The Origin of the Mind/Body/Emotion Split

Anne Wilson Schaef, *When Society Becomes an Addict* (Harper & Row, 1987).

Riane Eisler, Ph.D., *The Chalice and the Blade: Our History, Our Future* (Harper & Row, 1987).

Riane Eisler, Ph.D., *Sacred Pleasure: Sex, Myth, and the Politics of the Body* (HarperSanFrancisco, 1995).

Chapter 3: Inner Guidance

Jerry and Esther Hicks, *Ask and It Is Given: Learning to Manifest Your Desires* (Hay House, 2004).

Deena Spear (607-387-7787; www.singingwoods.org)

Deena is a vibrational and acoustical healer with a degree in neurobiology from

Cornell University who combines 29 years of experience as a violin maker with her training as an energy healer from the Barbara Brennan School of Healing.

Chapter 5: The Menstrual Cycle

Lara Owen, *Honoring Menstruation: A Time of Self-Renewal* (Crossing Press, 1998).

The Red Web Foundation (415-469-5425; www.theredweb.org)
The Red Web is dedicated to creating a positive view of the menstrual cycle (in its entirety from menarche through menopause) for girls and women through education and community. The group is also committed to women rediscovering meaning in their cycles because, as their website states, "When we learn how to live wisely with life-cycles, we learn to ground our self-esteem in profound internal wisdom. Body image and menstrual cycles are interlinking facets of women's total health and well-being."

Menstrual Cramps (Dysmenorrhea)

See chapter 17 resources for nutrition information.
For castor oil packs, please see page 800, under "Dysfunctional Uterine Bleeding (DUB)."

Menastil:
Menastil (available from Claire Ellen Products, 508-366-6311; www.menastil.com) is an effective and fast-acting topical roll-on product made from an extract of *Calendula* petals and other essential oils, and clinically tested under FDA guidelines.

Acupuncture:
Call the American Association of Oriental Medicine (866-455-7999 or 916-443-4770; www.aaom.org) to locate an acupuncturist near you.

Bupleurum (Xiao Yao Wan):
For menstrual cramps, Xiao Yao Wan is available through Quality Life Herbs (207-842-4929; www.qualitylifeherbs.com).

Premenstrual Syndrome (PMS)

Seasonal Affective Disorder/Light Therapy:
To purchase a full-spectrum light, contact **Light for Health** (800-468-1104 or 303-823-0274; www.lightforhealth.com).

Progesterone Cream:
Progesterone cream 2 percent is available from a number of different sources. I have personally used the following preparations and find them comparable in quality and effectiveness.

Pro-Gest, available from Emerson Ecologics (800-654-4432 or 603-656-9778; www.emersonecologics.com), is also widely available through pharmacies and health food stores.

Natural progesterone capsules are available through any formulary pharmacy. (See General Resources above.)

Chinese Herbal Supplements:

Xiao Yao Wan Plus (also available as Soothing Flow) is a Chinese nutritional supplement that helps women with either PMS or perimenopausal symptoms. This supplement contains the herb peaonia, a well-known female tonic. Available from Quality Life Herbs (207-842-4929; www.qualitylifeherbs.com).

Dysfunctional Uterine Bleeding (DUB)

Castor Oil Packs:

Castor oil packs are wonderful for healing menstrual problems, urinary tract infections, joint aches and pains, and abdominal distress. Applied to the upper chest, they also can relieve a cough. The usual treatment frequency is one hour three to five times a week. (Don't use them during the heaviest days of the menstrual period.) Used once per week, they are also good preventive medicine. They have been shown to increase immune system functioning.

A castor oil pack is wool flannel saturated with castor oil, applied directly to the skin. On the side opposite the skin, a plastic sheet goes over the pack, and a heat source is applied. We highly recommend a hot water bottle for this purpose; though a heating pad can be used, a nonelectrical source of heat is preferred. Once a castor oil pack is made up, it can be stored for months in a plastic bag and reused over and over, simply adding more oil as necessary.

Castor and flannel are available from Emerson Ecologics (800-654-4432 or 603-656-9778; www.emersonecologics.com).

Preparing Our Daughters

See chapter 5 resources for information on the Red Web Foundation.

Joan Morais, *A Time to Celebrate: A Celebration of a Girl's First Menstrual Period* (Lua Publishing, 2003); www.joanmorais.com.

Chapter 6: The Uterus

Endometriosis

Jeanne Blum, *Woman Heal Thyself: An Ancient Healing System for Contemporary Women* (Tuttle, 1995).

Endometriosis Treatment Program St. Charles Medical Center (541-383-6904; www.endometriosistreatment.org)

The Endometriosis Treatment Program in Bend, OR, is based on the pioneering surgical treatment of endometriosis developed by David Redwine, M.D. Women from throughout the United States and Canada have been treated for their endometriosis pain upon referral from their physicians. The program publishes a very informative newsletter three times per year.

The Endometriosis Association (414-355-2200; www.endometriosisassn.org)
This is a networking and educational organization for those with endometriosis.

Many medical centers have divisions devoted to the treatment of fibroids. Here are several examples.

Fibroids

Cleveland Clinic's Menstrual and Fibroid Treatment Center (800-223-2273, ext. 46601 or 216-444-6601; www.clevelandclinic.org/obgyn)
This new arm of the famed Cleveland Clinic was designed to give women minimally invasive options to treat menstrual aberrations and alternatives to hysterectomy. The center also gives patients access to groundbreaking clinical trials, clinical research opportunities, and education programs.

Johns Hopkins Fibroid Center (410-583-2749; http://womenshealth.jhmi. edu/gyn/conditions/fibroids.html)
This new fibroid treatment center specializes in state-of-the-art therapies and the rapid application of new research (such as magnetic resonance imaging [MRI]—guided high intensity ultrasound), with an emphasis on minimally invasive techniques.

See chapter 5 resources for natural progesterone and how to find an acupuncturist.

See General Resources above for formulary pharmacies.

Hysterectomy

See chapter 14 resources for labs that perform salivary hormone testing.

Nambudripad Allergy Elimination Technique (NAET), Devi S. Nambudripad, M.D., D.C., L.Ac., Ph.D. (714-523-8900; www.naet.com)
Dr. Nambudripad is an acupuncturist and chiropractor who has had extensive experience both personally and professionally treating allergies. She has developed a system of allergy treatment that "reprograms the brain" so that one can get rid of allergies without avoiding allergens completely. She has written a book called *Say Goodbye to Your Allergies* (Delta Publishing, 1993) and actively trains health care practitioners in her innovative techniques. NAET has also been reported to help fibroids, endometriosis, and numerous other conditions. Write or call to find a practitioner in your area.

Indole-3 Carbinol from Longevity Science is available through Emerson Ecologics (800-654-4432 or 603-656-9778; www.emersonecologics.com).

Chapter 7: The Ovaries

See chapter 5 resources for listing of full-spectrum light sources.

Genetic Counseling

If you've had a family member with ovarian cancer, you may want to determine whether or not you are at a high genetic risk. I'd recommend consulting with a genetics counselor or contacting the Gilda Radner Familial Ovarian Cancer Registry at the Roswell Park Cancer Institute (800-682-7426 or 716-845-4503; www.ovariancancer.com).

Chapter 8: Reclaiming the Erotic

See chapter 9 resources under "Stress Urinary Incontinence" for weighted cones for Kegel exercises.

See Dialectic Behavioral Therapy, chapter 8.

Chapter 9: Vulva, Vagina, Cervix, and Lower Urinary Tract

Vulvodynia

Oxalate Levels of Selected Foods is available for $12, including shipping (but California residents, please add tax) from the university bookstore at the University of California at San Diego (800-520-7323; www.bookstore.ucsd. edu). Low-oxalate recipes are also available from the **Vulvar Pain Foundation** (336-226-0704; www.vulvarpainfoundation.org).

National Vulvodynia Association (301-299-0775; www.nva.org)
    Provides a newsletter, support groups, and information services.

See chapter 6 resources for NAET.

Urinary Tract: Chronic, Recurrent UTI or Interstitial Cystitis

See chapter 6 resources for NAET, which works well for interstitial cystitis.

Stress Urinary Incontinence

Kegel Exercises:
    Weighted vaginal cones (including sets of cones having graduated weights) can be used for Kegel-type exercises to help alleviate urinary stress incontinence.

FemTone Weights are available from As We Change (800-203-5585 or 619-213-2200; www.aswechange.com).

Incontinence Pessaries:
    Mentor Corporation makes pessaries under the tradename EvaCare (800-525-0245; www.mentorcorp.com).

Proanthocyanidins

These powerful antioxidants are found in grape pips and pine bark. Recommendations: start with 1 mg per pound of body weight per day, divided into three doses. After two weeks, cut back to 40–80 mg per day. I recommend:

Proflavanol and Proflavanol 90, available from USANA (888-950-9595 or 905-264-9863; www.usana.com).

OPC Pine Gold and *OPC Grape Gold*, manufactured by Primary Source and available from Emerson Ecologics (800-654-4432 or 603-656-9778; www.emersonecologics.com).

Many excellent brands of OPCs are also available at pharmacies and natural food stores.

See General Resources above for formulary pharmacies.

Chapter 10: Breasts

For castor oil packs, see chapter 5 resources.

National Lymphedema Network (800-541-3259 or 510-208-3200; www.lymph-net.org)
A nonprofit information and networking organization to help those with lymphedema, either primary (the kind one is born with) or secondary (the kind one gets after an operation or injury, notably mastectomy and lymph node dissection). They publish a very helpful newsletter.

Breast Cancer

The Cancer Report: *The Latest Research in Psychoneuroimmunology (How Thousands Are Achieving Permanent Recoveries)* by John Voell and Cynthia Chatfield (Change Your World Press, 2005). (For more information on this research, visit www.cancer-report.com.)

The Moss Reports (800-980-1234 or 814-238-3367; www.cancerdecisions. com)
Ralph W. Moss, Ph.D., a former science writer and assistant director of public affairs at Memorial Sloan-Kettering Cancer Center in New York, has spent the last three decades independently evaluating the claims of various cancer treatments (both conventional and alternative). His reports, ordered online and delivered via e-mail, contain information on the most successful and innovative treatments.

Sanoviv Medical Institute (800-726-6848 or 801-954-7600; www.sanoviv. com)
This fully licensed medical facility along the Baja Coast of Mexico (about an hour from San Diego) combines both traditional and complementary medicine practices to treat the whole person, addressing physical, mental, and spiritual health. It offers everything from surgery to spa facilities. Although Sanoviv helps cancer patients, it also treats those with autoimmune diseases, including lupus, multiple sclerosis, diabetes, chronic fatigue, and neurodegenerative diseases such as Parkinson's and Alzheimer's.

Strang Cancer Prevention Center (212-794-4900; http://home.strang.org)
If you are concerned about your risk for breast (or other) cancer, I highly recommend the information available from Strang.

Coenzyme Q10:
I recommend **CoQuinone 30** from USANA (888-950-9595 or 905-264-9863; www.usana.com), which contains alpha lipoic acid in addition to coenzyme Q10. I also recommend **Pure Coenzyme Q-10** by Verified Quality, available from Emerson Ecologics (800-654-4432 or 603-656-9778; www.emersonecologics.com).

Chapter 11: Our Fertility

Candace De Puy, *The Healing Choice* (Simon & Schuster, 1997). I highly recommend this compassionate and enlightened book to all those who are seeking guidance and more in-depth healing information concerning abortion.

Birth Intuitive

Teresa Robertson, R.N., C.N.M., M.S.N. (303-258-3904; www.BirthIntuitive. com)
Teresa, a certified nurse midwife, has been involved in birth for more than twenty years and currently teaches women to connect with their unborn babies to alleviate pregnancy and birth complications. She offers classes and workshops and is available for phone or in-person consultations. I consider her work the obstetrics of the future, which involves connecting with your baby intuitively before it is born and working in partnership with the baby's consciousness.

Emergency Contraception

The Office of Population Research at Princeton University and the Association of Reproductive Health Professionals jointly operate a *hotline* (888-NOT2LATE) and website (www.not-2-late.com or http://ec.princeton.edu/) that gives consumer information about emergency contraception. The website also has an updated list of providers who prescribe emergency contraception in the U.S. and parts of Canada that is searchable by zip code.

Fertility

Randine A. Lewis, *The Infertility Cure: The Ancient Chinese Wellness Program for Getting Pregnant and Having Healthy Babies* (Little, Brown, 2004).

Julia Indichova, *Inconceivable: A Woman's Triumph Over Despair and Statistics* (Broadway Books, 2001).

Niravi B. Payne, M.S., and Brenda Lane Richardson, *The Whole Person Fertility Program: A Revolutionary Mind-Body Process to Help You Conceive* (Three Rivers Press, 1997).

Natural Family Planning

OVULATION METHOD

American Academy of Natural Family Planning St. John's Mercy Medical Center, Department of Fertility Care Service (314-569-6495; www.stl catholics.org). Uses Creighton Model Ovulation method.

Billings Ovulation Method Association (888-637-6371 or 651-699-8139; www.boma-usa.org)

Ovulite (800-923-9023; www.ovulite.com)
   Ovulite helps a woman determine her ovulation and fertility cycles based on the chemical content of her saliva. Ovulite allows a woman to take a small saliva sample to determine not only whether she is or is not fertile, but also if she is approaching ovulation or departing from ovulation. Accuracy rate of 98 percent.

Ovusoft Fertility Software (757-722-0991; www.ovusoft.com)
   I recommend this highly detailed and feature-rich software program that's made to correspond with the highly successful methods developed by Toni Weschler, M.P.H., author of *Taking Charge of Your Fertility* (HarperCollins, 2002). Ovusoft Fertility Software not only automates Toni's methodologies but also allows for individual preferences and personally tailored formatting, forecasting, charting, and reporting.

Breeches, Prematurity, and Other Pregnancy Complications

Lewis Mehl-Madrona, M.D., Ph.D, *Coyote Medicine* (Scribner, 1997).

Lewis Mehl-Madrona, M.D., Ph.D; www.drmadrona.com (Contact Dr. Mehl-Madrona via e-mail at coyotehealing@aol.com)
   Dr. Mehl-Madrona is available for personal consultation regarding selected pregnancy problems such as breech presentation. He also gives workshops nationwide.
   Also see resources for chapter 11 for information on Teresa Robertson, a certified nurse midwife who currently teaches women to connect with their unborn babies to alleviate pregnancy and birth complications.

Pregnancy Loss

Lorraine Ash, *Life Touches Life: A Mother's Story of Stillbirth and Healing* (NewSage, 2004).

The following websites offer a wide range of support options and resources for further information geared to women who have lost a child:
   Empty Cradles (www.empty-cradles.com)
   Silent Grief (www.silentgrief.com)
   Ob/Gyn.net (www.obgyn.net/women/loss/loss.htm)

Chapter 12: Pregnancy and Birthing

Doulas

Professional labor support professionals—or doulas—usually work well within the medical system. To locate one in your area, ask your doctor or midwife, or call the labor and delivery unit of your local hospital. You can also contact the organizations listed below.

DONA International (formerly known as Doulas of North America or DONA) (888-788-3662; 812-482-5077; www.dona.org)

Association of Labor Assistants and Childbirth Educators, or ALACE (888-222-5223 or 617-441-2500; www.alace.org)

Marshall Klaus, M.D., John Kennell, M.D., and Phyllis Klaus, C.S.W., *The Doula Book: How a Trained Labor Companion Can Help You Have a Shorter, Easier, and Healthier Birth* (Addison-Wesley, 1993). (Formerly titled *Mothering the Mother*.)

Pregnancy and Childbirth Education

CIMS (888-282-2467 or 904-285-1613; www.motherfriendly.org)

The Coalition for Improving Maternity Services (CIMS), a United Nations–recognized NGO, is a collaborative effort of numerous individuals, leading researchers, and more than fifty organizations representing over 90,000 members. CIMS promotes a wellness model of maternity care that will improve birth outcomes and substantially reduce costs; CIMS developed the Mother-Friendly Childbirth Initiative in 1996. A consensus document that has been recognized as an important model for improving the health care and well-being of children beginning at birth, the Mother-Friendly Childbirth Initiative has been translated into several languages and is gaining support around the world.

International Childbirth Education Association (952-854-8660; www. icea.org)

Ina May Gaskin, *Ina May's Guide to Childbirth* (Bantam, 2003).

Pilates and Pregnancy

Elizabeth Jones-Boswell, M.Ed., *Exercise for Pregnancy and Beyond: A Pilates-Based Approach for Women* (Jones-Boswell, Inc., 2006). For more information about this program to ease pregnancy's discomforts through Pilates, contact Elizabeth (509-443-6497; www.pilatesrehab.org), a mother of four and a Pilates master.

Chapter 13: Motherhood: Bonding with Your Baby

Postpartum Depression

Postpartum Support International (800-944-4PPD or 805-967-7636; www.post-partum.net)

Postpartum Support International is an education, referral, and advocacy group devoted to increasing awareness about and discussion of postpartum depression. Its website has lots of background information, as well as a bookstore, internet forums, and chat rooms, links to local support groups across the country, and a self-assessment test.

Vaginal Dryness

A number of excellent natural lubricants are available to supplement vaginal moisture during times of hormonal shifts, such as postpartum and perimenopausally. See chapter 14 resources.

Circumcision

National Organization of Circumcision Information and Resource Centers (415-488-9883; www.nocirc.org)

Doctors Opposing Circumcision (DOC) (www.doctorsopposingcircumci sion.org)

A nonprofit organization providing publications, videos, and a newsletter in order to educate practitioners and parents on how to stop perpetuating the practice of circumcision.

Circumcision Resource Center (617-523-0088; www.circumcision.org)

Focuses on circumcision as an American cultural practice and as a religious practice.

Ronald Goldman, Ph.D., *Circumcision: The Hidden Trauma* (Vanguard Publications, 1997).

Ronald Goldman, Ph.D., *Questioning Circumcision: A Jewish Perspective* (Vanguard Publications, 1988).

Kristen O'Hara, *Sex as Nature Intended It* (Turning Point Publications, 2002).

Thomas J. Ritter, *Say No to Circumcision: 40 Compelling Reasons Why You Should Respect His Birthright and Keep Your Son Whole* (Hourglass Book Publishing, 1996).

Breast-Feeding

La Leche League International (800-LALECHE or 847-519-7730; www.lalecheleague.org)

This organization provides accurate information and grassroots practical support for successful breast-feeding.

International Lactation Consultant Association (919-861-5577; www. ilca.org)
This organization of health professionals specializes in promoting, protecting, and supporting breast-feeding worldwide.

Chapter 14: Menopause

See also General Resources for formulary pharmacies and chapter 5 resources, particularly for 2-percent progesterone cream.

Christiane Northrup, M.D., *The Wisdom of Menopause* (Bantam Books, 2006).
Dr. Northrup's interactive website (www.drnorthrup.com) is the best place to find regularly updated information on her lectures and other resources. Dr. Northrup also welcomes your letters.

Barbara Hand Clow, *The Liquid Light of Sex: Kundalini, Astrology, and the Key Life Transitions* (Bear & Co., 1991).

Individualized Hormonal Support

Many physicians and formulary pharmacists work in partnership with their patients to provide individualized hormone replacement solutions. Ask your physician about this kind of customized care; he or she can call a local formulary pharmacy to consult with a knowledgeable pharmacist.

Salivary Hormone Testing for Adrenal Function:
Your doctor must order this testing and the result will be sent to your doctor. I recommend that you have your health care provider order a test known as the Adrenal Stress Index or the Temporal Adrenal Profile.

Diagnos-Techs, Inc. (800-878-3787 or 425-251-0596; www.diagnostechs. com)
This lab, established in 1987, was the first in the country to implement salivary-based hormone assessment into routine clinical practice. They offer a wide variety of salivary tests and panels, and the company website also offers a provider referral service.

Genova Diagnostics Great Smokies (800-522-4762 or 828-253-0621; www.gsdl.com)
Offers salivary and blood hormone testing as well as a wide range of other functional testing for bowel health, cardiovascular health, and more. Collection kits, articles, abstracts, and other publications regarding test methodology, clinical applications, and patient aids are available.

Erika Schwartz, M.D., *The 30-Day Natural Hormone Plan* (Warner Books, 2004) and *The Hormone Solution* (Warner Books, 2002).
Erika Schwartz, M.D. (866-373-7452 or 212-873-3420; www.drerika.com)
Dr. Schwartz is the founder of the International Hormone Institute, which does research about natural hormones and educates the public about their benefits. She offers online consultations in addition to personalized three-month programs for balancing hormones.

Vaginal Dryness

A number of excellent natural lubricants are available to supplement vaginal moisture during times of hormonal shifts, such as postpartum and perimenopausally.

My personal favorite is **Crème de la Femme** (available through www.drnorthrup.com), a carbohydrate-free, oil-based vaginal lubricant that can be used as a vehicle for delivery of natural hormones to vaginal tissue when necessary. (The hormones have to be placed in the cream by a formulary pharmacist.) Hormonal addition is appropriate for menopausal and perimenopausal women, but not postpartum women in most cases.

Thinning Hair

Shou Wu Pian is an effective supplement for supporting hair growth on the head for those experiencing perimenopausal or menopausal hair loss. Available through Quality Life Herbs (207-842-4929; www.qualitylifeherbs.com).

Chinese Herbal Nutritional Supplements

Joyful Change is a Chinese herbal formula that helps alleviate hot flashes, night sweats, low back pain, hot palms and soles of feet, constipation, and breakthrough bleeding. Take three tablets twice per day before meals. Available through Quality Life Herbs (207-842-4929; www.qualitylife herbs.com).

Women's Phase II supplement is a combination of dong quai, licorice root, burdock, motherwort, and wild yam. It has been clinically tested by Tori Hudson, N.D., a naturopathic expert on women's health. Take two to six caplets per day. Available through Emerson Ecologics (800-654-4432 or 603-656-9778 or www.emersonecologics.com).

Revival Soy Products. See resources for chapter 17.

Flax

The Flax Council of Canada (204-982-2115; www.flaxcouncil.ca) endeavors to provide general flax facts of interest to consumers, as well as more specialized information for nutritionists, dietitians, food producers, manufacturers, and flax growers.

FiProFlax (ground flax) is cold-milled by Health from the Sun from premium-quality flax with a high oil content, and is available from Emerson Ecologics (800-654-4432 or 603-656-9778; www.emersonecologics.com).

Whole Flax Seed from Cathy's Country Store is organically grown golden flax. Available from Emerson Ecologics (800-654-4432 or 603-656-9778; www.emersonecologics.com).

Dakota Flax Gold is an organic flaxseed grown at Heintzman Farms in South Dakota (888-333-5813 or 605-447-5823; www.heintzmanfarms.com). A "starter kit" is available that consists of three one-pound bags of flaxseed and an electric grinder.

Chapter 15: Steps for Creating Vibrant Health

Imagine Your Future
Step Nine
Healing from Sexual Abuse

Family Violence Prevention Fund (800-313-1310 or 415-252-8900; http://end-abuse.org)

The FVPF's website has research, statistics, and resources such as a detailed Personal Safety Plan.

National Center for Victims of Crime (800-394-2255 or 202-467-8700; www.ncvc.org)

This organization is the leading resource and advocacy organization for crime victims in the U.S. The center's website offers a comprehensive collection of online resources for crime victims in addition to an extensive database of service providers for referrals.

Chapter 16: Getting the Most Out of Your Medical Care

Guidance for Alternative Medical Care

Mary Morton and Michael Morton, *Five Steps to Selecting the Best Alternative Medicine: A Guide to Complementary and Integrative Health Care* (New World Library, 1996).

Preparing for Surgery

Jeanne Achterberg and Barbara Dossey, *Rituals of Healing* (Bantam, 1994).
Successful Surgery. Guided-imagery audio program by Belleruth Naparstek. Available from Health Journeys (800-800-8661 or 330-633-3831; www.health journeys.com).

Belleruth Naparstek's audiobooks combine healing imagery, powerful music, and the most current understanding of the mind/body connection to engage the imagination in the healing process. Topics include asthma, cancer, chemotherapy, depression, diabetes, general wellness, grief, headache, PMS, pain, stress, stroke, surgery, weight loss, and more.

Prepare for Surgery, Heal Faster. Book and relaxation/healing audio program by Peggy Huddleston (800-726-4173 or 303-487-4440; www.healfaster.com), available separately or as a combination.

Chapter 17: Nourishing Ourselves with Food

See chapter 5 resources for information about full-spectrum lighting.

See chapter 6 resources for information about NAET.

See chapter 14 resources for information about hormone and nutritional testing.

Pharmaceutical-Grade Multivitamins

USANA (888-950-9595 or 905-264-9863; www.usana.com)
USANA offers state-of-the-art vitamins and mineral supplements. Their Essentials combined with Proflavanol comprise an excellent basic nutritional program.

Emerson Ecologics (800-654-4432 or 603-656-9778; www.emersonecolog ics.com)
Emerson Ecologics is a full-service distributor of high-quality nutritional and health products, with education support for health care practitioners.

Protein Supplements and Meal Replacement Options

USANA (888-950-9595 or 905-264-9863; www.usana.com)
USANA offers both meal replacement shakes and snack bars that are high in protein and balanced to avoid glycemic stress.

Revival Soy Products (800-738-4825 or 336-722-2337; www.revivalsoy.com)
Revival is a delicious soy protein meal replacement drink that contains 1490 mg of soy per serving. Marketed through the medical profession, it was designed by a group of physicians who wanted to add to the clinical research database on the health benefits of soy. The chocolate variety tastes like Nestlé's Quik. Many women who have used this product regularly have experienced complete resolution of their menopausal symptoms. Revival's meal replacement shake mixes contain 20 g of protein and more than 160 mg of soy isoflavones per serving, the equivalent of six servings of soy. Gram for gram, Revival Soy contains more isoflavones than soy milk, for example, simply because it is formulated from whole, genetically pure soybeans to be six times more concentrated than most other soy products. Revival also carries soy bars in a number of flavors (including several low-carb varieties).

Notes

Chapter 1: The Patriarchal Myth:
The Origin of the Mind/Body/Emotion Split

1. Jamake Highwater, *Myth and Sexuality* (New York: Penguin, 1988), pp. 8–9.

2. Anne Wilson Schaef, *The Addictive Organization* (HarperSanFrancisco, 1988), p. 58.

3. S. Plichta and M. Falik, "Prevalence of Violence and Its Implications for Women's Health," *Women's Health Issues*, vol. 11 (2001), pp. 244–58.

4. National Consensus Guidelines on Identifying and Responding to Domestic Victimization in Health Care Settings, The Family Violence Prevention Fund, San Francisco (Sept. 2002).

5. M. A. Rodriguez, H. M. Bauer, E. McLoughlin, and K. Grumbach, "Screening and Intervention for Intimate Partner Abuse: Practices and Attitudes of Primary Care Physicians," *Journal of the American Medical Association*, vol. 282 (1999), pp. 468–74.

6. L. Heise, M. Ellsberg, and M. Gotemoeller, "Ending Violence Against Women," Population Reports, Series L, no. 11, Johns Hopkins University School of Public Health, Population Information Program, Baltimore (Dec. 1999); H. M. Bauer, P. Gibson, M. Hernandez, et al., "Intimate Partner Violence and High-Risk Sexual Behaviors Among Female Patients with Sexually Transmitted Diseases," *Sexually Transmitted Diseases*, vol. 29 (2002), pp. 411–16; N. Romero-Daza, M. Weeks, and M. Singer, " 'Nobody Gives a Damn If I Live or Die': Violence, Drugs, and Street-Level Prostitution in Inner-City Hartford, Connecticut," *Medical Anthropology*, vol. 22 (2003), pp. 233–59; R. M. Harris, P. W. Sharps, K. Allen, et al., "The Interrelationship Between Violence, HIV/AIDS, and Drug Use in Incarcerated Women," *Journal of Associated Nurses AIDS Care*, vol. 14 (2003), pp. 27–40; P. Braitstein, K. Li, M. Tyndall, et al., "Sexual Violence Among a Cohort of Injection Drug Users," *Social Science & Medicine*, vol. 57 (2003), pp. 561–69; R. J. Peters Jr., S. R. Tortolero, R. C. Addy, et al., "The Relationship Between Sexual Abuse and

Drug Use: Findings from Houston's Safer Choices 2 Program," *Journal of Drug Education*, vol. 33 (2003), pp. 49–59.

7. V. Felitti, R. Anda, D. Nordenberg, et al., "Relationship of Childhood Abuse and Household Dysfunction to Many of the Leading Causes of Death in Adults," *American Journal of Preventive Medicine*, vol. 14 (1998), pp. 245–58.

8. "Gender and Education for All: The Leap to Equality Summary Report," UNESCO Publishing, Paris (2003).

9. World Health Organization Fact Sheet #241 (June 2000).

10. Amelia Gentleman, "India Still Fighting to 'Save the Girl Child,'" *International Herald Tribune* (April 15, 2005).

11. Fadia Faqir, "Intrafamily Femicide in Defence of Honour: The Case of Jordan," *Third World Quarterly*, vol. 22, no. 1 (2001), pp. 65–82.

12. Nathan Morley, "New Report Blames Cyprus Government for Virtually Uncontrolled Trafficking of Women," *Voice of America* (Nov. 27, 2003).

13. "Gender and Education for All: The Leap to Equality Summary Report," UNESCO Publishing, Paris (2003).

14. Saniye Gulser Corat, "UNESCO and Violence Against Women." Presentation to UNESCO, New York (Mar. 1, 2005).

15. Simone de Beauvoir, *The Second Sex* (New York: Alfred A. Knopf, 1953).

16. Anne Wilson Schaef and Diane Fassel, *The Addictive Organization* (Harper-SanFrancisco, 1988), p. 58.

17. Data from Oxfam America, 115 Broadway, Boston, Massachusetts 02116.

18. B. Grad et al., "An Unorthodox Method of Treatment on Wound Healing in Mice," *International Journal of Parapsychology*, vol. 3 (Spring 1961), pp. 5–24. This well-designed study showed that wound healing in mice was speeded up significantly (p. <.01) when a self-styled healer passed hands over the animals' cage.

19. M. T. Stein, J. H. Kennell, and A. Fulcher, "Benefits of a Doula Present at the Birth of a Child," *Journal of Developmental and Behavioral Pediatrics*, vol. 25 (5 Suppl.), (Oct. 2004), pp. S89–92; M. T. Stein, J. H. Kennell, and A. Fulcher, "Benefits of a Doula Present at the Birth of a Child," *Journal of Developmental and Behavioral Pediatrics*, vol. 24, no. 3 (June 2003), pp. 195–98; J. H. Kennell and M. H. Klaus, "Continuous Nursing Support During Labor," *Journal of the American Medical Association*, vol. 289, no. 2 (Jan. 8, 2003), pp. 175–76; M. H. Klaus, J. H. Kennell, S. S. Robertson, and R. Sosa, "Effects of Social Support During Parturition in Maternal and Infant Mortality," *British Medical Journal*, vol. 293 (1986), pp. 585–87; M. H. Klaus, J. H. Kennell, G. Berkowitz, and P. Klaus, "Maternal Assistance and Support in Labor: Father, Nurse, Midwife, or Doula?" *Clinical Consultation in Obstetrics and Gynecology*, vol. 4 (Dec. 1992); M. Klaus, J. Kennell, and P. Klaus, *Mothering the Mother: How a Doula Can Help You Have a Shorter, Easier, and Healthier Birth* (New York: Addison-Wesley, 1993), p. 25.

20. Stephen Hall, "Cheating Fate," *Health*, vol. 6, no. 2 (Apr. 1992), p. 38. Every doctor has seen at least a few cases of "spontaneous remission," and every year these cases are reported in the medical literature. Far too often, instead of being studied, they are ignored. Their existence flies in the face of the medical belief system.

21. Thomas E. Andreoli et al., *Cecil: Essentials of Medicine*, 2d ed. (Philadelphia: W. B. Saunders and Co., 1990), pp. 422–23.

22. K. Hartmann, M. Viswanathan, R. Palmieri, G. Gartlehner, J. Thorp, Jr., and K. N. Lohr, "Outcomes of Routine Episiotomy: A Systematic Review," *Journal of the American Medical Association*, vol. 293, no. 17 (May 4, 2005), pp. 2141–48.

23. Anne Wilson Schaef, *When Society Becomes an Addict* (Harper-SanFrancisco, 1987), p. 72.

24. Clarissa Pinkola Estes, *Women Who Run with the Wolves: Myths and Stories of the Wild Woman Archetype* (New York: Ballantine, 1992), p. 3.

25. Patricia Reis, "The Women's Spirituality Movement: Ideas Generated and Questions Asked." Presentation to feminist seminar, Proprioception Writing Center, Maine (Dec. 3, 1990).

Chapter 2: Feminine Intelligence and a New Mode of Healing

1. Stephanie Field et al., *Science News*, vol. 127, no. 301; reported in *Brain/Mind Bulletin*, Dec. 9, 1985.

2. Marshall H. Klaus and John H. Kennell, *Parent/Infant Bonding*, 2d ed. (St. Louis: C. V. Mosby Co., 1982).

3. L. F. Berman and S. L. Syme, "Social Networks, Host Resistance, and Mortality: A Nine-Year Follow-up of Almeda County Residents," *American Journal of Epidemiology*, vol. 109 (1978), pp. 186–204.

4. Jeanne Achterberg, *Imagery in Healing: Shamanism and Modern Medicine* (Boston: Shambhala, 1985).

5. V. J. Felitti, R. F. Anda, D. Nordenberg, D. F. Williamson, A. M. Spitz, V. Edwards, M. P. Koss, and J. S. Marks, "Relationship of Childhood Abuse and Household Dysfunction to Many of the Leading Causes of Death in Adults. The Adverse Childhood Experiences (ACE) Study," *American Journal of Preventive Medicine*, vol. 14, no. 4 (May 1998), pp. 245–58.

6. Michael Gershon, *The Second Brain* (New York: HarperCollins, 1998).

7. Candace Pert, *Molecules of Emotion: Why You Feel the Way You Feel* (New York: Scribner, 1997).

8. Larry Dossey, *Healing Words: The Power of Prayer and the Practice of Medicine* (San Francisco: HarperSanFrancisco, 1993).

9. Quoted from personal notes of 1991 lecture series, Mystery School Program, at which Jean Houston was the facilitator.

10. Anne Moir and David Jessel, *Brain Sex* (New York: Carol Publishing Co., a Lyle Stuart Book, 1991), p. 195.

11. Robert Bly and Deborah Tannen, "Where Are Women and Men Today," *New Age*, Jan–Feb. 1992, p. 32.

12. S. J. Schleifer et al., "Depression and Immunity: Lymphocyte Function in Ambulatory Depressed Patients, Hospitalized Schizophrenic Patients, and Patients

Hospitalized for Herniorrhaphy," *Archives of General Psychiatry*, vol. 42 (1985), pp. 129–33.

13. J. K. Kiecolt-Glaser et al., "Stress, Loneliness, and Changes in Herpes Virus Latency," *Journal of Behavioral Medicine*, vol. 8, no. 3 (1985), pp. 249–60.

14. The following autoimmune diseases affect women much more frequently than men: Systemic lupus erythematosus—90 percent of sufferers are women. Myasthenia gravis—85 percent are women. Autoimmune thyroid disease—80 percent are women. Rheumatoid arthritis—75 percent are women. Multiple sclerosis—70 percent are women.

15. S. F. Maier et al., "Opiate Antagonists and Long-Term Analgesic Reaction Induced by Inescapable Shock in Rats," *Journal of Comparative Physiology and Psychology*, vol. 4 (Dec. 1980), pp. 1177–83; M. L. Laudenslager, "Coping and Immunosuppression: Inescapable but Not Escapable Shock Suppresses Lymphocyte Proliferation," *Science*, Aug. 1983, pp. 568–70; Steven E. Locke et al., "Life Change Stress, Psychiatric Symptoms and Natural Killer Cell Activity," *Psychosomatic Medicine*, vol. 46, no. 5 (1984), pp. 441–53; B. S. Linn et al., "Degree of Depression and Immune Responsiveness," *Psychosomatic Medicine*, vol. 44 (1982), p. 128.

16. R. J. Weber and C. B. Pert, "Opiatergic Modulation of the Immune System," in E. E. Muller and Andrea R. Genazzani, eds., *Central and Peripheral Endorphins* (New York: Raven Press, 1984), p. 35.

17. R. L. Roessler et al., "Ego Strength, Life Changes, and Antibody Titers," paper presented at the annual meeting of the American Psychosomatic Society, Dallas, Texas, Mar. 25, 1979.

18. B. R. Levy, M. D. Slade, S. R. Kunkel, and S. V. Kasl, "Longevity Increased by Positive Self-Perceptions of Aging," *Journal of Personality and Social Psychology*, vol. 83, no. 2 (Aug. 2002), pp. 261–70.

19. Ellen Langer, *Mindfulness* (Reading, MA: Addison-Wesley, 1989), pp. 100–13.

20. Maude Guerin, "Psychosocial Lecture Notes," Department of Obstetrics and Gynecology, Michigan State University School of Medicine, Lansing, MI, 1991.

21. Elisabeth Kübler-Ross, *On Death and Dying* (New York: Macmillan, 1969).

Chapter 3: Inner Guidance

1. Stephen Sullivan, "Inhibition of Salivary and Lacrimal Secretion by an Enkephalin Analogue," *American Journal of Psychiatry*, vol. 139, no. 3 (Mar. 1982), pp. 385–86.

2. W. G. Frey et al., "Effect of Stimulus on the Composition of Tears," *American Journal of Ophthalmology*, vol. 92, no. 4 (1982), pp. 559–67.

3. Olga and Ambrose Worrall, *The Gift of Healing* (Columbus, OH: Ariel Press, 1985). The work of Olga Worrall, a world-renowned intuitive healer, was studied and documented by physicians at Johns Hopkins School of Medicine. The book is available from Ariel Press, P.O. Box 30975, Columbus, OH 43230. Her work is currently being carried on by Dr. Robert Leichtman. Edgar Cayce is another well-known medical intuitive.

4. Marilyn Ferguson, "Commentary: Waking up in the Dark," *Brain/Mind and Common Sense*, Apr. 1993, p. 3.

5. E. R. McDonald, S. A. Wiedenfeld, A. Hillel, C. L. Carpenter, and R. A. Walter, "Survival in Amyotrophic Lateral Sclerosis: The Role of Psychological Factors," *Archives of Neurology*, vol. 51, no. 1 (Jan. 1994), pp. 17–23.

6. Fox, quoted in Michael Toms, "Renegade Priest: An Interview with Matthew Fox," *The Sun*, issue 89 (Aug. 1991), p. 10.

Chapter 4: The Female Energy System

1. Graham Bennette, "Psychic and Cellular Aspects of Isolation and Identity Impairment in Cancer," *Annals of the New York Academy of Science*, vol. 131 (1972), pp. 352–63.

2. C. E. Wenner and S. Weinhouse, "Diphosphopyridine Nucleotide Requirements of Oxidations by Mitochondria of Normal and Neoplastic Tissues," *Cancer Research*, vol. 12 (1952), pp. 306–7.

3. I am talking about common patterns here. Some illnesses are mysterious—almost archetypal—and don't fit the personal patterns I describe in this section.

4. D. B. Clayson, *Chemical Carcinogenesis* (London: Churchill Publishers, 1962).

5. Caroline B. Thomas and K. R. Duszynski, "Closeness to Parents and the Family Constellation in Prospective Study of Five Disease States: Suicide, Mental Illness, Malignant Tumor, Hypertension, Coronary Heart Disease," *Johns Hopkins Medical Journal*, vol. 134 (1974), pp. 251–70.

6. Personal communication from a colleague.

7. See Norm Shealy and Caroline Myss, *The Creation of Health* (Walpole, NH: Stillpoint Publications, 1988), and also C. Myss, *Anatomy of the Spirit* (New York: Harmony Books, 1996), which goes into much more detail on the human energy system. Dr. Shealy, a neurosurgeon who founded the American Holistic Medical Association, has done extensive research on energy medicine with Caroline Myss. A world-renowned medical intuitive, Myss needs to know only the name and age of an individual to be able to give a full diagnostic reading; the individual can be located anywhere in the world. For several years, Caroline assisted me in clinical practice with energy readings on my own patients, whose physical conditions were correlated with energy anatomy. Her concepts formed the original basis for this chapter. In the revised edition, I was assisted in updating the material by Mona Lisa Schulz, M.D., Ph.D., who is both a psychiatrist and a behavioral neuroscientist with an extensive research background. She is also a practicing medical intuitive and the research editor for *Health Wisdom for Women*.

8. G. A. Bachman et al., "Childhood Sexual Abuse and Consequences in Adult Women," *Obstetrics and Gynecology*, vol. 71, no. 4 (1988), pp. 631–41.

9. R. C. Reiter et al., "Correlation Between Sexual Abuse and Somatization in Women with Somatic and Nonsomatic Pain," *American Journal of Obstetrics and Gynecology*, vol. 165, no. 1 (1991), p. 104.

10. Scientific studies supporting this premise include M. Tarlau and M. A. Smalheiser, "Personality Patterns in Patients with Malignant Tumors of the Breast and

Cervix," *Psychosomatic Medicine*, vol. 13 (1951), p. 117. In this study of women with cervical cancer, most of the subjects had uniformly negative feelings toward heterosexual relations. Most of them had a higher incidence of premarital sexual experiences, and nearly 75 percent had had multiple marriages ending in divorce or separation.

11. Colin A. Ross, "Childhood Sexual Abuse and Psychosomatic Symptoms in Irritable Bowel Syndrome," *Journal of Child Sexual Abuse*, vol. 14, no. 1 (2005), pp. 27–38; P. Salmon, K. Skaife, and J. Rhodes, "Abuse, Dissociation, and Somatization in Irritable Bowel Syndrome: Towards an Explanatory Model," *Journal of Behavioral Medicine*, vol. 26, no. 1 (Feb. 2003), pp. 1–18; Sarah Payne, "Sex, Gender, and Irritable Bowel Syndrome: Making the Connections," *Gender Medicine*, vol. 1, no. 1 (Aug. 2004), pp. 18–28; J. M. Lackner, G. D. Gudleski, and E. B. Blanchard, "Beyond Abuse: The Association Among Parenting Style, Abdominal Pain, and Somatization in IBS Patients," *Behaviour Research and Therapy*, vol. 42, no. 1 (Jan. 2004), pp. 41–56; D. A. Drossman, Y. Ingel, B. A. Vogt, J. Leserman, W. Lin, J. K. Smith, and W. Whitehead, "Alterations of Brain Activity Associated with Resolution of Emotional Distress and Pain in a Case of Severe Irritable Bowel Syndrome," *Gastroenterology*, vol. 124, no. 3 (Mar. 2003), pp. 754–61; A. Ali, B. B. Toner, N. Stuckless, R. Gallop, N. E. Diamant, M. I. Gould, and E. I. Vidins, "Emotional Abuse, Self-Blame, and Self-Silencing in Women with Irritable Bowel Syndrome," *Psychosomatic Medicine*, vol. 62, no. 1 (Jan.–Feb. 2000), pp. 76–82.

12. "The differences in body image scores between the body-exterior cancer group and the body-interior cancer group seem to reflect basic differences in personality orientation." S. Fisher and S. E. Cleveland, "Relationship of Body Image to Site of Cancer," *Psychosomatic Medicine*, vol. 18, no. 4 (1956), p. 309.

13. Tarlau and Smalheiser, "Personality Patterns" (see note 10).

14. J. I. Wheeler and B. M. Caldwell, "Psychological Factors in Breast Cancer: A Preliminary Study of Some Personality Trends in Patients with Cancer of the Breast," *Psychosomatic Medicine*, vol. 17 (1955), p. 96; A. H. Labrum, "Psychological Factors in Gynecologic Cancer," *Primary Care*, vol. 3, no. 4 (1976), pp. 811–24.

Chapter 5: The Menstrual Cycle

1. E. Hartman, "Dreaming Sleep (the D State) and the Menstrual Cycle," *Journal of Nervous and Mental Disease*, vol. 143 (1966), pp. 406–16; E. M. Swanson and D. Foulkes, "Dream Content and the Menstrual Cycle," *Journal of Nervous and Mental Disease*, vol. 145, no. 5 (1968), pp. 358–63.

2. F. A. Brown, "The Clocks: Timing Biological Rhythms," *American Scientist*, vol. 60 (1972), pp. 756–66; M. Gauguelin, "Wrangle Continues of Pseudoscientific Nature of Astrology," *New Scientist*, Feb. 25, 1978; W. Menaker, "Lunar Periodicity in Human Reproduction: A Likely Unit of Biological Time," *American Journal of Obstetrics and Gynecology*, vol. 77, no. 4 (1959), pp. 904–14; E. M. Dewan, "On the Possibility of the Perfect Rhythm Method of Birth Control by Periodic Light Stimulation," *American Journal of Obstetrics and Gynecology*, vol. 99, no. 7 (1967), pp. 1016–19.

3. R. P. Michael, R. W. Bonsall, and P. Warner, "Human Vaginal Secretion and Volatile Fatty Acid Content," *Science*, vol. 186 (1974), pp. 1217–19; W. B. Cutler, "Human Sex-Attractant Pheromones: Discovery Research, Development, and Application in Sex Therapy," *Psychiatric Annals*, vol. 29 (1999), pp. 54–59.

4. Charles Wira, "Mucosal Immunity: The Primary Interface Between the Patient and the Outside World," in "The ABC's of Immunology," course syllabus, Dartmouth Hitchcock Medical Center, September 20–21, 1996.

5. E. Hampson and D. Kimura, "Reciprocal Effects of Hormonal Fluctuations on Human Motor and Perceptual Skills," *Behavioral Neuroscience*, vol. 102 (1988), pp. 456–59.

6. Wira, "Mucosal Immunity" (see note 4).

7. Demetra George, *Mysteries of the Dark Moon: The Healing Power of the Dark Goddess* (HarperSanFrancisco, 1992), pp. 70–71.

8. Menaker, "Lunar Periodicity" (see note 2).

9. Lunar data adapted from Caroline Myss.

10. Hartman, "Dreaming Sleep," and Swanson and Foulkes, "Dream Content" (see note 1).

11. M. Altemus, B. E. Wexler, and N. Boulis, "Neuropsychological Correlates of Menstrual Mood Changes," *Psychosomatic Medicine*, vol. 51 (1989), pp. 329–36.

12. Therese Benedek and Boris Rubenstein, "Correlations Between Ovarian Activity and Psychodynamic Processes: The Ovulatory Phase," *Psychosomatic Medicine*, vol. 1, no. 2 (1939), pp. 245–70.

13. Bernard C. Gines, "Cultural Hypnosis of the Menstrual Cycle," *New Concepts of Hypnosis* (London: George Allen Press, 1953).

14. Diane Ruble, "Premenstrual Symptoms: A Reinterpretation," *Science*, vol. 197 (July 15, 1977), pp. 291–92.

15. For further information, see Riane Eisler, *The Chalice and the Blade: Our History, Our Future* (HarperSanFrancisco, 1988) and Marija Gimbutas, *Goddesses and Gods of Old Europe, 7000 to 35 B.C.* (Berkeley and Los Angeles: University of California Press, 1982). The degradation of women's wisdom took place gradually. By the time European settlers arrived in what would become the United States, native tribes were mixed in their approach to women. Some degraded them and their bodily processes, setting them apart in shame, while others revered women's wisdom.

16. Credit for the term *offices of womanhood* goes to Tamara Slayton. See also Brooke Medicine Eagle, "Women's Moontime: A Call to Power," *Shaman's Drum*, vol. 4 (Spring 1986), p. 21.

17. P. L. Brown and W. M. O'Neil, cited in P. Shuttle and P. Redgrove, *The Wise Wound* (New York: Grove, 1986).

18. Quoted by Dr. Ronald Norris at lecture on PMS (Rockland, ME, Nov. 1982).

19. R. Loudall, P. Snow, and J. Johnson, "Myths about Menstruation: Victims of Our Folklore," *International Journal of Women's Studies*, vol. 1 (1984), p. 70; W. M. O'Neil, *Time and the Calendars* (Manchester, UK: Manchester University Press, 1976); P. L. Brown, *Megaliths, Myths and Men: An Introduction to Astro-Archeology* (London: Blandford Press, 1976).

20. Dr. John Goodrich, lecture on adolescent gynecology, Maine Medical Center, Portland, ME, July 29, 1992.

21. Quoted from Tampax box insert, given to me by Gina Orlando.

22. A. H. DeCherney, "Hormone Receptors and Sexuality in the Human Female," *Journal of Women's Health and Gender-Based Medicine*, vol. 9, supplement 1 (2000), pp. S9–13.

23. For an in-depth discussion of postpartum sexuality, please see my book *Mother-Daughter Wisdom* (New York: Bantam, 2005), pp. 99–100.

24. Cutler, "Human Sex-Attractant Pheromones" (see note 3).

25. M. K. McClintock, "Menstrual Synchrony and Suppression," *Nature*, vol. 299 (1971), pp. 244–45.

26. M. C. P. Rees, A. Anderson, et al., "Prostaglandins in Menstrual Fluid in Menorrhagia and Dysmenorrhea," *British Journal of Obstetrics and Gynecology*, vol. 91 (1984), p. 673.

27. K. M. Fairfield, D. J. Hunter, G. A. Colditz, C. S. Fuchs, D. W. Cramer, F. E. Speizer, W. C. Willett, and S. E Hankinson, "A Prospective Study of Dietary Lactose and Ovarian Cancer," *International Journal of Cancer*, vol. 110, no. 2 (June 10, 2004), pp. 271–77.

28. Z. Harel, F. M. Biro, R. K. Kottenhahn, and S. L. Rosenthal, "Supplementation with Omega-3 Fatty Acids in the Management of Dysmenorrhea in Adolescents," *American Journal of Obstetrics and Gynecology*, vol. 174 (1996), pp. 1335–38.

29. G. E. Abraham, "Nutritional Factors in the Etiology of the Premenstrual Tension Syndromes," *Journal of Reproductive Medicine*, vol. 28, no. 7 (1983), pp. 446–64.

30. F. Facchinetti et al., "Magnesium Prophylaxis of Menstrual Migraine," *Headaches*, vol. 31 (1991), pp. 298–304; F. Facchinetti et al., "Oral Magnesium Successfully Relieves Premenstrual Mood Changes," *Obstetrics and Gynecology*, vol. 78, no. 2 (Aug. 1991), pp. 177–81.

31. E. B. Butler and E. McKnight, "Vitamin E in the Treatment of Primary Dysmenorrhea," *Lancet*, vol. 1 (1955), pp. 844–47.

32. Joseph M. Helms, "Acupuncture for the Management of Primary Dysmenorrhea," *Obstetrics and Gynecology*, vol. 69, no. 1 (Jan. 1987), pp. 51–56.

33. The diagnosis of "liver stagnation" or "blocked liver *chi*" is supported by the fact that the herbs mentioned have been shown to normalize elevated liver enzymes. Margaret Naeser, "Outline Guide to Chinese Herbal Patent Medicines in Pill Form—with Sample Pictures of the Boxes: An Introduction to Chinese Medicine," available from Boston Chinese Medicine Society, P.O. Box 5747, Boston, MA 02114.

34. During the menstrual cycle, excess epinephrine released via stress (known as autonomic overdrive) may disrupt the natural autonomic nervous system balance. E. W. Winenman, "Autonomic Balance Changes During the Human Menstrual Cycle," *Psychophysiology*, vol. 8, no. 1 (1971), pp. 1–6.

35. There is no uniformly agreed-upon definition of PMS in the medical literature, so many of the studies on the incidence of this disorder disagree. Regardless of medical definition, the experience of thousands of women around their menstrual cycle is one

of emotional and physical suffering. F. L. Reid and S. S. Yen, "Premenstrual Syndrome," *American Journal of Obstetrics and Gynecology*, vol. 139 (1981), p. 86.

36. Ronald Norris, "Progesterone for Premenstrual Tension," *Journal of Reproductive Medicine*, vol. 28, no 8 (Aug. 1983), pp. 509–15.

37. D. L. Jakubowicz, E. Godard, and J. Dewhurst, "The Treatment of Premenstrual Tension and Mefanamic Acid: Analysis of Prostaglandin Concentration," *British Journal of Obstetrics and Gynaecology*, vol. 91 (1984), p. 78.

38. In one study, PMS patients consumed five times more dairy products than controls without PMS. The excess calcium intake from the dairy products may hinder magnesium absorption. G. S. Goci and G. E. Abraham, "Effect of Nutritional Supplement...on Symptoms of Premenstrual Tension," *Journal of Reproductive Medicine*, vol. 83 (1982), pp. 527–31.

39. A. M. Rossignol, "Caffeine-Containing Beverages and Premenstrual Syndrome in Young Women," *American Journal of Public Health*, vol. 75, no. 11 (1985), pp. 1335–37.

40. B. L. Snider and D. F. Dietman, "Pyridoxine Therapy for Premenstrual Acne Flare," *Archives of Dermatology*, vol. 110 (July 1974); G. E. Abraham and J. T. Hargrove, "Effect of Vitamin B on Premenstrual Tension Syndrome: A Double Blind Crossover Study," *Infertility*, vol. 3 (1980), p. 155; M. S. Biskind, "Nutritional Deficiency in the Etiology of Menorrhagia Cystic Mastitis, Premenstrual Syndrome, and Treatment with Vitamin B Complex," *Journal of Clinical Endocrinology and Metabolism*, vol. 3 (1943), pp. 227–334; R. W. Engel, "The Relation of B Complex Vitamins and Dietary Fat to the Lipotropic Action of Choline," *Journal of Biological Chemistry*, vol. 37 (1941), p. 140.

41. D. G. Williams, "The Forgotten Hormone," *Alternatives*, vol. 4, no. 6 (1991), p. 11.

42. B. L. Denrefer et al., "Progesterone and Adenosine 3,5' Monophospate Formation by Isolated Corpora Lutea of Different Ages: Influence of Human Chorionic Gonadotropin and Prostaglandins," *Journal of Clinical Endocrinology and Metabolism*, vol. 3 (1943), pp. 227–34.

43. B. R. Goldin et al., "Estrogen Excretion Patterns and Plasma Levels in Vegetarian and Omnivorous Women," *New England Journal of Medicine*, vol. 307 (1982), pp. 1542–47; B. R. Goldin et al., "Effect of Diet on Excretion of Estrogens in Pre- and Post-Menopausal Women," *Cancer Research*, vol. 41 (1981), pp. 3771–73.

44. G. E. Abraham, "Nutritional Factors in the Etiology of the Premenstrual Tension Syndromes," *Journal of Reproductive Medicine*, vol. 28 (1983), p. 446; M. Lubran and G. Abraham, "Serum and Red Cell Magnesium Levels in Patients with Premenstrual Tension," *American Journal of Clinical Nutrition*, vol. 34 (1982), p. 2364; G. E. Abraham and J. T. Hargrove, "Effect of Vitamin B on Premenstrual Tension Syndrome: A Double Blind Crossover Study," *Infertility*, vol. 3 (1980), p. 155; Facchinetti et al., "Oral Magnesium" (see note 30).

45. R. S. Landau et al., "The Effect of Alpha Tocopherol in Premenstrual Symptomatology: A Double-Blind Trial," *Journal of the American College of Nutrition*, vol. 2 (1983), pp. 115–23; M. R. Werback, *Nutritional Influences on Illness* (Tarzana, CA: Third Line Press, 1988).

46. Lubran and Abraham, "Serum and Red Cell Magnesium Levels" (see note 44); Facchinetti et al., "Oral Magnesium" (see note 30).

47. B. L. Parry et al., "Morning vs. Evening Bright Light Treatment of Late Luteal Phase Dysphoric Disorder," *American Journal of Psychiatry*, vol. 146 (1991), p. 9.

48. J. Ott, *Health and Light* (New York: Pocket Books, 1978); Z. Kime, *Sunlight Could Save Your Life* (Penryn, CA: World Health Publications, 1980, available by writing to World Health Publications, P.O. Box 400, Penryn, CA 95663); Jacob Liberman, *Light: Medicine of the Future* (Santa Fe: Bear and Co., 1991); M. D. Rao, B. Muller-Oerlinghausen, and H. P. Volz, "The Influence of Phototherapy on Serotonin and Metatonin in Nonseasonal Depression," *Pharmacopsychiatry*, vol. 23 (1990), pp. 155–58; J. E. Blundell, "Serotonin and Appetite," *Neuropharmacology*, vol. 23, no. 128 (1984), pp. 1537–51.

49. M. Steiner et al., "Fluoxetine in the Treatment of Premenstrual Dysphoria," *New England Journal of Medicine*, vol. 332, no. 23 (1995), pp. 1529–34.

50. P. Muller, presentation at the First International Symposium of Magnesium Deficit in Human Pathology, 1971; Abraham, "Nutritional Factors in the Etiology of the Premenstrual Tension Syndromes" (see note 29); Facchinetti, "Magnesium Prophylaxis of Menstrual Migraine" (see note 30).

51. Kim Dirke et al., "The Influence of Dieting on the Menstrual Cycle of Healthy Young Women," *Journal of Clinical Endocrinology and Metabolism*, vol. 60, no. 6 (1985), pp. 1174–79.

52. I. Goodale, A. Domar, and H. Benson, "Alleviation of Premenstrual Syndrome Symptoms with the Relaxation Response," *Obstetrics and Gynecology*, vol. 75, no. 4 (Apr. 1990), pp. 649–89.

53. Terry Oleson and William Flocco, "Randomized Controlled Study of Premenstrual Symptoms Treated with Ear, Hand, and Foot Reflexology," *Obstetrics and Gynecology*, vol. 82 (1993), pp. 901–11; Jeanne Blum, *Woman Heal Thyself* (Boston: Charles Tuttle, 1995).

54. J. Prior et al., "Conditioning Exercise Decreases Premenstrual Symptoms: A Prospective Controlled Six-Month Trial," *Fertility and Sterility*, vol. 47 (1987), pp. 402–9.

55. Parry, "Morning vs. Evening" (see note 47). For a full discussion of light therapy, see Liberman, *Light: Medicine of the Future* (see note 48).

56. Controlled trials of natural progesterone that have been reported in the gynecological literature *do not* bear out my experience here. I think that this is because diet, exercise, and supplements have not been part of these studies, and also because women in these studies have not been taught how to think about their PMS as a signal that their lives are out of balance.

57. A. J. Rapkin, M. Morgan, L. Goldman, D. Brann, D. Simone, and V. B. Mahesh, "Progesterone Metabolite Allopregnanolone in Women with Premenstrual Syndrome," *Obstetrics and Gynecology*, vol. 90, no. 5 (Nov. 1997), pp. 709–14; E. S. Arafat, J. T. Hargrove, W. S. Maxon, et al., "Sedative and Hypnotic Effects of Oral Administration of Micronized Oral Progesterone May Be Medicated Through Its Metabolites," *American Journal of Obstetrics and Gynecology*, vol. 159 (1988), p. 1203; Andrew Herzog, "Intermittent Progesterone Therapy and Frequency of Complex Partial Seizures in Women with Menstrual Disorders," *Neurology*, vol. 36 (1986), pp. 1607–10.

58. Data based on report from independent testing of over-the-counter progesterone and yam creams, performed by Aeron LifeCycles Laboratory, 1933 Davis Street, Suite 310, San Leandro, CA 94577, 1-800-631-7900.

59. For years, those interested in PMS have batted around the idea of a "meno-toxin" present in women around the time of their periods because of this Jekyll-and-Hyde phenomenon and also because skin breakouts were worse premenstrually.

60. A. Barbarino, L. De Marinis, G. Follis, et al., "Corticotrophin-Releasing Hormone Inhibition of Gonadotropin Secretion During the Menstrual Cycle," *Metabolism*, vol. 38 (1989), pp. 504–6; I. Nagata, K. Kota, K. Seki, and K. Furuya, "Ovulatory Disturbances: Causative Factors Among Japanese Women Student Nurses in a Dormitory," *Journal of Adolescent Health Care*, vol. 7 (1986), pp. 1–5; M. R. Soules, R. I. McLachlan, E. K. Marit, et al., "Luteal Phase Deficiency: Characterization of Reproductive Hormones over the Menstrual Cycle," *Journal of Clinical Endocrine Metabolism*, vol. 69 (1989), pp. 804–12.

61. S. Zuckerman, "The Menstrual Cycle," *Lancet* (June 18, 1949), pp. 1031–35.

62. Cystic and adenomatous hyperplasia of the endometrium is very common after periods of amenorrhea or anovulation. It is a benign condition if there is no atypia of the cells. A good gynecological pathologist can make a prediction as to how dangerous this condition is, depending upon the nature of the cells present on the specimen.

63. Clomid has an estrogenlike structure. Its presence in the first half of the menstrual cycles causes the hypothalamus to put out increased levels of the hormones LH and FSH, thus stimulating the ovary to produce an egg.

64. A. J. Hartz, P. N. Baroriak, A. Wong, et al., "The Association of Obesity with Infertility and Related Menstrual Abnormalities in Women," *International Journal of Obesity*, vol. 3 (1979), pp. 57–73.

65. Dewan, "Perfect Rhythm Method of Birth Control" (see note 2).

66. D. M. Lithgow and W. M. Polizer, "Vitamin A in the Treatment of Menorrhagia," *South African Medical Journal*, vol. 51 (1977), p. 191; T. Fumii, "The Clinical Effects of Vitamin E on Purpura Due to Vascular Defects," *Journal of Vitaminology*, vol. 18 (1972), pp. 125–30.

67. J. D. Cohen and H. W. Rubin, "Functional Menorrhagia: Treatment with Bioflavonoids and Vitamin C," *Current Therapeutic Research*, vol. 2 (1960), p. 539.

68. C. Benedetto, "Eicosanoids in Primary Dysmenorrhea, Endometriosis and Menstrual Migraines," *Gynecological Endocrinology*, vol. 3, no. 1 (1989), pp. 71–94; A. Anderson et al., "Reduction of Menstrual Blood Loss by Prostaglandin-Synthetase Inhibitors," *Lancet*, 1967, p. 774.

69. Hugh O'Connor and Adam Magos, "Endometrial Resection for the Treatment for Menorrhagia," *New England Journal of Medicine*, vol. 335 (1996), pp. 151–56.

70. Rachael O'Neil, "A Modern Day Tribal Menarche Ceremony," *The Red Web Foundation Newsletter*, vol. 2, no. 4 (Fall 2005), pp. 1–3.

71. I was introduced to this concept by Tamara Slayton.

Chapter 6: The Uterus

1. While doing the research for this book, I was amazed by the lack of data on the uterus itself, separate from childbearing. The silence on the organ speaks volumes.

2. Celso-Ramon Garcia and Winnifred Cutler, "Preservation of the Ovary: A Reevaluation," *Fertility and Sterility*, vol. 42, no. 4 (Oct. 1984), pp. 510–14.

3. Lisa Lepine et al., "Hysterectomy Surveillance—United States, 1980–1993," *Centers for Disease Control and Prevention Surveillance Summaries*, Morbidity and Mortality Weekly Report 1997, vol. 46, no. SS-04 (Aug. 8, 1997), pp. 1–16.

4. Homa Keshavarz et al., "Hysterectomy Surveillance—United States, 1994–1999," *Centers for Disease Control and Prevention Surveillance Summaries*, Morbidity and Mortality Weekly Report 2002, vol. 51, no. SS-05 (July 12, 2002), pp. 1–8.

5. W. Cutler and E. Genovese-Stone, "Wellness in Women After 40 Years of Age: The Role of Sex Hormones and Pheromones," *Disease-A-Month*, vol. 44, no. 9 (Sept. 1998), p. 526.

6. All statistics from Thomas G. Stoval, "Hysterectomy," in Jonathan S. Berek, Eli Adashi, and Paula Hillars, eds., *Novak's Gynecology*, 12th ed. (Baltimore, MD: Williams and Wilkins, 1996), p. 727.

7. J. C. Gambone and R. C. Reiter, "Nonsurgical Management of Chronic Pelvic Pain: A Multidisciplinary Approach," *Clinical Obstetrics and Gynecology*, vol. 33 (1990), pp. 205–11; R. C. Reiter and J. C. Gambone, "Demographic and Historic Variables in Women with Idiopathic Chronic Pelvic Pain," *Obstetrics and Gynecology*, vol. 75 (1990), pp. 428–32.

8. Reiter and Gambone, "Demographic and Historic Variables" (see note 7).

9. Information from Caroline Myss.

10. Dr. Isaac Schiff (Chairman of the Department of Gynecology at Massachusetts General Hospital) at Grand Rounds, Maine Medical Center, Portland, ME, 1993.

11. Nancy Petersen and B. Hasselbring, "Endometriosis Reconsidered," *Medical Self Care*, May–June 1987.

12. David B. Redwine, "The Distribution of Endometriosis in the Pelvis by Age Groups and Fertility," *Fertility and Sterility*, vol. 47 (Jan. 1987), p. 173.

13. Supporting evidence can be found in Vaughan Bancroft, C. A. Williams, and M. Elstein, "Minimal/Mild Endometriosis and Infertility: A Review," *British Journal of Obstetrics and Gynaecology*, vol. 96, no. 4, pp. 454–50. The role of minimal or mild endometriosis in the etiology of infertility remains unclear, but an increased prostanoid content and macrophage activity in peritoneal fluid may exert an effect by a variety of mechanisms, including altered tubal motility, sperm function, and early embryo wastage. Ovarian function may be altered in a variety of ways, including many subtle abnormalities detectable only by detailed investigation. Autoimmune phenomena may also be contributory.

14. John Sampson, "Peritoneal Endometriosis Due to the Menstrual Dissemination of Endometrial Tissue into the Peritoneal Cavity," *American Journal of Obstetrics and Gynecology*, vol. 14 (1927), pp. 422–69.

15. This theory is based on the work of Dr. David Redwine, who along with Nancy

Petersen, R.N., is the founder of the St. Charles Medical Center endometriosis treatment program in Bend, Oregon.

16. Petersen and Hasselbring, "Endometriosis Reconsidered" (see note 11). See also David Redwine, "Age-Related Evolution in Color Appearance of Endometriosis," *Fertility and Sterility*, vol. 48, no. 6 (Dec 1987), pp. 1062–63; David Redwine, "Is Microscopic Peritoneal Endometriosis Invisible?" *Fertility and Sterility*, vol. 50, no. 4 (Oct. 1988), pp. 665–66.

17. Norbert Gleicher, "Is Endometriosis an Autoimmune Disease?" *Obstetrics and Gynecology*, vol. 70, no. 1 (July 1987); E. Surry and J. Halme, "Effect of Peritoneal Fluid from Endometriosis Patients on Endometrial Stromal Cell Proliferation in Vitro," *Obstetrics and Gynecology*, vol. 76, no. 5, part 1 (Nov. 1990), pp. 792–98; S. Kalma et al., "Production of Fibronection by Peritoneal Macrophages and Concentration of Fibronection in Peritoneal Fluid from Patients With or Without Endometriosis," *Obstetrics and Gynecology*, vol. 72 (July 1988), pp. 13–19; J. Halme, S. Becker, and S. Haskil, "Altered Maturation and Function of Peritoneal Macrophages: Possible Role in Pathogenesis of Endometriosis," *American Journal of Obstetrics and Gynecology*, vol. 156 (1987), p. 783; J. Halme, M. G. Hammond, J. F. Hulka, et al., "Retrograde Menstruation in Healthy Women and in Patients with Endometriosis," *Obstetrics and Gynecology*, vol. 64 (1984), pp. 13–18.

18. Christiane Northrup, *Mother-Daughter Wisdom* (New York: Bantam, 2005), p. 234.

19. Conventional insurance is set up to cover only certain treatment modalities and often does not cover relatively inexpensive measures to maintain health. Much has been written about the politics of medical treatment, a topic that is beyond the scope of this book. Though all of us end up paying for very expensive conventional medical treatments such as GnRH agonists, individuals with insurance don't bear this cost *directly* and therefore don't want to pay for modalities that aren't covered by insurance.

20. H. Koike, T. Egawa, M. Lhytsuka, et al., "Correlation Between Dysmenorrheic Severity and Prostaglandin Production in Women with Endometriosis," *Prostaglandins, Leukotrines, Essential Fatty Acids*, vol. 46 (1992), pp. 133–37.

21. D. Mills, "The Nutritional Status of the Endometriosis Patient," Institute for Optimum Nutrition project, Sept. 1991, reported in Nance Edwards Merrill, *Endometriosis Association Newsletter*, vol. 17, nos. 5–6 (1996).

22. Francis Hutchins Jr., "Uterine Fibroids: Current Concepts in Management," *Female Patient*, vol. 15 (Oct. 1990), p. 29.

23. A. D. Feinstein, "Conflict over Childbearing and Tumors of the Female Reproduction System: Symbolism in Disease," *Somatics* (Fall/Winter 1983).

24. R. C. Reiter, P. C. Wagner, and J. C. Gambone, "Routine Hysterectomy for Large Asymptomatic Leiomyomata: A Reappraisal," *Obstetrics and Gynecology*, vol. 79, no. 4 (Apr. 1992), pp. 481–84.

25. An entire body of literature on the healing power of sound is available. Each chakra, for example, is associated with a certain vibration. Healers who use sound may suggest that a person sing certain tones or listen to specially designed music. For more information about this treatment, read: W. David, *The Harmonics of Sound, Color, and Vibration: A System for Self-Awareness and Evolution* (Marina

del Rey, CA: DeVorss and Co., 1985); Kay Gardner, *Sounding the Inner Landscape* (Stonington, ME: Caduceus Publications, 1990).

26. A. J. Friedman et al. "A Randomized Double-Blood Trial of Gonadotropin... in the Treatment of Leiomyomata Uteki, *Fertility and Sterility*, vol. 49 (1987), p. 404.

27. Progestin hormone, in the form of Provera or Aygestin, can be taken daily on days fourteen to twenty-eight of the menstrual cycle to decrease excess buildup of endometrial tissue inside the uterus. This treatment sometimes works like a D&C and in fact is sometimes called a "medical D&C." I recommend this approach for those women whose heavy bleeding is unaffected by dietary change or for whom dietary change is impractical. It is sometimes used in addition to other therapies, such as acupuncture. Each case is individualized.

28. Alan de Cherney, M.D., chairman of the Department of Obstetrics and Gynecology, Tufts University Medical Center, Boston, MA, is a pioneer in this surgery and has trained physicians throughout the country in this technique.

29. L. Bradley and J. Newman, "Uterine Artery Embolization for Treatment of Fibroids: From Scalpel to Catheter," *The Female Patient*, vol. 25 (2000), pp. 71–78.

30. K. J. Carlson, B. Z. Miller, and F. J. Fowler, "The Maine Women's Health Study: I. Outcomes of Hysterectomy," *Obstetrics and Gynecology*, vol. 83 (1994), pp. 556–65.

31. Susan Rako, *The Hormone of Desire* (New York: Harmony Books, 1996).

32. L. Zussman et al., "Sexual Response After Hysterectomy-Oophorectomy: Recent Studies and Reconsideration of Psychogenesis," *American Journal of Obstetrics and Gynecology*, vol. 140, no. 7 (Aug. 1, 1981), pp. 725–29.

33. Carlson, Miller, and Fowler, "Outcomes of Hysterectomy" (see note 30).

34. J. P. Roovers, J. G. van der Bom, C. H. van der Vaart, and A. P. Heintz, "Hysterectomy and Sexual Wellbeing: Prospective Observational Study of Vaginal Hysterectomy, Subtotal Abdominal Hysterectomy, and Total Abdominal Hysterectomy," *British Medical Journal*, vol. 327, no. 7418 (Oct. 4, 2003), pp. 774–78.

35. B. Ranney and S. Abu-Ghazaleh, "The Future Function and Control of Ovarian Tissue Which Is Retained in Vivo During Hysterectomy," *American Journal of Obstetrics and Gynecology*, vol. 128 (1977), p. 626; N. Siddle, P. Sarrel, and M. Whitehead, "The Effect of Hysterectomy on the Age of Ovarian Failure: Identification of a Subgroup of Women and Premature Loss of Ovarian Function and Literature Reviews," *Fertility and Sterility*, vol. 47 (1987), p. 94.

36. B. J. Parys et al., "The Effects of Simple Hysterectomy on Vesicourethral Function," *British Journal of Urology*, vol. 64 (1989), pp. 594–99; S. J. Snooks et al., "Perineal Nerve Damage in Genuine Stress Urinary Incontinence," *British Journal of Urology*, vol. 42 (1985), pp. 3–9; C. R. Wake, "The Immediate Effect of Abdominal Hysterectomy and Intervesical Pressure and Detrusor Activity," *British Journal of Obstetrics and Gynaecology*, vol. 87 (1980), pp. 901–2: A. G. Hanley, "The Late Urological Complications of Total Hysterectomy," *British Journal of Urology*, vol. 41 (1969), pp. 682–84.

37. J. H. Manchester et al., "Premenopausal Castration and Documented Coronary

Atherosclerosis," *American Journal of Cardiology*, vol. 28 (1971), pp. 33–37; A. B. Ritterband et al., "Gonadal Function and the Development of Coronary Heart Disease," *Circulation*, vol. 27 (1963), pp. 237–87.

38. Shiatsu massage is a type of massage that uses pressure on acupuncture meridians to stimulate the flow of *chi* in the body.

39. Because of the size and location of the fibroids, she was not a candidate for endometrial ablation.

40. Stanley West, *The Hysterectomy Hoax* (New York: Doubleday, 1994); Harold Goldfarb, *The No-Hysterectomy Option* (New York: John Wiley and Sons, 1990).

Chapter 7: The Ovaries

1. J. Johnson, J. Canning, T. Kaneko, J. K. Pru, and J. L. Tilly, "Germline Stem Cells and Follicular Renewal in the Postnatal Mammalian Ovary," *Nature*, vol. 428, no. 6979 (Mar. 11, 2004), pp. 145–50.

2. R. H. Asch and R. Greenblatt, "Steroidogenesis in the Postmenopausal Ovary," *Clinical Obstetrics and Gynecology*, vol. 4, no. 1 (1977), p. 85.

3. E. R. Novak, B. Goldberg, and G. S. Jones, "Enzyme Histochemistry of the Menopausal Ovary Associated with Normal and Abnormal Endometrium," *American Journal of Obstetrics and Gynecology*, vol. 93 (1965), p. 669; C. R. Garcia and W. Cutler, "Preservation of the Ovary: A Reevaluation," *Fertility and Sterility*, vol. 42, no. 4 (Oct. 1985), pp. 510–14.

4. K. P. McNatty et al., "The Production of Progesterone, Androgens, and Estrogens by Granulosa Cells, Thecal Tissue, and Stromal Tissue by Human Ovaries in Vitro," *Journal of Clinical Endocrinology and Metabolism*, vol. 49 (1979), p. 687.

5. B. Dennefors et al., "Steroid Production and Responsiveness to Gonadotropin in Isolated Stromal Tissue of Human Postmenopauseal Ovaries," *American Journal of Obstetrics and Gynecology*, vol. 136 (1980), p. 997; G. Mikhail, "Hormone Secretion of Human Ovaries," *Gynecological Investigation*, vol. 1 (1970), p. 5; B. B. Sherwin and M. M. Gelfand, "The Role of Androgen in the Maintenance of Sexual Functioning in Oophorectomized Women," *Psychosomatic Medicine*, vol. 49 (1987), p. 397.

6. Mantak Chia and Maneewan Chia, *Cultivating Female Sexual Energy: Healing Love Through the Tao* (Huntington, NY: Healing Tao Books, 1986), available from Healing Tao Books, 2 Creskill Place, Huntington, NY 11743.

7. Frank P. Paloucek and John B. Graham, "The Influence of Psychosocial Factors on the Prognosis in Cancer of the Cervix," *Annals of the New York Academy of Sciences*, vol. 125 (1966), pp. 815–16.

8. I. Gerendai, W. Rotsztejn, et al., "Unilateral Ovariotomy-Induced Luteinizing Hormone-Releasing Hormone Content Changes in the Two Halves of the Mediobasal Hypothalamus," *Neuroscience Letters*, vol. 9 (1978), pp. 333–36.

9. J. R. Givens, "Reproduction and Hormonal Alterations in Obesity," in P. Bjorntorp and B. Brodoff, eds., *Obesity*, (New York: Lippincott, 1992).

10. R. L. Barbieri et al., "Insulin Stimulates Androgen Accumulation in Incubations

of Ovarian Stroma Obtained from Women with Hyperandrogenism," *Journal of Clinical Endocrinology and Metabolism*, vol. 62 (1986), p. 904.

11. R. J. Chang, R. M. Nakamura, H. L. Judd, and S. A. Kaplan, "Insulin Resistance in Non-Obese Patients with Polycystic Ovarian Syndrome," *Journal of Clinical Endocrinology and Metabolism*, vol. 61 (1985), p. 946; C. A. Stuart et al., "Insulin Resistance with Acanthosis Nigricans: The Role of Obesity and Androgen Excess," *Metabolism*, vol. 35 (1986), p. 197.

12. K. Kelly et al., "Psychodynamic Psychological Correlates with Secondary Amenorrhea," *Psychosomatic Medicine*, vol. 16 (1954), p. 129; M. M. Gill, "Functional Disturbances in Menstruation," *Bulletin of the Menninger Clinic*, vol. 7 (1943), p. 12.

13. T. B. Clarkson, M. R. Adams, J. R. Kaplan, C. A. Shively, and D. R. Koritnik, "From Menarche to Menopause: Coronary Artery Atherosclerosis and Protection in Cynomolgus Monkeys," *American Journal of Obstetrics and Gynecology*, vol. 160, no. 5, part 2 (May 1989), pp. 1280–85.

14. T. Piotrowski, Psychogenic Factors in Anovulatory Women," *Fertility and Sterility*, vol. 13 (1962), p. 11; T. Loftus, "Psychogenic Factors in Anovulatory Women: Behavioral and Psychoanalytic Aspects of Anovulatory Amenorrhea," *Fertility and Sterility*, vol. 13 (1962), p. 20.

15. W. Menaker, "Lunar Periodicity in Human Reproduction: A Likely Unit of Biological Time," *American Journal of Obstetrics and Gynecology*, vol. 77, no. 4 (1959), pp. 905–14; F. M. DeWan, "On the Possibility of the Fact of the Rhythm Method of Birth Control by Periodic Light Stimulation," *American Journal of Obstetrics and Gynecology*, vol. 99, no. 7 (1967), pp. 1016–19.

16. R. A. DeFronzo, "The Triumvirate: B-Cell, Muscle, Liver: A Collusion Responsible for NIDDM," *Diabetes*, vol. 37 (1983), pp. 667–87; G. W. Mitchell and J. Rogers, "The Influence of Weight Reduction on Amenorrhea in Obese Women," *New England Journal of Medicine*, vol. 249 (1953), pp. 835–37.

17. Though some might argue that all cysts should therefore be removed when they are first diagnosed and are relatively small, I disagree. Not all cysts grow rapidly, and not all cysts replace all normal ovarian tissue. And of course, some cysts go away on their own.

18. B. S. Centerwall, "Premenopausal Hysterectomy," *American Journal of Obstetrics and Gynecology*, vol. 139 (1981), p. 38; R. Punnonen and L. Raurama, "The Effect of Long-Term Oral Oestriol Succinate Therapy on the Skin of Castrated Women," *Annals of Gynaecology*, vol. 66 (1977), p. 214.

19. W. B. Cutler, "Human Sex-Attractant Pheromones: Discovery, Research, Development, and Application in Sex Therapy," *Psychiatric Annals*, vol. 29 (1999), pp. 54–59.

20. J. G. Annegers et al., "Ovarian Cancer: Reappraisal of Residual Ovaries," *American Journal of Obstetrics and Gynecology*, vol. 97 (1967), p. 124; G. V. Smith, "Ovarian Tumors," *American Journal of Surgery*, vol. 95 (1958), p. 336; V. S. Counselor et al., "Carcinoma of the Ovary Following Hysterectomy," *American Journal of Obstetrics and Gynecology*, vol. 69 (1955), p. 538; R. H. Grogan, "Reappraisal of Residual Ovaries," *American Journal of Obstetrics and Gynecology*, vol. 97 (1967), p. 124.

21. Theodore Sperof, "A Risk-Benefit Analysis of Elective Bilateral Oophorectomy:

Effect of Changes in Compliance with Estrogen Therapy on Outcome," *American Journal of Obstetrics and Gynecology* (Jan. 1991), pp. 165–74.

22. D. W. Cramer and B. L. Harlow, "Author's Response to Progress in Nutritional Epidemiology of Ovarian Cancer," *American Journal of Epidemiology*, vol. 134, no. 5 (1991), pp. 460–61; D. W. Cramer et al., "Galactose Consumption and Metabolism in Relationship to Risks for Ovarian Cancer," *Lancet*, vol. 2 (1989), pp. 66–71; D. W. Cramer, "Lactose Persistence and Milk Consumption as Determinants of Ovarian Cancer Risk," *American Journal of Epidemiology*, vol. 130 (1989), pp. 904–10; D. W. Cramer et al., "Dietary Animal Fat and Relationship to Ovarian Cancer Risk," *Obstetrics and Gynecology*, vol. 63, no. 6 (1984), pp. 833–38.

23. C. J. Mettlin and M. S. Diver, "A Case-Control Study of Milk-Drinking and Ovarian Cancer Risk," *American Journal of Epidemiology*, vol. 132 (1990), pp. 871–75; C. J. Mettlin, "Invited Commentary: Progress in Nutritional Epidemiology of Ovarian Cancer," *American Journal of Epidemiology*, vol. 134, no. 5 (1991), pp. 457–59.

24. K. M. Fairfield, D. J. Hunter, G. A. Colditz, C. S. Fuchs, D. W. Cramer, F. E. Speizer, W. C. Willett, and S. E. Hankinson, "A Prospective Study of Dietary Lactose and Ovarian Cancer," *International Journal of Cancer*, vol. 110, no. 2 (June 10, 2004), pp. 271–77.

25. D. W. Cramer, W. R. Welsh, R. E. Scully, and C. A. Wojciechowski, "Ovarian Cancer and Talc: A Case-Control Study," *Cancer*, vol. 50 (1982), pp. 372–76; W. J. Henderson, T. C. Hamilton, and K. Griffiths, "Talc in Normal and Malignant Ovarian Tissue," *Lancet*, vol. 1 (1979), p. 499.

26. G. E. Egli and M. Newton, "The Transport of Carbon Particles in the Human Female Reproductive Tract," *Fertility and Sterility*, vol. 12 (1961), pp. 151–55.

27. B. L. Harlow et al., "The Influence of Lactose Consumption on the Association of Oral Contraceptive Pills and Ovarian Cancer Risk," *American Journal of Epidemiology*, vol. 134, no. 5 (1991), pp. 445–61.

28. B. V. Stadel, "The Etiology and Prevention of Ovarian Cancer," *American Journal of Obstetrics and Gynecology*, vol. 123 (1975), pp. 772–74.

29. K. Helzisouer et al., "Serum Gonadotrophins and Steroid Hormones and the Development of Ovarian Cancer," *Journal of the American Medical Association*, vol. 274, no. 24 (Dec. 27, 1995), pp. 1926–30.

30. S. E. Hankinson et al., "Tubal Ligation, Hysterectomy, and Risk of Ovarian Cancer: A Prospective Study," *Journal of the American Medical Association*, Dec. 15, 1993; A. S. Whittemore, R. Harris, J. Intyre, and the Collaborative Ovarian Cancer Group, "Characteristics Relating to Ovarian Cancer Risk: Collaborative Analysis of 12 U.S. Case-Control Studies. Part II: Invasive Epithelial Ovarian Cancers in White Women," *American Journal of Epidemiology*, vol. 136 (1992), pp. 1184–1203.

31. Rebecca Ferrini, "Screening Asymptomatic Women for Ovarian Cancer: American College of Preventive Medicine Practice Policy Statement," *American Journal of Preventive Medicine*, vol. 13, no. 6 (Nov./Dec. 1997), pp. 444–46.

32. Ibid.

33. C. Granai, "Sounding Board: Ovarian Cancer: Unrealistic Expectations," *New England Journal of Medicine*, vol. 327, no. 3 (1993), pp. 197–200.

34. S. J. Skates and D. E. Singer, "Quantifying the Potential Benefit of CA-125 Screening for Ovarian Cancer," *Journal of Clinical Epidemiology*, vol. 44 (1991), pp. 365–80; M. M. Schapira, D. B. Matchar, and M. J. Young, "The Effectiveness of Ovarian Cancer Screening: A Decision-Analysis Model," *Annals of Internal Medicine*, vol. 118 (1993), pp. 838–43.

35. S. Campbell, V. Bhan, J. Royston, et al., "Screening for Early Ovarian Cancer," *Lancet*, vol. 1 (1988), pp. 710–11.

36. E. Andolf, E. Svalenius, and B. Astedt, "Ultrasonography for the Early Detection of Ovarian Cancer," *British Journal of Obstetrics and Gynaecology*, vol. 93 (1986), pp. 1286–89.

37. Gilda Radner, a well-known comedienne and wife of actor Gene Wilder, died of familial ovarian cancer. To prevent this from happening to others, Wilder has publicized the genetic risk for those who have this disease in their families, usually in first-degree relatives on the mother's side of the family.

38. J. K. Tobachman et al., "Intra-Abdominal Carcinomatosis after Prophylactic Oophorectomy in Ovarian Cancer Prone Families," *Lancet*, vol. 2 (1982), p. 795; Elvio Silva and Rosemary Jenkins, "Serious Carcinoma in Endometrial Polyps," *Modern Pathology*, vol. 3, no. 2 (1990), pp. 120–22.

39. S. L. Parker, T. Tong, S. Bolden, and P. A. Wingo, "Cancer Statistics, 1997," *CA: A Cancer Journal for Clinicians*, vol. 47 (1997), pp. 5–27.

40. Denise Grady, "Gain Reported in Combating Ovary Cancer," *The New York Times*, Jan. 5, 2006, pp. 1–3.

41. Brendan O'Regan and Caryle Hirshberg, *Spontaneous Remission: An Annotated Bibliography* (Petaluma, CA: Institute of Noetic Sciences, 1993).

Chapter 8: Reclaiming the Erotic

1. Gina Ogden, *Women Who Love Sex* (New York: Pocket Books, 1994).

2. Josephine Lowdes Sevely, *Eye's Secrets: A New Theory of Female Sexuality* (New York: Random House, 1987), pp. 89–90.

3. Caroline Muir and Charles Muir, *Tantra: The Art of Conscious Loving* (San Francisco: Mercury House, 1989). The Muirs teach that finding the sacred spot is often difficult for a woman to accomplish alone. Even if she does locate it, it may be very difficult for her to stimulate it herself, which is the only way to access its healing power and its sexual and spiritual potential. Nevertheless, you can try to locate it in the following way: squat with two fingers inside the vagina, press your fingers upward toward the navel while pressing down on the pubic bone with the other hand. If you can manage to stimulate or massage the area, the spot will swell. You may then be able to feel it between your fingers. For most women, this part of their awakening process requires the loving touch of a partner who respects the vulnerable nature of this spot.

Following the first edition of this book, I received a letter from Robert Svoboda, the first Westerner to graduate from a college of Ayurvedic medicine in India. As a student of the tantric tradition, with a deep understanding of its complexities and subtleties, he pointed out that to equate tantric yoga only with "enjoyable sex," as the Muirs do in their book, is to misunderstand and misrepresent this field. Though I find the Muirs' work helpful, I do not want to mislead my readers into thinking that it represents true tantric yoga. For further reading on tantric yoga, see Douglas Renfrew Brooks, *The Secret of the Three Cities: An Introduction to Hindu Sakta Tantrism* (Chicago: University of Chicago Press, 1990).

4. Muir and Muir, *Tantra*, p. 74 (see note 3).

5. T. M. Hines, "The G-Spot: A Modern Myth," *American Journal of Obstetrics and Gynecology*, vol. 185, no. 2 (Aug. 2001), pp. 359–62.

6. J. K. Davidson, Sr., C. A. Darling, and C. Conway-Welch, "The Role of the Grafenberg Spot and Female Ejaculation in the Female Orgasmic Response: An Empirical Analysis," *Journal of Sex & Marital Therapy*, vol. 15, no. 2 (Summer 1989), pp. 102–20.

7. Naura Hayden, *How to Satisfy a Woman Every Time and Have Her Beg for More* (New York: Biblio-Phile, 1980). Though I don't agree with everything in this book, it's a very practical guide for satisfactory heterosexual lovemaking. A good book to give to a male partner, it can be obtained by writing to Biblio-Phile at P.O. Box 5189, New York, NY 10022.

8. Paula Brown Doress and Diana Laskin Siegal, *Ourselves Growing Older* (New York: Simon & Schuster, 1987).

9. H. B. Van de Weil, W. C. Schultz, et al., "Sexual Functioning Following Treatment of Cervical Cancer," *European Journal of Gynecologic Oncology* (1988), pp. 275–81.

10. So-called natural male sexual needs are also deeply influenced by the culture. Barbara Hand Clow, in *The Liquid Light of Sex* (Santa Fe, NM: Bear and Co., 1991), points out that many men in this culture achieve erection via their third-chakra power centers. But erection achieved in this way is a form of power over others, and erections maintained through their chakra energy are the basis of rape, which is not about sexuality at all but about power and dominance. Caroline Myss says that in this culture, the size of a man's wallet and the size of his erections are related. When a man is able to clear his lower chakras of negativity, his erections are achieved more through fourth-chakra or heart energy. Then the act of intercourse becomes an act of sharing, caring, and love. The orgasm achieved in this way is symbolic of this man's love not only for the woman he's with but for creation itself.

11. Aaron Glatt, S. Zinner, and W. McCormack, "The Prevalence of Dyspareunia," *Obstetrics and Gynecology*, vol. 75, no. 3 (March 1990), pp. 433–36.

12. "A View from Above: The Dangerous World of Wannabes," *Time*, Nov. 25, 1991, p. 77.

13. "A View from Above" (see note 12).

14. J. E. Darroch, D. J. Landry, and S. Oslak, "Age Difference Between Sexual Partners in the United States," *Family Planning Perspectives*, vol. 31, no. 4 (July–August 1999).

15. Bill Albert, Laura Lippman, Kerry Franzetta, Erum Ikramullah, Julie Dombrowski Keith, Rebecca Shwalb, Suzanne Ryan, and Elizabeth Terry-

Humen, *Freeze Frame: A Snapshot of America's Teens,* National Campaign to Prevent Teen Pregnancy, (Sept. 2005) p. 21.

16. Barbara Walker, *The Women's Encyclopedia of Myths and Secrets* (HarperSanFrancisco, 1983), pp. 1049–51. Scholarly research on the whole issue of the virgin birth has been done. "In ancient times impregnation by a ghost used to be 'the acceptable explanation for pregnancy in most pagan countries where the sexual act was part of the fertility rites,' so Christians thought impregnation by spirits was still credible, whether the alleged father was a dead hero, a devil, an incubus, or even—in some sects—the Holy Ghost again." R. Holmes, *Witchcraft in History* (Secaucus, NJ: Citadel Press, 1974); quoted in Walker, *The Women's Encyclopedia,* p. 1050.

17. Barbara G. Walker, *The Woman's Encyclopedia of Myths and Secrets* (San Francisco: Harper & Row, 1983), pp. 1051–52.

18. Elizabeth Cady Stanton, *The Original Feminist Attack on the Bible* (New York: Arno Press, 1974), p. 114; quoted in Walker, *The Women's Encyclopedia,* p. 1051 (see note 16).

19. Barbara Walker points out that the Hebrew Gospels designated Mary by the word *mah,* mistakenly translated as "virgin" but really meaning "young woman." See also Esther Harding, *Women's Mysteries, Ancient and Modern* (New York: Rider and Co., 1955).

20. Women's sense of smell is more acute than men's. A smell can evoke an entire stream of memories, either positive or negative. Smell is the longest-remembered sense. A particular smell evokes associated memories more than the senses of vision, hearing, and touch. The olfactory center is located in the brain in an area that is intimately connected with memory function.

21. Part of normal dolphin life is being sexual with each other. Male dolphins often wrap their penis around a female's lower body, playfully—not to procreate but simply to communicate. Male dolphins sometimes do this when they are communicating with humans, too. This happened to my sister once—she described her dolphin encounter as an ecstatic experience.

22. Mantak Chia and Maneewan Chia, *Cultivating Female Sexual Energy: Healing Love Through the Tao* (Huntington, NY: Healing Tao Books, 1986); available from Healing Tao Books, 2 Creskill Place, Huntington, NY 11743.

23. Riane Eisler, *Sacred Pleasure: Sex, Myth, and the Politics of the Body* (HarperSanFrancisco, 1995), p. 15.

24. National Geographic Channel, "Totally Wild," May 25, 2005.

25. W. Cutler and E. Genovese-Stone, "Wellness in Women After 40 Years of Age: The Role of Sex Hormones and Pheromones," *Disease-A-Month,* vol. 44, no. 9 (September 1998), p. 526.

26. Antonio Damasio, "Brain Trust," *Nature,* vol. 435 (June 2, 2005), pp. 571–72.

27. Bud Berkeley, *Foreskin: A Closer Look* (Boston: Alyson Publications, 1993), p. 188.

28. Josephine Lowndes Sevely, *Eve's Secrets: A New Theory of Female Sexuality* (New York: Random House, 1987), p. 17; William H. Masters and Virginia E. Johnson, *Human Sexual Response* (Boston: Little, Brown, 1966), p. 46.

29. K. O'Hara and J. O'Hara, "The Effect of Male Circumcision on the Sexual

Enjoyment of the Female Partner," *British Journal of Urology*, vol. 83, supplement 1 (Jan. 1999), pp. 79–84.

30. I have replaced the repugnant term *masturbation* with the term *self-love*, or as a friend of mine calls it, "being your own best friend."

Chapter 9: Vulva, Vagina, Cervix, and Lower Urinary Tract

1. Riane Eisler, *Sacred Pleasure: Sex, Myth, and the Politics of the Body* (HarperSanFrancisco, 1995), p. 225; Robert Stoller, *Sexual Excitement: The Dynamics of Erotic Life* (New York: Pantheon Books, 1979), pp. 6, 23, and 26.

2. See the book by the Body Shop Team, *Mamamoto: A Celebration* (New York: Viking, 1992), p. 78.

3. T. R. Nansel et al., "The Association of Psychosocial Stress and Bacterial Vaginosis in a Longitudinal Cohort," *American Journal of Obstetrics and Gynecology*, vol. 194, no. 2 (Feb. 2006), pp. 381–86.

4. R. J. Hafner, S. L. Stanton, and J. Guy, "A Psychiatric Study of Women with Urgency and Urge Incontinence," *British Journal of Urology*, vol. 49 (1977), pp. 211–14; L. R. Staub, H. S. Ripley, and S. Wolf, "Disturbance of Bladder Function Associated with Emotional States," *Journal of the American Medical Association*, vol. 141 (1949), p. 1139.

5. A. J. Macaulay et al., "Psychological Aspects of 211 Female Patients Attending a Urodynamic Unit," *Journal of Psychosomatic Research*, vol. 31, no. 1 (1991), pp. 1–10; D. L. P. Rees and N. Farhoumand, "Psychiatric Aspects of Recurrent Cystitis in Women," *British Journal of Urology*, vol. 49 (1977), pp. 651–58.

6. M. Tarlau and M. A. Smalheiser, "Personality Patterns in Patients with Malignant Tumors of the Breast and Cervix," *Psychosomatic Medicine*, vol. 13 (1951), p. 117. Women with cervical cancer characteristically experienced an early rejection; the patients grew up in homes lacking a male figure due to the death or desertion of the father.

7. James H. Stephenson and William Grace, "Life Stress and Cancer of the Cervix," *Psychosomatic Medicine*, vol. 14, no. 4 (1954), pp. 287–94.

8. A. Schmale and H. Iker, "Psychological Setting of Uterine Cervical Cancer," *Annals of the New York Academy of Sciences,* vol. 125 (1966), pp. 807–13.

9. M. H. Antoni and K. Goodkin, "Host Moderator Variables in the Promotion of Cervical Neoplasia: I. Personality Facets," *Journal of Psychosomatic Research*, vol. 32, no. 3 (1988), pp. 327–28.

10. K. Goodkin et al., "Stress and Hopelessness in the Promotion of Cervical Intraneoplasia to Invasive Squamous? Cell Carcinoma of the Cervix," *Journal of Psychosomatic Research*, vol. 30, no. 1 (1986), pp. 67–76.

11. L. Koutsky, "Epidemiology of Genital Human Papillomavirus Infection," *The American Journal of Medicine*, vol. 102, no. 5A (May 5, 1997), pp. 3–8.

12. J. Buscema, "The Predominance of Human Papilloma Virus—Type 16 in Vulvar Neoplasia," *Obstetrics and Gynecology*, vol. 71, no. 4 (1988), pp. 601–5.

13. R. Kiecolt-Glasser, J. K. Glaser, C. E. Speicher, and J. E. Holliday, "Stress,

Loneliness, and Changes in Herpes Virus Latency," *Journal of Behavioral Medicine*, vol. 8, no. 3 (1985), pp. 249–60.

14. To diagnose warts that aren't visible, or so-called flat warts, the penis must be bathed in vinegar and then viewed through some sort of magnifying lens. Only then will the flat white warts be obvious to those who know what to look for. Treatment issues for men are exactly the same as for women.

15. For more information about podofilox, you or your doctor can write to Oclassen Pharmaceuticals, Inc., 100 Pelican Way, San Rafael, CA 94901.

16. L. Sadler, A. Saftlas, W. Wang, M. Exeter, J. Whittaker, L. McCowan, "Treatment for Cervical Intraepithelial Neoplasia and Risk of Preterm Delivery," *Journal of the American Medical Association*, vol. 291, no. 17 (May 5, 2004), pp. 2100–6.

17. Two studies note that many patients have effectively used hypnosis to relieve warts. See R. H. Rulison, "Warts: A Statistical Study of 921 Cases," *Archives of Dermatology and Syphilology*, vol. 46 (1942), pp. 66–81; and M. Ullman, "On the Psyche and Warts. II: Hypnotic Suggestion and Warts," *Psychosomatic Medicine*, vol. 22 (1960), pp. 68–76.

18. N. Whitehead et al., "Megaloblastic Changes in Cervical Epithelium: Association of Oral Contraceptive Therapy and Reversal with Folic Acid," *Journal of the American Medical Association*, vol. 226 (1993), pp. 1421–24; J. N. Orr, "Localized Deficiency of Folic Acid in Cervical Epithelial Cells May Promote Cervical Dysplasia and Eventually Carcinoma of the Cervix," *American Journal of Obstetrics and Gynecology*, vol. 151 (1985), pp. 632–35; J. Lindenbaum et al., "Oral Contraceptive Hormones, Eolate Metabolism, and Cervical Epithelium," *American Journal of Clinical Nutrition*, Apr. 1975, pp. 346–53; S. L. Romney et al., "Plasma Vitamin C and Uterine Cervical Dysplasia," *American Journal of Obstetrics and Gynecology*, vol. 151, no. 7 (1985), pp. 976–80; S. L. Romney et al., "Retinoids in the Prevention of Cervical Dysplasia," *American Journal of Obstetrics and Gynecology*, vol. 141, no. 8 (1981), pp. 890–94; S. Wassertheil-Smaller et al., "Dietary Vitamin C and Uterine Cervical Dysplasia," *American Journal of Epidemiology*, vol. 114, no. 5 (1981), pp. 714–24; C. LaVecchia et al., "Dietary Vitamin A and the Risk of Invasive Cervical Cancer," *International Journal of Cancer*, vol. 34 (1985), pp. 319–22; P. Ramsnamy and R. Natarajan, "Vitamin B_6 Status in Patients with Cancer of the Uterine Cervix," *Nutrition and Cancer*, vol. 6 (1984), pp. 176–80; E. Dawson et al., "Serum Vitamin and Selenium Changes in Cervical Dysplasia," *Federal Proceedings*, vol. 43 (1984), p. 612.

19. Louise Hay, *I Love My Body* (Farmingdale, NY: Coleman Publishing, 1985), p. 49.

20. D. T. Fleming et al., "Herpes Simplex Virus Type 2 in the United States, 1976 to 1994," *New England Journal of Medicine*, vol. 337, no. 16 (Oct. 16, 1997), pp. 1105–11; L. Stanberry et al., "New Developments in the Epidemiology, Natural History and Management of Genital Herpes," *Antiviral Research*, vol. 42, no. 1 (May 1999), pp. 1–14; A. J. Nahmias et al., "Sero-Epidemiological and Sociological Patterns of Herpes Simplex Virus Infection in the World," *Scandinavian Journal of Infectious Diseases, Supplementum*, vol. 69 (1990), pp. 19–36.

21. G. J. Mertz, S. L. Rosenthal, and L. R. Stanberry, "Is Herpes Simplex Virus Type 1 (HSV-1) Now More Common Than HSV-2 in First Episodes of Genital Herpes?" *Sexually Transmitted Diseases*, vol. 30, no. 10 (Oct. 2003), pp. 801–2; A. Wald et al., "Oral Shedding of Herpes Simplex Virus Type 2," [published erratum appears

in *Sex Transm Infect*, vol. 80, no. 6 (Dec. 2004), pp. 546] *Sexually Transmitted Infections*, vol. 80, no. 4 (Aug. 2004), pp. 272–76; R. Engelberg et al., "Natural History of Genital Herpes Simplex Virus Type 1 Infection," *Sexually Transmitted Diseases*, vol. 30, no. 2 (Feb. 2003), pp. 174–77.

22. Wald et al., "Frequent Genital Herpes Simplex Virus 2 Shedding in Immunocompetent Women: Effect of Acyclovir Treatment," *The Journal of Clinical Investigation*, vol. 99, no. 5 (March 1997), pp. 1092–97.

23. L. Koutsky et al., "Underdiagnosis of Genital Herpes by Current Clinical and Viral-Isolation Procedures," *New England Journal of Medicine*, vol. 326, no. 23 (1992), pp. 1533–39.

24. H. C. Taylor, "Vascular Congestion and Hyperemia," *American Journal of Obstetrics and Gynecology*, vol. 57, no. 22 (1949), p. 22; M. E. Kemeny et al., "Psychological and Immunological Predictors of Genital Herpes Recurrence," *Psychosomatic Medicine*, vol. 52 (1989), p. 195–208.

25. A Wald et al., "Reactivation of Genital Herpes Simplex Virus Type 2 Infection in Asymptomatic Seropositive Persons," *New England Journal of Medicine*, vol. 342, no. 12 (March 23, 2000), pp. 844–50.

26. Z. A. Brown et al., "Genital Herpes Complicating Pregnancy," *Obstetrics and Gynecology*, vol. 106, no. 4 (October 2005), pp. 845–56.

27. K. M. Stone et al., "Pregnancy Outcomes Following Systemic Prenatal Acyclovir Exposure: Conclusions from the International Acyclovir Pregnancy Registry, 1984–1999," *Birth Defects Research Part A, Clinical and Molecular Teratology*, vol. 70, no. 4 (April 2004), pp. 201–7.

28. Z. A. Brown et al., "Effect of Serologic Status and Cesarean Delivery on Transmission Rates of Herpes Simplex Virus from Mother to Infant," *Journal of the American Medical Association*, vol. 289, no. 2 (Jan. 8, 2003), pp. 203–9.

29. J. J. van Everdingen, M. F. Peeters, and P. ten Have, "Neonatal Herpes Policy in The Netherlands: Five Years After a Consensus Conference," *Journal of Clinical Investigation*, vol. 21, no. 5 (1993), pp. 371–75.

30. M. A. Adefumbo and B. H. Lau, "Allium Sativum (Garlic): A Natural Antibiotic," *Medical Hypothesis*, vol. 12, no. 3 (1983), pp. 327–37.

31. There are a number of brands of garlic on the market: Kyolic (by the Wakunga Company) and Garlicin (by Murdock) are two that Women to Women often recommends.

32. R. H. Wolbling and K. Leonhardt, "Local Therapy of Herpes Simplex with Dried Extract from *Melissa Officinalis*," *Phytomedicine*, vol. 1 (1994), pp. 25–31; R. A. Cohen et al., "Antiviral Activity of *Melissa Officinalis* (Lemon Balm Extract)," *Proceedings of the Society for Experimental Biology and Medicine*, vol. 117 (1964), pp. 431–34; F. C. Herrmann Jr. and L. S. Kucera, "Antiviral Substances in Plants of the Mint Family (*Labiatae*). II. Nontannin Polyphenol of *Melissa Officinalis*," *Proceedings of the Society for Experimental Biology and Medicine*, vol. 124, no. 3 (1967), pp. 869–74; Z. Dimitrova et al., "Antiherpes Effect of *Melissa Officinalis* L. Extracts," *Acta Microbiologica Bulgarica* (Sofia), vol. 29 (1993), pp. 65–75.

33. Not all products labeled "tea tree oil" are equally effective. I've used Melaleuca oil or Melagel from the Melaleuca Company; see also Richard Bruse, *Melaleuca:*

Nature's Antiseptic (1989), Sunnyside Health Center, 8800 S. E. Sunnyside Rd., Suite 111, Clackamus, Oregon 97015; 503-654-8225.

34. G. Eby, "Use of Topical Zinc to Prevent Recurrent Herpes Simplex Infection: Review of Literature and Suggested Protocols," *Medical Hypothesis*, vol. 17 (1985), pp. 157–65; G. T. Terezhabny et al., "The Use of a Water-Soluble Bioflavonoid Ascorbic Acid Complex in the Treatment of Recurrent Herpes Labialis," *Oral Surgery Oral Medicine and Oral Pathology*, vol. 45 (1978), pp. 56–62; G. R. B. Skinner, "Lithium Ointment for Genital Herpes," *Lancet*, vol. 2 (1983), p. 288; E. F. Finnerty, "Topical Zinc in the Treatment of Herpes Simplex," *Cutis*, vol. 37, no. 2 (Feb. 1986), pp. 130–31.

35. R. S. Griffith et al., "Multicentered Study of Lysine Therapy of HSV Infection," *Dermatological*, vol. 156 (1978), pp. 157–67; M. A. McCune et al., "Treatment of Recurrent Herpes Simplex Infections with L-Lysine Monohydrochloride," *Cutis*, vol. 34 (1984), pp. 366–73; D. D. Schmeisser et al., "Effect of Excess Lysine on Plasma Lipids in the Chick," *Journal of Nutrition*, vol. 113 (1983), pp. 1777–83; D. J. Thein and W. C. Hurt, "Lysine as a Prophylactic Agent in the Treatment of Recurrent Herpes," *Oral Surgery*, vol. 58 (1984), pp. 659–66; J. H. DiGiovanni and H. Blank, "Failure of Lysine in Frequently Recurrent Herpes Simplex Infection," *Archives of Dermatology*, vol. 120 (1984), pp. 48–51.

36. Antoni and Goodkin, "Host Moderator Variables" (see note 9); Goodkin et al., "Stress and Hopelessness" (see note 10).

37. "Pap Smear Screening for Cervical Cancer," *Maine Cancer Perspectives*, vol. 2, no. 2 (April 1996).

38. Damaris Christensen, "New Cervical Test 'More Effective' Than Pap Smear," *Medical Tribune*, Dec. 12, 1996.

39. J. D. Oriel, "Sex and Cervical Cancer," *Genitourinary Medicine*, vol. 64 (1988), pp. 81–89; C. LaVecchia, A. Decarli, A. Fosoli, et al., "Oral Contraceptives and Control Study," *British Journal of Cancer*, vol. 54 (1986), p. 311; J. J. Schlesselman, "Cancer of the Breast and Reproductive Tract in Relation to Use of CC's," *Contraception*, vol. 40 (1989), p. 1.

40. N. Potischman and L. Brinton, "Nutrition and Cervical Neoplasia," *Cancer Causes and Control*, vol. 7 (1996), pp. 113–26.

41. Pap smears are taken even after the cervix has been removed in a hysterectomy. This is especially important for women who have had a prior history of an abnormal Pap smear.

42. Therapeutic touch, a system of healing with the hands, has been very well studied, and its beneficial effects have been well documented by Delores Kreiger, Ph.D., a nurse at Columbia University. Marcelle Pick, a cofounder of Women to Women, has studied with Dr. Kreiger.

43. I feel that chlamdydia *may* also be a normal inhabitant of the vagina in some women and that it may cause problems only when there's an imbalance. Chlamydia is like the buzzard flying around the dying calf, as far as I'm concerned, though many of my colleagues would disagree.

44. C. Wira and C. Kaushic, "Mucosal Immunity in the Female Reproductive Tract: Effect of Sex Hormones on Immune Recognition and Responses," in H. Kiyono,

P. L. Ogra, and J. R. McGhee, eds., *Mucosal Vaccines* (New York: Academic Press, 1996), pp. 375–88.

45. Gardiner-Caldwell SynerMed, "The Role of Reduced Regimens in the Management of Vulvovaginitis," *Medical Monitor*, vol. 1, no. 1 (Apr. 1991), available from Gardiner-Caldwell SynerMed, P.O. Box 458, Califon, NJ 07830.

46. Mary Ryan Miles, Linda Olsen, and Alvin Rogers, "Recurrent Vaginal Candidiasis: Importance of an Intestinal Reservoir," *Journal of the American Medical Association*, vol. 238, no. 17 (Oct. 24, 1977), pp. 1836–37.

47. Genova Diagnostics in Asheville, NC. See Resources.

48. Miles, Olsen, and Rogers, "Recurrent Vaginal Candidiasis" (see note 46).

49. D. Steward et al., "Psychosocial Aspects of Chronic, Clinically Unconfirmed Vulvovaginitis," *Obstetrics and Gynecology*, vol. 76, no. 5, part 1 (Nov. 1990), pp. 852–56.

50. S. Mathur et al., "Anti-Ovarian and Anti-Lymphocyte Antibodies in Patients with Chronic Vaginal Candidiasis," *Journal of Reproductive Immunology*, vol. 2 (1980), pp. 247–62.

51. C. Fordham von Reyn, M.D., "HIV and Acquired Immunodeficiency Syndrome," lecture, Sept. 21, 1996, Dartmouth Medical School, Lebanon, NH.

52. There are also known cases of persons infected with HIV for over ten years who have no evidence of either declining levels of CD4+ T lymphocytes or AIDS. A. R. Lifson et al., "Long-Term Human Immunodeficiency Virus Infection in Asymptomatic Homosexual and Bisexual Men with Normal CD4+ Lymphocyte Counts: Immunologic and Virologic Characteristics," *Journal of Infectious Disease*, vol. 163 (1991), pp. 959–65.

53. Frank Pittman, "Frankly Speaking," *Psychology Today*, Sept.–Oct. 1996, p. 60.

54. F. J. Palella Jr. et al., "Declining Morbidity and Mortality Among Patients with Advanced Human Immunodeficiency Virus Infection. HIV Outpatient Study Investigators," *New England Journal of Medicine*, vol. 338, no. 13 (March 26, 1998), pp. 853–60.

55. Caroline Myss, *AIDS, Passageway to Transformation* (Walpole, MA: Stillpoint Publications, 1985).

56. Niro Markoff, who went from HIV positive to HIV negative, now teaches internationally. Her story and her teaching are available in *Why I Survive AIDS* (New York: Simon & Schuster, 1991). Bob Owen, *Roger's Recovery from AIDS* (Cannon Beach, OR: Davar Press, 1987) also documents a case of reversal from HIV positive to HIV negative. It is available by writing to Davar Press, P.O. Box 1100, Cannon Beach, OR 97110.

57. S. M. Hammer, "Clinical Practice, Management of Newly Diagnosed HIV Infection," *New England Journal of Medicine*, vol. 353, no. 16 (Oct. 20, 2005), pp. 1702–10.

58. A tape of this panel presentation can be ordered from the American Holistic Medical Association (AHMA, 4101 Lake Boone Trail, Suite 201, Raleigh, NC 27607; (919) 787-5181). See also Laurence Badgley, *Healing AIDS Naturally* (San Bruno, CA: Human Energy Press, 1987); available from Human Energy Press, Suite D, 370 West San Bruno Avenue, San Bruno, CA 94066.

59. W. W. Fawzi et al., "A Randomized Trial of Multivitamin Supplements and HIV Disease Progression and Mortality," *New England Journal of Medicine*, vol. 351, no. 1 (July 1, 2004), pp. 23–32.

60. C. B. Furlonge et al., "Vulvar Vestibulitis Syndrome: A Clinicopathological Study," *British Journal of Obstetrics and Gynaecology*, vol. 98 (1991), pp. 703–6.

61. Eduard Friedrick, "Vulvar Vestibulitis Syndrome," *Journal of Reproductive Medicine*, vol. 32, no. 2 (Feb. 1987), pp. 110–14.

62. T. Warner et al., "Neuroendocrine Cell-Axonal Complexes in the Minor Vestibular Gland," *Journal of Reproductive Medicine*, vol. 41 (1996), pp. 397–402.

63. C. C. Solomons, M. H. Melmed, and S. M. Heitler, "Calcium Citrate for Vestibulitis," *Journal of Reproductive Medicine*, vol. 36, no. 12 (1991), pp. 879–82.

64. Dr. McNamara's study uses the USANA brands Essential and Proflavanol.

65. Donna E. Stewart et al., "Psychological Aspects of Chronic Clinically Unconfirmed Vulvovaginitis," *Obstetrics and Gynecology*, vol. 76 (1990), pp. 852–56; Donna E. Stewart et al., "Vulvodynia and Psychological Distress," *Obstetrics and Gynecology*, vol. 84, no. 4 (Oct. 1994), pp. 587–90.

66. E. A. Walker et al., "Medical and Psychiatric Symptoms in Women with Childhood Sexual Abuse," *Psychosomatic Medicine*, vol. 54 (1992), pp. 658–64.

67. Howard Glazer, "Treatment of Vulvar Vestibulitis Syndrome with Electromyographic Biofeedback of Pelvic Floor Musculature," *Journal of Reproductive Medicine*, vol. 4, no. 4 (1995), pp. 283–90.

68. Benson Horowitz, M.D., Grand Rounds presentation, Maine Medical Center, July 24, 1996.

69. Ibid.

70. M. M. Karram, "Frequency, Urgency, and Painful Bladder Syndromes," in M. D. Walters and M. M. Karram, eds., *Clinical Urogynecology* (St. Louis: Mosby, 1993), pp. 285–98.

71. E. M. Messing and T. A. Stamey, "Interstitial Cystitis: Early Diagnosis, Pathology, and Treatment," *Urology*, vol. 12 (1978), page 381.

72. National Kidney and Urologic Diseases Information Clearinghouse website (http://kidney.niddk.nih.gov/kudiseases/pubs/interstitialcystitis/).

73. A. E. Sobota, "Inhibition of Bacterial Adherence by Cranberry Juice: Potential Use for the Treatment of Urinary Tract Infections," *Journal of Urology*, vol. 131 (1984), pages 1013–16; P. N. Papas et al., "Cranberry Juice in the Treatment of Urinary Tract Infections," *Southwestern Medicine*, vol. 47A (1966), pp. 17–30; D. R. Schmidt and A. E. Sobota, "An Examination of the Antiadherence Activity of Cranberry Juice on Urinary and Non-Urinary Bacterial Isolates," *Microbios*, vol. 55, nos. 224–225 (1988), pp. 173–81.

74. J. Avorn et al., "Reduction of Bacteria and Pyuria After Ingestion of Cranberry Juice," *Journal of the American Medical Association*, vol. 271 (1994), pp. 751–54.

75. V. Frohne, "Untersuchungen zur Frage der Garbdesfuzierenden Wirkungen von Barentraubenblatt-Extracten," *Planta Medica*, vol. 18 (1970), pp. 1–25.

76. R. Raz, W. Stamm, et al., "A Controlled Trial of Intravaginal Estriol in Post-Menopausal Women with Recurrent Urinary Tract Infections," *New England Journal of Medicine*, vol. 329 (1993), pp. 753–56.

77. D. C. H. Tchou et al., "Pelvic Floor Musculature Exercises in Treatment of Anatomical Urinary Stress Incontmence," *Physical Therapy*, vol. 68 (1988), pp. 652–55; K. Bo et al., "Pelvic Floor Muscle Exercises for the Treatment of Female Stress Incontinence: Effects of Two Different Degrees of Pelvic Floor Muscle Exercises," *Neurological Urodynamics*, vol. 11 (1990), pp. 107–113; and P. A. Burns et al., "A Comparison of Effectiveness of Biofeedback and Pelvic Muscle Exercise Treatment in the Treatment of Stress Incontinence in Older Community-Dwelling Women," *Journal of Gerontology*, vol. 48, no. 4 (1993), pp. 167–74.

78. N. Bhatia et al., "Urodynamic Effects of a Vaginal Pessary in Women with Stress Urinary Incontinence," *American Journal of Obstetrics and Gynecology*, vol. 147 (1983), p. 876; and A. Diokno, "The Benefits of Conservative Management for SUI," *Contemporary ObGyn*, March 1997, pp. 128–42.

Chapter 10: Breasts

1. C. Chen, "Adverse Life Events and Breast Cancer: A Case-Controlled Study," *British Medical Journal*, vol. 311 (Dec. 9, 1995), pp. 1527–30.

2. S. Geyer, "Life Events Prior to Manifestation of Breast Cancer: A Limited Prospective Study Covering Eight Years Before Diagnosis," *Journal of Psychosomatic Research*, vol. 35 (1991), pp. 355–63.

3. A. Ramirez et al., "Stress and Relapse of Breast Cancer," *British Medical Journal*, vol. 298 (1989), pp. 291–93.

4. In the nineteenth century, the unusual case history studies of Herbert Snow likened breast and uterine cancer with a history of a "troubled mind and chronic anxiety." Particularly evident in the women he studied was the loss of a significant relationship as the precipitating factor in the manifestation of a tumor. See Herbert Snow, *The Proclivity of Women to Cancerous Disease* (London 1883).

     In this century, M. Tarlau and M. A. Smalheiser found that the typical pattern for women with breast cancer was that their father had been absent psychologically; for women with cervical cancer, the father had been absent due to death or desertion. See M. Tarlau and M. A. Smalheiser, "Personality Patterns in Patients with Malignant Tumors of the Breast and Cervix," *Psychosomatic Medicine*, vol. 13 (1951), p. 117. They also found that women with breast cancer uniformly had negative feelings about their sexuality, had adapted by denying their sexuality, and often had negative feelings about heterosexual relationships as such. Women with cervical cancer, by contrast, had less negative feelings about their sexuality. The breast cancer patients were much more likely to have remained in an unsatisfactory marriage, while many of the cervical cancer patients were divorced or had been married several times.

     A study by Bacon and colleagues found that many women with breast cancer frequently were unable to discharge or deal appropriately with their anger, aggressiveness, or hostility. Often these women covered up such feelings with a facade of pleasantness. Women with breast cancer frequently responded with "denial and unrealistic sacrifice" to resolve hostile conflict with their mothers. See C. L. Bacon et al., "A Psychosomatic Survey of Cancer of the Breast," *Psychosomatic Medicine*, vol. 14, no. 6 (1952), pp. 453–59.

See also C. B. Bahnson, "Stress and Cancer: The State of the Art," *Psychosomatics*, vol. 22, no. 3 (1981), pp. 207–20.

5. Sandra Levy et al., "Perceived Social Support and Tumor Estrogen Progesterone Receptor Status as Predictors of Natural Killer Cell Activity in Breast Cancer Patients," *Psychosomatic Medicine*, vol. 51 (1990), pp. 73–85.

6. A. Bremond, G. Kune, and C. Bahnson, "Psychosomatic Factors in Breast Cancer Patients: Results of a Case Control Study," *Journal of Psychosomatic Obstetrics and Gynecology*, vol. 5 (1986), pp. 127–36.

7. K. W. Pettingale et al., "Serum IgA Levels and Emotional Expression in Breast Cancer Patients," *Journal of Psychosomatic Research*, vol. 21 (1977), p. 395.

8. D. B. Thomas et al., "Randomized Trial of Breast Self-Examination in Shanghai: Final Results," *Journal of the National Cancer Institute*, vol. 94, no. 19 (Oct. 2, 2002), pp. 1445–57.

9. S. M. Love, R. S. Gelman, and W. J. Sile, "Fibrocystic 'Disease' of the Breast: A Non-Disease," *New England Journal of Medicine*, vol. 307 (1982), p. 1010.

10. P. E. Preece et al., "Importance of Mastalgia in Operable Breast Cancer," *British Medical Journal*, vol. 284 (1982), pp. 1299–1300; and L. E. Hughes and D. J. Webster, "Breast Pain and Modularity," in *Benign Disorders and Disease of the Breast* (London, Bailliere Tindale, 1989).

11. G. Plu-Bureau et al., "Cyclic Mastalgia as a Marker of Breast Cancer Susceptibility: Results of a Case Control Study Among French Women," *British Journal of Cancer*, vol. 65 (1992), pp. 945–49; and J. R. Harris et al., "Breast Cancer," part 1, *New England Journal of Medicine*, vol. 327 (1992), pp. 319–28.

12. P. L. Jenkins et al., "Psychiatric Illness in Patients with Severe Treatment-Resistant Mastalgia," *General Hospital Psychiatry*, vol. 15 (1993), pp. 55–57.

13. N. Boyd, "Effect of a Low-Fat, High-Carbohydrate Diet on Symptoms of Cyclical Mastopathy," *The Lancet*, vol. 2 (1988), p. 128; D. Rose et al., "Effect of a Low-Fat Diet on Hormone Levels in Women with Cystic Breast Disease. I: Serum Steroids and Gonadotropins," *Journal of the National Cancer Institute*, vol. 78 (1987), p. 623; D. Rose et al., "Effect of a Low-Fat Diet on Hormone Levels in Women with Cystic Breast Disease. II: Serum Radioimmunoassayable Prolactin and Growth Hormone and Bioactive Lactogenic Hormones," *Journal of the National Cancer Institute*, vol. 78 (1987), p. 627.

14. M. Woods, "Low-Fat, High-Fiber Diet and Serum Estrone Sulfate in Premenopausal Women," *American Journal of Clinical Nutrition*, vol. 49 (1989), p. 1179; D. Ingram, "Effect of Low-Fat Diet on Female Sex Hormone Levels," *Journal of the National Cancer Institute*, vol. 79 (1987), p. 1225; and H. Aldercreutz, "Diet and Plasma Androgens in Postmenopausal Vegetarian and Omnivorous Women and Postmenopausal Women with Breast Cancer," *American Journal of Clinical Nutrition*, vol. 49 (1989), p. 433; A. Tavani et al., "Consumption of Sweet Foods and Breast Cancer Risk in Italy," *Annals of Oncology*, (Oct. 25, 2005) [Epub ahead of print].

15. Rose et al., "Serum Steroids and Gonadotropins" (see note 13).

16. K. J. Chang et al., "Influences of Percutaneous Administration of Estradiol and Progesterone on Human Breast Epithelial Cell Cycle in Vivo," *Fertility and Sterility*, vol. 63 (1995), pp. 785–91.

17. D. Bagga et al., "Dietary Modulation of Omega-3/Omega-6 Polyunsaturate Fatty Acid Ratios in Patients with Breast Cancer," *Journal of the National Cancer Institute*, vol. 89, no. 15 (1997), pp. 1123–31.

18. R. S. London et al., "The Effect of Alpha-Tocopherol on Premenstrual Symptomatology," *Cancer Research*, vol. 41 (1981), pp. 3811–16; R. S. London et al., "The Effect of Alpha-Tocopherol on Premenstrual Symptomatology: A Double-Blind Study," *Journal of American College Nutrition*, vol. 3 (1984), pp. 351–56; R. S. London et al., "The Role of Vitamin E in Fibrocystic Breast Disease," *Obstetrics and Gynecology*, vol. 65 (1982), pp. 104–6; A. A. Abrams, "Use of Vitamin E for Chronic Cystic Mastitis," *New England Journal of Medicine*, vol. 272 (1965), pp. 1080–81.

19. B. A. Eskin et al., "Mammary Gland Dysplasia in Iodine Deficiency," *Journal of the American Medical Association*, vol. 200 (1967), pp. 115–19.

20. P. E. Mohr et al., "Serum Progesterone and Prognosis in Operable Breast Cancer," *British Journal of Cancer*, vol. 73 (1996), pp. 1552–55.

21. R. Harris, "Effectiveness: The Next Question for Breast Cancer Screening," *Journal of the National Cancer Institute*, vol. 97, no. 14 (July 20, 2005), pp. 1021–23.

22. D. A. Berry et al., "Effect of Screening and Adjuvant Therapy on Mortality from Breast Cancer," *New England Journal of Medicine*, vol. 353, no. 17 (Oct 27, 2005), pp. 1784–92.

23. J. G. Elmore et al., "Ten-Year Risk of False Positive Screening Mammograms and Clinical Breast Exams," *New England Journal of Medicine*, vol. 338, no. 16 (April 16, 1998), pp. 1089–96.

24. P. C. Gotzsche and O. Olsen, "Is Screening for Breast Cancer with Mammography Justifiable?" *The Lancet*, vol. 355, no. 9198 (Jan. 8, 2000), pp. 129–34; P. C. Gotzsche and O. Olsen, "Cochrane Review on Screening for Breast Cancer with Mammography," *The Lancet*, vol. 358, no. 9290 (Oct. 20, 2001), pp. 1340–42.

25. Andrew M. D. Wolf, "Share the Burden of Uncertainty with Patients," *Consultant*, vol. 43, no. 9 (August 2003), pp. 1102–03.

26. A. B. Miller et al., "Canadian National Breast Screening Study-2: 13-Year Results of a Randomized Trial in Women Aged 50–59 Years," *Journal of the National Cancer Institute*, vol. 92, no. 18 (Sept. 20, 2000), pp. 1490–99.

27. K. Kerlikowske et al., "Continuing Screening Mammography in Women Aged 70 to 79 Years: Impact on Life Expectancy and Cost-Effectiveness," *Journal of the American Medical Association*, vol. 282, no. 22 (Dec. 8, 1999), pp. 2156–63.

28. J. P. van Netten et al., "Physical Trauma and Breast Cancer," *The Lancet*, vol. 343, no. 8903 (Apr. 16, 1994), pp. 978–79.

29. C. Baines, "Rethinking Breast Screening—Again," *British Medical Journal*, vol. 331 (2005), p. 1031.

30. A. T. Stavros et al., "Solid Breast Nodules: Use of Sonography to Distinguish Between Benign and Malignant Lesions," *Radiology*, vol. 195 (1995), pp. 123–34; E. Staren, "Breast Ultrasound for Surgeons," *American Surgeon*, vol. 62 (1996), pp. 109–12.

31. Gina Kolata, "Breast Cancer Screening Under 50: Experts Disagree if Benefit Exists," *New York Times*, Dec. 14, 1993, p. C–1; W. Gilbert Welch and William

Black, "Advances in Diagnostic Imaging," *New England Journal of Medicine*, vol. 328 (Apr. 1993), pp. 1237–42; M. Nielson et al., "Breast Cancer and Atypia Among Young Middle-Aged Women: A Study of 110 Medical-Legal Autopsies," *British Journal of Cancer*, vol. 56 (1987), pp. 814–19. An unpublished autopsy study with similar findings was done at Cook County Hospital in Chicago (personal communication with Kate Havens, M.D.).

32. V. Ernster et al., "Incidence of and Treatment for Ductal Carcinoma In Situ of the Breast," *Journal of the American Medical Association*, vol. 275, no. 12 (March 27, 1996), pp. 913–18.

33. G. Arpino, R. Laucirica, and R. M. Elledge, "Premalignant and In Situ Breast Disease: Biology and Clinical Implications," *Annals of Internal Medicine*, vol. 143, no. 6 (Sept. 20, 2005), pp. 446–57.

34. C. I. Li et al., "Age-specific Incidence Rates of In Situ Breast Carcinomas in Histologic Type, 1980 to 2001," *Cancer Epidemiology, Biomarkers & Prevention*, vol. 14, no. 4 (April 2005), pp. 1012–15.

35. National Center for Health Statistics, *Vital Statistics of the United States*, 1987, vol. 2, *Mortality, Part A*, DHHS Publication no. (PHS) 90-1101 (Washington, DC: U.S. Government Printing Office, 1990).

36. The following chemicals have been implicated: the pesticides DDT, heptachlor, and atrazine, several polycyclic aromatic hydrocarbons (PAHs), petroleum by-products, dioxin, and polychlorinated biphenyls (PCBs). See also Janet Ralof, "Ecocancer: Do Environmental Factors Underlie a Breast Cancer Epidemic?," *Science News*, vol. 144 (July 3, 1993), pp. 1013.

37. Samuel Epstein, M.D., letter to Dr. David Kessler, commissioner of the FDA, Feb. 14, 1994, cited in Barbara Joseph, *My Healing from Breast Cancer* (New Canaan, CT: Keats, 1996), p. 7.

38. P. Buell, "Changing Incidence of Breast Cancer in Japanese-American Women," *Journal of the National Cancer Institute*, vol. 51 (1973), pp. 1479–83; L. Kinlen, "Meat and Fat Consumption and Cancer Mortality: A Study of Strict Religious Orders in Britain," *The Lancet*, 1982, pp. 946–49; W. Willett et al., "Dietary Fat and Risk of Breast Cancer," *New England Journal of Medicine*, vol. 316, no. 22 (1987).

39. D. J. Hunter et al., "Cohort Studies of Fat Intake and the Risk of Breast Cancer: A Pooled Analysis," *New England Journal of Medicine*, vol. 334 (1996), pp. 356–61.

40. S. Franceschi et al., "Intake of Macronutrients and Risk of Breast Cancer," *The Lancet*, vol. 347 (1996), pp. 1351–56.

41. S. Seely and D. F. Horrobin, "Diet and Breast Cancer: The Possible Connection with Sugar Consumption," *Medical Hypotheses*, vol. 3 (1983), pp. 319–27; K. K. Carol, "Dietary Factors in Immune-Dependent Cancer," in M. Winick, ed., *Current Concepts in Nutrition*, vol. 6, *Nutrition and Cancer* (New York: John Wiley and Sons, 1977), pp. 25–40; S. K. Hoeh and K. K. Carroll, "Effects of Dietary Carbohydrate in the Incidence of Mammary Tumors Induced in Rates by 7, 12-Dimethylbenzanthracene," *Nutrition and Cancer*, vol. 1, no. 3 (1979), pp. 27–30; R. Kazer, "Insulin Resistance, Insulin-Like Growth Factor I and Breast Cancer: A Hypothesis," *International Journal of Cancer*, vol. 62 (1995), pp. 403–6.

42. M. H. Holl et al., "Gut Bacteria and Aetiology of Cancer of the Breast," *The Lancet*,

vol. 2 (1971), pp. 172–73; R. E. Hughes, "Hypothesis: A New Look at Dietary Fiber in Human Nutrition," *Clinical Nutrition*, vol. 406 (1986), pp. 81–86.

43. H. Aldercreutz et al., "Dietary Phytoestrogens and the Menopause in Japan," *The Lancet*, vol. 339 (1992), pp. 1233; H. P. Lee et al., "Dietary Effects of Breast Cancer Risk in Singapore," *The Lancet*, vol. 337 (May 18, 1991), pp. 1197–1200.

44. N. N. Ismael, "A Study of Menopause in Malaysia," *Maturitas*, vol. 19 (1994), pp. 205–9.

45. L. J. Lu et al., "Decreased Ovarian Hormones During a Soya Diet: Implications for Breast Cancer Prevention," *Cancer Research*, vol. 60, no. 15 (Aug 1, 2000), pp. 4112–21; N. B. Kumar et al., "The Specific Role of Isoflavones on Estrogen Metabolism in Premenopausal Women," *Cancer*, vol. 94, no. 4 (Feb 15, 2002), pp. 1166–74; C. Nagata et al., "Decreased Serum Estradiol Concentration Associated with High Dietary Intake of Soy Products in Premenopausal Japanese Women," *Nutrition and Cancer*, vol. 29, no. 3 (1997), pp. 228–33.

46. T. Hirano et al., "Antiproliferative Activity of Mammalian Lignan Derivatives Against the Human Breast Carcinoma Cell Line ZR-75-1," *Cancer Investigations*, vol. 8 (1990), pp. 595–602.

47. H. Aldercreutz et al., "Excretion of the Lignans Enterolactone and Enterodiol and of Equol in Omnivorous and Vegetarian Women and in Women with Breast Cancer," *The Lancet*, vol. 2 (1992), pp. 1295–99.

48. J. Michnovicz and H. Bradlow, "Altered Estrogen Metabolism and Excretion in Humans Following Consumption of Indole-3-Carbinol," *Nutrition and Cancer*, vol. 16 (1991), pp. 59–66.

49. K. P. McConnell et al., "The Relationship Between Dietary Selenium and Breast Cancer," *Journal of Surgical Oncology*, vol. 5 no. 1 (1980), pp. 67–70.

50. L. C. Clark, G. F. Combs, B. W. Turnbull, et al., "Effects of Selenium Supplementation for Cancer Prevention in Patients with Carcinoma of the Skin," *Journal of the American Medical Association*, vol. 276 (1996), pp. 1957–63.

51. T. T. Kellis and L. E. Vickery, "Inhibition of Human Estrogen Synthetase (Aromatase) by Flavonoids," *Science*, vol. 255 (1984), pp. 1032–34. The bioflavonoids compete for estrogen as a substrate in fat metabolism.

52. B. Goldin and J. Gorsbach, "The Effect of Milk and Lactobacillus Feeding on Human Intestinal Bacterial Enzyme Activity," *American Journal of Clinical Nutrition*, vol. 39 (1984), pp. 756–61. *Lactobacillus acidophilus* inhibits beta glucuronidase, the fecal bacterial enzyme responsible for deconjugating liver-conjugated estrogen.

53. R. R. Brown et al., "Correlation of Serum Retinol Levels with Response to Chemotherapy in Breast Cancer," *American Journal of Obstetrics and Gynecology*, vol. 148, no. 3, pp. 309–12.

54. K. Lockwood et al., "Partial and Complete Regression of Breast Cancer in Patients in Relation to Dosage of Coenzyme Q10," *Biochemical and Biophysical Research Communications*, vol. 199, no. 3 (1994), pp. 1504–8.

55. Rosenberg et al., "Breast Cancer and Alcoholic Beverage Consumption," *The Lancet*, vol. 1 (1982), p. 267.

56. I. Kato et al., "Alcohol Consumption in Cancers of Hormone Related Organs in Females," *Japan Journal of Clinical Oncology*, vol. 19, no. 3 (1989), pp. 202–7.

57. I. Thune et al., "Physical Activity and the Risk of Breast Cancer," *New England Journal of Medicine*, vol. 336 (1997), pp. 1269–75.

58. B. Rockhill et al., "A Prospective Study of Recreational Physical Activity and Breast Cancer Risk," *Archives of Internal Medicine*, vol. 159, no. 19 (Oct 25, 1999), pp. 2290–96.

59. P. K. Verkasalo et al., "Sleep Duration and Breast Cancer: A Prospective Cohort Study," *Cancer Research*, vol. 65, no. 20 (Oct. 15, 2005), pp. 9595–600.

60. E. S. Schernhammer et al., "Rotating Night Shifts and Risk of Breast Cancer in Women Participating in the Nurses Health Study," *Journal of the National Cancer Institute*, vol. 93, no. 20 (Oct. 17, 2001), pp. 1563–68.

61. D. E. Blask et al., "Melatonin-Depleted Blood from Premenopausal Women Exposed to Light at Night Stimulates Growth of Human Breast Cancer Xenografts in Nude Rats," *Cancer Research*, vol. 65, no. 23 (Dec. 1, 2005), pp. 11174–84.

62. E. S. Schernhammer et al., "Urinary Melatonin Levels and Breast Cancer Risk," *Journal of the National Cancer Institute*, vol. 97, no. 14 (July 20, 2005), pp. 1084–87.

63. S. Narod et al., "Familial Breast-Ovarian Cancer Locus on Chromosome 17q12a23," *The Lancet*, vol. 338 (July 13, 1991), pp. 82–83.

64. M. B. Fitzgerald et al., "Germ Line BrCa 1 Mutations in Jewish and Non-Jewish Women with Early Onset Breast Cancer," *New England Journal of Medicine*, vol. 334, no. 3 (1996), pp. 143–49; F. S. Collins, "BrCa 1: Lots of Mutations, Lots of Dilemmas," *New England Journal of Medicine*, vol. 334, no. 3 (1996), pp. 186–88; A. A. Langston, "BrCa 1 Mutations in Population-Based Sample of Young Women with Breast Cancer," *New England Journal of Medicine*, vol. 334, no. 3 (1996), pp. 137–42.

65. S. B. Haga et al., "Genomic Profiling to Promote a Healthy Lifestyle: Not Ready For Prime Time," *Nature Genetics*, vol. 34, no. 4 (Aug. 2003), pp. 347–50.

66. Soma Johnson, *Wildfire: Igniting the She-volution* (Albuquerque, NM: Wildfire Books), p. 38.

67. Breast cancer, in the conventional sense, can recur anytime. That's why no conventional doctor would consider Monica "cured." They would say that she is "in remission." Whatever one calls it, I like the way she looks and is living her life.

68. For a fascinating account of the breast implant controversy, see the "Chronology of Silicone Breast Implants" page on the website for the PBS show *Frontline* at www.pbs.org/wgbh/pages/frontline/implants/cron.html.

69. L. A. Brinton, et al., "Cancer Risk at Sites Other Than the Breast Following Augmentation Mammoplasty," *Annals of Epidemiology*, vol. 11, no. 4 (May 2001), pp. 248–56.

70. Implant statistics cited in Marsha Angell, "Shattuck Lecture—Evaluating the Health Risks of Breast Implants: The Interplay of Medical Science, the Law, and Public Opinion," *New England Journal of Medicine*, vol. 334, no. 23 (1996), pp. 1513–18.

71. L. A. Brinton et al., "Mortality Among Augmentation Mammoplasty Patients," *Epidemiology*, vol. 12, no. 3 (May 2001), pp. 321–26.

72. V. C. Koot et al., "Total and Cause Specific Mortality Among Swedish Women with Cosmetic Breast Implants: Prospective Study," *British Medical Journal*, vol. 326, no. 7388 (March 8, 2003), pp. 527–28.

73. J. S. Hasan, "Psychological Issues in Cosmetic Surgery: A Functional Overview," *Annals of Plastic Surgery*, vol. 44, no. 1 (Jan. 2000), pp. 89–96.

74. Personal communication from Mona Lisa Schulz, M.D., Ph.D., who researched the area thoroughly prior to having bilateral reconstructions herself after the diagnosis of breast cancer.

75. "Saline-Filled Breast Implant Surgery: Making an Informed Decision," patient labeling for saline-filled breast implants, Mentor Corporation (updated Jan. 2004); "Making an Informed Decision: Saline-Filled Breast Implant Surgery; 2004 Update," Patient labeling for saline-filled breast implants, INAMED Corporation (updated Nov. 2004).

76. Schulz (see note 74).

77. Nancy Hurst, "Lactation After Augmentation Mammoplasty," *Obstetrics and Gynecology*, vol. 87, no. 1 (1996), pp. 30–34.

78. A. R. Staib and D. R. Logan, "Hypnotic Stimulation of Breast Growth," *American Journal of Clinical Hypnosis* (Apr. 1977), and R. D. Willard, "Breast Enlargement Through Visual Imagery and Hypnosis," *American Journal of Clinical Hypnosis* (Apr. 1977); J. E. Williams, "Stimulation of Breast Growth by Hypnosis," *Journal of Sex Research*, vol. 10, no. 4 (1974), pp. 316–26; L.M. LeCron, "Breast Development Through Hypnotic Suggestion," *Journal of the American Society of Psychosomatic Dentistry and Medicine*, vol. 16, no. 2 (1969), pp. 58–62.

79. S. Levy et al., "Survival Hazards Analysis in First Recurrent Breast Cancer Patients: 7-Year Follow-Up," *Psychosomatic Medicine*, vol. 50 (1988), pp. 520–88.

Chapter 11: Our Fertility

1. David Chamberlain, *The Mind of Your Newborn Baby* (Berkeley, CA: North Atlantic Books, 1998).

2. I met a woman OB/GYN physician from China who told me she had performed twenty thousand abortions in her career. In China, only one child per couple is allowed—sometimes not even one. Abortion is commonly used for birth control. If a couple has more than one child, the parents may lose a job or be subject to other sanctions. As a result, Chinese couples now selectively abort female fetuses, and now an entire generation of young men do not have enough women their age for wives—a fact that, although tragic, seems a cruel kind of justice.

3. Carroll Smith-Rosenberg, *Disorderly Conduct: Visions of Gender in Victorian America* (New York: Oxford University Press, 1986).

4. In a society in which there is so much incest and rape, sexual behavior is often distorted, starting in childhood. Any woman who has recovered from sexual abuse will

tell you that having multiple sexual partners and sexual "acting out" are among the consequences of sexual abuse. I'm not blaming these women. I'm merely suggesting that we need to start the healing process somewhere.

5. Available from Kris Bercov, P.O. Box 3586, Winter Park, FL 32790; 407- 628-0095. Price: $5.00 plus $1.00 shipping. Volume discounts available.

6. Smith-Rosenberg, *Disorderly Conduct* (see note 3).

7. Smith-Rosenberg, *Disorderly Conduct*, page 218 (see note 3).

8. M. Melbye, J. Wohlfahrt, et al., "Induced Abortion and the Risk of Breast Cancer," *New England Journal of Medicine*, vol. 336 (1996), pp. 81–85.

9. Gladys McGarey, *Born to Live* (Phoenix, AZ: Gabriel Press, 1980), p. 54. This book is currently out of print but should be available again in the near future. For more information, contact Gladys McGarey, M.D., Scottsdale Holistic Medical Group, 7350 Statson, Suite 128, Scottsdale, AZ 85251; 602-990-1528.

10. "Preven Emergency Contraceptive Kit—the first and only emergency contraceptive product—approved by the FDA," press release from Gynetics, Inc. (Somerville, NJ; Sept. 2, 1998).

11. J. Trussell, F. Stewart, F. Guest, and R. A. Hatcher, "Emergency Contraceptive Pills: A Simple Proposal to Reduce Unintended Pregnancies," *Family Planning Perspectives*, vol. 24, no. 6 (Nov–Dec 1992), pp. 269–73.

12. S. F. Wood, "Women's Health and the FDA," *New England Journal of Medicine*, vol. 353, no. 16 (Oct. 20, 2005), pp. 1650–51.

13. R. Hatcher et al., *Contraceptive Technology* (New York: Irvington Publishers, 1991).

14. M. K. Horwitt et al., "Relationship Between Levels of Blood Lipids, Vitamins C, A, E, Serum Copper, and Urinary Excretion of Tryptophan Metabolites in Women Taking Oral Contraceptive Therapy," *American Journal of Clinical Nutrition*, vol. 28 (1975), pp. 403–12; K. Amatayakul, "Vitamin Metabolism and the Effects of Multivitamin Supplementation in Oral Contraceptive Users," *Contraception*, vol. 30, no. 2 (1984), pp. 179–96; and J. L. Webb, "Nutritional Effects of Oral Contraceptive Use," *Journal of Reproductive Health*, vol. 25, no. 4 (1980), p. 151.

15. A. M. Kaunitz, "Oral Contraceptives," in Thomas G. Stovall and Frank W. Ling, eds., *Gynecology for the Primary Care Physician* (Philadelphia: Current Medicine, 1999).

16. I. F. Godsland et al., "The Effects of Different Formulations of Oral Contraceptive Agents on Lipid and Carbohydrate Metabolism," *New England Journal of Medicine*, vol. 323, no. 20 (Nov. 15, 1990), pp. 1375–81.

17. V. Cogliano et al., "Carcinogenicity of Combined Oestrogen-Progestagen Contraceptives and Menopausal Treatment," *Lancet Oncology*, vol. 6, no. 8 (August 2005), pp. 552–53.

18. Collaborative Group on Hormonal Factors in Breast Cancer, "Breast Cancer and Hormonal Contraceptives: Further Results," *Contraception*, vol. 54, no. 3 suppl. (Sept. 1996), pp. 1S–106S.

19. C. Panzer et al., "Impact of Oral Contraceptives on Sex Hormone Binding Globulin and Androgen Levels: A Retrospective Study in Women with Sexual Dysfunction," *Journal of Sexual Medicine*, vol. 3, no. 1 (January 2006), pp. 104–13.

20. U.S. Food and Drug Administration, "FDA Updates Labeling for Ortho Evra Contraceptive Patch," Nov. 10, 2005. Available online at www.fda.gov/bbs/topics/news/2005/NEW01262.html

21. Quoted from Joan Morais flyer, used by permission of the author.

22. My introduction to the true scope of science backing natural family planning came when I heard Dr. Joseph Stanford speak at the 1993 annual meeting of the American Holistic Medical Association in Kansas City, Kansas. The research that is cited in this section was graciously provided to me by Dr. Stanford, who currently teaches in the Department of Family and Preventive Medicine, University of Utah, 50 North Medical Drive, Salt Lake City, Utah 84132.

23. The rhythm method relies on calendar estimates of the fertility period rather than physiologic signs of fertility. It is much less reliable than the methods discussed in the text.

24. Observation of vaginal mucus discharge to determine time of fertility was originally developed by two physicians, John and Evelyn Billings. Hence, this method is sometimes referred to as the Billings method.

25. T. W. Hilgers, A. I. Bailey, and A. M. Prebil, "Natural Family Planning IV: The Identification of Postovulatory Infertility," *Obstetrics and Gynecology*, vol. 58, no. 3 (1981), pp. 345–50.

26. T. W. Hilgers, "The Medical Applications of Natural Family Planning: A Contemporary Approach to Women's Health Care" (Omaha, NE: Pope Paul VI Institute Press, 1991); T. W. Hilgers, "The Statistical Evaluation of Natural Methods of Family Planning," *International Review of Natural Family Planning*, vol. 8, no. 3 (Fall 1984), pp. 226–64; J. Doud, "Use-Effectiveness of the Creighton Model of NFP," *International Review of Natural Family Planning*, vol. 9, no. 54 (1985).

27. Thomas Hilgers et al., "Cumulative Pregnancy Rates in Patients with Apparently Normal Fertility and Fertility-Focused Intercourse," *Journal of Reproductive Medicine*, vol. 37, no. 10 (Oct. 1992), pp. 864–66.

28. Quote taken from lecture handout of J. Stanford, annual meeting of the American Holistic Medical Association, March 13, 1993. Study cited is in T. W. Hilgers, "The Medical Applications of Natural Family Planning" (see note 26).

29. G. Freundl et al., "Demographic Study on the Family Planning Behavior of the German Population: The Importance of Natural Methods," *International Journal of Fertility*, vol. 33 (1988), suppl. pp. 54–58.

30. A. Wilcox and C. Weinberg, "Timing of Sexual Intercourse in Relation to Ovulation: Effects on the Probability of Conception, Survival of Pregnancy, and Sex of Baby," *New England Journal of Medicine*, vol. 333 (1995), pp. 1517–21.

31. H. Klaus, "Natural Family Planning: A Review," *Obstetrics and Gynecology Survey*, vol. 37, no. 2 (Feb. 1982), pp. 128–50; T. W. Hilgers, A. M. Prebil, "The Ovulation Method: Vulvar Observations as an Index of Fertility and Infertility," *Obstetrics and Gynecology*, vol. 53, no. 1 (Jan. 1979), pp. 12–22; World Health Organization, "A Prospective Multicentre Trial of the Ovulation Method of Natural Family Planning: I. The Teaching Phase," *Fertility and Sterility*, vol. 362 (Aug. 1981), pp. 152–58.

32. T. W. Hilgers, G. F. Abraham, and D. Cavanagh, "Natural Family Planning. I. The

Peak Symptom and Estimated Time of Ovulation," *American Journal of Obstetrics and Gynecology*, vol. 52, no. 5 (Nov. 1978), pp. 575–82.

33. Material for this section was obtained from Dr. Joseph Stanford.

34. J. F. Cattanach and B. J. Milne, "Post-Tubal Sterilization Problems Correlated with Ovarian Steroidogenesis," *Contraception*, vol. 38, no. 5 (1988); J. Donnez, M. Wauters, and K. Thomas, "Luteal Function After Tubal Sterilization," *Obstetrics and Gynecology*, vol. 57, no. 1 (1981); M. M. Cohen, "Long-Term Risk of Hysterectomy After Tubal Sterilization," *American Journal of Epidemiology*, vol. 125 (1987).

35. S. Sumiala et al., "Salivary Progesterone Concentration After Tubal Sterilization," *Obstetrics and Gynecology*, vol. 88 (1996), pp. 792–96.

36. A. Domar et al., "The Prevalence and Predictability of Depression in Infertile Women," *Fertility and Sterility*, vol. 58 (1992), pp. 1158–63; A. Domar et al., "The Psychological Impact of Infertility: A Comparison with Patients with Other Medical Conditions," *Journal of Psychosomatic Obstetrics and Gynecology*, vol. 14 (1993), pp. 45–52.

37. I. Gerhard et al., "Prolonged Exposure to Wood Preservatives Induces Endocrine and Immunologic Disorders in Women," *American Journal of Obstetrics and Gynecology*, vol. 165, no. 2 (Aug. 1991), pp. 487–88; P. Thompkins, "Hazards of Electromagnetic Fields to Human Reproduction," *Fertility and Sterility*, vol. 53, no. 1 (Jan. 1990), pp. 185.

38. A. Stagnaw-Green et al., "Detection of At Risk Pregnancy by Means of Highly Sensitive Assays for Thyroid Autoantibodies," *Journal of the American Medical Association*, vol. 269, no. 11 (Sept. 19, 1990), pp. 1422–25; and O. B. Christiansen et al., "Autoimmunity and Spontaneous Abortion," *Human Reproduction* [Denmark], vol. 4, no. 8 (1989), pp. 913–17.

39. M. Stauber, "Psychosomatic Problems of Childless Couples," *Archives of Gynecology and Obstetrics*, vol. 245, nos. 1–4 (1989), pp. 1047–50.

40. L. Jeker et al., "Wish for a Child and Infertility: A Study of 116 Couples. I. Interview and Psychodynamic Hypotheses," *International Journal of Fertility*, vol. 33, no. 6 (1988), pp. 411–20.

41. T. Shevell et al., "Assisted Reproductive Technology and Pregnancy Outcome," *Obstetrics and Gynecology*, vol. 106, no. 5 (Nov. 2005), pp. 1039–1045.

42. Ellen Hopkins, "Tales from the Baby Factory," *New York Times Magazine* (Mar. 15, 1992).

43. P. Kemeter, "Studies on Psychosomatic Implications of Infertility: Effects of Emotional Stress on Fertilization and Implantation in In Vitro Fertilization," *Human Reproduction*, vol. 3, no. 3 (April 1988), pp. 341–52.

44. F. Facchinetti et al., "An Increased Vulnerability to Stress Is Associated with a Poor Outcome of In Vitro Fertilization—Embryo Transfer Treatment," *Fertility and Sterility*, vol. 67 (1997), pp. 309–14.

45. Karl Menninger, "Somatic Correlations with the Unconscious Repudiation of Femininity in Women," *Journal of Nervous and Mental Disease*, vol. 89 (1939), p. 514; Therese Benedek and Boris Rubenstein, "Correlations Between Ovarian Activity and Psychodynamic Processes: The Ovulatory Phase," *Psychosomatic*

Medicine, vol. 1, no. 2 (1939), pp. 245–70; A. Mayer, "Sterility in Women as a Result of Functional Disturbance," *Journal of the American Medical Association*, vol. 105 (1935), p. 1474; Kemeter, "Studies on Psychosomatic Implications of Infertility" (see note 343).

46. Havelock Ellis, *Studies in the Psychology of Sex* (Philadelphia: Davis and Co., 1928); T. H. Van de Veld, *Fertility and Sterility in Marriage* (New York: Covic Fried, 1931).

47. H. F. Dunbar, *Emotions and Bodily Changes* (New York: Columbia University Press, 1935), p. 595; R. L. Dickerson, "Medical Analysis of 1000 Marriages," *Journal of the American Medical Association*, vol. 97 (1931), p. 529; C. C. Norris, "Sterility in the Female Without Gross Pathology," *Surgery, Gynecology, and Obstetrics*, vol. 15 (1912), p. 706.

48. D. H. Hellhammer et al., "Male Infertility, Relationships Among Gonadotropins, Sex Steroids, Seminal Parameters, and Personality Attitudes," *Psychosomatic Medicine*, vol. 47, no. 1 (1985), pp. 58–66.

49. A. M. Brkovich and W. A. Fisher, "Psychological Distress and Infertility: Forty Years of Research," *Journal of Psychosomatic Obstetrics and Gynaecology*, vol. 19, no. 4 (Dec. 1998), pp. 218–28.

50. A. D. Domar et al., "The Mind/Body Program for Infertility: A New Behavioral Treatment Approach for Women with Infertility," *Fertility and Sterility*, vol. 53., no. 2 (Feb. 1990), pp. 246–9.

51. Some of this material was originally published in the June 1997 issue of Christiane Northrup's newsletter, *Health Wisdom for Women*.

52. D. R. Meldrum, "Female Reproductive Aging—Ovarian and Uterine Factors," *Fertility and Sterility*, vol. 59, vol. 1 (Jan. 1993), p. 1–5; C. Wood, I. Calderon, and A. Crombie, "Age and Fertility: Results of Assisted Reproductive Technology in Women Over 40 Years," *Journal of Assisted Reproduction and Genetics*, vol. 9, no. 5 (Oct. 1992), p. 482–4; S. L. Tan, et al., "Cumulative Conception and Livebirth Rates After In-Vitro Fertilisation," *The Lancet*, vol. 339, no. 8806 (June 1992), p. 1390–4.

53. W. J. Kennedy, *Edinburgh Medical Journal*, vol. 27 (1882), p. 1086.

54. Personal communication from Brant Secunda.

55. J. Johnson et al., "Germline Stem Cells and Follicular Renewal in the Postnatal Mammalian Ovary," *Nature*, vol. 428, no. 6979 (March 11, 2004), pp. 145–50.

56. B. E. Hamilton et al., "Births: Preliminary Data for 2003," *National Vital Statistics Report*, vol. 53, no. 9 (Nov. 23, 2004), pp. 1–17.

57. S. K. Henshaw, "Unintended Pregnancy in the United States," Family Planning Perspectives, vol. 30, no. 1 (Jan–Feb. 1998), pp. 24–9, 46.

58. H. Benson, "Stress, Anxiety and the Relaxation Response," *Behavioral Biology in Medicine: A Monograph Series*, No. 3. (So. Norwalk, CT: Meducation, 1985), pp. 1–28.

59. While the pregnancy rate for other infertile couples seeking medical treatment is between 17 and 25 percent, the pregnancy rate in Dr. Domar's program is 44 percent, with 37 percent taking home a baby (some pregnancies end in miscarriage). "The Goddess of Fertility," *Boston Magazine*, March 1997, pp. 57–117.

60. Facchinetti et al., "An Increased Vulnerability to Stress" (see note 44).

61. Harry Fisch with Stephen Braun, *The Male Biological Clock: The Startling News About Aging. Sexuality, and Fertility in Men* (New York: Free Press, 2005), p. xiii.

62. J. Pei et al., "Quantitative Evaluation of Spermatozoa Ultrastructure After Acupuncture Treatment for Idiopathic Male Infertility," *Fertility and Sterility*, vol. 84, no. 1 (July 2005), pp. 141–47.

63. Fisch, p. xiv (see note 61).

64. E. Dewan, "On the Possibility of a Perfect Rhythm Method of Birth Control by Periodic Light Stimulation," *American Journal of Obstetrics and Gynecology*, vol. 99, no. 7 (Dec. 1, 1967), pp. 1016–19. See also notes for chapter 5, The Menstrual Cycle.

65. E. R. Gonzalez, "Sperm Swim Singly After Vitamin C Therapy," *Journal of the American Medical Association*, vol. 20 (1983), p. 2747; T. R. Haroma et al., "Zinc, Plasma Androgens, and Male Sterility," letter to the editor, *The Lancet*, vol. 3 (1977), pp. 1125–26; M. Igarashi, "Augmentative Effects of Ascorbic Acid upon Induction of Human Ovulation in Clomiphene Ineffective Anovulatory Women," *International Journal of Fertility*, vol. 22, no. 3 (1977), pp. 68–73; D. W. Dawson, "Infertility and Folate Deficiency," case reports, *British Journal of Obstetrics and Gynaecology*, vol. 89 (1982), p. 678.

66. J. Hargrove and E. Guy, "Effect of Vitamin B_6 on Infertility in Women with Premenstrual Tension Syndrome," *Infertility*, vol. 2, no. 4 (1979), pp. 315–22.

67. L. M. Westphal et al., "A Nutritional Supplement for Improving Fertility in Women: A Pilot Study," *Journal of Reproductive Medicine*, vol. 49, no. 4 (Apr. 2004), pp. 289–93.

68. D. E. Stewart et al., "Infertility and Eating Disorders," *American Journal of Obstetrics and Gynecology*, vol. 163 (1990), pp. 1196–99.

69. *2002 Assisted Reproductive Technology Success Rates: National Summary and Fertility Clinic Reports*, Centers for Disease Control and Prevention, U.S. Department of Health and Human Services.

70. Lucia Cappachione, *The Wisdom of Your Other Hand* (North Hollywood, CA: Newcastle Publishing Co., 1990).

71. For more information, write Whitney Oppersdorff at the following address: RFD 2, Box 606, Lincolnville, ME 04849.

72. A. Blau et al., "The Psychogenic Etiology of Premature Births," *Psychosomatic Medicine*, vol. 25 (1963), p. 201; Robert J. Weil, "The Problem of Spontaneous Abortion," *American Journal of Obstetrics and Gynecology*, vol. 73 (1957), p. 322.

73. L. Fenster et al., "Caffeinated Beverages, Decaffeinated Coffee, and Spontaneous Abortion," *Epidemiology*, vol. 8., no. 5 (Sept. 1997), pp. 515–23.

74. Robert J. Weil and C. Tupper, "Personality, Life Situation, Communication: A Study of Habitual Abortion," *Psychosomatic Medicine*, vol. 22, no. 6 (1960), pp. 448–55.

75. Weil and Tupper, "Personality" (see note 74).

76. E. R. Grimm, "Psychological Investigation or Habitual Abortion," *Psychosomatic Medicine*, vol. 24, no. 4 (1962), pp. 370–78.

77. R. L. VandenBergh, "Emotional Illness in Habitual Aborters Following Suturing of Incompetent Cervical Os," *Psychosomatic Medicine*, vol. 28, no. 3 (1966), pp. 257–63.

78. "Chapter 10: Ectopic Pregnancy," in F. Gary Cunningham et al., eds., *Williams Obstetrics, 22nd edition* (New York: McGraw Hill Professional, 2005), pp. 254–55.

79. Jennifer Ehrle Macomber, Erica H. Zielewski, Kate Chambers, and Rob Geen, "Foster Care Adoption in the United States: An Analysis of Interest in Adoption and a Review of State Recruitment Strategies," Urban Institute, Washington, D.C., November 2005.

80. Union of Concerned Scientists, 26 Church Street, Cambridge, MA 02238: 617-547-5552.

Chapter 12: Pregnancy and Birthing

1. Thomas R. Verny and Pamela Weintraub, *Tomorrow's Baby: The Art and Science of Parenting from Conception Through Infancy* (New York: Simon & Schuster, 2002), p. 29.

2. Peter W. Nathanielsz, *Life in the Womb: The Origin of Health and Disease* (Ithaca, NY: Promethean Press, 1999).

3. U.S. Department of Health, Education, and Welfare, the National Center for Health Statistics, *Wanted and Unwanted Births by Mothers 15–44 Years of Age: United States, 1973* (Washington, DC: U.S. Government Printing Office, 1973); advance data from *Vital and Health Statistics*, no. 9 (Aug. 10, 1977); National Institutes of Health, Institute of Child Health and Human Development, research reports (Nov. 1992), available from NICHD Office of Research Reporting, building 31, room 2A312, National Institutes of Health, Bethesda, MD 01892; (310) 496-5133; M. D. Muylder et al., "A Women's Attitude Toward Pregnancy: Can It Predispose Her to Preterm Labor?" *Journal of Reproductive Medicine*, vol. 37, no. 4 (Apr. 1992); R. Newton and L. Hunt, "Psychosocial Stress in Pregnancy and Its Relationship to Low Birth Weight," *British Medical Journal*, vol. 288 (1984), p. 1191.

4. Ronald Meyers, "Maternal Anxiety and Fetal Death," *Psychoneuroimmunology in Reproduction* (New York: Elsevier/North-Holland Biomedical Press, 1979), pp. 555–73.

5. L. E. Mehl et al., "The Role of Hypnotherapy in Facilitating Normal Birth," in P. G. Fedor-Freburgh and M. L. V. Vogel, eds., *Encounter with the Unborn: Perinatal Psychology and Medicine* (Park Ridge, NJ: Parthenon, 1988), pp. 189–207; I. E. Mehl, "Hypnosis in Preventing Premature Labor," *Journal of Prenatal and Perinatal Psychology*, vol. 8 (1988), pp. 234–240; A. Omer, "Hypnosis and Premature Labor," *Journal of Psychosomatic Medicine*, vol. 57 (1986), pp. 454–60.

6. R. L. VandenBerge et al., "Emotional Illness in Habitual Aborters Following Suturing of the Incompetent Cervical Os," *Psychosomatic Medicine*, vol. 28, no. 3 (1966), pp. 257–63.

7. G. Berkowitz and S. Kasl, "The Role of Psychosocial Factors in Spontaneous Preterm Delivery," *Journal of Psychosomatic Research*, vol. 27 (1983), p. 283;

R. Newton et al., "Psychosocial Stress in Pregnancy and Its Relation to the Onset of Premature Labour," *British Medical Journal*, vol. 2 (1979), p. 411; A. Blau et al., "The Psychogenic Etiology of Premature Births: A Preliminary Report," *Psychosomatic Medicine*, vol. 25 (1963), p. 201.

8. V. Laukaran and C. van Den Berg, "The Relationship of Maternal Attitude to Pregnancy Outcomes and Obstetric Complications: A Cohort Study of Unwanted Pregnancies," *American Journal of Obstetrics and Gynecology*, vol. 139 (1981), p. 596; R. McDonald, "The Role of Emotional Factors in Obstetric Complications," *Psychosomatic Medicine*, vol. 30 (1968), p. 222; M. D. De Muylder, "Psychological Factors and Preterm Labour," *Journal of Reproductive Psychology*, vol. 7 (1989), p. 55.

9. R. Myers, "Maternal Anxiety and Fetal Death," in L. Zichella and P. Pancheri, eds., *Psychoneuroendocrinocology and Reproduction* (New York: Elsevier, 1979).

10. L. E. Mehl, "A Psychosocial Prenatal Intervention to Reduce Alcohol, Smoking, and Stress and Improve Birth Outcome Among Minority Women," obtainable from Lewis Mehl-Medrona, M.D., Ph.D., 16 Quail Run, South Burlington, VT 05403; 800-931-8584.

11. H. P. Schobel et al., "Preeclampsia: A State of Sympathetic Overactivity," *New England Journal of Medicine*, vol. 335, no. 20 (1996), pp. 480–85; H. J. Passloer, "Angstlich—Feindseliges Verhalten als Prakursor einer Schaumangerschaf-stinduzierten Hypertonic (SIJ)," *A. Guburtsh Perinat.*, vol. 195 (1991), pp. 137–42.

12. E. Muller-Tyl and B. Wimmer-Puchinger, "Psychosomatic Aspects of Toxemia," *Journal of Psychosomatic Obstetrics and Gynecology*, vol. 1, nos. 3–4 (1982), pp. 111–17; C. Ringrose, "Psychosomatic Influence in the Genesis of Toxemia of Pregnancy," *Canadian Medical Association Journal*, vol. 84 (1961), p. 647; and A. J. Cooper, "Psychosomatic Aspects of Pre-eclamptic Toxemia," *Journal of Psychosomatic Research*, vol. 2 (1958), p. 241.

13. R. L. McDonald, "Personality Characteristics in Patients with Three Obstetric Complications," *Psychosomatic Medicine*, vol. 27, no. 4 (1965), pp. 383–90.

14. C. Cheek and E. Rossi, *Mind-Body Hypothesis* (New York: W. W. Norton, 1989).

15. L. Mehl, "Hypnosis and Conversion of the Breech to the Vertex Position," *Archives of Family Medicine*, vol. 3 (1994), pp. 881–87.

16. Katz et al., "Catecholamine Levels in Pregnant Physicians and Nurses: A Pilot Study of Stress and Pregnancy," *Obstetrics and Gynecology*, vol. 77, no. 3 (Mar. 1991), pp. 338–41.

17. J. A. McGregor et al., "The Omega-3 Story: Nutritional Prevention of Preterm Birth and Other Adverse Pregnancy Outcomes," *Obstetrical and Gynecological Survey*, vol. 56, no. 5 suppl. 1 (May 2001), pp. S1–13.

18. E. B. Da Fonseca et al., "Prophylactic Administration of Progesterone by Vaginal Suppository to Reduce the Incidence of Spontaneous Preterm Birth in Women at Increased Risk: A Randomized Placebo-Controlled Double-Blind Study," *American Journal of Obstetrics and Gynecology*, vol. 188, no. 2 (Feb. 2003), pp. 419–24; P. J. Meis et al., "Prevention of Recurrent Preterm Delivery by 17 Alpha-Hydroxyprogesterone Caproate," *New England Journal of Medicine*, vol. 348, no. 24 (June 12, 2003), pp. 2379–85.

19. N. Mamelle et al., "Prevention of Preterm Birth in Patients with Symptoms of

Preterm Labor—The Benefits of Psychologic Support," *American Journal of Obstetrics and Gynecology*, vol. 177, no. 4 (1977), pp. 947–52.

20. T. Field et al., "Pregnant Women Benefit from Massage Therapy," *Journal of Psychosomatic Obstetrics and Gynaecology*, vol. 20, no. 1 (Mar. 1999), pp. 31–38; T. Field, "Labor Pain Is Reduced by Massage Therapy," *Journal of Psychosomatic Obstetrics and Gynaecology*, vol. 18, no. 4 (Dec. 1997), pp. 286–91.

21. D. A. Oren et al., "An Open Trial of Morning Light Therapy for Treatment of Antepartum Depression," *American Journal of Psychiatry*, vol. 159, no. 4 (April 2002), pp. 666–69.

22. K. C. Johnson and B. A. Daviss, "Outcomes of Planned Home Births with Certified Professional Midwives: Large Prospective Study in North America," *British Medical Journal*, vol. 330, no. 7505 (June 18, 2005), p. 1416.

23. Centers for Disease Control and Prevention, "State-Specific Maternal Mortality Among Black and White Women—United States, 1987–1996," *Morbidity and Mortality Weekly Report*, vol. 48, no. 23 (June 18, 1999).

24. Judith Levit, *Brought to Bed: Childbearing in America, 1750–1950* (New York: Oxford University Press, 1988).

25. R. Sosa et al., "The Effect of Supportive Companions on Perinatal Problems, Length of Labor, and Mother-Infant Interaction," *New England Journal of Medicine*, vol. 303 (1980), pp. 597–600; M. H. Klaus, J. H. Kennell, S. S. Robertson, and R. Sosa, "Effects of Social Support During Parturition in Maternal and Infant Mortality," *British Medical Journal*, vol. 293 (1986), pp. 585–87; M. H. Klaus, J. H. Kennell, G. Berkowitz, and P. Klaus, "Maternal Assistance and Support in Labor: Father, Nurse, Midwife, or Doula?" *Clinical Consultation in Obstetrics and Gynecology*, vol. 4 (Dec. 1992).

26. Robert M. Sapolsky, *Why Zebras Don't Get Ulcers* (New York: W. H. Freeman, 1994), pp. 116–22.

27. F. T. Kapp et al., "Some Psychological Factors in Prolonged Labor Due to Inefficient Uterine Action," *Comparative Psychiatry*, vol. 4 (1963), p. 9; L. Gunter, "Psychopathology and Stress in the Life Experience of Mothers of Premature Infants," *American Journal of Obstetrics and Gynecology*, vol. 86 (1963), p. 333; A. Davids and S. Devault, "Maternal Anxiety During Pregnancy and Childbirth Abnormalities," *Journal of Psychosomatic Medicine*, vol. 24 (1972), p. 464.

28. Questions provided here are part of the American College of Obstetricians and Gynecologists Domestic Violence Screening Program.

29. J. J. Oat et al., "Characteristics and Motives of Women Choosing Elective Induction of Labor," *Journal of Psychosomatic Research*, vol. 30, no. 3 (1986), pp. 375–80.

30. Cited in Gayle H. Peterson, *Birthing Normally: A Personal Approach to Childbirth* (Berkeley, CA: Mindbody Press), appendix 2, p. 181. See also Lewis Mehl, Gayle Peterson, et al., "Complications of Home Delivery: Analysis of a Series of 287 Deliveries from Santa Cruz, California," *Birth and Family Journal*, vol. 2, no. 4 (1975), pp. 123–31; and Gayle Peterson, Lewis Mehl, et al., "Outcome of 1146 Elective Home Births," *Journal of Reproductive Medicine*, vol. 19, no. 3 (1977), pp. 281–90.

31. Peggy O'Mara, "The Community of Normal Birth: What Does It Look Like? How

Do You Find It?" Keynote address of the annual conference of Association for Pre- & Perinatal Psychology and Health (APPPAH), November 2005, San Diego, CA.

32. Data are from the Houston Healthcare Coalition, Houston, TX (1986); personal communications with Dr. Bethany Hays.

33. D. A. Luthy, K. K. Shy, et al., "Effects of Electronic Fetal Heart Rate Monitoring as Compared with Periodic Auscultation on the Neurologic Development of Premature Infants," *New England Journal of Medicine* (Mar. 1, 1990), pp. 588–93.

34. S. Gardner, "When Your Patient Demands a C-Section," *OBG Management* (Nov. 1991).

35. M. H. Hall, "Commentary: Confidential Enquiry into Maternal Death," *British Journal of Obstetrics and Gynaecology*, vol. 97, no. 8 (Aug. 1990), pp. 752–53; N. Schuitemaker et al., "Maternal Mortality After Cesarean Section in the Netherlands," *Acta Obstetricia et Gynecologica Scandinavica*, vol. 76, no. 4 (1997), pp. 332–34.

36. E. L. Shearer, "Cesarean Section: Medical Benefits and Costs," *Social Science & Medicine*, vol. 37, no. 10 (1993), pp. 1223–31; American College of Obstetricians and Gynecologists, Task Force on Cesarean Delivery Rates, *Evaluation of Cesarean Delivery* (Washington, DC: ACOG, 2000).

37. S. M. Miovich et al., "Major Concerns of Women After Cesarean Delivery," *Journal of Obstetric, Gynecologic, and Neonatal Nursing*, vol. 23, no. 1 (1994), pp. 53–59.

38. E. R. Declercq et al., *Listening to Mothers: Report of the First National U.S. Survey of Women's Childbearing Experiences* (New York: Maternity Center Association/ Harris Interactive Inc., Oct. 2002).

39. M. Lydon-Rochelle et al., "Association Between Method of Delivery and Maternal Rehospitalization," *Journal of the American Medical Association*, vol. 283, no. 18 (2000), pp. 2411–16.

40. J. Jolly, J. Walker, and K. Bhabra, "Subsequent Obstetric Performance Related to Primary Mode of Delivery," *British Journal of Obstetrics and Gynaecology*, vol. 106, no. 3 (1999), pp. 227–32.

41. J. M. Crane et al., "Neonatal Outcomes with Placenta Previa," *Obstetrics and Gynecology*, vol. 93, no. 4 (1999), pp. 541–44.

42. March of Dimes, medical references: preterm birth. http://www.marchofdimes.com/professionals/14332_1157.asp

43. M. A. Van Ham, P. W. van Dongen, and J. Mulder, "Maternal Consequences of Caesarean Section. A Retrospective Study of Intra-Operative and Postoperative Maternal Complications of Caesarean Section During a 10-Year Period," *European Journal of Obstetrics, Gynecology, and Reproductive Biology*, vol. 74, no. 1 (1997), pp. 1–6.

44. D. J. Annibale et al., "Comparative Neonatal Morbidity of Abdominal and Vaginal Deliveries After Uncomplicated Pregnancies," *Archives of Pediatrics & Adolescent Medicine*, vol. 149, no. 8 (1995), pp. 862–67.

45. E. M. Levine et al., "Mode of Delivery and Risk of Respiratory Diseases in Newborns," *Obstetrics and Gynecology*, vol. 97, no. 3 (2001), pp. 439–42.

46. K. Hartmann et al., "Outcomes of Routine Episiotomy: A Systematic Review," *Journal of the American Medical Association*, vol. 293, no. 17 (May 4, 2005), pp. 2141–48.

47. P. Shiono et al., "Midline Episiotomies: More Harm than Good," *American Journal of Obstetrics and Gynecology*, vol. 75, no. 5 (May 1990), pp. 765–70.

48. Walker et al., "Epidural Anesthesia, Episiotomy, and Obstetric Laceration," *American Journal of Obstetrics and Gynecology*, vol. 77, no. 5 (May 1991), pp. 668–71.

49. J. Ecker et al., "Is There a Benefit to Episiotomy at Operative Vaginal Delivery: Observations over 10 Years in a Stable Population," *American Journal of Obstetrics and Gynecology*, vol. 176 (1997), pp. 411–14.

50. Hartmann, "Outcomes of Routine Episiotomy" (see note 46).

51. J. Press et al., "Mode of Delivery and Pelvic Floor Dysfunction: A Systematic Review of the Literature on Urinary and Fecal Incontinence and Sexual Dysfunction by Mode of Delivery," Medscape Ob/Gyn & Women's Health, Clinical Update (posted Jan. 17, 2006); available at http://www.medscape.com/viewprogram/4989.

52. James Thorpe et al., "The Effect of Continuous Epidural Anesthesia on Cesarean Sections for Dystocia in Primiparous Patients," *American Journal of Obstetrics and Gynecology* (Sept. 1989); H. Kaminski, A. Stafl, and J. Aiman, "The Effect of Epidural Analgesia on the Frequency of Instrumental Obstetric Delivery," *American Journal of Obstetrics and Gynecology*, vol. 69, no. 5 (May 1987); L. Fusi, P. J. Steer, M. J. A. Maresh, and R. W. Bears, "Maternal Pyrexia Associated with the Use of Epidural Analgesia in Labour," *The Lancet*, vol. 1, no. 8649 (1989), pp. 1250–51.

53. E. Lieberman et al., "Association of Epidural Analgesia with Cesarean Delivery in Nulliparas," *Obstetrics and Gynecology*, vol. 88 (1996), pp. 993–1000; Shiv Sharma et al., "Cesarean Delivery: A Randomized Trial of Epidural versus Patient-Controlled Meperidine Analgesia during Labor," *Anesthesiology*, vol. 87, no. 3 (1997), pp. 487–94; David Chestnut, "Epidural Analgesia and the Incidence of Cesarean Section," *Anesthesiology*, vol. 87, no. 3 (1997), pp. 472–76.

54. E. Lieberman et al., "Changes in Fetal Position During Labor and Their Association with Epidural Analgesia," *Obstetrics and Gynecology*, vol. 105, no. 5 Pt 1 (May 2005), pp. 974–82.

55. E. Lieberman, "Epidural Analgesia, Intrapartum Fever, and Neontal Sepsis Evaluation," *Pediatrics*, vol. 99, no. 1 (1997), 415–19.

56. Jeanne Achterberg, *Women as Healer* (Boston: Shambhala, 1990), p. 126.

57. Known as the McRoberts Maneuver, this can be demonstrated by bringing your legs up into a "squatting position" while lying on your back.

58. M. Klaus, J. Kennell, and P. Klaus, *Mothering the Mother: How a Doula Can Help You Have Shorter, Easier, and Healthier Birth* (New York: Addison-Wesley, 1993), p. 25.

59. Jacqueline Stenson, "Number of C-Sections Must Be Reduced," *Medical Tribune* (May 2, 1996).

60. Reported in *Medical Tribune* (Mar. 21, 1996).

61. M. B. Landon et al., "Maternal and Perinatal Outcomes Associated with a Trial of Labor After Prior Cesarean Delivery," *New England Journal of Medicine*, vol. 351, no. 25 (Dec. 16, 2004), pp. 2581–89.

62. Membranes rarely rupture from pelvic examinations. Perhaps mine did because of

an unusual umbilical cord insertion on the membranes, known as a villamentous insertion. Or maybe they were just ready to go!

63. As we will see, being "distracted" in the middle of a process as important as labor may not be the best approach.

64. Vicki Noble, *Shakti Woman* (San Francisco: Harper and Row, 1992).

Chapter 13: Motherhood: Bonding with Your Baby

1. Marshall H. Klaus and John H. Kennell *Maternal-Infant Bonding* (St. Louis: C.V. Mosby Company, 1976).

2. Marshall H. Klaus and John H. Kennell, *Parent-Infant Bonding* (St. Louis, MO: CV Mosby Company, 1982).

3. C. M. Huhn et al., "Tactile-Kinesthetic Stimulation Effects on Sympathetic and Adrenocortical Function in Preterm Infants," *Journal of Pediatrics*, vol. 119, no. 3 (1991), pp. 434–40.

4. Actually, the first studies on putting babies in incubators were done on premature babies who weren't expected to live and who therefore had been "discarded" by their mothers. Martin Cooney, a pioneer in neonatal care, put a group of these infants in incubators and toured with them, even to the Chicago World's Fair, where he had an attraction called "Live Babies in Incubator"; its receipts were second only to those of Sally Rand the Fan Dancer. Once he got the babies to a certain weight, he tried to give them back to their mothers, but the mothers didn't want them, having formed no emotional tie with them. This information is from Kennell and Marshall, *Maternal-Infant Bonding* (see note 1).

5. G. M. Morley, "Cord Closure: Can Hasty Clamping Injure the Newborn?" *OBG Management*, vol. 10, no. 7 (1998), pp. 29–36; S. Kinmond et al., "Umbilical Cord Clamping and Preterm Infants: A Randomised Trial," *British Medical Journal*, vol. 306, no. 6871 (1993), pp. 172–75. If a blood pressure gauge is placed on an unclamped umbilical cord, it will pick up pressure rises as high as 60 mm Hg with each uterine contraction. This indicates that these contractions are intimately involved in the transfer of placental blood through the cord. A striking pressure rise, which persists through the first few hours of life, is also evident in the baby's vena cava and right atrium of the heart. All studies on this indicate a significantly higher systemic pressure in infants who have been clamped late (90 percent in the first nine hours) and conversely, a significant drop in those early-clamped infants (70 percent of systemic by the second hour, and almost 50 percent of systemic by the fourth hour). (A. J. Moss and M. Monset-Couchard, "Placental Transfusion; Early versus Late Clamping of the Umbilical Cord," *Pediatrics*, vol. 40, no. 1 [July 1967], pp. 109–126.) The placental blood normally belongs to the infant, and his or her failure to get this blood is equivalent to submitting the newborn to a severe hemorrhage at birth. The time of cord clamping may be involved in the pathogenesis of idiopathic respiratory distress syndrome (the earlier clamped, the more respiratory distress). (S. Saigal et al., "Placental Transfusion and Hyperbilirubinemia in the Premature," *Pediatrics*, vol. 49, no. 3 [March 1972], pp. 406–419.) Placental blood acts as a source of nourishment that protects infants against the breakdown of body protein. (Q. B. De Marsh et

al., "The Effect of Depriving the Infant of Its Placental Blood," *Journal of the American Medical Association*, vol. 116, no. 23 [June 7, 1941], pp. 2568–73.] Studies have shown that immediate cord clamping prolongs the average duration of the third stage and greatly increases maternal blood loss. (S. Z. Walsh, "Maternal Effects of Early and Late Clamping of the Umbilical Cord," *The Lancet*, vol. 1, no. 7550 [May 11, 1968], pp. 996–97.)

6. Shaila Kulkarni Misri, *Pregnancy Blues: What Every Woman Needs to Know About Depression During Pregnancy* (New York: Delacorte Press, 2005).

7. H. Vinamaki et al., "Evolution of Postpartum Mental Health," *Journal of Psychosomatic Obstetrics and Gynecology*, vol. 18 (1997), pp. 213–19; D. D. Affonso and G. Domino, "Postpartum Depression: A Review," *Birth*, vol. 11, no. 4 (Winter 1984), pp. 231–35.

8. K. Dalton, "Successful Prophylactic Progesterone for Idiopathic Post-Natal Depression," *International Journal of Prenatal Studies* (1989), pp. 322–27.

9. D. Sichel et al., "Prophlactic Estrogen in Recurrent Postpartum Affective Disorder," *Society of Biological Psychiatry*, vol. 38 (1995), pp. 814–18.

10. George Denniston, "Unnecessary Circumcision," *Female Patient*, vol. 17 (July 1992), p. 13.

11. Data on the effects of circumcision are available from the Circumcision Resource Center, attn. Ronald Goldman, P.O. Box 232, Boston, MA 02133; (617) 523-0088.

12. July/August 1995 issue of the *Baby Friendly Hospital Initiative Newsletter*, cited by Elizabeth Baldwin in "So Why Do We Have Breastfeeding Legislation?" *New Beginnings: La Leche League's Breastfeeding Journal*, vol. 13, no. 2 (March/April 1996), p. 43.

13. A. Lucas et al., "Breast Milk and Subsequent Intelligence Quotient in Children Born Preterm," *The Lancet* (Feb. 1, 1992), pp. 261–64.

14. A solution to this might be the visualization procedure mentioned at the end of the section on breast augmentation in chapter 10.

15. Ellen Goodman, "Search for Father Dominating Lives," *Portland Press Herald* (Apr. 10, 1992), syndicated from *Boston Globe*.

16. Nancy McBrine Sheehan, 11 Fox Run, East Sandwich, MA 02537; used here with the author's permission.

Chapter 14: Menopause

1. Tamara Slayton, *Reclaiming the Menstrual Matrix: Evolving Feminine Wisdom— A Workbook* (Petaluma, CA: Menstrual Health Foundation, 1990), p. 41.

2. Slayton, *Reclaiming the Menstrual Matrix*, p. 41 (see note 1).

3. J. C. Prior et al., "Spinal Bone Loss and Ovulatory Disturbances," *New England Journal of Medicine*, vol. 323 (1990), pp. 1221–27.

4. C. Longscope, R. Hunter, and C. Franz, "Steroid Secretion by the Postmenopausal Ovary," *American Journal of Obstetrics and Gynecology*, vol. 138 (1980), pp. 6540–68; C. Longscope, C. Bourget, and C. Flood, "The Production and Aromatization of Dehydroepiandrosterone in Postmenopausal Women," *Maturitas*,

vol. 4 (1982), pp. 325–32; C. Longscope, W. Jaffe, and G. Griffing, "Production Rates of Androgens and Oestrogens in Post-Menopausal Women," *Maturitas*, vol. 3 (1981), pp. 215–23.

5. W. M. Jeffries, "Cortisol and Immunity," *Medical Hypotheses*, vol. 34 (1991), pp. 198–208; J. P. Kahn et al., "Salivary Cortisol: A Practical Method for Evaluation of Adrenal Function," *Biological Psychiatry*, vol. 23 (1988), pp. 335–49; M. H. Laudet et al., "Salivary Cortisol: A Practical Approach to Assess Pituitary-Adrenal Function," *Journal of Clinical Endocrinology and Metabolism*, vol. 66 (1988), pp. 343–48; R. F. Vining and R. A. McGinley, "The Measurement of Hormones in Saliva: Possibilities and Pitfalls," *Journal of Steroid Biochemistry*, vol. 27, nos. 1–3 (1987), pp. 81–94.

6. E. Barrett-Connor et al., "A Prospective Study of Dehydroepiandrosterone Sulfate, Mortality, and Cardiovascular Disease," *New England Journal of Medicine*, vol. 315, no. 24 (1986), pp. 1519–24; R. E. Bulbrook et al., "Relation Between Urinary Androgen and Corticoid Excretion and Subsequent Breast Cancer," *The Lancet*, vol. 2, no. 7721 (1971), pp. 395–98; S. E. Monroe and K. M. J. Menon, "Changes in Reproductive Hormone Secretion During the Climacteric and Post-Menopausal Periods," *Clinical Obstetrics and Gynecology*, vol. 20 (1977), pp. 113–22; W. Regelson et al., "Hormonal Intervention: 'Buffer Hormones' or 'State Dependency': The Role of DHEA, Thyroid Hormone, Estrogen, and Hypophysectomy in Aging," *Annals of the New York Academy of Sciences*, vol. 521 (1988), pp. 260–73. A recent study of postmenopausal women age sixty to seventy using DHEA skin cream showed that after a year of treatment, the women experienced a 10-percent decrease in body fat, a 10 percent increase in muscle mass, decreased blood sugar levels, decreased insulin levels, and a decrease in cholesterol. Their vaginal tissue also showed a thickening similar to that seen with estrogen, but there was no increase in stimulation of the uterine lining. There was also an increase in bone density. Unfortunately, these women also experienced a 70-percent increase in the oiliness of their skin, which resulted in acne—an effect that could probably be reduced with somewhat lower doses. See R. Sahelian, "Landmark One-Year DHEA Study," *Health Counselor*, vol. 9, no. 2 (1997), pp. 46–47.

7. Ralph Golan, *Optimal Wellness* (New York: Ballantine, 1995), specifically chapter 11, "Adrenal Exhaustion," pp. 197–207; E. Olya, *The New Definition of Stress Evaluation Adrenal Stress Index* (Kent, WA: Diagnos-Techs, 1991); Laudet et al., "Salivary Cortisol" (see note 5); Kahn et al., "Salivary Cortisol" (see note 5); J. B. Jemmott et al., "Academic Stress, Power, Motivation, and Decrease in Salivary IgA Secretion Rate," *The Lancet* (June 1983), pp. 1400–2; F. Horst and J. Born, "Evidence for the Entrainment of Nocturnal Cortisol Secretion and Sleep Process in Human Beings," *Neuroendocrinology*, vol. 53 (1991), pp. 171–76; J. W. Tintera, "The Hypoadrenocortical State and Its Management," *New York Journal of Medicine*, vol. 55, no. 13 (July 1, 1955).

8. R. McCraty et al., "The Impact of a New Emotional Self-Management Program on Stress, Emotions, Heart Rate Variability, DHEA and Cortisol," *Integrative Physiological and Behavioral Sciences*, vol. 33, no. 3 (April–June 1998). An updated "Research Overview" provides more information on the many studies the Institute of HeartMath has done and is presently involved with. Available from the Institute of HeartMath, P.O. Box 1463, Boulder Creek, CA 95006, (931) 338-8500.

9. J. Hargrove and E. Eisenberg, "Menopause," *Medical Clinics of North America*, vol. 79, no. 6 (1995), pp. 1337–56.

10. C. B. Coulam, "Premature Gonadal Failure," *Fertility and Sterility*, vol. 38, no. 645 (1982); C. B. Coulam, S. C. Adamson, and J. F. Annegers, "Incidence of Premature Ovarian Failure," *American Journal of Obstetrics and Gynecology*, vol. 67, no. 4 (1986); R. des Moraes et al., "Autoimmunity and Ovarian Failure," *American Journal of Obstetrics and Gynecology*, vol. 112, no. 5 (1972); H. J. Gloor, "Autoimmune Oophoritis," *American Journal of Clinical Pathology*, vol. 81 (1984), pp. 105–9; M. Leer, B. Patel, M. Innes, et al., "Secondary Amenorrhea Due to Autoimmune Ovarian Failure," *Australia and New Zealand Journal of Obstetrics and Gynecology*, vol. 20 (1980), pp. 177–79; T. Miyake et al., "Acute Oocyte Loss in Experimental Autoimmune Oophoritis as a Possible Model of Premature Ovarian Failure," *American Journal of Obstetrics and Gynecology*, vol. 158, no. 1 (1988); T. Miyake et al., "Evidence of Autoimmune Etiology in Some Premature Menopause," *ObGyn News* (Nov. 1981).

11. J. Pfenninger, "Sex and the Maturing Female," *Mature Health* (Jan.–Feb. 1987), pp. 12–15.

12. L. Zussman et al., "Sexual Response After Hysterectomy-Oophorectomy: Recent Studies and Reconsideration of Psychogenesis," *American Journal of Obstetrics and Gynecology*, vol. 140, no. 7 (1981), pp. 725–29.

13. L. C. Swartzman, "Impact of Stress on Objectively Recorded Menopausal Hot Flashes and on Flush Report Bias," *Health Psychology*, vol. 9 (1990), pp. 529–45.

14. F. Grodstein, J. E. Manson, and M. J. Stampfer, "Hormone Therapy and Coronary Heart Disease: The Role of Time Since Menopause and Age at Hormone Initiation," *Journal of Women's Health (Larchmont)*, vol. 15, no. 1 (Jan./Feb. 2006), pp. 35–44.

15. B. R. Bhavnani and A. Cecutti, "Pharmacokinetics of 17b-Dihydroequilin Sulfate and 17b-Dihydroequilin in Normal Postmenopausal Women," *Journal of Clinical Endocrinology and Metabolism*, vol. 78 (1994), pp. 197–204.

16. A. Follingstad, "Estriol, the Forgotten Hormone," *Journal of the American Medical Association*, vol. 239, no. 1 (1978), pp. 29–39; H. Lemon, "Clinical and Experimental Aspects of the Anti-Mammary Carcinogenic Activity of Estriol," *Frontiers of Hormonal Research*, vol. 5, no. 1 (1977), pp. 155–73; H. Lemon, "Estriol Prevention of Mammary Carcinoma Induced by 7, 12-Dimethyibenzathracene and Procarbazine," *Cancer Research*, vol. 35 (1975), pp. 1341–53; H. Lemon, "Oestriol and Prevention of Breast Cancer," *The Lancet*, vol. 1, no. 802 (1973), pp. 546–47; H. Lemon, "Pathophysiologic Considerations in the Treatment of Menopausal Patients with Oestrogens: The Role of Oestriol in the Prevention of Mammary Cancer," *Acta Endocrinologica*, vol. 233, Suppl. (1980), pp. 17–27; H. Lemmon, H. Wortiz, L. Parsons, et al., "Reduced Estriol Excretion in Patients with Breast Cancer Prior to Endocrine Therapy," *Journal of the American Medical Association*, vol. 196 (1966), pp. 1128–36; B. G. Wren and J. A. Eden, "Do Progesterones Reduce the Risk of Breast Cancer? A Review of the Evidence," *Menopause: The Journal of the North American Menopause Society*, vol. 3, no. 1 (1996), pp. 4–12; M. van Haaften, G. H. Donker, A. A. Haspeis, et al., "Oestrogen Concentrations in Plasma, Endometrium, Myometrium, and Vagina of Postmenopausal Women, and Effects of Vaginal Oestriol (E3) and Oestradiol (E2) Applications," *Journal of Steroid Biochemistry*, vol. 4A (1989), pp. 647–53.

17. M. Melamed et al., "Molecular and Kinetic Basis for the Mixed Agonist/Antagonist Activity of Estriol," *Molecular Endocrinology*, vol. 11, no. 12 (Nov. 1997), pp. 1868–78.

18. L. Rajkumar et al., "Prevention of Mammary Carcinogenesis by Short-Term Estrogen and Progestin Treatments," *Breast Cancer Research*, vol. 6, no. 1 (2004), pp. R31–37.

19. S. Granberg et al., "The Effects of Oral Estriol on the Endometrium in Postmenopausal Women," *Maturitas*, vol. 42, no. 2 (June 25, 2002), pp. 149–56.

20. K. Takahashi et al., "Efficacy and Safety of Oral Estriol for Managing Postmenopausal Symptoms," *Maturitas*, vol. 34, no. 2 (Feb. 15, 2000), pp. 169–77; K. Takahashi et al., "Safety and Efficacy of Oestriol for Symptoms of Natural or Surgically Induced Menopause," *Human Reproduction*, vol. 15, no. 5 (May 2000), pp. 1028–36.

21. R. Punnonen and L. Raurama, "The Effect of Longterm Oral Oestriol Succinate Therapy on the Skin of Castrate Women," *Annals of Gynecology*, vol. 66 (1977), p. 214.

22. Hargrove and Eisenberg, "Menopause" (see note 9).

23. Hargrove and Eisenberg, "Menopause" (see note 9).

24. J. Hargrove et al., "Menopausal Hormone Replacement Therapy with Continuous Daily Oral Micronized Estradiol and Progesterone," *Obstetrics and Gynecology*, vol. 73, no. 4 (1989), pp. 606–12.

25. Quote in A. Voda, M. Dinnerstein, and C. R. O'Donnell, eds., *Changing Perspectives on Menopause* (Austin: University of Texas Press, 1982).

26. J. K. Brown and V. Kerns, eds., *In Her Prime: A New View of Middle-Aged Women* (Amherst, MA: Bergin and Garvey, 1985).

27. F. Kronenberg and J. A. Downey, "Thermoregulatory Physiology of Menopausal Hot Flashes: A Review," *Canadian Journal of Physiological Pharmacology*, vol. 65 (1987), pp. 1312–24.

28. R. S. Finkler, "The Effect of Vitamin E in the Menopause," *Journal of Clinical Endocrinology and Metabolism*, vol. 9 (1949), pp. 89–94.

29. C. J. Smith, "Non-Hormonal Control of Vasomotor Flushing in Menopausal Patients," *Chicago Medicine*, vol. 67, no. 5 (1964), pp. 193–95.

30. C. A. B. Clemetson, S. J. DeCarol, G. A. Burney, et al., "Estrogens in Food: The Almond Mystery," *International Journal of Gynecology and Obstetrics*, vol. 15 (1978), pp. 515–21; S. O. Elakovich and J. Hampton, "Analysis of Couvaestrol, a Phytoestrogen, in Alpha Tablets Sold for Human Consumption," *Journal of Agricultural and Food Chemistry*, vol. 32 (1984), pp. 173–75.

31. H. Aldercrueutz et al., "Dietary Phyto-Oestrogens and the Menopause in Japan," *The Lancet*, vol. 339 (1992), p. 1233; M. J. Messina, V. Persky, K. D. R. Setchel, et al., "Soy Intake and Cancer Risk: A Review of the In Vitro and In Vivo Data," *Nutrition and Cancer*, vol. 21 (1994), pp. 113–31; and G. Wilcox et al., "Oestrogenic Effects of Plant Foods in Postmenopausal Women," *British Medical Journal*, vol. 301 (1990), pp. 905–6.

32. K. Dupree et al., "Effects of Soy on Quality of Life in Post-Menopausal Women," The Endocrine Society Annual Meeting 2005, San Diego, CA, June 4–7.

33. M. Murray, "HRT vs Remifemin in Menopause," *American Journal of Natural Medicine*, vol. 3, no. 4 (1996), pp. 7–10; G. Warnecke, "Beeinflussing Klimakterischer Beschwerden durch ein Phytotherapeutikum [Influencing Menopausal Symptoms with a Phytotherapeutic Agent]," *Medwelt*, vol. 36 (1985), pp. 871–74.

34. I. I. Bukham and O. I. Kirillov, "Effect of Eleutherococus on Alarm-Phase of Stress," *Annual Review of Pharmacology*, vol. 8 (1969), pp. 113–21; A. Milewiez, E. Gejdel, et al., "Vitex Agnus Castus Extract in the Treatment of Luteal Phase Defects Due to Hyperprolactinemia: Results of a Randomized Placebo-Controlled Double-Blind Study," *Arzneimittel-Forschung/Drug Research*, vol. 43 (1993), pp. 752–56; D. B. Mowrey, *The Scientific Validation of Herbal Medicine* (New Canaan, CT: Keats, 1986); G. Sliutz, P. Speiser, et al., "Agnus Castus Extracts Inhibit Prolactin Secretion of Rat Pituitary Cells," *Hormone and Metabolic Research*, vol. 2 (1993), pp. 253–55.

35. J. R. Lee, *What Your Doctor May Not Tell You About Menopause* (New York: Warner Books, 1996).

36. A. D. Domar and H. Dreher, *Healing Mind, Healthy Woman* (New York: Henry Holt and Co., 1996), pp. 291–92; Swartzman, "Impact of Stress" (see note 13); R. R. Freedman and S. Woodward, "Behavioral Treatment of Menopausal Hot Flashes: Evaluation by Ambulatory Monitoring," *American Journal of Obstetrics and Gynecology*, vol. 167 (1992), pp. 436–39; L. C. Swartzman, R. Edelberg, and E. Kemmann, "The Menopausal Hot Flush: Symptom Reports and Concomitant Physical Changes," *Journal of Behavioral Medicine*, vol. 13 (1990), pp. 15–30; D. W. Stevenson and D. J. Delprato, "Multiple Component Self-Control Program for Menopausal Hot Flashes," *Journal of Behavior Therapy and Experimental Psychology*, vol. 14, no. 2 (1983), pp. 137–40.

37. S. Weed, *Menopausal Years: The Wise Women's Way: Alternative Approaches for Women 30–90* (Woodstock, NY: Ash Tree Publishing, 1992).

38. M. Bygdeman and M. L. Swahn, "Replens versus Dienoestrol Cream in Symptomatic Treatment of Vaginal Atrophy in Postmenopausal Women," *Maturitas*, vol. 23 (1996), pp. 256–63.

39. Susan Rako, M.D., *The Hormone of Desire: The Truth About Sexuality, Menopause, and Testosterone* (New York: Harmony, 1996).

40. V. L. Handa, "Vaginal Administration of Low-Dose Conjugated Estrogens: Systemic Absorption and Effects of the Endometrium," *Obstetrics and Gynecology*, vol. 84 (1994), pp. 215–18; G. M. Heimer and E. L. E. Englund, "Effects of Vaginally Administered Oestriol on Postmenopausal Urogenital Disorders: A Cytohormonal Study," *Maturitas*, vol. 3 (1992), pp. 171–79; C. S. Iosif, "Effects of Protracted Administration of Estriol on the Lower Urinary Tract in Postmenopausal Women," *Archives of Gynecology and Obstetrics*, vol. 3, no. 251 (1992), pp. 115–20; A. L. Kirkengen, P. Anderson, E. Gjersoe, et al., "Oestriol in the Prophylactic Treatment of Recurrent Urinary Tract Infections in Postmenopausal Women," *Scandinavian Journal of Primary Health Care*, (June 1992), pp. 139–42; R. Ruz and W. Stamm, "A Controlled Trial of Intravaginal Estriol in Post-Menopausal Women with Recurrent Urinary Tract Infections," *New England Journal of Medicine*, vol. 329, no. 11 (1993), pp. 753–56. M. van Haaften et al., "Oestrogen Concentrations in Plasma, Endometrium, Myometrium, and Vagina of Postmenopausal Women, and Effects of Vaginal Oestriol (E3) and Oestradiol (E2) Applications," *Journal of Steroid Biochemistry*, vol. 4A (1989), pp. 647–53.

41. L. Avioli, "Osteoporosis: A Growing National Health Problem," *Female Patient*, vol. 17 (1992), pp. 25–28; W. A. Wallace, "The Increasing Incidence of Fractures of the Proximal Femur: An Orthopaedic Epidemic," *The Lancet*, vol. 1, no. 833 (June 25, 1993), p. 1413.

42. W. S. Browner et al., "Mortality Following Fractures in Older Women: The Study of Osteoporotic Fracture," *Archives of Internal Medicine*, vol. 156 (1996), pp. 1521–25; P. Dargen-Molina et al., "Fall-Related Factors and Risk of Hip Fracture: The EPI-DOX Prospective Study," *The Lancet*, vol. 348 (1996), pp. 148–49.

43. L. S. Harkness et al., "Decreased Bone Resorption with Soy Isoflavone Supplementation in Postmenopausal Women," *Journal of Women's Health (Larchmont)*, vol. 13, no. 9 (Nov. 2004), pp. 1000–7; M. Mori et al., "Soy Isoflavone Tablets Reduce Osteoporosis Risk Factors and Obesity in Middle-Aged Japanese Women," *Clinical and Experimental Pharmacology and Physiology*, vol. 31, supplement 2 (Dec. 2004), pp. S39–41; M. Mori et al., "Soy Isoflavones Improve Bone Metabolism in Postmenopausal Japanese Women," *Clinical and Experimental Pharmacology and Physiology*, vol. 31, supplement 2 (Dec. 2004), pp. S44–46; E. Nikander et al., "Effects of Phytoestrogens on Bone Turnover in Postmenopausal Women with a History of Breast Cancer," *Journal of Clinical Endocrinology and Metabolism*, vol. 89, no. 3 (March 2004), pp. 1207–12.

44. D. Michaelson, C. Stratakis, L. Hill, et al., "Bone Mineral Density in Women with Depression," *New England Journal of Medicine*, vol. 335 (1996), pp. 1176–81.

45. C. E. Cann, M. C. Martin, and R. B. Jaffe, "Decreased Spinal Mineral Content in Amenorrheic Women," *Journal of the American Medical Association*, vol. 25, no. 5 (1984), pp. 626–29; J. S. Lindberg, M. R. Powell, et al., "Increased Vertebral Bone Mineral in Response to Reduced Exercise in Amenorrheic Runners," *Western Journal of Medicine*, vol. 146 (1987), pp. 39–42; R. Marcus et al., "Menstrual Function and Bone Mass in Elite Women Distance Runners," *Annals of Internal Medicine*, vol. 102 (1985), pp. 158–63; J. C. Prior, "Spinal Bone Loss and Ovulatory Disturbances," *New England Journal of Medicine*, vol. 323 (1990), pp. 1221–27.

46. M. Hernandez-Avila et al., "Caffeine, Moderate Alcohol Intake, and Risk of Fracture of the Hip and Forearm in Middle-Aged Women," *American Journal of Clinical Nutrition*, vol. 54 (1991), pp. 157–63; D. E. Nelson, R. W. Suttin, J. A. Langois, et al., "Alcohol as a Risk Factor for Fall Injury Events Among Elderly Persons Living in the Community," *Journal of the Geriatric Society*, vol. 40 (1992), pp. 658–61; H. D. Nelson et al., "Smoking, Alcohol, and Neuromuscular and Physical Function of Older Women," *Journal of the American Medical Association*, vol. 272, no. 24 (1994), pp. 1909–13.

47. D. C. Bauer et al., "Factors Associated with Appendicular Bone Mass in Older Women," *Archives of Internal Medicine*, vol. 118, no. 9 (1993), pp. 657–65; D. P. Kiel et al., "Caffeine and the Risk of Hip Fracture: The Framingham Study," *Biological Psychiatry*, vol. 23 (1988), pp. 335–49.

48. B. Dawson-Hughes et al., "Effect of Vitamin D Supplementation on Wintertime and Overall Bone Loss in Healthy Postmenopausal Women," *Annals of Internal Medicine*, vol. 115, no. 17 (1991), pp. 505–12.

49. H. I. Abdalla, D. M. Hart, E. Purdee, et al., "Prevention of Bone Mineral Loss in Postmenopausal Women by Norethisterone," *Obstetrics and Gynecology*, vol. 66

(1985), pp. 789–92; J. Dequeker and E. De Muylder, "Long-Term Progestogen Treatment and Bone Remodeling in Premenopausal Women; A Longitudinal Study," *Maturitas*, vol. 4 (1982), pp. 309–13; R. Lindsay, D. M. Hart, D. Purdee, et al., "Comparative Effectiveness of Estrogen and a Progestogen on Bone Loss in Postmenopausal Women," *Clinical Science and Molecular Medicine*, vol. 54 (1978), pp. 93–95; J. McCann and N. Horwitz, "Provera Alone Builds Bone," *Medical Tribune*, July 1987, pp. 4–5; J. C. Prior et al., "Progesterone as a Bone-Tropic Hormone," *Endocrine Reviews*, vol. 11 (1990), pp. 386–98; B. L. Riggs, J. Jowsery, P. J. Kelly, et al., "Effect of Sex Hormones in Bone in Primary Osteoporosis," *Journal of Clinical Investigations*, vol. 48 (1969), pp. 1065–72; F. G. R. Snow and C. Anderson, "The Effect of 17-Beta Estradiol and Progestogen on Trabecular Bone Remodeling in Oophorectomized Dogs," *Calcification Tissue*, vol. 39 (1986), pp. 198–205.

50. A. K. Banerjee, P. J. Lane, and F. W. Meichen, "Vitamin C and Osteoporosis in Old Age," *Age and Aging*, vol. 7, no. 1 (1978), pp. 16–18.

51. F. H. Nielsen, "Studies on the Relationship Between Boron and Magnesium Which Possibly Affects the Formation and Maintenance of Bones," *Magnesium Trace Elements*, vol. 9, no. 2 (1990), pp. 61–91; J. U. Reginster et al., "Preliminary Report of Decreased Serum Magnesium in Post-Menopausal Osteoporosis," *Magnesium*, vol. 8, no. 2 (1989), pp. 106–9.

52. T. L. Holbrook et al., "Dietary Calcium and Risk of Hip Fracture: A 14-Year Prospective Population Study," *The Lancet*, vol. 2 (1988), pp. 1046–49; H. Spencer et al., "Absorption of Calcium in Osteoporosis," *American Journal of Medicine*, vol. 37 (1964), pp. 223–24.

53. F. H. Nielsen et al., "Effects of Dietary Boron on Mineral, Estrogen, and Testosterone Metabolism in Post-Menopausal Women," *Federation of American Societies for Experimental Biology Journal*, vol. 1 (1987), pp. 394–97.

54. U. Hartmann et al., "Low Sexual Desire in Midlife and Older Women: Personality Factors, Psychosocial Development, Present Sexuality," *Menopause*, vol. 11, no. 6, pt. 2 (Nov./Dec. 2004), pp. 726–40; R. Basson, "Recent Advances in Women's Sexual Function and Dysfunction," *Menopause*, vol. 11, no. 6, pt. 2 (Nov./Dec. 2004), pp. 714–25; *NAMS Supplement—Update on Sexuality at Menopause and Beyond: Normative, Adaptive, Problematic, Dysfunctional*, North American Menopause Society, vol. 11, no. 6 (Nov. 2004), pp. 708–86; P. Sarrel and M. I. Whitehead, "Sex and Menopause: Defining the Issues," *Maturitas*, vol. 7 (1985) pp. 217–24; R. H. van Lunsen and E. Laan, "Genital Vascular Responsiveness and Sexual Feelings in Midlife Women: Psychophysiologic, Brain, and Genital Imaging Studies," *Menopause*, vol. 11, no. 6, pt. 2 (Nov./Dec. 2004), pp. 741–48.

55. B. Zumoff, B. W. Strain, L. K. Miller, and W. Roser, "24-Hour Mean Plasma Testosterone Concentration Declines with Age in Normal Premenopausal Women," *Journal of Clinical Endocrinology and Metabolism*, vol. 80, no. 4 (1995), pp. 1429–30.

56. G. A. Bachmann, "Correlates of Sexual Desire in Postmenopausal Women," *Maturitas*, vol. 7, no. 3 (1985), p. 211, cited in David Youngs, "Common Misconceptions About Sex and Depression During Menopause: A Historical Perspective," *Female Patient*, vol. 17 (1992), pp. 25–28; Pfenninger, "Sex and the Maturing Female" (see note 11); J. R. Wilson, "Sexuality in Aging," in J. J. Sciarra, ed., *Gynecology and Obstetrics* (Philadelphia: Lippincott, 1987), pp. 1–12.

57. Bachmann, "Correlates of Sexual Desire" (see note 56).

58. Harry Fisch with Stephen Braun, *The Male Biological Clock: The Startling News About Aging, Sexuality, and Fertility in Men* (New York: Free Press, 2005).

59. Mantak Chia and Maneewan Chia, *Cultivating Female Sexual Energy: Healing Love Through the Tao* (Huntington, NY: Healing Tao Books, 1986); available from Healing Tao Books, 2 Creskill Place, Huntington, NY 11743.

60. Personal communication with Dr. Alan Gaby (a specialist in nutritional medicine); personal communication with David Zava, Ph.D., Aeron Lifecycles Lab.

61. J. K. Meyers, M. M. Weissman, and G. L. Tischler, "Six-Month Prevalence of Psychiatric Disorder in Three Communities," *Archives of General Psychiatry*, vol. 41 (1984), p. 959.

62. S. M. McKinlay, J. B. McKinlay, and D. J. Bramblilla, "Health Status and Utilization Behavior Associated with Menopause," *American Journal of Epidemiology*, vol. 125 (1987), p. 110.

63. M. Murray, "HRT vs. Remifemin in Menopause," *American Journal of Natural Medicine*, vol. 3, no. 4 (1996), pp. 7–10; Warnecke, "Beeinflussing" (see note 33).

64. S. Hozl, L. Demisch, and B. Gollnik, "Investigations About Antidepressive and Mood Change Effects of *Hypericum Perforatum*," *Planta Medica*, vol. 55 (1989), p. 643.

65. Marian Van Eck McCain, *Transformation Through Menopause* (Amherst, MA: Bergin and Garvey, 1991).

66. Marguerite Holloway, "The Estrogen Factor," *Scientific American* (June 1992).

67. S. E. File et al., "Eating Soya Improves Human Memory," *Psychopharmacology* (Berl), vol. 157, no. 4 (Oct. 2001), pp. 430–36; S. E. File et al., "Cognitive Improvement After 6 Weeks of Soy Supplements in Postmenopausal Women Is Limited to Frontal Lobe Function," *Menopause*, vol. 12, no. 2 (March 2005), pp. 193–201; R. Duffy et al., "Improved Cognitive Function in Postmenopausal Women After 12 Weeks of Consumption of a Soya Extract Containing Isoflavones," *Pharmacology, Biochemistry, and Behavior*, vol. 75, no. 3 (June 2003), pp. 721–29.

68. K. J. Chang et al., "Influences of Percutaneous Administration of Estradiol and Progesterone on Human Breast Epithelial Cell Cycle in Vivo," *Fertility and Sterility*, vol. 63, no. 4 (April 1995), pp. 785–91; M. J. Foidart et al., "Estradiol and Progesterone Regulate the Proliferation of Human Breast Epithelial Cells," *Fertility and Sterility*, vol. 69, no. 5 (May 1998), pp. 963–69.

69. J. C. Prior, "Perimenopause: The Complex Endocrinology of the Menopausal Transition," *Endocrine Reviews*, vol. 19, no. 4 (Aug. 1998), pp. 397–428.

70. S. Franceschi, A. Gavero, A. Decarli, et al., "Intake of Macronutrients and Risk of Breast Cancer," *The Lancet*, vol. 347 (1996), pp. 1351–56; A. Tavam et al., "Consumption of Sweet Foods and Breast Cancer Risk in Italy," *Annals of Oncology* (Oct. 2005) [Epub ahead of print].

71. E. Ginsburg, N. Mello, et al., "Effects of Alcohol Ingestion on Estrogens in Postmenopausal Women," *Journal of the American Medical Association*, vol. 276, no. 21 (1996), pp. 1747–51.

72. M. Eades and M. D. Eades, *Protein Power* (New York: Dutton, 1995). Both the Eadeses and the Hellers have done groundbreaking research on the effects of diet,

excessive fat, and insulin on health. Both teams are available for consultation with physicians, and their books are excellent practical guides for patients and physicians alike.

73. J. Jeppesen et al., "Effects of Low-Fat, High-Carbohydrate Diets on Risk Factors for Ischemic Heart Disease in Postmenopausal Women," *American Journal of Clinical Nutrition*, vol. 65 (1997), pp. 1027–33.

74. M. Kearney et al., "William Heberden Revisited: Postprandial Angina Interval—Interval Between Food and Exercise and Meal Consumption Are Important Determinants of Time of Onset of Ischemia and Maximal Exercise Tolerance," *Journal of the American College of Cardiology*, vol. 29 (1997), pp. 302–7.

75. B. M. Altura et al., "Cardiovascular Risk Factors and Magnesium: Relationships to Atherosclerosis, Ischemic Heart Disease, and Hypertension," *Magnesium and Trace Elements*, vol. 10 (1991–92), pp. 182–92; R. DeGronzo and E. Ferrannini, "Insulin Resistance: A Multifaceted Syndrome Responsible for NIDDM, Obesity, Hypertension, Dyslipidemia, and Atherosclerotic Cardiovascular Disease," *Diabetes Care*, vol. 14, no. 3 (1991), pp. 173–94; A. Ferrara et al., "Sex Differences in Insulin Levels in Older Adults and the Effect of Body Size, Estrogen Replacement Therapy, and Glucose Tolerance Status: The Rancho Bernardo Study, 1984–87," *Diabetes Care*, vol. 18, no. 2 (1995), pp. 220–25; J. M. Gaziano, "Antioxidant Vitamins and Coronary Artery Disease Risk," *American Journal of Medicine*, vol. 97 (1994), pp. 3A–18S, 21S; J. Hallfrisch et al., "High Plasma Vitamin C Associated with High Plasma HDL and HDL(2) Cholesterol," *American Journal of Clinical Nutrition*, vol. 60 (1994), pp. 100–5; M. Modan et al., "Hyperinsulinemia: A Link Between Hypertension, Obesity, and Glucose Intolerance," *Journal of Clinical Investigation*, vol. 75 (1985), pp. 809–17; H. Morrison et al., "Serum Folate and Risk of Fatal Coronary Heart Disease," *Journal of the American Medical Association*, vol. 275, no. 24 (1996), pp. 1893–96; R. A. Riemersma et al., "Risk of Angina Pectoris and Plasma Concentrations of Vitamins A, E, C, and Carotene," *The Lancet*, vol. 337 (1991), pp. 1–5; M. Stampfer et al., "Vitamin E Consumption and the Risk of Coronary Heart Disease in Women," *New England Journal of Medicine*, vol. 328 (1993), pp. 1444–49; D. Steinberg et al., "Antioxidants in the Prevention of Human Atherosclerosis," *Circulation*, vol. 85, no. 6 (1972), pp. 2338–43; D. A. Street et al., "A Population Based Case Control Study of the Association of Serum Antioxidants and Myocardial Infarction," *American Journal of Epidemiology*, vol. 124 (1991), pp. 719–20.

76. M. Daviglus et al., "Fish Consumption and the 30-Year Risk of Fatal Myocardial Infarction," *New England Journal of Medicine*, vol. 336 (April 10, 1997), pp. 1046–53.

77. D. L. Bachman et al., "Incidence of Dementia and Probable Alzheimer's Disease in a General Population: The Framingham Study," *Neurology*, vol. 43, no. 3 pt. 1 (Mar. 1993), pp. 515–19.

78. L. E. Hebert et al., "Alzheimer Disease in the U.S. Population: Prevalence Estimates Using the 2000 Census," *Archives of Neurology*, vol. 60, no. 8 (Aug. 2003), pp. 1119–22.

79. S. D. Edland et al., "Dementia and Alzheimer Disease Incidence Rates Do Not Vary

by Sex in Rochester, Minn.," *Archives of Neurology*, vol. 59, no. 10 (Oct. 2002), pp. 1589–93.

80. M. A. Espeland et al., "Conjugated Equine Estrogens and Global Cognitive Function in Postmenopausal Women: Women's Health Initiative Memory Study," *Journal of the American Medical Association*, vol. 291, no. 24 (June 23, 2004), pp. 2959–68.

81. D. Snowden et al., "Linguistic Ability in Early Life and Cognitive Function and Alzheimer's Disease in Late Life," *Journal of the American Medical Association*, vol. 275, no. 7 (1996), pp. 528–32.

82. V. Henderson et al., "Estrogen Replacement Therapy in Older Women: Comparisons Between Alzheimer's Disease Cases and Nondemented Control Subjects," *Archives of Neurology*, vol. 51 (1994), pp. 896–900; H. Honjo, Y. Ogina, K. Tanaka, et al., "An Effect of Conjugated Estrogen to Cognitive Impairment in Women with Senile Dementia, Alzheimer's Type: A Placebo-Controlled Double Blind Study," *Journal of the Japanese Menopause Society*, vol. 1 (1993), pp. 167–71; T. Ohkura, K. Isse, K. Akazawa, et al., "Evaluation of Estrogen Treatment in Female Patients with Dementia of the Alzheimer's Type," *Endocrine Journal*, vol. 41 (1994), pp. 361–71; A. Paganini-Hill and V. W. Henderson, "Estrogen Deficiency and Risk of Alzheimer's Disease in Women," *American Journal of Epidemiology*, vol. 140 (1994), pp. 256–61.

83. M. Freedman, J. Knoefel, et al., "Computerized Axial Tomography in Aging," in M. L. Albert, ed., *Clinical Neurology of Aging* (New York: Oxford University Press, 1984); U. Lehr and R. Schmitz-Scherzer, "Survivors and Non-Survivors: Two Fundamental Patterns of Aging," in H. Thomas, ed; *Patterns of Aging* (Basel: S. Karger, 1976); A. L. Benton, P. J. Eslinger, and A. R. Damasio, "Normative Observations on Neuropsychological Test Performance in Old Age," *Journal of Clinical Neuropsychiatry*, vol. 3 (1981), pp. 33–42

84. P. H. Evans, J. Klinowski, and E. Yano, "Cephaloconiosis: A Free Radical Perspective on the Proposed Particulate-Induced Etiopathogenesis of Alzheimer's Dementia and Related Disorders," *Medical Hypotheses*, vol. 34 (1991), pp. 209–19; I. Rosenberg and J. Miller, "Nutritional Factors in Physical and Cognitive Functions of Elderly People," *American Journal of Clinical Nutrition*, vol. 55 (1992), pp. 1237S–1243S; R. N. Strachan and J. G. Henderson, "Dementia and Folate Deficiency," *Quarterly Journal of Medicine*, vol. 36 (1967), pp. 189–204.

85. J. F. Flood, J. E. Morley, and E. Roberts, "Memory-Enhancing Effects in Male Mice of Pregnenolone and Steroids Metabolically Derived from It," *Proceedings from the National Academy of Sciences*, vol. 89 (Mar. 1992), pp. 1567–71: C. R. Mevril et al., "Reduced Plasma DHEA Concentrations in HIV Infection and Alzheimer's Disease," in M. Kalimi and W. Regelson, eds., *The Biological Role of Dehydroepiandrosterone* (New York: de Gruyter, 1990), pp. 101–5; W. Regelson et al., "Dehydroepiandrosterone (DHEA)—The 'Mother Steroid.' I. Immunologic Action," *Annals of the New York Academy of Sciences*, vol. 719 (1994), pp. 553–63; S. S. C. Yen et al., "Replacement of DHEA in Aging Men and Women: Potential Remedial Effects," *Annals of the New York Academy of Sciences*, vol. 774 (1995), pp. 128–42.

86. Weed, from an introductory flyer for *Menopausal Years* (see note 37).

Chapter 15: Steps for Creating Vibrant Health

1. Exercise adapted from a workshop author participated in with Annie Gill O'Toole, author of the book *Choosing Life*, which contains many other helpful exercises for achieving health. Available from Lighthouse International, 22 Stacey Rd., Marlborough, MA 01752; 508-624-7735.

2. This teaching is from Abraham, who teaches through Esther Hicks. I've consistently found the Abraham teachings to be very practical material for living joyfully. For more information, write Abraham Hicks Publications, P.O. Box 690070, San Antonio, TX 78269.

3. Leslie Kussman, personal communication (May 6, 1992), before filming *Harbour of Hope*, a documentary about those who have healed from chronic or terminal illness. For information write Aquarius Production, 31 Martin Road, Wellesley, MA 02181; 617-237-0608.

4. Joe Dominguez and Vicki Robin, *Your Money or Your Life* (New York: Viking, 1992); Joe Dominguez, "Transforming Your Relationship with Money and Creating Financial Independence," brochure; write to New Road Map Foundation, P.O. Box 15981, Seattle, WA 98115.

5. At one of my workshops a woman from Atlanta told me that her woman's group simply calls this deep work "the process." She had never heard of Anne Wilson Schaef or her work.

6. Naomi Wolf has documented the tragic aspects of this in *The Beauty Myth* (New York: Morrow, 1990).

7. Frances Scovel Shinn, *The Game of Life and How to Play It* (Marina del Rey, CA: DeVorss and Co., 1925).

8. Patricia Reis, author of *Through the Goddess* (Freedom, CA: Crossing Press, 1991), worked with us at Women to Women for four years, teaching us the deep patterns held in women's psyches and bodies.

9. An in-depth approach to this is available in Vicki Noble, *Shakti Woman* (HarperSanFrancisco, 1992).

10. For more information, write to the Proprioceptive Writing Center, P.O. Box 833333, Portland, ME 04102; 207-772-1847.

11. Dream incubation is adapted from the work of Patricia Reis.

12. D. Spiegel, J. Bloom, H. D. Kraemer, et al., "Effects of Psychosocial Treatment on Survival of Patients with Metastatic Breast Cancer," *The Lancet*, vol. 2 (1989), pp. 888–91; D. Spiegel, "A Psychosocial Intervention and Survival Time of Patients with Metastatic Breast Cancer," *Advances*, vol. 7, no. 3 (1991), pp. 10–19.

13. Boston Women's Health Book Collective, *The New Our Bodies, Ourselves* (New York: Simon & Schuster, Inc., 1984); Riane Eisler, *The Chalice and the Blade: Our History, Our Future* (HarperSanFrancisco, 1988).

14. F. Luskin and B. Bland, "Stanford–Northern Ireland Hope 2 Project," unpublished manuscript, Stanford University, Palo Alto, CA (Feb. 2001).

15. R. McCraty et al., "The Effects of Emotions on Short-Term Power Spectrum Analysis of Heart Rate Variability," *American Journal of Cardiology*, vol. 76, no. 14 (Nov. 15, 1995), pp. 1089–93; Doc Lew Childre, *Women Lead with*

Their Hearts: A White Paper, obtainable from the Institute of HeartMath, P.O. Box 1463, Boulder Creek, CA 95006; (831) 338-8500; website: www.hearthealth.org.

16. Stephen Levine, *Guided Meditations, Explorations and Healings* (New York: Doubleday, 1991), p. 324.

17. David Ehrenfeld, *The Arrogance of Humanism*, quoted in Richard Sandor, "The Attending Physician," *Sun*, vol. 4 (Sept. 1, 1991), p. 4.

18. Quoted in Jerry Hicks and Esther Hicks, *A New Beginning*, parts I and II (see note 2).

Chapter 16: Getting the Most Out of Your Medical Care

1. Norman Cousins, *Anatomy of an Illness as Perceived by the Patient* (New York: Bantam, 1979), pp. 49–50.

2. H. Benson et al., "The Placebo Effect: A Neglected Asset in the Care of Patients," *Journal of the American Medical Association*, vol. 232, no. 12 (June 23, 1975); A. B. Carter, The Placebo: Its Use and Abuse," *Lancet* (Oct. 17, 1973), p. 823; B. Blackwell et al., "Demonstration to Medical Students of Placebo Responses and Non-Drug Factors," *The Lancet*, vol. 2 (June 1972), p. 1279; S. Wolf, H. K. Beecher, "The Powerful Placebo," *Journal of the American Medical Association*, vol. 159 (1955), pp. 1602–6.

3. J. B. Moseley, et al., "A Controlled Trial of Arthroscopic Surgery for Osteoarthritis of the Knee," *New England Journal of Medicine*, vol. 347, no. 2 (July 11, 2002), pp. 81–88.

4. G. Null, C. Dean, M. Feldman, and D. Rasio, "Death by Medicine," Nutrition Institute of America (Oct. 2000); Ray D. Strand, *Death by Prescription* (Nashville: Thomas Nelson Publishers, 2003).

5. These steps adapted from a supplement to C. Northrup's *Health Wisdom for Women* newsletter.

6. Irving Kirsch, Thomas J. Moore, et al., "The Emperor's New Drugs: An Analysis of Antidepressant Medication Data Submitted to the U.S. Food and Drug Administration," *Prevention & Treatment*, vol. 5, no. 1 (July 2002), p. 23.

7. Peggy Huddleston, *Prepare for Surgery, Heal Faster* (Cambridge, MA: Angel River Press, 1996).

8. The sense of the word *heroic* in this context is from the philosophy of Susun Weed, a wise woman herbalist who associates the heroic tradition with allopathic medicine.

9. *Gentle Visions: A Pre-Operative Relaxation Program*, 1991, 1992. For more information or to order, write to Healing Images, P.O. Box 2972, Framingham Center Station, Framingham, MA 01701.

10. This entire section is adapted from an article in the April 1996 issue of C. Northrup's *Health Wisdom for Women* newsletter. An extensive bibliography of the studies that support these steps can be found in Huddleston, *Prepare for Surgery* (see note 7).

11. One summer, while climbing Mount Katahdin, I ran a stick through my shin. Not

only did it hurt, it left an ugly gash that I knew would leave a scar. I grieved for my leg, even as my brother joked, "What do you care? You're not a model—you don't need your legs to look good for anything."

Chapter 17: Nourishing Ourselves with Food

1. During medical school, one of the surgeons I studied with performed intestinal by-pass surgery on women (and men) who were morbidly obese. Though they lost weight quickly, postoperatively many were unable to adjust to their new size and continued to think and feel fat.

2. M. Mackensie, "A Cultural Study of Weight: America vs. Western Samoa," *Radiance,* vol. 3, no. 3 (Summer/Fall 1986), pp. 23–25; cited in K. Johnson and T. Ferguson, *Trusting Ourselves: The Sourcebook of Psychology for Women* (New York: Atlantic Monthly Press, 1990).

3. V. J. Felitti et al., "Relationship of Childhood Abuse and Household Dysfunction to Many of the Leading Causes of Death in Adults. The Adverse Childhood Experiences (ACE) Study," *American Journal of Preventive Medicine,* vol. 14, no. 4 (May 1998), pp. 245–58.

4. V. J. Felitti, "Long-Term Medical Consequences of Incest, Rape, and Molestation," *Southern Medicine Journal,* vol. 84 (1991), pp. 328–31; I. Clearly-Merker, "Childhood Sexual Abuse as an Antecedent to Obesity," *Bariatrician* (Spring 1991), pp. 17–22; D. A. Drossman, J. Leserman, G. Nachman, et al., "Sexual and Physical Abuse in Women with Functional or Organic Gastrointestinal Disorders," *Annals of Internal Medicine,* vol. 113 (1990), pp. 828–33.

5. L. Lissner et al., "Variability of Body Weight and Health Outcomes in the Framingham Population," *New England Journal of Medicine,* vol. 324 (1991), pp. 1839–44.

6. The scenario of the overachieving, driven adolescent girl is a setup for anorexia. It's estimated that 50 percent of prep school girls are bulimic or anorexic to some extent. Marion Woodman's *Addiction to Perfection: The Still Unravished Bride* (Toronto: Inner City Press, 1982) is a beautiful exploration of the depth issues represented by eating disorders.

7. A. Tavani et al., "Consumption of Sweet Foods and Breast Cancer Risk in Italy," *Annals of Oncology* (Oct. 25, 2005) [Epub ahead of print].

8. See the extensive bibliography of the medical literature in National Academy of Sciences, *Diet, Nutrition, and Cancer* (Washington, D.C.: National Academy Press, 1982), pp. 73–105.

9. B. MacMahan et al., "Urine Estrogen Profiles in Asian and North American Women," *International Journal of Cancer,* vol. 14 (1974), pp. 161–67; L. E. Dickinson et al., "Estrogen Profiles of Oriental and Caucasian Women in Hawaii," *New England Journal of Medicine,* vol. 291 (1974), pp. 1211–13; D. A. Snowden, letter to the editor, *Journal of the American Medical Association,* vol. 3, no. 254 (1985), pp. 356–57; D. W. Cramer et al., "Dietary Animal Fat and Relationship to Ovarian Cancer Risk," *Obstetrics and Gynecology,* vol. 63, no. 6 (1984), pp. 833–38; T. McKenna, "Pathogenesis and Treatment of Polycystic Ovary Syndrome," *New England Journal of Medicine,* vol. 318 (1988), p. 558; D. Polson,

"Polycystic Ovaries—A Common Finding in Normal Women," *The Lancet,* vol. 1 (1988), p. 870.

10. P. Hill, "Diet, Lifestyle, and Menstrual Activity," *American Journal of Clinical Nutrition,* vol. 33 (1980), p. 1192.

11. A. Sanchez, "A Hypothesis on the Etiologic Role of Diet on the Age of Menarche," *Medical Hypotheses,* vol. 7 (1981), p. 1339; S. Schwartz, "Dietary Influences on Growth and Sexual Maturation in Premenarchal Rhesus Monkeys," *Hormones and Behavior,* vol. 22 (1988), p. 231.

12. C. Leigh Broadhurst, "Nutrition and Non-Insulin Dependent Diabetes Mellitus from an Anthropological Perspective," *Alternative Medicine Review,* vol. 2, no. 5 (1997), pp. 378–399.

13. S. B. Eaton, S. B. Eaton III, M. J. Konner, and M. Shostak, "An Evolutionary Perspective Enhances Understanding of Human Nutritional Requirements," *Journal of Nutrition,* vol. 126, no. 6 (June 1996), pp. 1732–40; S. B. Eaton, S. B. Eaton III, and M. J. Konner, "Paleolithic Nutrition Revisited: A Twelve-Year Retrospective on Its Nature and Implications," *European Journal of Clinical Nutrition,* vol. 51, no. 4 (April 1997), pp. 207–16; Michael Crawford and David Marsh, *Nutrition and Evolution* (New Caanan, CT: Keats Publishing, 1995).

14. Joseph Mercola, *The No-Grain Diet* (New York: Dutton, 2003), p. 3.

15. Studies cited in Philip Lipetz's *The Good Calorie Diet* (New York: HarperCollins, 1994), p. 72. This book has more helpful, scientifically documented information on the differences between carbohydrates than anything else I've found.

16. Raphael Melmed et al., "The Influence of Emotional State on the Mobilization of Marginal Pool Leukocytes and Insulin-Induced Hypoglycemia: A Possible Role for Eicosanoids as Major Mediators of Psychosomatic Processes," *Annals of the New York Academy of Sciences,* vol. 296 (1987), pp. 467–76.

17. Mary Catherine Bateson, *Composing a Life* (New York: Plume, 1989), p. 200.

18. Statistics from Kerry O'Nell, "*The Famine Within* Probes Women's Pursuit of Thinness," review of Katherine Gilday's film *The Famine Within, Christian Science Monitor,* Aug. 31, 1992.

19. L. K. G. Hsu, "The Treatment of Anorexia Nervosa," *American Journal of Psychiatry,* vol. 143 (1986), p. 573.

20. J. E. Mitchell, M. E. Seim, E. Clon, et al., "Medical Complications and Medical Management of Bulimia," *Annals of Internal Medicine,* vol. 71 (1987).

21. R. E. Frisch, "The Right Weight: Body Fat, Menarche, and Ovulation," *Baillieres Clinical Obstetrics and Gynecology,* vol. 4, no. 3 (Sept. 1990), pp. 419–39.

22. Michael Eades and Mary Dan Eades, *Protein Power* (New York: Bantam, 1996).

23. M. Nelson et al., "Effects of High-Intensity Strength Training on Multiple Risk Factors for Osteoporitic Fractures: A Randomized Controlled Trial," *Journal of the American Medical Association,* vol. 272, no. 24 (Dec. 28, 1994), pp. 1909–14.

24. Margaret Bullitt-Jonas, *Holy Hunger: A Memoir of Desire* (New York: A. A. Knopf, 1999), p. 119.

25. Personal communication with Dr. Michael Eades, who has reviewed the existing literature on this topic and shared it with me.

26. A. Wayler, E. Queiroz, N. S. Scrimshaw, F. H. Steinke, W. M. Rand, and V. R.

Young, "Nitrogen Balance Studies in Young Men to Assess the Protein Quality of an Isolated Soy Protein in Relation to Meat Proteins," *Journal of Nutrition*, vol. 113, no. 12 (Dec. 1983), pp. 2485–91.

27. N. Istfan, E. Murray, M. Janghorbani, and V. R. Young, "An Evaluation of the Nutritional Value of a Soy Protein Concentrate in Young Adult Men Using the Short-Term N-Balance Method," *Journal of Nutrition*, vol. 113, no. 12 (Dec. 1983), pp. 2516–23; V. R. Young, A. Wayler, C. Garza, F. H. Steinke, E. Murray, W. M. Rand, and N. S. Scrimshaw, "A Long-Term Metabolic Balance Study in Young Men to Assess the Nutritional Quality of an Isolated Soy Protein and Beef Proteins," *American Journal of Clinical Nutrition*, vol. 39, no. 1 (Jan. 1984), pp. 8–15.

28. V. R. Young, M. Puig, E. Queiroz, N. S. Scrimshaw, and W. M. Rand, "Evaluation of the Protein Quality of an Isolated Soy Protein in Young Men: Relative Nitrogen Requirements and Effects of Methionine Supplementation," *American Journal of Clinical Nutrition*, vol. 39, no. 1 (Jan. 1984), pp. 16–24; A. Y. Zezulka and D. H. Calloway, "Nitrogen Retention in Men Fed Varying Levels of Amino Acids from Soy Protein With or Without Added L-Methionine," *Journal of Nutrition*, vol. 106, no. 2 (Feb. 1976), pp. 212–21.

29. A. Baglieri, S. Mahe, S. Zidi, J. F. Huneau, F. Thuillier, P. Marteau, and D. Tome, "Gastro-Jejunal Digestion of Soya-Bean-Milk Protein in Humans," *British Journal of Nutrition*, vol. 72, no. 4 (Oct. 1994), pp. 519–32; F. Mariotti, S. Mahe, R. Benamouzig, C. Luengo, S. Dare, C. Gaudichon, and D. Tome, "Nutritional Value of [15N]-Soy Protein Isolate Assessed from Ileal Digestibility and Postprandial Protein Utilization in Humans," *Journal of Nutrition*, vol. 129, no. 11 (Nov. 1999), pp. 1992–97; C. Gaudichon, S. Mahe, R. Benamouzig, C. Luengo, H. Fouillet, S. Dare, M. Van Oycke, F. Ferriere, J. Rautureau, and D. Tome, "Net Postprandial Utilization of [15N]-Labeled Milk Protein Nitrogen Is Influenced by Diet Composition in Humans," *Journal of Nutrition*, vol. 129, no. 4 (April 1999), pp. 890–95.

30. "Lean Beef Shown to Be as Healthy as Chicken and Fish," *Food Chemistry News*, vol. 32, no 39 (1990), p. 6 cited in Jeffrey Bland, letter to the editor, *New England Journal of Medicine*, vol. 326, no. 3 (1992), p. 200.

31. J. F. Balch, *Prescription for Nutritional Healing* (New York: Avery Publications, 1990).

32. M. Studer et al., "Effect of Different Antilipidemic Agents and Diets on Mortality: A Systematic Review," *Archives of Internal Medicine*, vol. 165, no. 7 (April 11, 2005), pp. 725–30.

33. A. Leaf and P. C. Weber, "Cardiovascular Effects of N-3 Fatty Acids," *New England Journal of Medicine*, vol. 318, no. 9 (March 3, 1988), pp. 549–57; E. B. Schmidt, K. Varming, N. Svaneborg, and J. Dyerberg, "N-3 Polyunsaturated Fatty Acid Supplementation (Pikasol) in Men with Moderate and Severe Hypertriglyceridaemia: A Dose-Response Study," *Annals of Nutrition & Metabolism*, vol. 36, no. 5–6 (1992), pp. 283–87; F. B. Hu, E. Cho, K. M. Rexrode, C. M. Albert, and J. E. Manson, "Fish and Long-Chain Omega-3 Fatty Acid Intake and Risk of Coronary Heart Disease and Total Mortality in Diabetic Women," *Circulation*, vol. 107, no. 14 (April 15, 2003), pp. 1852–57; P. J. Skerrett and C. H. Hennekens, "Consumption of Fish and Fish Oils and Decreased Risk of Stroke," *Preventive Cardiology*, vol. 6, no. 1 (Winter 2003), pp. 38–41.

34. R. L. McLennon, "Reversal of Arrhythmogenic Effects of Long-Term Saturated Fatty Acid Intake by Dietary N3 and N6 Polyunsaturated Fatty Acids," *American Journal of Clinical Nutrition*, vol. 51 (1980), pp. 53–58; D. Kim et al., "Dietary Fish Oil Added to Hyperlipidemic Diet for Swine Results in Reduction in Excessive Numbers of Monocytes Attached to Arterial Epithelium," *Arteriosclerosis*, vol. 81 (1991), pp. 209–16; C. J. Diskin et al., "Fish Oil to Prevent Intimal Hyperplasia and Thrombosis," *Nephron*, vol. 55 (1990), pp. 445–47.

35. U. N. Das et al., "Benzo(a)pyrene and Gamma Radiation Induced Genetic Damage in Mice May Be Prevented by GLA but Not Arachidonic Acid," *Nutrition Research*, vol. 5 (1985), pp. 101–5.

36. D. Horrobin et al., "Omega-6 Fatty Acids May Reverse Carcinogenesis by Restoring Natural PGE-1 Metabolism," *Medical Hypotheses*, vol. 6 (1980), pp. 469–86; J. J. Jarkowski and W. T. Cave, "Dietary Fish Oil May Inhibit Development of Breast Cancer," *Journal of the National Cancer Institute*, vol. 74 (1985), pp. 1145–50.

37. J. M. Kremer, "N-3 Fatty Acid Supplements in Rheumatoid Arthritis," *American Journal of Clinical Nutrition*, vol. 71, no. 1 Suppl. (Jan. 2000), pp. 349S–51S.

38. R. L. Weank et al., "Effect of Low Saturated Fat Diet in Early and Late Cases of Multiple Sclerosis," *The Lancet*, vol. 336 (1990), pp. 1145–50.

39. M. G. Enig et al., "Dietary Fat and Cancer Trends: A Critique," *Federal Proceedings*, vol. 37 (1978), pp. 25–30.

40. G. Abraham, "Primary Dysmenorrhea," *Clinical Obstetrics and Gynecology*, vol. 21, no. 1 (1978), pp. 139–45.

41. T. A. Barringer et al., "Effect of a Multivitamin and Mineral Supplement on Infection and Quality of Life. A Randomized, Double-Blind, Placebo-Controlled Trial," *Annals of Internal Medicine*, vol. 138, no. 5 (March 4, 2003), pp. 365–71.

42. B. Villeponteau, R. Cockrell, and J. Feng, "Nutraceutical Interventions May Delay Aging and the Age-Related Diseases," *Experimental Gerontology*, vol. 35, no. 9–10 (Dec. 2000), pp. 1405–17.

43. E. R. Miller III, "Meta-Analysis: High-Dosage Vitamin E Supplementation May Increase All-Cause Mortality," *Annals of Internal Medicine*, vol. 142, no. 1 (Jan. 4, 2005), p. 37–46.

44. C. D. Morris and S. Carson, "Routine Vitamin Supplementation to Prevent Cardiovascular Disease: A Summary of the Evidence for the U.S. Preventive Services Task Force," *Annals of Internal Medicine*, vol. 139, no. 1 (July 1, 2003), pp. 56–70.

45. M. J. Stampfer et al., "Vitamin E Consumption and the Risk of Coronary Disease in Women," *New England Journal of Medicine*, vol. 328, no. 20 (May 20, 1993), pp. 1444–49.

46. R. M. Bostick et al., "Reduced Risk of Colon Cancer with High Intakes of Vitamin E: The Iowa Women's Health Study," *Cancer Research*, vol. 53, no. 18 (Sept. 15, 1993), pp. 4230–37.

47. P. P. Zandi, "Reduced Risk of Alzheimer Disease in Users of Antioxidant Vitamin Supplements: The Cache County Study." *Archives of Neurology*, vol. 61, no. 1 (Jan. 2004), pp. 82–88.

48. M. Lu, "Prospective Study of Dietary Fat and Risk of Cataract Extraction Among

US Women," *American Journal of Epidemiology*, vol. 161, no. 10 (May 15, 2005), pp. 948–59.

49. Christiane Northrup, *The Wisdom of Menopause* (New York: Bantam Books, 2001).

50. M. R. Malinow et al., "The Effects of Folic Acid Supplementation on Plasma Total Homocysteine Are Modulated by Multivitamin Use and Methylenetetrahydrofolate Reductase Genotypes," *Arteriosclerosis, Thrombosis, and Vascular Biology*, vol. 17, no. 6 (June 1997), pp. 1157–62.

51. M. F. Bellamy et al., "Oral Folate Enhances Endothelial Function in Hyperhomocysteinaemic Subjects," *European Journal of Clinical Investigation*, vol. 29, no. 8 (Aug. 1999), pp. 659–62; A. Bronstrup et al., "Effects of Folic Acid and Combinations of Folic Acid and Vitamin B-12 on Plasma Homocysteine Concentrations in Healthy, Young Women," *American Journal of Clinical Nutrition*, vol. 68, no. 5 (1998), pp. 1104–10.

52. A. Vahratian et al., "Multivitamin Use and Risk of Preterm Birth," *American Journal of Epidemiology*, vol. 160, no. 9 (Nov. 1, 2004), pp. 886–92.

53. R. A. Anderson and S. Koslovsky, "Chromium Intake, Absorption, and Excretion of Subjects Consuming Self-Selected Diets," *American Journal of Clinical Nutrition*, vol. 41 (1985), pp. 1177–80.

54. W. Mestz et al., "Present Knowledge of the Role of Chromium," *Fedéral Proceedings*, vol. 33 (1974), pp. 2275–83.

55. Interestingly, breast milk contains 300 mg of calcium per quart, while cow's milk contains 1,200 mg per quart. Yet the breast-fed infant absorbs more calcium than the infant fed cow's milk. More isn't necessarily better. Source: William Manahan, *Eat for Health* (Tiburon, CA: H. J. Kramer, 1988), p. 164.

56. Frank Oski, *Don't Drink Your Milk* (Syracuse, NY: Mollica Press, 1983); available from Teach Services, Route 1, Box 182, Brushton, NY 12916; 800-367-1844.

57. Daniel Cramer et al., "Galatose Consumption and Metabolism in Relation to the Risk of Ovarian Cancer," *The Lancet,* vol. 2, no. 8654 (July 8, 1989), pp. 66–71.

58. T. Colin Campbell, quoted in "More on the Dietary Fat and Breast Cancer Link," *NABCO News*, vol. 4, no. 3 (July 1990), pp. 1–2; available from National Alliance of Breast Cancer Organizations (NABCO), 2nd floor, 1180 Avenue of the Americas, New York, NY 10036; 212- 719-0154.

59. Manahan, *Eat For Health* (see note 55). Dentists point out that the first place osteoporosis shows up is in the lower jaw, and that osteoporosis is linked with periodontal disease, the leading cause of adult tooth loss.

60. T. Colin Campbell, "Nutrition, Environment, and Health Project: Chinese Academy of Preventive Medicine-Cornell-Oxford," reported in Nathaniel Mead, "The Champion Diet," *East West* (Sept. 1990), p. 46.

61. B. Dawson-Hughes et al., "Effect of Vitamin D Supplementation on Wintertime and Overall Bone Loss in Healthy Postmenopausal Women," *Annals of Internal Medicine*, vol. 115, no. 17 (1991), pp. 505–12.

62. M. F. Holick, "Vitamin D Deficiency: What a Pain It Is," *Mayo Clinic Proceedings*, vol. 78, no. 12 (Dec 2003), pp. 1457–9.

63. R. D. Jackson et al., "Calcium Plus Vitamin D Supplementation and the Risk of

Fractures," *New England Journal of Medicine*, vol. 354, no. 7 (Feb. 16, 2006), pp. 669–83.

64. Bone metabolism also requires vitamin C, vitamin D, and a number of trace minerals, including zinc, silica, copper, boron, and manganese. All of these substances, working synergistically, form bone.

65. M. Grossman, J. Kirsner, and I. Gillespie, "Basal and Histalog-Stimulated Gastric Secretion in Control Subjects and Patients with Peptic Ulcer or Gastric Cancer," *Gastroenterology*, vol. 45 (1963), pp. 15–26.

66. R. Recker, "Calcium Absorption and Achlorhydria," *New England Journal of Medicine*, vol. 313 (1985), pp. 70–73; M. J. Nicar and C. Y. C. Pak, "Calcium Bioavailability from Calcium Carbonate and Calcium Citrate," *Journal of Clinical Endocrinology and Metabolism*, vol. 61 (1985), pp. 391–93.

67. Personal communication with Jeffrey Bland.

68. D. Michaelson et al., "Bone Mineral Density in Women with Depression," *New England Journal of Medicine*, vol. 335 (1996), pp. 1176–81.

69. Sources for this table are U.S. Department of Agriculture, *Composition of Foods*, handbooks no. 8 and 456 (Washington, D.C.: U.S. Government Printing Office, 1963); J. A. Duke and A. A. Atchley, *Handbook of Proximate Analysis—Tables of Higher Plants* (Boca Raton: CRC Press, 1986); Leonard Jacobs, article in *East/West Journal*, May 1985); John Lee, "Osteoporosis Reversal: The Role of Progesterone," *International Clinical Nutrition Review*, vol. 10 (1990), pp. 384–91; Judith Cooper Madlener, *The Sea Vegetable Book* (New York: Clarkson N. Potter, 1977); Nutrition Search, Inc., John Kirschmann, Dir. Comp., *Nutrition Almanac*, rev. ed. (New York: McGraw-Hill, 1979); U.S. Department of Agriculture, *Nutritive Value of Foods*, Handbook no. 72 (Washington, D.C.: U.S. Government Printing Office, 1971); Mark Pedersen, *Nutritional Herbology* (Bountiful, UT: Pederson, 1987); and Maine Coast Sea Vegetables Co., Shore Road, Franklin, ME 04634.

70. These recipes are from Susun Weed, *Menopausal Years: The Wise Woman's Way: Alternative Approaches for Women 30–90* (Woodstock, NY: Ash Tree Publishing, 1992). A wide variety of sources are listed in Weed's *Healing Wise: A Wise Woman's Herbal* (Woodstock, NY: Ash Tree Publishing, 1992).

71. M. J. Eisenberg, "Magnesium Deficiency and Sudden Death," *American Heart Journal*, vol. 124, no. 2 (1992), pp. 544–49; P. D. Turlapaty and B. M. Altura, "Magnesium Deficiency Produces Spasms in Coronary Arteries: Relationship to Etiology of Sudden Death Ischemic Heart Disease," *Science*, vol. 208, no. 4440 (April 11, 1980), pp. 198–200; B. M. Altura, "Sudden Death Ischemic Heart Disease and Dietary Magnesium Intake: Is the Target Site Coronary Vascular Smooth Muscle?" *Medical Hypotheses*, vol. 5, no. 8 (Aug. 1979), pp. 843–48.

72. B. S. Levine and J. W. Coburn, "Magnesium, the Mimic/Antagonist of Calcium," *New England Journal of Medicine*, vol. 310, no. 19 (May 10, 1984), pp. 1253–55.

73. Institute of Medicine, *Dietary Reference Intakes for Calcium, Phosphorus, Magnesium, Vitamin D, and Fluoride* (Washington, DC: National Academy Press, 1997).

74. M. DeVos, "Articular Disease and the Gut: Evidence of a Strong Relationship Between Spondylarthropathy and Inflammation of the Gut in Man," *Acta Clinica Belgica*, vol. 45, no. 10 (1990), pp. 20–24; and P. Jackson et al., "Intestinal

Permeability in Patients with Eczema and Food Allergy," *The Lancet*, vol. 1 (1981), p. 1285.

75. A. M. Larson et al., "Acetaminophen-Induced Acute Liver Failure: Results of a United States Multicenter, Prospective Study," *Hepatology*, vol. 42, no. 6 (Dec. 2005), pp. 1364–72.

76. A three-part series on common intestinal problems and holistic treatment for them is available in the April, May, and June 1997 issues of C. Northrup's *Health Wisdom for Women* newsletter.

77. I$_g$G levels are known to be altered in diseases related to intestinal dysbiosis and food allergies. I$_g$G is an immunoglobulin that is involved with the body's response to outside elements such as pollen, animal dander, grass, wheat, etc., which are not usually harmful to our bodies. However, in those people who are chronically stressed either emotionally or physically, the I$_g$G levels are elevated, creating the possibility for hyperimmune response, which results in reactions to normally occurring environmental substances. In some people, the I$_g$G levels are decreased, resulting in immunosuppression and therefore increased susceptibility to colds, etc.

78. The lab Women to Women uses for this is ImmunoLaboratories, Fort Lauderdale, FL; 800-231-9197.

79. T. Shirakawa et al., "Lifestyle Effect on Total I$_g$G: Lifestyles Have a Cumulative Impact of Controlling Total I$_g$G Levels," *Allergy*, vol. 46 (1991), pp. 561–69; I. Waxman, "Case Records of the MGH: A 59–Year–Old Woman with Abdominal Pain and an Abnormal CT Scan," *New England Journal of Medicine*, vol. 329, no. 5 (1993), pp. 343–49.

80. Data from *Brain/Mind Bulletin* (Dec. 1988).

81. Thomas Petros, article in *Physiology and Behavior*, vol. 41 (1991), pp. 25–30.

82. W. C. Willett et al., "Moderate Alcohol Consumption and the Risk of Breast Cancer," *New England Journal of Medicine*, vol. 316, no. 19 (May 7, 1987), pp. 1174–80.

83. J. A. Ewing, "Detecting Alcoholism. The CAGE Questionnaire," *Journal of the American Medical Association*, vol. 252, no. 14 (Oct. 12, 1984), pp. 1905–7.

84. L. D. Johnson, P. M. O'Malley, J. G. Bachman, and J. E. Schulenberg, Ann Arbor, MI. "Decline in Teen Smoking Appears to Be Nearing Its End," University of Michigan News and Information Services, Dec. 19, 2005 [On-line]. Available: www.monitoringthefuture.org.

85. Ibid.

86. Statistics from ASH—Action on Smoking and Health, 2013 H Street, N.W., Washington, D.C., 20006; 202-659-4310.

87. F. Clavel-Chapelon et al., "Smoking Cessation Rates Four Years After Treatment by Nicotine Gum and Acupuncture," *Preventive Medicine*, vol. 26, no. 1 (1997), pp. 25–28.

88. B. Haglund et al., "Cigarette Smoking as a Risk Factor for Sudden Infant Death Syndrome," *American Journal of Public Health*, vol. 80 (199), pp. 29–32.

89. R. A. Riemersma et al., "Risk of Angina Pectoris and Plasma Concentration of Vitamins A, C, E and Carotene," *The Lancet* vol. 337 (1991), pp. 1–5.

90. S. E. Moner, "Acupuncture and Addiction Treatment," *Journal of Addictive Disease*, vol. 15, no. 3 (1996), pp. 79–100.

91. Saul Miller, *Food for Thought: A New Look at Food and Behavior* (New York: Prentice-Hall, 1979).

92. Alexander Schauss, *Diet, Crime, and Delinquency* (Berkeley, CA: Parker House, 1980).

93. R. M. Nerem, M. J. Levesque, and J. T. Cornill, "Social Environment as a Factor in Diet-Induced Atherosclerosis," *Science*, vol. 208, no. 4451 (1980), pp. 1474–76.

94. Melvin Morse, *Transformed by the Light* (New York: Villard, 1992).

Chapter 18: The Power of Movement

1. Brian Swimme, *The Universe Is a Green Dragon* (Bear and Company, 1983), p. 106.

2. Many of the following studies were found in R. A. Anderson, *Wellness Medicine* (Lynnwood, WA: American Health Press 1987).

3. *Body Bulletin* (Emmaus, PA: Rodale Press, Jan. 1984).

4. I. Thune et al., "Physical Activity and the Risk of Breast Cancer," *New England Journal of Medicine*, vol. 336 (1997), pp. 1269–75.

5. Belloc and Breslow, "Relationship of Physical Fitness and Health Status," *Preventive Medicine*, vol. 1, no. 3 (1972), pp. 109–21.

6. Martha Gulati et al., "The Prognostic Value of a Nomogram of Exercise Capacity in Women," *New England Journal of Medicine*, vol. 353, no. 5 (Aug 4, 2005), pp. 468–75.

7. P. J. Harvey et al., "Exercise as an Alternative to Oral Estrogen for Amelioration of Endothelial Dysfunction in Postmenopausal Women," *American Heart Journal*, vol. 149, no. 2 (Feb. 2005), pp. 291–97.

8. R. J. Young, "Effects of Regular Exercise on Cognitive Functioning and Personality," *British Journal of Sports Medicine*, vol. 13, no. 3 (1979), pp. 110–17; B. Gutin, "Effect of Increase in Physical Fitness on Mental Ability Following Physical and Mental Stress," *Research Quarterly*, vol. 37, no. 2 (1966), pp. 211–20.

9. Archana Singh-Manoux et al., "Effects of Physical Activity on Cognitive Functioning in Middle Age: Evidence from the Whitehall II Prospective Cohort Study," *American Journal of Public Health*, vol. 95, no. 12 (Dec. 2005), pp. 2252–58.

10. M. S. Bahrke, "Exercise, Meditation and Anxiety Reduction," *American Corrective Therapy Journal*, vol. 33, no. 2 (1979), pp. 41–44; J. W. Collingswood and L. Willet, "The Effects of Physical Training Upon Self-Concept and Body Attitude," *Journal of Clinical Psychology*, vol. 27, no. 3 (1971), pp. 411–12.

11. R. Prince et al., "Prevention of Postmenopausal Osteoporosis: A Comparative Study of Exercise, Calcium Supplementation and Hormone Replacement Therapy," *New England Journal of Medicine*, vol. 325, no. 17 (1991), pp. 1189–1204; J. F. Aloia et al., "Prevention of Involution Bone Mass by Exercise," *Annals of Internal Medicine*, vol. 89, no 3 (1978), pp. 351–58; Consensus Development Conference on Osteoporosis, National Institutes of Health (Washington, DC, 1989).

12. S. J. Griffin and J. Trinder, "Physical Fitness, Exercise, and Human Sleep," *Psychophysiology*, vol. 15, no. 5 (1978), pp. 447–50.

13. J. Morgan et al., "Psychological Effects of Chronic Physical Activity," *Medical Science Sports*, vol. 2, no. 4 (1970), pp. 213–17.

14. S. P. Helmrich et al., "Physical Activity and Reduced Occurrence of Non-Insulin-Dependent Diabetes Mellitus," *New England Journal of Medicine*, vol. 325, no. 3 (July 18, 1991).

15. J. Prior, "Conditioning Exercise Decreases Premenstrual Symptoms: A Prospective, Controlled 6-Month Trial," *Fertility and Sterility*, vol. 47, no. 402 (1987).

16. B. P. Worth et al., "Running Through Pregnancy," *Runner's World* (Nov. 1978), pp. 54–59.

17. I have found that The Firm aerobic workout with weights is very effective if you have the time to do it. Each workout lasts from forty-five to sixty minutes, and you can feel results in your body after only five or so workouts, doing three workouts per week on average. To order a five-minute preview, call 1-800-THE FIRM. My favorites are volumes 4, 5, and 6. I'd recommend that you begin with volume 6. The USANA L-E-A-N videos are also excellent. To order see USANA listing in resources.

18. H. H. Jones et al., "Humeral Hypertrophy in Response to Exercise," *Journal of Bone and Joint Surgery*, vol. 59, no. 2 (1977), pp. 204–8; N. K. Dalen and E. Olsson, "Bone Mineral Content and Physical Activity," *Acta Orthopaedica Scandinavia*, vol. 45, no. 2 (1974), pp. 170–74.

19. M. Nelson et al., "Effects of High-Intensity Strength Training on Multiple Risk Factors for Osteoporitic Fractures: A Randomized Controlled Trial," *Journal of the American Medical Association*, vol. 272, no. 24 (1994), pp. 1909–14. The program Nelson used has been adapted for home use and is available in her book, *Strong Women Stay Young* (New York: Bantam, 1997).

20. Jin Putai, "Changes in Heart Rate, Noradrenaline, Cortisol, and Mood During Tai Chi," *Journal of Psychosomatic Research*, vol. 33, no. 2 (1989), pp. 197–206.

21. S. L. Wolf, H. X. Barnhart, and N. G. Kutner, "Reducing Frailty and Falls in Older Persons: An Investigation of Tai Chi and Computerized Balance Training," *Journal of the American Geriatric Society*, vol. 44 (1996), pp. 489–97.

22. I'm a big fan of model-mugging—the training that helps women develop a strategy for surviving an attack.

23. Ann Ray Martin and Valerie Gladstone, "The Quickest Fixes," *Longevity* (May 1991), pp. 48, 49.

24. R. Markus et al., "Menstrual Function and Bone Mass in Elite Women Distance Runners: Endocrine and Metabolic Features," *Annals of Internal Medicine*, vol. 102 (1985), pp. 158–63.

25. N. A. Rigotti et al., "Osteoporosis in Women with Anorexia Nervosa," *New England Journal of Medicine*, vol. 311 (1989), pp. 1601–5.

26. L. L. Schweiger et al., "Caloric Intake, Stress, and Menstrual Function in Athletes," *Fertility and Sterility*, vol. 49 (1988), pp. 447–50.

27. B. L. Drinkwater et al., "Bone Mineral Density After Resumption of Menses in Amenorrheic Athletes," *Journal of the American Medical Association*, vol. 256 (1986), pp. 380–82; J. S. Lindberg et al., "Increased Vertebral Bone Mineral in

Response to Reduced Exercise in Amenorrheic Runners," *Western Journal of Medicine*, vol. 146 (1987), pp. 39–47.

28. Nancy Lane, M.D., "Exercise and Bone Status," *Complementary Medicine* (May/June 1986).

Chapter 19: Healing Ourselves, Healing Our World

1. C. W. Birky, "Relaxed Cellular Controls and Organelle Heredity," *Science*, vol. 222 (1983), pp. 466–75; M. C. Corballis and M. J. Morgan, "On the Biological Basis of Human Laterality," *Journal of Behavioral Science*, vol. 2 (1978), pp. 261–336; Norman Geschwind and Albert Galaburda, "Cerebral Lateralization, Biological Mechanisms, and Pathology," *Archives of Neurology*, vol. 42, no. 6 (1985), pp. 521–52.

2. *The Burning Tree* is a documentary film that chronicles the burning of nine million women and their sympathizers as witches during the Middle Ages. For more information, write to the filmmaker, Donna Reed, Direct Cinema, P. O. Box 10003, Santa Monica, CA 90410; 310-396-4774, 800-525-4000. For more information on this subject, see Starhawk, *The Spiral Dance: A Rebirth of the Ancient Goddess* (Harper-SanFrancisco, 1979).

3. Rupert Sheldrake, *The Presence of the Past: Morphic Resonance and the Habits of Nature* (London: Collins, 1988) and *A New Science of Life* (Boston: Houghton Mifflin, 1981). Sheldrake's theory concerns "morphic units," which can be regarded as forms of energy. "Although these aspects of form and energy can be separated conceptually they are always associated with one another. No morphic unit can have energy without form, and no material form can exist without energy." The characteristic form of a given morphic unit is determined by the form of previous similar systems that act upon it across time and space, in a process of "morphic resonance" through "morphogenic fields." This influence depends on the system's three-dimensional structures and patterns of vibration.

   For example, thousands of rats are trained to perform a new task in a laboratory in London. If Sheldrake's theory holds, then at a later time and in laboratories somewhere else, similar rats should be able to learn and carry out the same task more quickly. That's because the initial rats have changed the "morphogenic field" around rat learning. This effect should take place in the absence of any known physical connection or communication between the two laboratories.

   Evidence that this effect actually occurs has been reported by Ager et al., "Fourth (Final) Report on a Test of McDougall's Lamarckian Experiment in the Training of Rats," *Journal of Experimental Biology*, vol. 3 (1954), pp. 304–21.

4. *Ms.* (Jan–Feb 1992), cover.

5. Audre Lorde, *Burst of Light* (Ithaca, NY: Firebrand Books, 1988), p. 131. According to her book, Lorde had metastases of breast cancer to her liver, diagnosed in 1984. In 1992, she was named the poet laureate of New York State. Usually a tumor that has metastasized to the liver gives the person six months to live. Lorde lived nine years after this diagnosis.

6. Annie Rafter, a nurse practitioner, is one of the original founders of Women to Women. She currently practices in Santa Fe, N.M.

7. This thought had a bit of accuracy in it. Medical students are notorious for starting to experience the symptoms of the patients they are around when they're just
   learning about different diseases. My personal boundaries were not very well
   placed in the past, and I have "taken home" too much of what goes on in the office. Since I'm in the energy field associated with fibroids all day long and am quite
   empathetic with my patients, my energy field has undoubtedly been influenced by
   theirs—and I still have to take responsibility for this condition and learn and
   grow from it.

Index

Page numbers of illustrations appear in italics

About the Author

Christiane Northrup, M.D., trained at Dartmouth Medical School and Tufts New England Medical Center. She is a board-certified obstetrician/gynecologist with more than twenty years of clinical and medical teaching experience. As past president of the American Holistic Medical Association, and past Clinical Assistant Professor of Obstetrics and Gynecology through the University of Vermont College of Medicine's program at Maine Medical Center, she appreciates the need for a partnership between the best of conventional and complementary medicine. Dr. Northrup is the author of the number-one *New York Times* best-selling book *The Wisdom of Menopause* and *Mother-Daughter Wisdom*—a Quill Award nominee in 2005. She is the editor of the monthly e-letter *Women's Health Wisdom* and the *Dr. Christiane Northrup* bimonthly newsletter. She has hosted five successful public television specials and her work has been featured on *The Oprah Winfrey Show*, *The Today Show*, *Nightly News with Tom Brokaw*, *The View*, and *Good Morning America*. She lives in Maine.